COLPOSCOPY

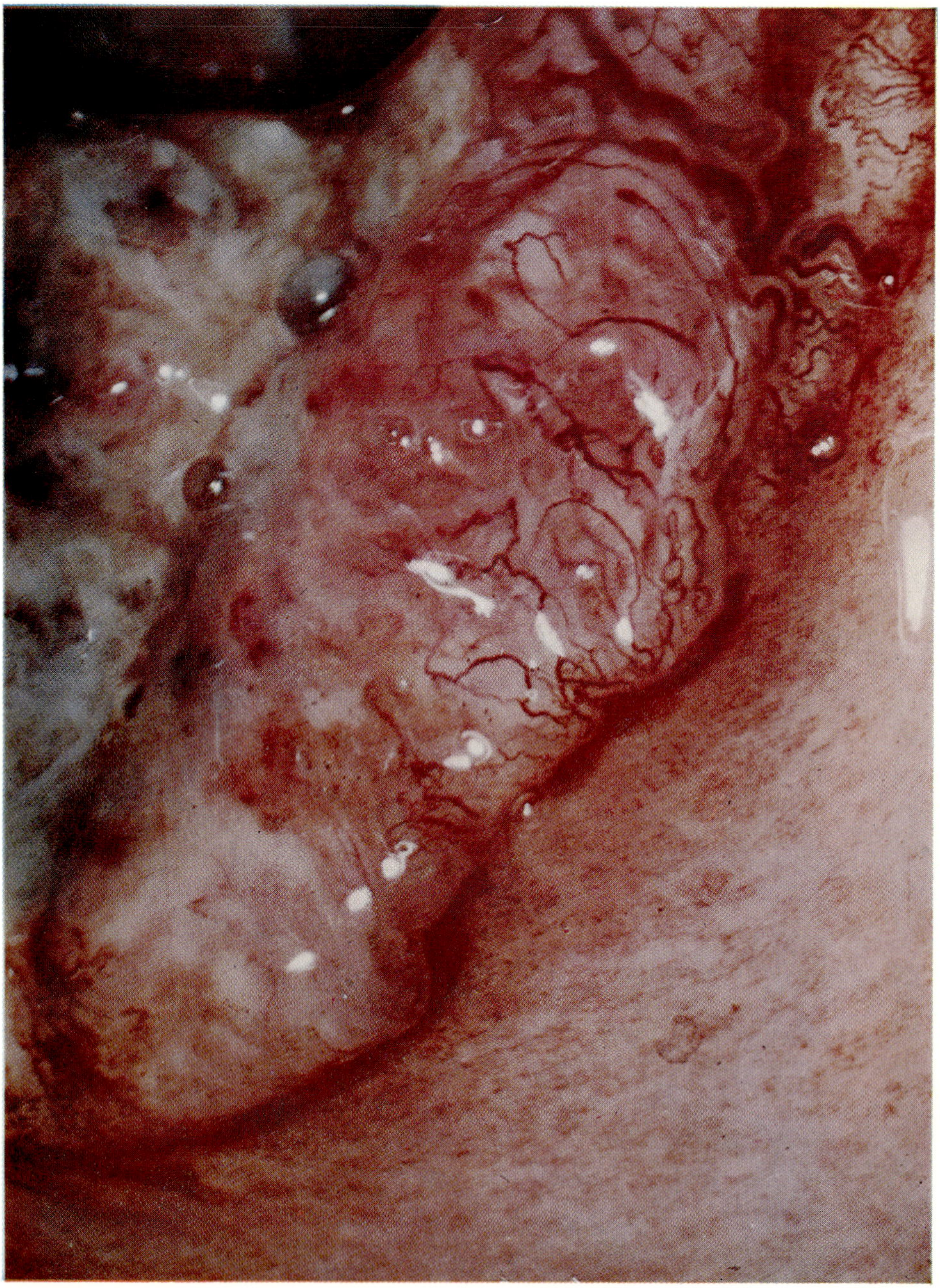

COLPOSCOPY

A SCIENTIFIC AND PRACTICAL APPROACH TO THE CERVIX AND VAGINA IN HEALTH AND DISEASE

Second Edition

By

MALCOLM COPPLESON, M.D.
(Syd.), F.A.G.O., F.R.C.O.G.
King George V Memorial Hospital
Royal Prince Alfred Hospital
Sydney, Australia

ELLIS PIXLEY, M.B.
(Qld.), F.A.G.O., F.R.C.O.G.
King Edward Memorial Hospital
Perth, Australia

BEVAN REID, M.D. (Syd),
B.V.Sc., D.T.M. and H.
Queen Elizabeth II Research Institute for
Mothers and Infants
The University of Sydney
Sydney, Australia

With Contributions by

ADOLF STAFL, M.D., Ph.D.
Medical College of Wisconsin
Milwaukee, Wisconsin

DUANE E. TOWNSEND, M.D.
University of Southern California
School of Medicine
Los Angeles, California

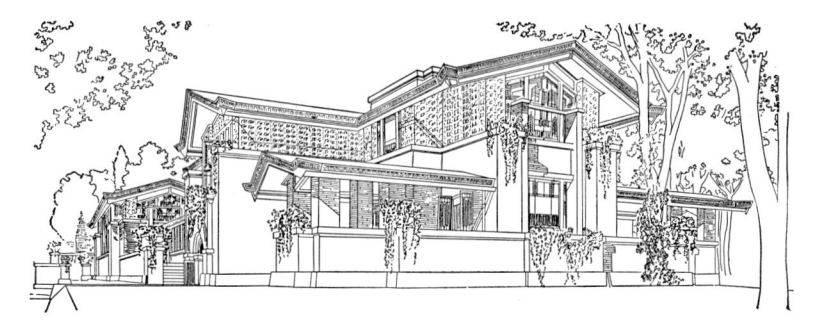

CHARLES C THOMAS · PUBLISHER
Springfield · Illinois · U.S.A.

Published and Distributed Throughout the World by
CHARLES C THOMAS • PUBLISHER
Bannerstone House
301-327 East Lawrence Avenue, Springfield, Illinois, U.S.A.

This book is protected by copyright. No part of it may be reproduced in any manner without written permission from the publisher.

© 1971, 1978, by CHARLES C THOMAS • PUBLISHER
ISBN 0-398-03761-2
Library of Congress Catalog Card Number: 77-25338

First Edition, First Printing, 1971
First Edition, Second Printing, 1975
First Edition, Third Printing, 1976
Second Edition, 1978

With THOMAS BOOKS careful attention is given to all details of manufacturing and design. It is the Publisher's desire to present books that are satisfactory as to their physical qualities and artistic possibilities and appropriate for their particular use. THOMAS BOOKS will be true to those laws of quality that assure a good name and good will.

Library of Congress Cataloging in Publication Data
Coppleson, Malcolm.
   Colposcopy.

   (American lecture series; publication no. 1020)
   Bibliography: P. 440
   Includes index.
   1. Colposcopy. I. Pixley, Ellis, joint author. II. Reid, Bevan, joint author. III. Title.
RG107.5.C6C66 1978   618.1′4′0754   77-25338
ISBN 0-398-03761-2

Printed in the United States of America
C-1

Publication Number 1020
AMERICAN LECTURE SERIES®

A Monograph in
The BANNERSTONE DIVISION *of*
AMERICAN LECTURES IN GYNECOLOGY AND OBSTETRICS

Edited by
LAMAN A. GRAY, A.B., M.D., F.A.C.S., F.A.C.O.G.
Professor of Obstetrics and Gynecology
University of Louisville School of Medicine
Louisville, Kentucky

FOREWORD

In 1971 a new book entitled *Colposcopy, A Scientific and Practical Approach to the Cervix in Health and Disease* appeared in this country by the authors Malcolm Coppleson, M.D., Ellis Pixley, M.B., and Bevan Reid, M.D., all of Australia. In the past seven years this book has required three printings and is now appearing with extensive revisions and additions as a second edition. America was ready for this book with its perennial curiosity which extends as thoroughly into the scientific community as into every other phase of life in this country.

After Hinselmann used his first colposcope some fifty years ago the application of the method to study the cervix by means of this relatively small magnification was limited almost entirely to the gynecologists of the continent of Europe. The large and famous gynecologic clinics had their colposcopes, which were demonstrated regularly, but their use was never enthusiastically received by the visiting American gynecologic surgeons. Many of the American professors in the past two generations, and many today, have felt that this instrument cannot see sufficiently into the endocervix to make it of great value. However, now it is appearing more obviously that the transformation zone in the vast majority of women can be visualized, except in the occasional younger woman and, unfortunately more commonly, in the woman after 60 years of age.

In this country, which gave birth to the cytologic diagnostic criteria which indicate abnormal changes in the cervix uteri, cytology has been relied upon almost totally to determine the presence of preclinical cancer and dysplasia of the cervix. While we have thought that the degree of error in accuracy of diagnosis after the first cytologic examination was 5 percent or less, it is beginning to appear that the false negatives may extend to 10 percent of patients who truly have an early lesion.

This book, *Colposcopy*, appeared at just the right time. It has become the standard of excellence in the use of this method in this country. Undoubtedly all involved will be interested in the second edition which contains much new material as well as important revisions, both large and small. The changes of meanings from only a few words can clarify a situation a great deal. Not only the many changes throughout this book, along with fresh comments on problem situations, are important, but in addition there are two new chapters by Adolph Stafl, M.D., and Duane Townsend, M.D., among our most authoritative contributors to diagnosis by means of colposcopy in America. These chapters deal particularly with the DES problems.

The young resident in training today will have developed a reasonable skill in the use of the colposcope and will carry it with him into the practice of gynecology. The method has been more thoroughly introduced into this country by the book by Coppleson, Pixley and Reid than by any other stimulus.

Every now and then a book comes along which proves itself exceedingly popular and it is accepted by the medical profession with great interest. Mr. Charles C Thomas once told me that his publication of a small book on general surgery by John Homans of Boston astounded him because of the sudden and widespread acceptance of that book. As a medical student it was one of my treasured purchases. Now another book which fills a need and stands on its merit has become our standard of excellence in the use of colposcopy. Colposcopic findings again have been correlated with microscopic disease. The clinical methodology offered by these authors encompasses sound conservative techniques of treatment.

LAMAN A. GRAY, SR., M.D.
Editor for Obstetrics and Gynecology

PREFACE TO THE SECOND EDITION

NEARLY A DECADE has passed since this book was conceived and written. The appearance of a second edition became necessary with the rate of advance of the field of knowledge on several important fronts. First, there has been an overall trend toward increasingly conservative methods of management of cervical intraepithelial neoplasia necessitating a revision and rewriting of the aims and descriptions of these methods. We are aware of criticism of the possibilities for under treatment of invasive cancer that inexpert and inappropriate use of the colposcopic method may allow. Accordingly, great care has been taken to provide guidance in order to avoid this error. Second, an increase in the occurrence of vaginal lesions associated with the maternal use of diethylstilboestrol prompted a full-scale treatment of the subject of the ontogeny and colposcopic morphology of the vagina preparatory to chapters by two distinguished American authors on the specific appearances so induced. Third, a new chapter on the occurrence of atypical appearances of doubtful or physiological significance became necessary as part of a critical evaluation of the colposcopic method. Fourth, the participation of some of the authors in numerous teaching programmes, seminars and the like at all levels of student seniority over the past seven years gave us first hand knowledge of the most common problems which arise in learning about the subject. This knowledge permits a comprehensive assembly of its many aspects into a more polished story.

In addition to four new chapters, extensive rewriting and revision of the text of the first edition means that little of the book remains in its original prose. The illustrations have changed both by extensive replacing of older photographs and the addition of nearly a hundred new illustrations.

We have hopefully set out to answer all questions which arise in a comprehensive study of colposcopy by descriptions and discussions whose accuracy is warranted by our close association with the several clinical, teaching and research aspects of the whole field.

PREFACE TO THE FIRST EDITION

THE COLPOSCOPE was invented through the labours of Hans Hinselmann in Hamburg over forty years ago. By virtue of the combination of a knowledge of optics and great curiosity about the origins of cervical cancer, he constructed an instrument capable of magnifying the image upon which a powerful light source was focussed. His main purpose was the discovery of a primary focus of the cancer. Instead of the simple nodule he suspected, he found a profusion of quite novel appearances which, with the aid of biopsy, were shown to represent variations in the pattern of the cervical epithelia. A glimpse of the pictures which follow in this book will indicate the range of these variations and perhaps give some idea of the complex task faced by this pioneer as he slowly and painstakingly categorised them in a series of papers over the next twenty years. Through him we learned to look for the origins of clinical cancer not in a focus, but in a sheet of epithelium, a concept which opened the way to a much clearer understanding.

The use of the instrument spread quickly throughout the continent of Europe helped by such disciples as Mestwerdt, Limburg, Wespi, Navratil, Antoine, Bret, Coupez, Cramer and many others, all of whom added refinements and modifications to Hinselmann's original concepts. More recently some newer potential of the technique has been realised. Koller and Kolstad in Norway have produced some beautiful photographs of the cervix by variations in the optics. They have used some of these photographs to quantitate the capillary vascular bed of the organ which they have been able to correlate with some aspects of carcinogenesis.

In Australia we have also developed the use of the instrument as a valuable research ally in attempting to define the natural history of the cervix. The pictorial record of this development lent itself to collation as a book.

This book is in many respects, an amplification of a chapter and the continuation of an approach developed in a companion volume, *Preclinical Carcinoma of the Cervix, Origin, Nature and Management* (Coppleson and Reid, 1967), to which the reader is referred for a more profound treatment of the practical as well as the more academic and abstruse aspects of the field.

ACKNOWLEDGEMENTS

A PUBLICATION of this kind has upon it the stamp of others than its authors. Friends and family, teachers and typists, and a thousand encounters in hospital corridors, scientific meetings and teaching sessions are all present somewhere between its covers. Mention cannot be made of all, but those who are not formally acknowledged will know their page, their conceptual contribution and technical participation.

It is befitting to acknowledge again a debt to Sir John Stallworthy in whose department at Oxford, England, one of us first looked down a colposcope over twenty years ago and whose encouragement has continued unabated in the interim. Our special thanks are directed towards the editor of the American Lecture Series of which this book forms part. At a time when the method had little acceptance Dr. Laman Gray invited the senior author to introduce the topic to an American audience through this influential series. It is comforting to see how his gamble has paid off in the now widespread and safe place that the subject now enjoys on the American scene. We continue to recognise his encouragement and guidance.

Much of the routine assembly of the book was accomplished at the King George V Hospital, Sydney and the Department of Obstetrics and Gynaecology, University of Sydney where encouragement and facilities were generously extended respectively by colleagues of the Visiting Medical Staff and by Professor R. P. Shearman. Dr. Colin Laverty, Chief of the Department of Pathology at King George V Hospital, deserves special thanks for advice, lengthy discussions, as well as for the provision of several of the microphotographs. For much active assistance in the Colposcopy Clinic at the same hospital, we thank Dr. Richard Reid and Miss Margaret Arnold. The illustrations are the skilful work of the Departments of Illustration, the University of Sydney and the Royal Prince Alfred Hospital under the direction respectively of Mr. Ken Clifford and Mr. Brian Magee. The drawings were made by Miss Julie Eichorn and Miss Fiona Pixley, daughter of the author. The typing of the manuscript was done by Mrs. Shirley Bottrell, Mrs. Judy Shade and Miss Pat Neill. Our thanks are due to all for their valuable help and sustained labours.

We have also received encouragement, advice and assistance over the years from Dr. William Chanen, Royal Womens Hospital, Melbourne, who has pioneered the entry and use of the instrument in that city, from Dr. Frank Pacey, Senior Cytologist, Institute of Clinical Pathology and Medical Research, Lidcombe, N.S.W., and from Mr. Walter Schroeder of Sydney.

It is difficult to overrate the influence of our frequent visits to the United States of America over the past seven years on the development and maturation of many of our viewpoints. Our special patrons in this country were Doctors Duane Townsend of Los Angeles, Adolf Stafl of Milwaukee, Joseph Scott of Miami and John Marlow of Washington, who have been our hosts, guides, philosophers and friends. As illustrative of this influence is our inclusion of Drs. Stafl and Townsend as guest authors. We are indebted to them for making this contribution to the book.

We also owe a debt for a less formal but very real contribution from numerous people in North America. Such has been the extent of contact at courses, meetings, symposia, lectures and the like that it has proved difficult to compile an exhaustive list. For this valuable dialogue we thank: Jim Abell, Joseph Ballina, John Bise, Lawrence Borow, Philip Brooks, Louis Burke, William Christopherson, Leonard Cibley, Bill Creasman, Arch Dillard, Philip DiSaia, Val Clark Donahue, Lawrence Donohue, Charles Dungar, John W. Greene, Jr., Earl Greenwald, William Hart, Arthur Herbst, Arthur Hertig, Lewis Hicks, Lorna Johnson, Howard W. Jones, Jr., Leo Koss, Philip Krupp, Leo Lagasse, Warren Lang, John L. Lewis, Jr., Gordon Lickrish, Michael Liebermann, Barbara Mathews, Dick Mattingly, Paul Morrow, Jack van Nagell, Lester Odell, Donald Ostergard, James Park, A. D. de Petrillo, John Queenan, Jim Reagan, Ralph Richart, Marvin Rodney, Milton Roy, William Russell, Edward Savage, Fred Schlichting, Albrecht Schmitt, George Schneider, Robert Scully, Hugh Shingleton, Mojmir Sonek, Jose Torres, Harold Tovell, George Trombetta, Carlos Vence, Alma Young, Maclyn Wade, Jim Walsh, James Weatherholt, Winston Weese, George Wied, George Wilbanks, Cecil Wright, Roland Zwick.

Colposcopy has now become world wide in its coverage and we have travelled extensively in many other countries. It is a pleasure to record our indebtedness to our foreign colleagues. Dr. Albert Singer originally from Sydney, now in Sheffield, and an adviser to the first edition of this book, and Dr. Joe Jordan of Birmingham are old established colleagues whose advice, cooperation and friendship we have valued for many years. Professor Per Kolstad, Oslo, Professor Erich Burghardt, Graz, Dr. James Maclean, Buenos Aires and Professor Santiago Dexeus, Barcelona have all influenced our views. Valuable discussions have been held with other leading exponents in various countries. In particular we acknowledge:

Prof. J. P. Rieper, Brazil; Drs. R. Cartier and F. Coupez, France; Drs. H. K. Bauer, G. Herbeck, F. Menken, Prof. G. Mestwerdt and Dr. W. Walz, Germany; Dr. S. Noda, Japan; Prof. H. Green and Dr. W. A. McIndoe, New Zealand; Drs. M. Borja and A. Padilla-Cruz, Philippines; Prof. W. A. van Niekerk, South Africa; Prof. F. Bonilla Musoles, Spain; and Prof. H. J. Wespi, Switzerland.

Acknowledgments

We thank Pergamon Press for permission to reproduce a few illustrations from an earlier book, *Preclinical Carcinoma of the Cervix, Origin, Nature and Management.*

The publishers, Charles C Thomas, have rendered ready and willing assistance with the same enterprise to which we had been accustomed during the preparation of the first edition. We record our special thanks to Mr. Payne Thomas and to Mr. William Bried, for courtesy, help, advice and solicitude in our attempt to present the material in the best possible way.

MALCOLM COPPLESON
ELLIS PIXLEY
BEVAN REID

CONTENTS

Page

Foreword vii
Preface ix
Acknowledgments xiii

PART I
INTRODUCTION

Chapter
1. THE CASE FOR COLPOSCOPY 5

PART II
SCIENTIFIC BASIS OF COLPOSCOPY

2. DEFINITIONS 15
3. TOPOGRAPHY OF THE CERVICAL EPITHELIA (LOCATION OF PRECLINICAL CERVICAL CARCINOMA AND DYSPLASIA) 68
4. NATURAL HISTORY OF SQUAMOUS METAPLASIA AND THE TRANSFORMATION ZONE 76
5. THE TISSUE BASIS OF COLPOSCOPIC APPEARANCES 120

PART III
TECHNIQUE

6. THE TECHNIQUE OF COLPOSCOPY 167

PART IV
COLPOSCOPIC MORPHOLOGY

7. COLPOSCOPIC APPEARANCES OF THE ORIGINAL EPITHELIA 193
8. COLPOSCOPIC APPEARANCES OF THE TYPICAL TRANSFORMATION ZONE . 209
9. COLPOSCOPIC APPEARANCES OF THE ATYPICAL TRANSFORMATION ZONE . 226
10. COLPOSCOPIC APPEARANCES OF OVERT CANCER 262
11. COLPOSCOPIC APPEARANCES OF MISCELLANEOUS CONDITIONS . . . 278

PART V
RECENT ADVANCES

12. THE VAGINA 307
13. VAGINAL ADENOSIS 331
    Adolf Stafl

Chapter	Page
14. The Cervix and Vagina of Women Exposed to Synthetic Non-steroidal Oestrogens 341	
Duane E. Townsend	

PART VI
DIFFICULTIES OF COLPOSCOPIC INTERPRETATION

15. Atypical Colposcopic Appearances of Doubtful or Physiological Significance 357	

PART VII
PRACTICAL USES OF COLPOSCOPY

16. The Uses of Colposcopy 389	
References 437	
Bibliography 440	
Index 471	

COLPOSCOPY

PART I

Introduction

Chapter 1

THE CASE FOR COLPOSCOPY

THE EXTENSIVE UPSURGE of interest in the use of colposcopy for the diagnosis and management of preclinical cervical and vaginal cancer has necessitated a complete revision of the tone of this introductory chapter. Since 1971, when the first edition of this book was published, the use of colposcopy, especially in the United States of America, has burgeoned to such an extent that the apologetic overtones of the previous introduction seem quite inapposite today. In spite of some elements of disapproval that recur from time to time, the successful installation and popularity of the method have guaranteed it an established place in gynaecological practice.

The reasons for the re-emergence of the technique stem from the almost complete break between the new colposcopy and that of its European founders practised half a century ago. The break is concerned most with concepts which the newer use of the colposcope has generated on the subject of the life history of the cervical covering layers and the intimate connection of this life history with the origin of cervical squamous cancer. An easily grasped unfolding story of great attraction to students has replaced a more pedantic and rigorous classification of static pictures of the earlier masters. If seeing is believing, the gynaecologist has been converted through his own insight afforded by the use of the colposcope.

The major aims of the book are threefold: First, to promote colposcopy as a clinical discipline, neither dependent nor independent of its fellow disciplines of exfoliative cytology and histology, yet capable of permitting sound judgement in some of the most vexed problems of the cervix. Colposcopy is the method par excellence for enabling the clinician to appreciate the physiology and pathology of the cervix in a fashion not approached by any other method.

Second, this volume also provides a contemporary atlas of colposcopy, incorporating significant advances in the understanding of the natural history of cervical epithelia. This is important as a basis for understanding aspects of both precarcinoma and carcinoma. The approach is different from the traditional atlases and descriptions of disease appearing in the early German literature.

Third, the aim is to present a scheme for detection and management of the cervical cancer precursors and early cancer and to describe other practical uses of colposcopy. It was our conviction when writing the first edition of this book that much management of cervical lesions at that time was imbalanced, illogical, and too radical. The cause, we believed, was that the clinician had abdicated his traditional captaincy of the management team in favour of others less directly concerned, such as the pathologist or exfoliative cytologist. It remains our conviction today that a similar state persists in centres where colposcopy has not yet been introduced. However, the recent upswing in the use of the instrument encouraging the more widespread use of a more conservative approach to the precursors of cervical cancer, an appraisal requiring great detail for its correct execution, has necessitated a complete rewriting of the section on treatment.

At this stage, few would question the necessity of the colposcopic approach in individualisation of conservative treatment for cervical intraepithelial neoplasia. Its value in an individualised approach to preclinical invasive cancer is presently not appreciated, and we can anticipate a similar advance in this more controversial area. The combined colposcopic-histological discipline has greatly assisted the gynaecologist in the exclusion of preclinical invasive cancer but has not yet made a commensurate impact on the individualisation of treatment. The woman with symptomless invasive cancer, without sign, is still managed exclusively by procedures based on the opinion of the histopathologist, but problems result (p. 414).

The major reason for the appearance of the first edition of this book was the recognition of the central importance of colposcopy in a decade of study of the normal and diseased cervix. This importance seemed to require an expansion beyond a single chapter accorded it in another book in which these researches were reported (Coppleson and Reid, 1967).

Profitable as our extensive studies with exfoliative cytology, light microscopy, ultramicroscopy, autoradiography, cytochemistry, and tissue culture have been, we have found no more satisfactory way of viewing critical changes than by the use of the colposcope. Again and again, when confronted with the problems of diagnosis, management, or research, we turn to the instrument and the unique advantages it confers.

For a variety of reasons ranging from clinical practice to pure research, we have examined colposcopically more than 25,000 human cervices and categorised the findings. The recorded series includes foetal and prepubertal females, virgin and promiscuous adolescents, and women in pregnancy, the reproductive years, and after the menopause. Photographic records have been kept, sometimes sequential of one organ through a number of years, which has enabled constant study, contrast, and reappraisal. This material forms the basis of this book.

It became obvious early in the course of our investigations that traditional concepts failed to explain the things we saw. Efforts to determine the reasons for these discrepancies brought us gradually but forcibly to the conclusion that many present-day concepts and descriptions of the cervix in health and disease were inadequate. The traditional concepts have provided neither key nor rationale to an obviously complex situation and have delayed clarification of many accessible factors related to the natural history of the precursors of cervical cancer.

Traditional concepts have been built up largely on disciplines concerned with events at the microscopic and ultrastructural levels. There has been a hiatus in that zone from the naked eye, which is singularly unsuitable as a means of studying the organ, to the low power of the microscope. Highly useful as the microscopic approach has been to this, as to many other organ studies, there is no doubt that its value is enhanced when combined with careful observation at those intermediate magnifications provided by the colposcope. A new and picturesque world is revealed, any part of which can then be examined by excision biopsy and microscopy. The colposcopic scrutiny may be sequential, allowing the emergence of concepts with respect to dynamic and chronological aspects of behaviour of tissue. Short-lived but active phases, which can do so much to clarify events in the life history of the cervical epithelia, may be identified.

This colposcopic approach led to the development of revised concepts, the most important of which has been the newer understanding of the biology of the transformation zone. The metamorphosis of this zone lies at the heart of the subject and remains the key to any attempt at comprehension of the cervical epithelia.

The academic advance has promoted reason and rhyme in the interpretation of the images derived from the colposcope. Earlier writings represented cervical epithelia in stasis rather than in movement, a movement which traces a remarkable life history. Unfolding of the life history produces new concepts, and in turn, these have allowed a better understanding by the gynaecologist of the significance of changes in appearance of the organ.

Furthermore, the attraction of critical minds to the subject, which is obligatory for any academic approach, is reflected in the rapid incorporation of the discipline into university departments and counters the older arguments that the method was not sufficiently scientific. Particularly, sister disciplines such as pathology have become involved, establishing a bridge between clinician and pathologist that had been unavailable in their absence.

It is not surprising then that a substantial part of the work is devoted to the transformation zone and its fortunes as the basis of an understanding of the natural history of cervical cancer.

In the light of a wider acceptance of the colposcopic technique, many of its earlier criticisms become of historical interest. We might well reflect on why such a valuable technique as colposcopy has so slowly and with misgivings entered the English-speaking world. It is probable that the advent of exfoliative cytology to the diagnostic scene was initially the major factor. As a result, perhaps of national and parochial attitudes, an almost universal misconception arose that the techniques of colposcopy and exfoliative cytology were in opposition, and their possible complementary value received scant consideration. To the gynaecologist, the facility of taking the smear and obtaining a report is appealing. On the other hand, some knowledge of gynaecological pathology is an obligatory complement to the understanding of the colposcopic image.

Language difficulties, the necessity of learning new and unfamiliar terms, the lack of teachers, the difficulty of self-tuition, the paucity of sufficient scientific papers in English on the subject, and the frank disapproval of the technique by some eminent gynaecologists and pathologists in the United States and in the United Kingdom have been other factors. It is also probable that the teaching of colposcopy has frequently been too rigidly dogmatic and orthodox and based on false concepts of cervical physiology. Presently, the paraphernalia of modern teaching, intensive courses including live patient sessions, video display, and so forth, has displaced the schoolroom-like pedantry of the older colposcopy and doubtless is responsible for much of the verve currently accompanying the rapid spread of its use. It seems only too apparent to the authors that the gusto which is so typical of the American approach to new knowledge could only have occurred when the technique made inroads into the United States.

Traditional colposcopic terminology with its ponderous and pedagogic nomenclature and its many variations of atypical appearances appears to have confused rather than enlightened the subject. Much of the fearsome jargon and attendant misconceptions have now been eliminated by a crisp new terminology. This terminology has followed on the newer concepts on transformation zone physiology and so in turn has been a major force in the renaissance in the colposcopic method.

From discussions with many physicians unfamiliar with the method, we find four other major criticisms of colposcopy frequently advanced.

The first criticism is that the technique is too impractical, too complex, and too expensive. Many antagonists of the method are under the impression that colposcopy, to be useful, must be a routine part of all gynecological examinations. Although such programs are regarded by many continental authorities as valuable, we do not share their opinion and list our more practical indications later. With skill and practice, the procedure is little more time consuming than the introduction of a speculum and taking of a smear. Complexity is insufficient argument on which to condemn a method merely on the grounds of a short apprenticeship. Concerning expense, the cost of the instrument is not a major item in the overall budget for treating cervical disease.

The second and more important criticism is that "the instrument cannot see into the cervical canal," and as "most preclinical carcinomas are endocervical," the method can be of little use. The fallacy is immediately obvious to the colposcopist and is dealt with later (Chap. 3).

The third criticism is that colposcopy denies essential information because cancer has only limited surface representation. Way (1968) has aptly expressed this view "beauty is skin deep, but cancer is not." This is far from the truth. The neoplasm starts in the epithelium, is for many years confined to it, and once it extends beyond this level, is usually associated with even more conspicuous surface abnormalities of contour, bleeding, and ulceration. Striking appearances of early neoplasia, evident when colposcopic magnification is applied, are illustrated later.

The final criticism, unacceptably presumptuous, is that no further useful information can be obtained by the method. There is a deep-rooted impression in the minds of many clinicians that the problems of preclinical carcinoma of the cervix can be resolved by the combined use of exfoliative cytology and biopsy. Some revision of this attitude is emerging from reports in the literature on the occurrence of high false negative rates, inability to eradicate cervical cancer despite intensive smear campaigns, and so forth. The difficulty of interpretation of cellular and tissue specimens and the subjectivity and fallibility of these diagnostic methods is usually ignored by many clinicians. Yet, the thoughtful practitioner is left in doubt about the authority with which these methods are presently vested. To counter such comments on the "uselessness of colposcopy" or a minimal concession that "it may help to define the best site for biopsy," Chapter 16 discusses those uses of the technique, which indicates the extent of additional valuable information available to the gynaecologist.

There is a new criticism of colposcopy. The use of the colposcope has found expression in the extensive trend towards conservatism in management of preclinical cervical cancer and related lesions. Many lesions are now being managed by physical methods of destruction, such as cyrosurgery, electrodiathermy, and surgical laser application as office procedures in some centres, whereas similar lesions are being treated by hysterectomy in others. The pace of emergence of this conservative management is such that it is not surprising that warnings have been issued from some authoritative gynaecological oncologists. A widely circulated technical bulletin from the American College of Obstetricians and Gynecologists (1976), in relegating colposcopy to a role secondary to conventional methods, implies that frank cancer can be missed. Doubtless these warnings are timely, especially as this conservatism, coupled with insufficient training and experience, may lead to gross mismanagement of serious lesions. The hazard of undertreatment of frank cancer is ever present.

The magnitude of the problem must await the appearance of sound clinical reports in the next few years, but in anticipation of such an imbalance, much of the prose of this book is directed toward the problems of excluding serious lesions. It is our opinion that the oversight of a serious lesion is not as probable on balance as is the potential for gross overtreatment of early lesions such as Stage 1A, Stage O, and dysplasia, in the absence of colposcopic oversight. The potential serious complications of radical irradiation and major surgery and the complications of cone biopsy and the attendant sterilisation of young women have to be discounted against management in the absence of colposcopy.

Experience in leading the uninitiated into the study of the uterine cervix by means of the colposcope has shown that students frequently pass through three well-defined phases. The first is one of excitement at the brilliant spectacle of living tissue in its natural state. The second, which starts after the first few months, is one of disappointment. The beginner, encouraged to take biopsies from most atypical areas as he recognises them, finds relatively few significant cases of preclinical carcinoma or even major dysplasias. At the seat of this disappointment is his failure to realise an expected close correlation between colposcopy and other methods of studying the same tissue, exfoliative cytology and histology. Unless the unwary student recognises that it is especially in the case of the lesser atypical appearances that the cytologist and histopathologist fail to confirm his discovery and report a normal or low-grade abnormality at most, he enters the third phase. There is understandably a waning of enthusiasm, the entry of doubts as to the real value and the eventual abandonment of the idea. Our especial resolve is to encourage the student to recognise the potential of colposcopy and to gain satisfaction from the assured and confident approach towards the understanding of cervical physiology and pathology which its continued use promotes.

A possible faltering by the student during the inductive phases poses the question of what constitutes an adequate training both in sequence and content. The optimum appears to be an initiation through textbook or atlas followed by a basic course of the type sponsored by the American Society of Colposcopy and Colpomicroscopy. A return to practice to consolidate this introductory formal training is best then followed by a further advanced course led by teachers of some experience in integrating colposcopy with histopathology and clinical gynaecology. The colposcopic method, through its direct visual function, then assumes its place as the pivot in such a front. A highly trained cadre of superspecialists with an involvement in research and development is envisaged as a component of such senior training.

The format of this manual follows a stratagem we have found to be most comprehensible to the beginner, to the consultant on a refresher course, as well as to the research investigator. It presents the subject as prosaically and pragmatically as possible, allowing an essentially pictorial subject to be expounded in pictures. In this way we reject rejoinders, "But you can't see more with the colposcope than with the naked eye." Where necessary, illustrations are supplemented with histological preparations of biopsies placing histology in perspective as frequently an ally, sometimes an enemy, but not necessarily authority.

PART II

Scientific Basis for Colposcopy

Chapter 2

DEFINITIONS
CLINICAL, ANATOMICAL, HISTOLOGICAL, COLPOSCOPIC, CYTOLOGICAL

IN GYNAECOLOGICAL LITERATURE, both historical and contemporary, much variation is encountered in terminology used to describe the cervix. Few, if any, systematic descriptions of the cervix uteri and its epithelia currently available withstand critical analysis, and few terms are precise. This inadequacy extends also to the nomenclature in the colposcopic literature of various countries, although recently attempts at standardisation are increasingly successful.

An abridged nomenclature used in our descriptions and discussions follows.

CLINICAL DEFINITIONS

Inspection of the cervix with the unaided eye allows the clinician to diagnose confidently the presence of *polyps, "follicles," condylomata,* and *overt cancer* and to recognise areas of *leukoplakia,* preferably termed *keratosis.*

The terms *erosion, erythroplakia, pseudoerosion, eversion, cervicitis, ectopy,* or even *ulceration* are used in reference to the common red area. *Healing, papillary,* and *follicular* forms are recognised. This traditional and clinically derived terminology is clearly erroneous and inappropriate. Indeed, appearances to which all of these terms can be applied can be found in the foetal cervix (Fig. 1). The material presented later warrants our dealing curtly at the outset with a taxonomy which is hallowed by general usage. Most of these terms may be abandoned. Erythroplakia is acceptable, to describe a red area for it is descriptive without being diagnostic, and does not suggest an abnormality as do conventional terms.

A smooth featureless pink surface surrounding the external os is designated *original squamous epithelium*. The presence of erythroplakia is recorded and its approximate distribution designated as *probably columnar epithelium with or without transformation zone*. White patches are recorded as *keratosis*. Structures and appearances recognised as *polyps, condyloma,* and *overt cancer* are sketched in terms of site and extent. Contact bleeding is noted.

16   *Colposcopy*

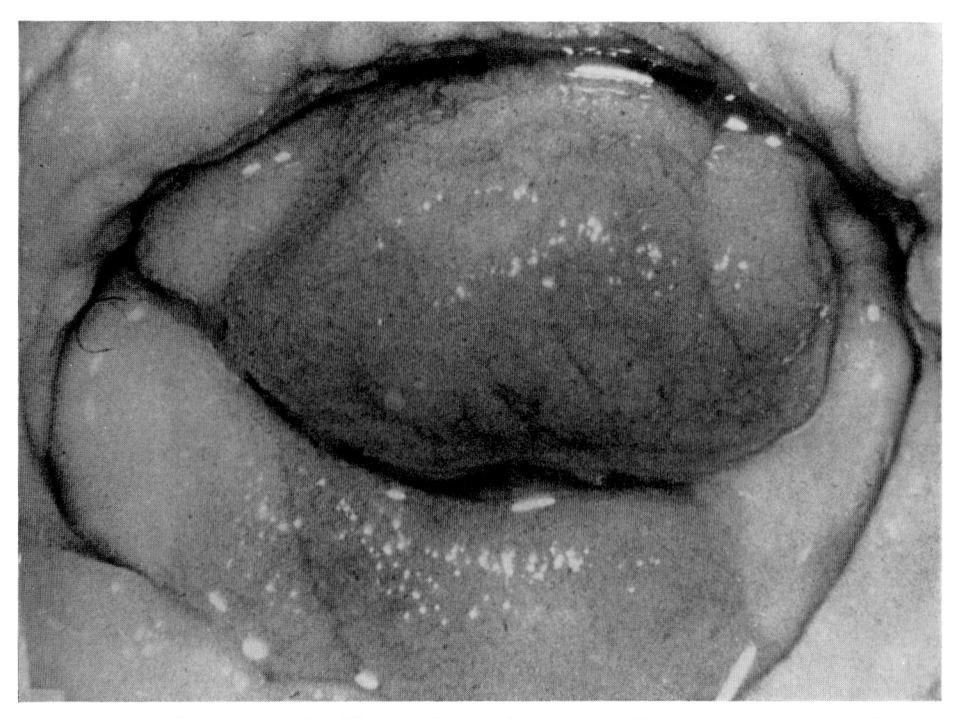

Figure 1. The human cervix. The study is of a preserved necropsy specimen from a day-old neonate. Supposedly adult features are recognisable. A transverse cervical os with lateral extensions is seen, and an extensive red area is present on the surface. Both features could be identified with the terms *laceration* and *erosion*, respectively, as used in descriptions of the adult organ. The occurrence of such features in the neonate emphasizes the fallacy in the use of these terms.

ANATOMICAL DEFINITIONS

Certain easily observed landmarks serve as the key reference points. They are used as the basis upon which illustrative, explanatory, and topographical concepts are developed.

Ectocervix

Ectocervix refers to the vaginal surface of the cervix, extending caudally from the external os to the reflection of the epithelium of the cervix on to the vaginal fornix (Fig. 2).

Endocervix

Endocervix refers to that portion of the cervix lined by epithelium extending cranially from the external os to the junction of its epithelium with the endometrium. This portion is also referred to as the *endocervical canal* (Fig. 2).

External os

When the vaginal walls are opposed, the anterior and posterior lips of the cervix come together, defining the external os usually as a transverse slit. With the introduction of the bivalve vaginal speculum, this relationship is disturbed. The lips are retracted, allowing a portion of the epithelium in the endocervical canal to be displayed. This is termed the *apparent* view. When the blades of the speculum are allowed to collapse upon the cervix, the epithelium returns to the canal and the appearance now constitutes the *real* view (Fig. 3A and B).

Original Squamocolumnar Junction

It has become necessary to refer to the *original squamocolumnar junction* in assisting the understanding of the origins and behaviour of the cervical epithelia. The original squamocolumnar junction can usually be identified in most subjects either with the colposcope or the microscope (Figs. 4 and 5). It is the line of demarcation separating original squamous epithelium from original columnar epithelium and is evident from the foetal stage onwards. In the majority of subjects, however, the original columnar epithelium has been replaced by metaplastic epithelium in its most distal portion, and the original squamocolumnar, now squamo-squamous junction, then separates the two types of squamous epithelium, original and metaplastic (Figs. 6 and 7).

New Squamocolumnar Junction

The line of demarcation separating the metaplastic squamous epithelium from the original columnar epithelium is the *new squamocolumnar junction*. It is thus on the cranial side of the original squamocolumnar junction, from which it is separated by metaplastic squamous epithelium (Fig. 6).

Eversion

Eversion is the dynamic process by which epithelial tissues of the lower portion of the endocervical canal may later become part of the covering of the ectocervix so that the original squamocolumnar junction is displaced caudally by the movement. No tissue destruction or replacement is involved. Eversion may be *apparent* when caused during speculum examination (Fig. 3A and B) or *real* as it can occur, for example, during pregnancy (*see* Figs. 73 to 76).

HISTOLOGICAL DEFINITIONS

Our studies of the cervical epithelium have enabled us to simplify the great number of terms characterising the confused literature on the his-

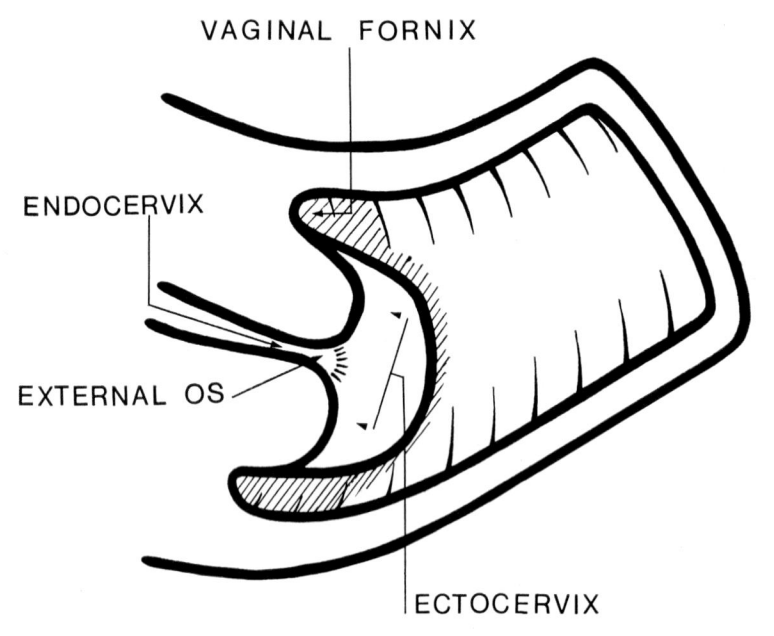

Figure 2. Line drawing of bisected cervix and adjacent vagina, showing anatomical landmarks.

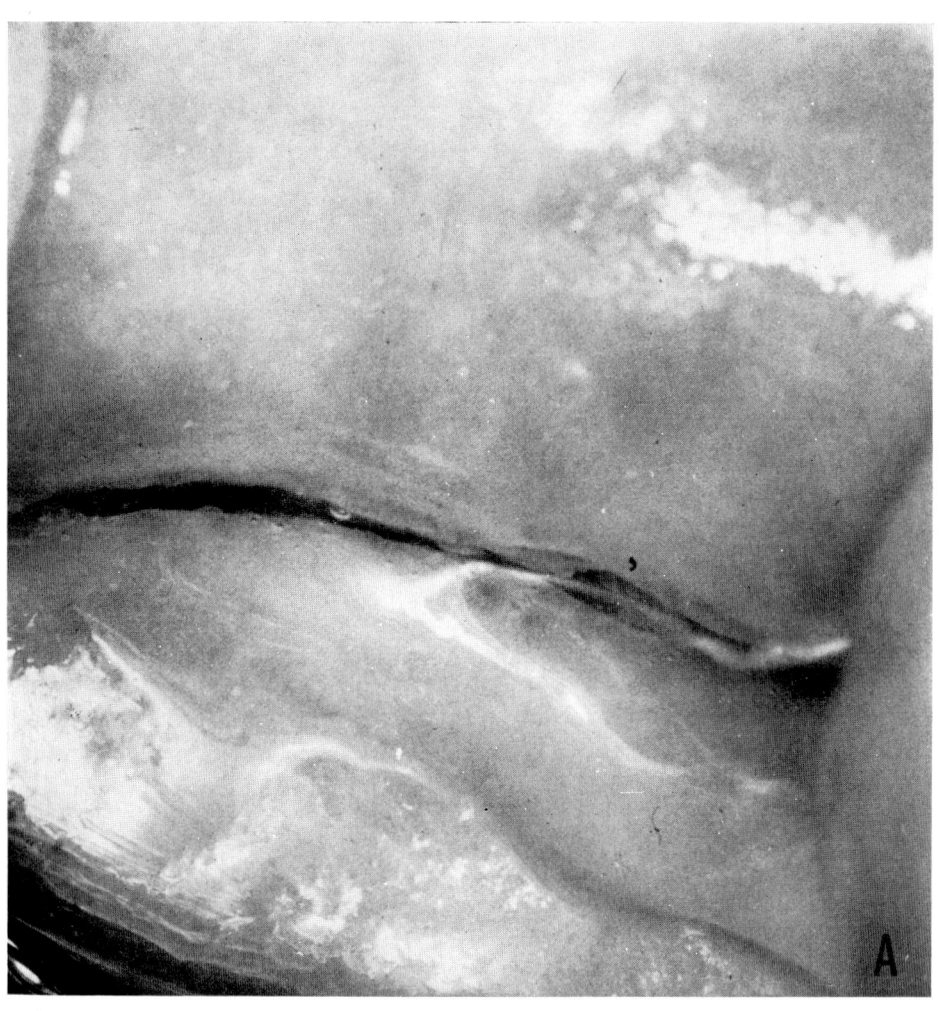

Figure 3A. Real study of cervix. Colpophotograph viewed with blades of speculum collapsed. No cervical canal epithelium is seen.

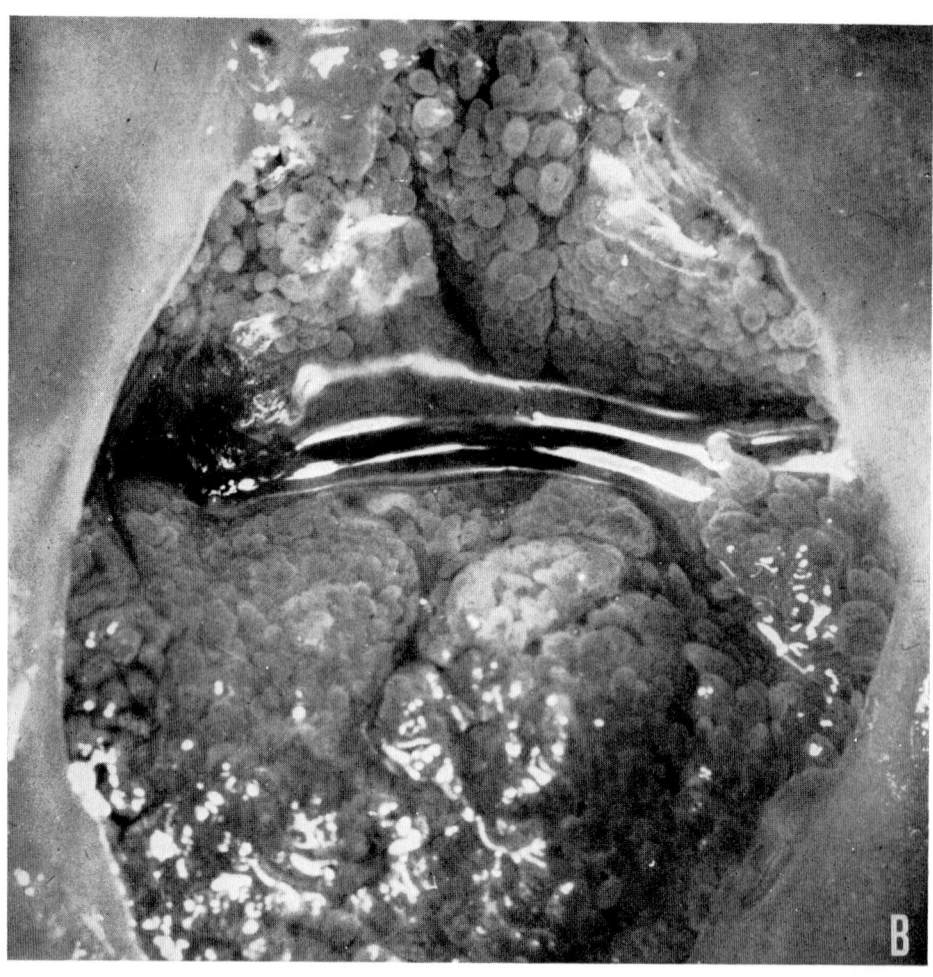

Figure 3B. Apparent study of cervix. Same cervix as Figure 3A. Speculum blades are widely separated, and an extensive area of canal epithelium is everted for inspection, both anteriorly and posteriorly.

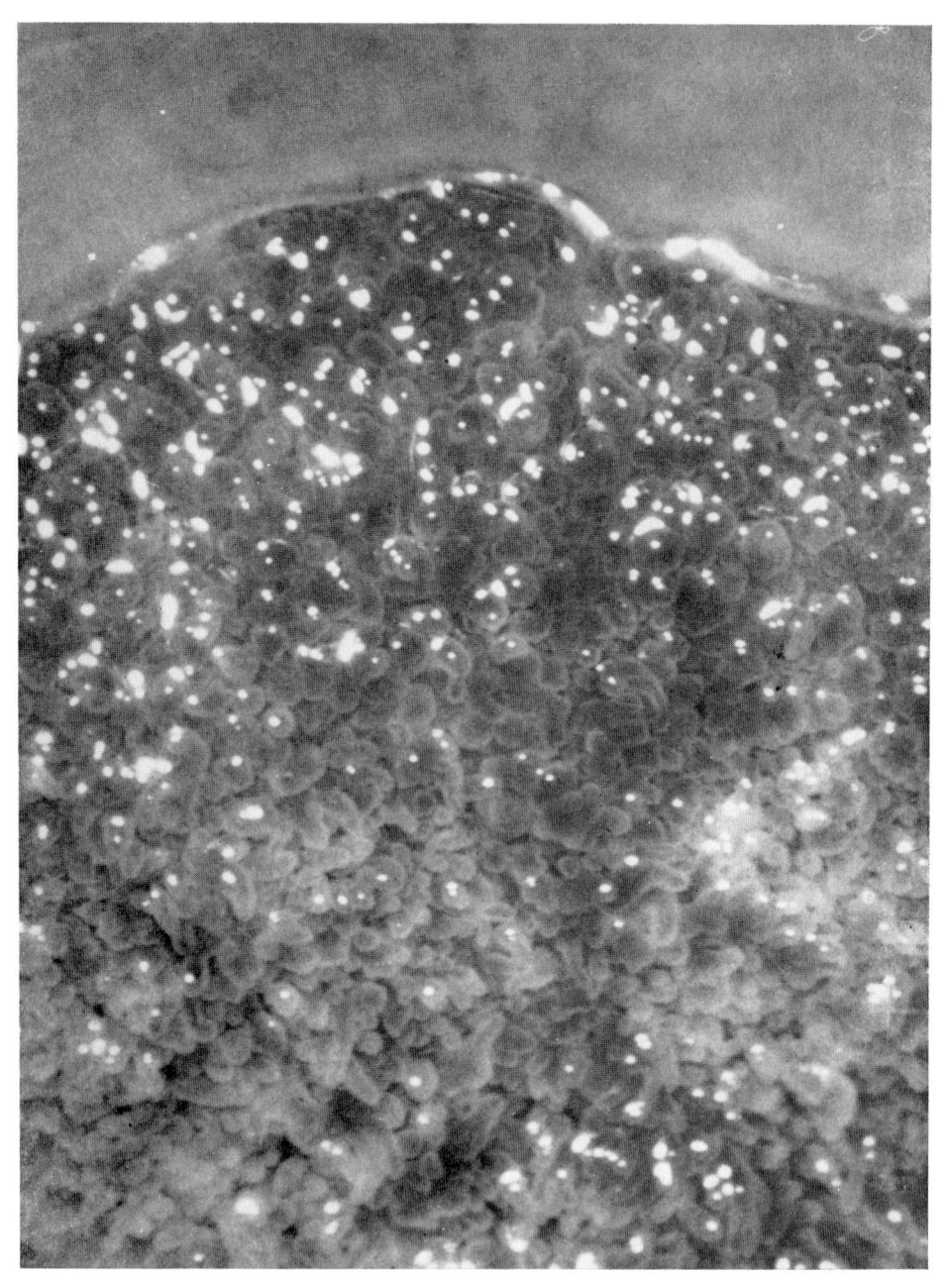

Figure 4. Original squamocolumnar junction. A distinct line across the upper quarter of the colpophotograph separates two types of epithelia: original squamous above and "grapelike" columnar below.

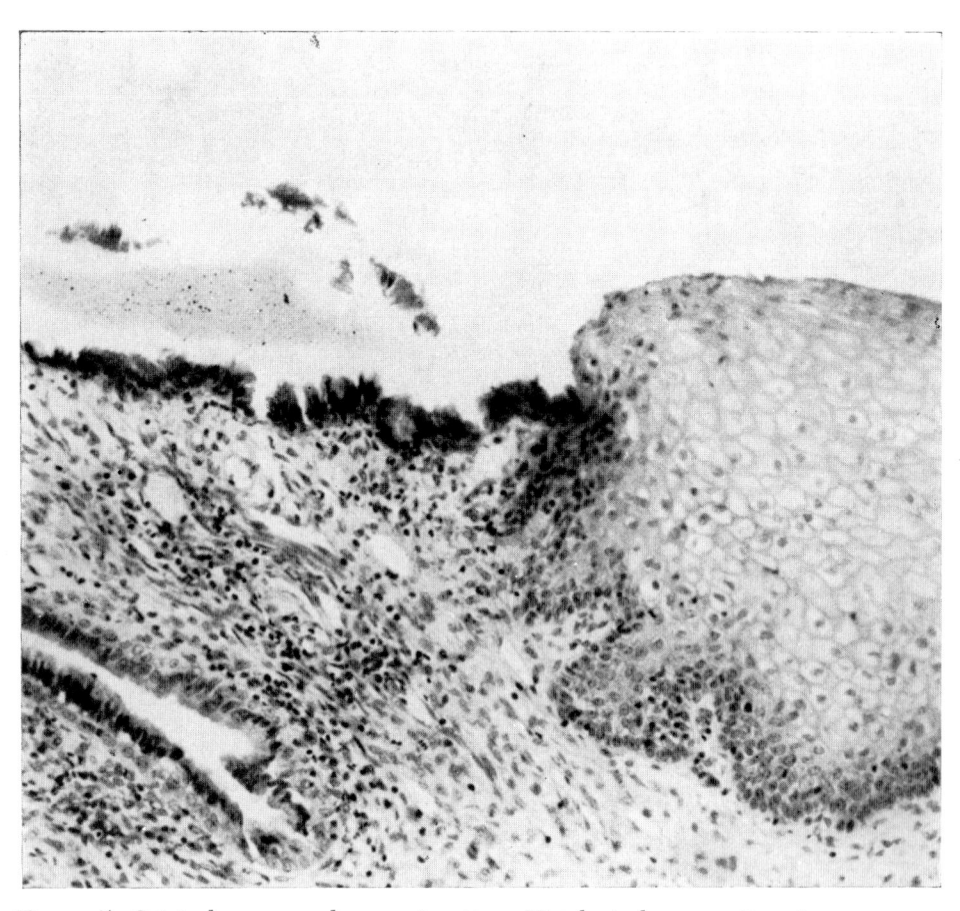

Figure 5. Original squamocolumnar junction. Histological preparation from an area similar to Figure 4. Multilayered squamous epithelium on the right adjoins single-layered columnar epithelium on the left.

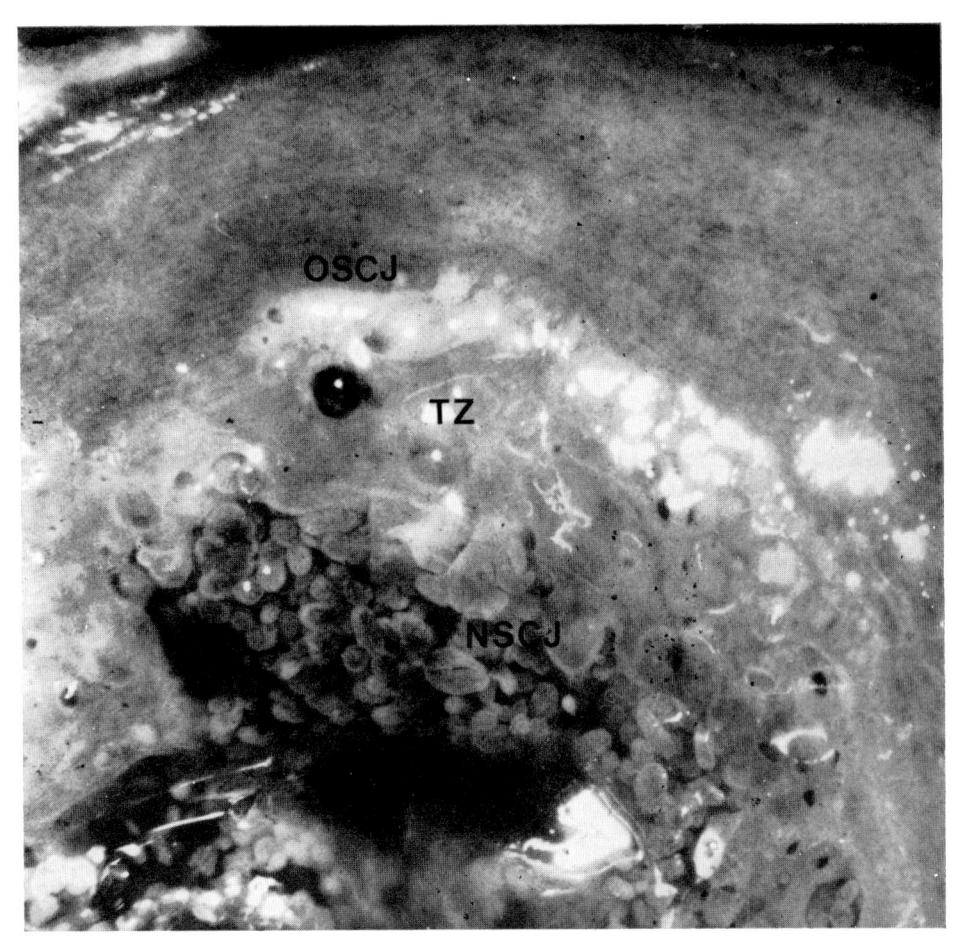

Figure 6. New squamocolumnar junction. This important boundary (NSCJ) marks the cephalic limit of the transformation zone (TZ). Usually visible, it is seen in this colpophotograph as an irregular border at the site where the columnar epithelium is confidently identified by its grapelike surface structure. The caudal limit of the transformation zone is the original squamocolumnar junction (OSCJ), which is now squamo-squamous.

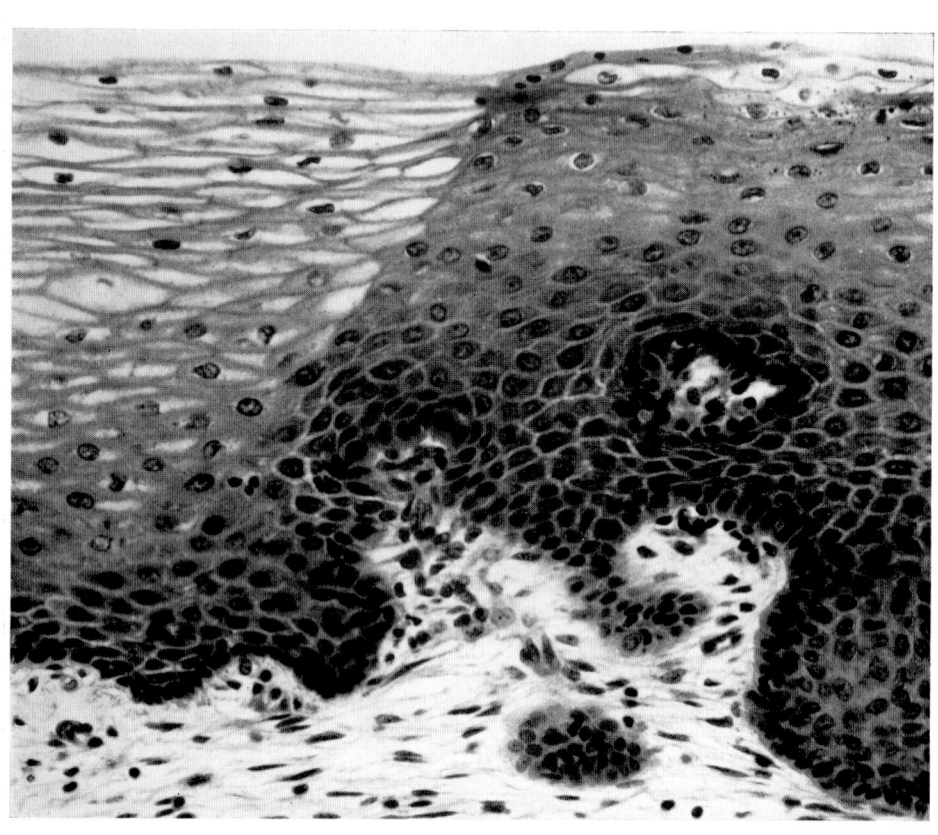

Figure 7. Original squamocolumnar junction (now squamosquamous junction). Histological preparation from area similar to Figure 6. An oblique line separates original squamous from new morphologically different epithelium on the right, which is metaplastic in origin.

tology of the area.* The assistance of colposcopy has been valuable in this regard. Almost invariably in every subject, squamous metaplasia, physiological or atypical, occurs in the caudal portion of the cervical columnar epithelium. This process of squamous metaplasia always occurs within the area cranial to the original squamocolumnar junction and continues to mature (p. 88) sporadically throughout the life of the individual. The recognition of this concept allows a simplified histological terminology.

Original Squamous Epithelium

An *original squamous* multilayered *epithelium,* with potential for keratin production, extends caudally from the original squamocolumnar junction as the covering of portion of the ectocervix, the vaginal fornix, and the vagina (Fig. 8).

Cervical Columnar Epithelium

Cervical columnar epithelium is a single-layered, mucus-producing epithelium continuous with the endometrium cranially and with either the original squamous epithelium or the metaplastic epithelium caudally (Fig. 9). Characteristically, it has clefts or glands and surface projections or villi.

The term *endocervical epithelium* is misleading, since it infers that columnar epithelium is exclusively within the cervical canal. This is erroneous at any stage of the life of the individual, and the term should be discarded.

Metaplastic Epithelium: (Physiological Metaplastic Epithelium)

A *metaplastic* multilayered *epithelium,* with potential for keratin production, is usually distinguishable from both types defined previously (Fig. 10). This epithelium, termed *physiological metaplastic epithelium,* gives rise to appearances which constitute the *typical transformation zone* and is encountered always cranial to the original squamocolumnar junc-

---

* In the comprehensive monograph on dysplasia and preclinical carcinoma (Gray, 1964), the following terms were encountered: active and undifferentiated immature metaplasia, adenomatous hyperplasia, anaplasia, atypical epithelium, atypical hyperplasia, atypical reserve cell hyperplasia, atypical metaplasia, basal cell hyperplasia, chronic endocervicitis, cystic cervicitis, dystrophic squamous epithelial lesions of the cervix, endocervicitis, epidermisation, epidermidalisation, epidermoid hyperplasia, glandular hyperplasia, immature metaplasia, intraglandular hyperplasia, indirect metaplasia, irregular dysplasis, papillary anaplasia, precancerous metaplasia, prickle cell hyperplasia, prickle cell hyperplasia with dysplasia, pseudoepitheliomatous hyperplasia, reserve cell anaplasia, reserve cell dysplasia, reserve cell hyperplasia, regular dysplasia, squamous prosoplasia, squamocolumnar prosoplasia, squamous metaplasia, subcylindrical cell hyperplasia, undifferentiated regenerative epithelium, *unruhig* epithelium.

tion, replacing a variable portion of the cervical columnar epithelium which originally occupied the site. Discrete sites of metaplastic epithelium occur apart from the main area.

Immature Metaplastic Epithelium

Immature metaplastic epithelium is multilayered, with a high cell density. The cytoplasm of its constituent cells is scant (Fig. 11). It represents the histological appearance of early phases of metaplasia. Some examples are difficult to distinguish from various forms of dysplasia and the full-thickness loss of differentiation characteristic of carcinoma in situ (Fig. 12). Large numbers of histological variations with increasing stratification and differentiation show progressive stages of maturation and are in part responsible for the confusion in terminology which has arisen.

Some stromal appearances accompanying various stages of maturity of physiological metaplasia are also frequently interpreted as a form of "cervicitis" or "chronic inflammation" (Fig. 13). Our understanding of the significance of these so-called inflammatory cells in the area is that they represent merely the cellular activity accompanying metaplasia and perhaps an as yet unspecified immunological response.

Dysplasia or Dysplastic Epithelium: (Atypical Metaplastic Epithelium)

Dysplasia or *dysplastic epithelium* is identical with the physiological metaplastic variety, except in a range of disorders of nuclear morphology. This identity of the histologically normal with the abnormal is stressed and seems to extend to all other features, such as topography. It arises on the cranial side of the original squamocolumnar junction and not from the original squamous epithelium. These epithelia exhibit cells of variable nuclear size, shape, chromatin content, and mitotic activity but retain some degree of squamous differentiation in their superficial layers.

MINOR DYSPLASIA: The disorder of nuclear structure and degree of undifferentiation involves half or less of the thickness of the epithelium (Fig. 14). When the disorder is just distinguishable on morphological grounds it is termed *abnormal epithelium* (Fig. 15).

MAJOR DYSPLASIA: The disorder involves more than half the thickness of the epithelium. Nuclear pleomorphism, hyperchromatism, and mitoses are more marked in this category (Fig. 16).

Carcinoma In Situ CIS (Stage O)

Carcinoma in situ is an epithelium identical with major dysplasia, except that the cellular disorder involves a full-thickness loss of differentiation (Fig. 17).

Cervical Intraepithelial Neoplasia

Cervical intraepithelial neoplasia (CIN) is a broad term covering all the precursors of squamous cancer (dysplasia and carcinoma in situ). A term of increasing popularity, its value lies in emphasising the graded continuity of the lesions. CIN 1, CIN 2, and CIN 3 are recognised and have an approximate correlation with minor dysplasia, major dysplasia, and carcinoma in situ.

Preclinical Invasive Carcinoma

Preclinical invasive carcinoma is not clinically evident following traditional inspection, palpation, probing, and endocervical curettage.

MICROINVASIVE CARCINOMA: This is identical with carcinoma in situ, except for the appearance of scattered small discrete foci of invasion through the basement membrane, whether from the surface epithelium or from that lining the cervical glands (Figs. 18 and 19). The depth of penetration into the stroma does not exceed 5 mm from the surface of the point of origin. The presence of lymphatic or vascular permeation does not exclude the diagnosis.

OCCULT INVASIVE CARCINOMA: This is diagnosed when the invasive foci are confluent and the depth of penetration into the stroma exceeds 5 mm. Such a lesion, in contradistinction to overt carcinoma, is not evident by classical clinical examination and is therefore defined as *occult*.

Preclinical Carcinoma

Carcinoma in situ and preclinical invasive carcinoma together constitute *preclinical carcinoma*.

Overt Carcinoma

Overt invasive carcinoma is obvious by clinical examination, usually in exophytic or ulcerative form. The histological appearances are similar to those found with occult invasive cancer but generally are more extensive in size and depth of penetration (Fig. 20).

Clinical and Histological Subdivisions of Stage I Cancer of the Cervix

Numerous classifications of Stage I carcinoma of the cervix (invasive cancer confined to the cervix) exist in the literature. These include the International Federation of Gynecology and Obstetrics (FIGO) "clinical" and numerous histological classifications. Few, if any, now use the term *preclinical invasive cancer* as just defined. Because of the authority of FIGO and our reticence to complicate further the nomenclature, it is necessary to justify the use of this term.

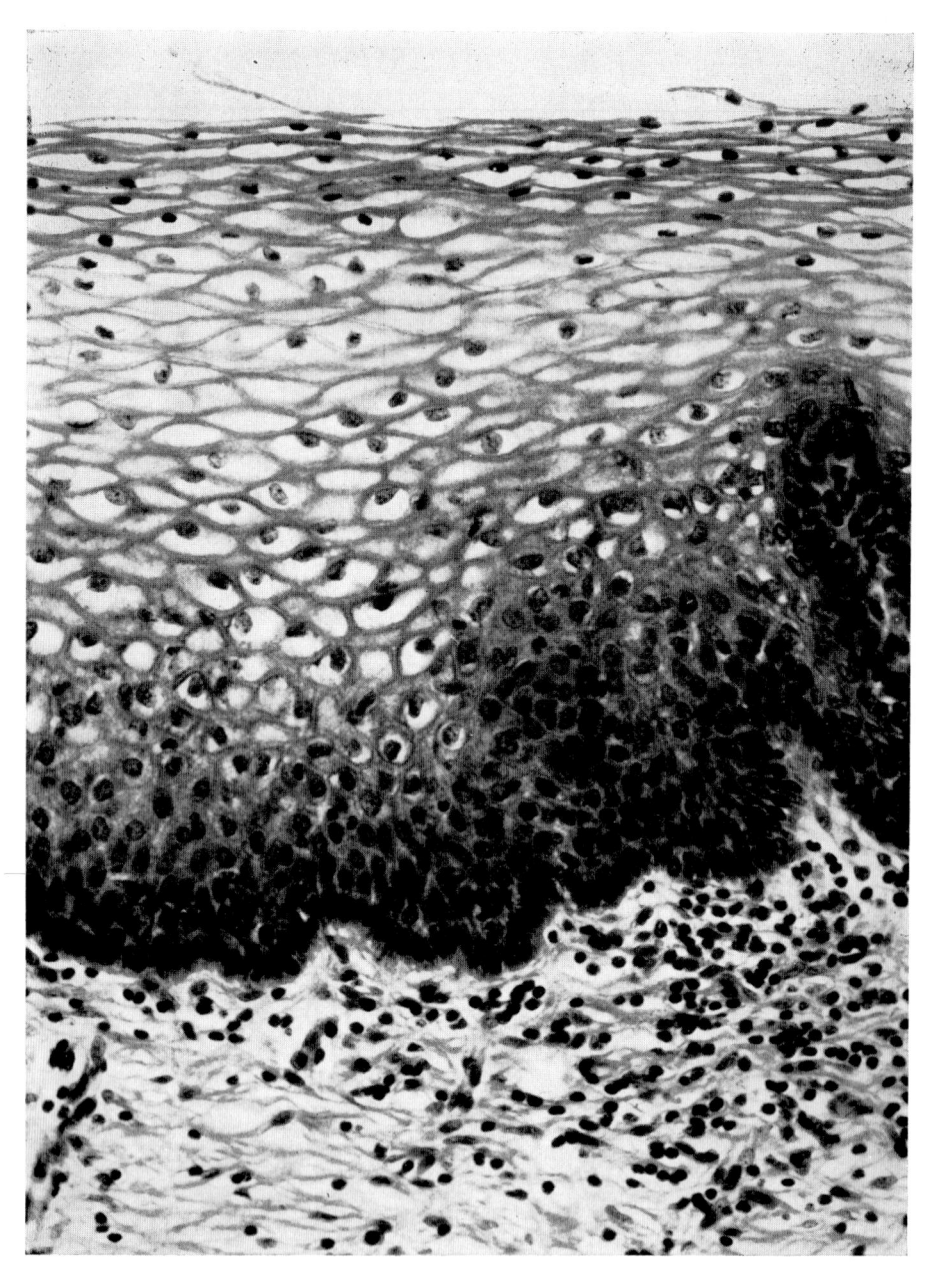

Figure 8. Original squamous epithelium. In the adult, fully differentiated multilayered epithelium with basal, parabasal, and prickle cells and superficial squames is present.

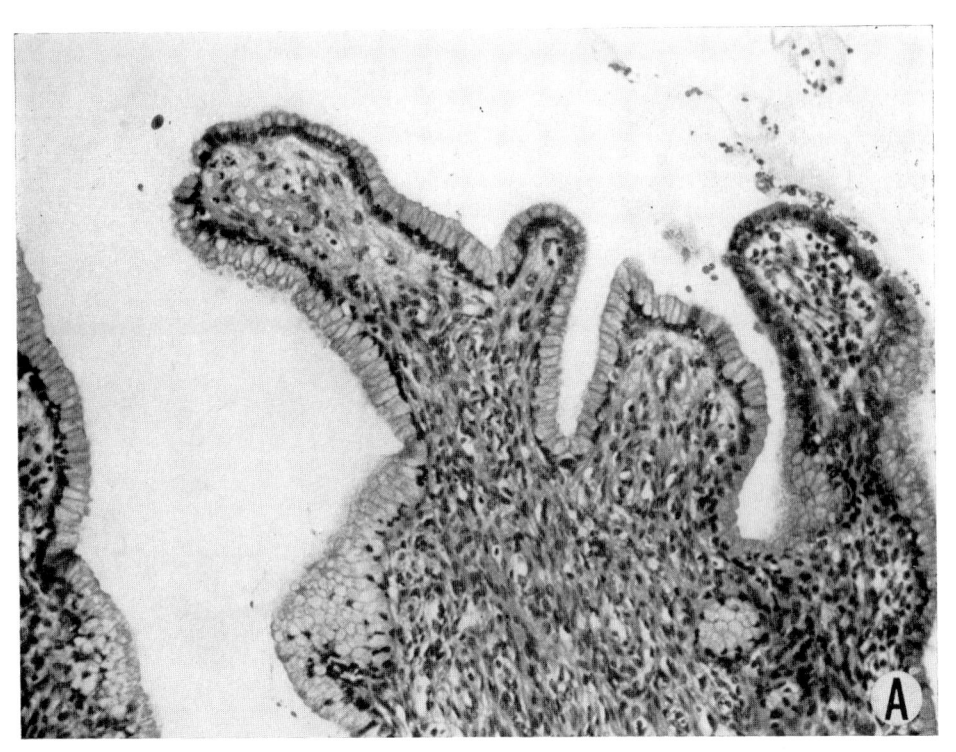

Figure 9A. Cervical columnar epithelium. (×150) In subjects of all ages, the single-layered, mucus-secreting epithelium overlying the stroma is disposed in villous and papillary surface projections. In this photograph, a cleft structure extends into the stroma.

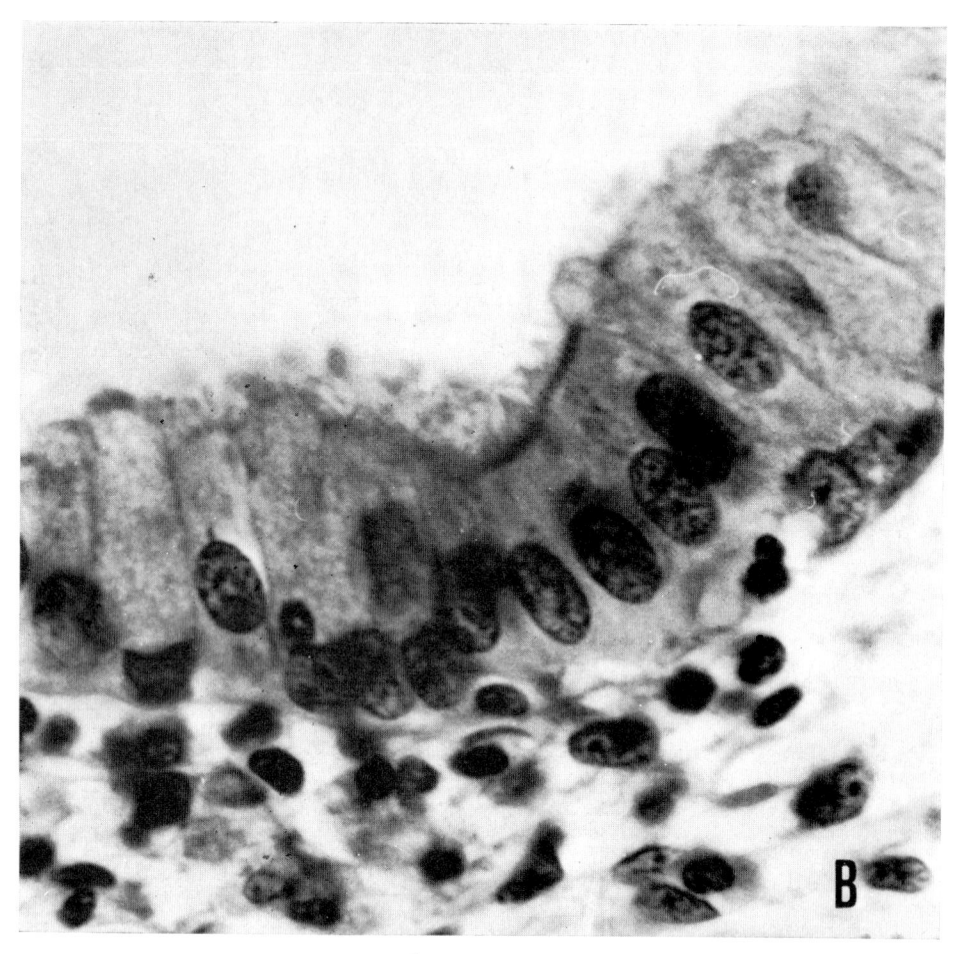

Figure 9B. Columnar epithelium. (×800)

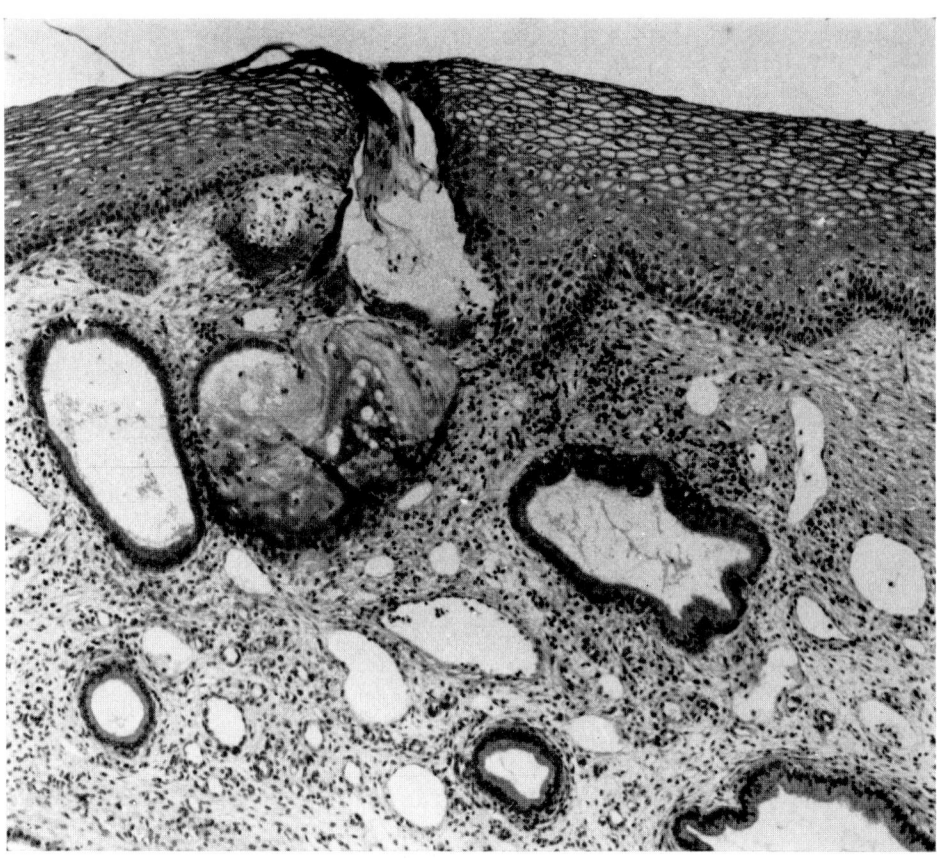

Figure 10. Metaplastic epithelium. Distinct from Figures 8 and 9, a multilayered, differentiated epithelium is seen overlying cervical glands. The metaplastic epithelium during its formation replaces similar columnar epithelium on the surface. Note the cleft opening in the centre, which would be recognisable colposcopically as a gland opening.

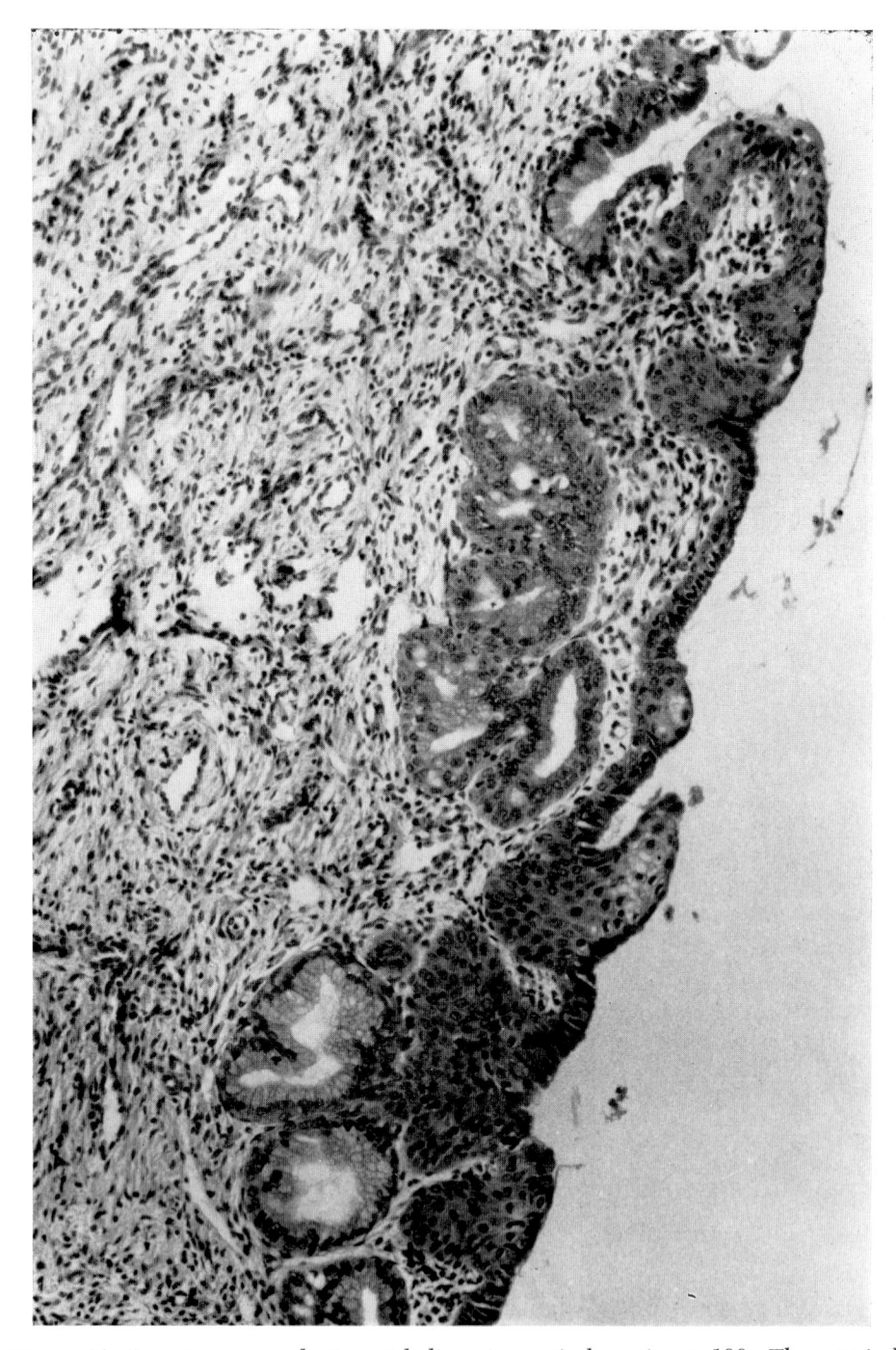

Figure 11. Immature metaplastic epithelium in vertical section ×100. The cervical canal is shown on the right of the photograph. During its initial phase, metaplastic epithelium seen here on the surface displays undifferentiated cells, especially in the lower third of the photograph. With maturity, the epithelium assumes the form seen in Figure 10. Lying deeper in the stroma are cervical glands indicating the columnar cell origin of the overlying epithelium.

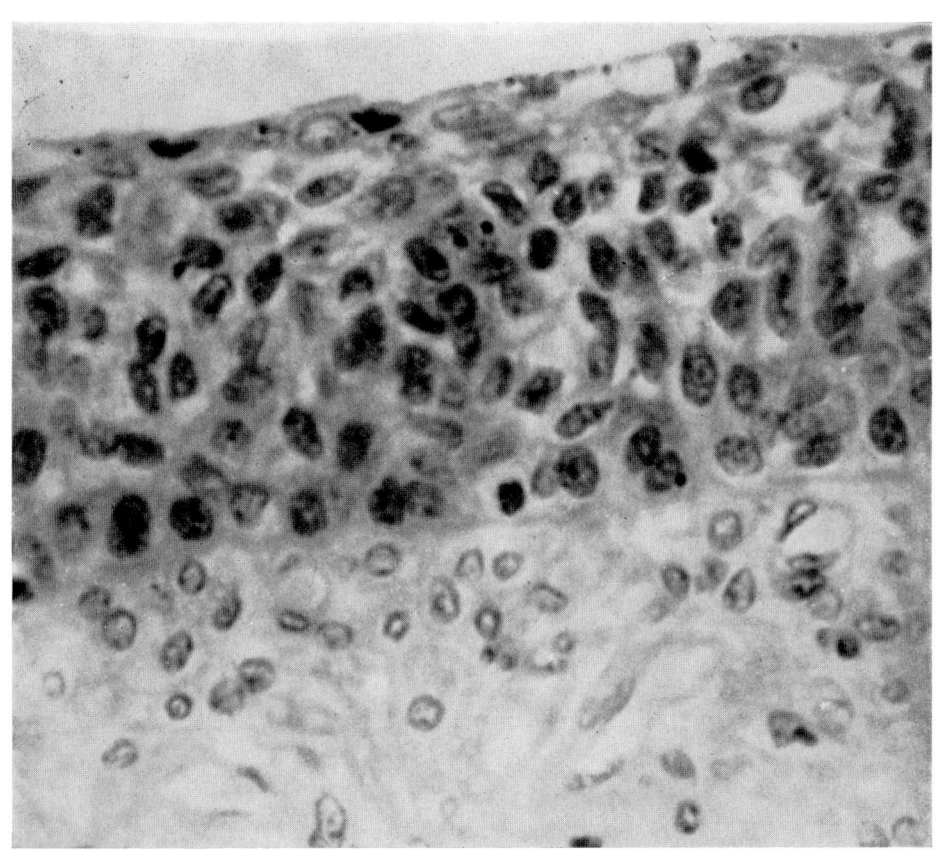

Figure 12. Immature metaplastic epithelium. Undifferentiated metaplastic squamous epithelium (six to ten cells thick) in a one-year-old girl. Absence of significant differentiation and lack of "polarisation" in this histological section indicates the difficulties of distinguishing such appearances from *in situ* carcinoma.

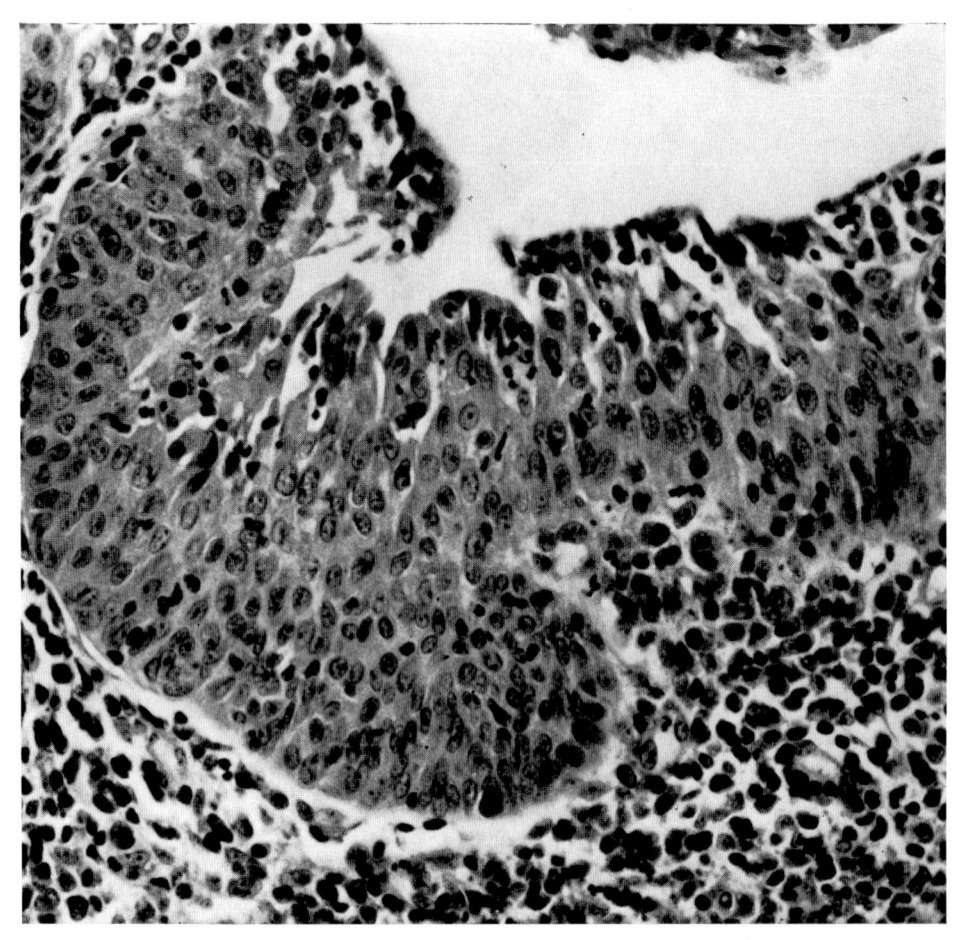

Figure 13. Chronic cervicitis. (×100) Collections of round cells in stroma adjacent to metaplastic epithelium. A few round cells have even infiltrated the epithelium. This appearance does not necessarily reflect response to infectious agents.

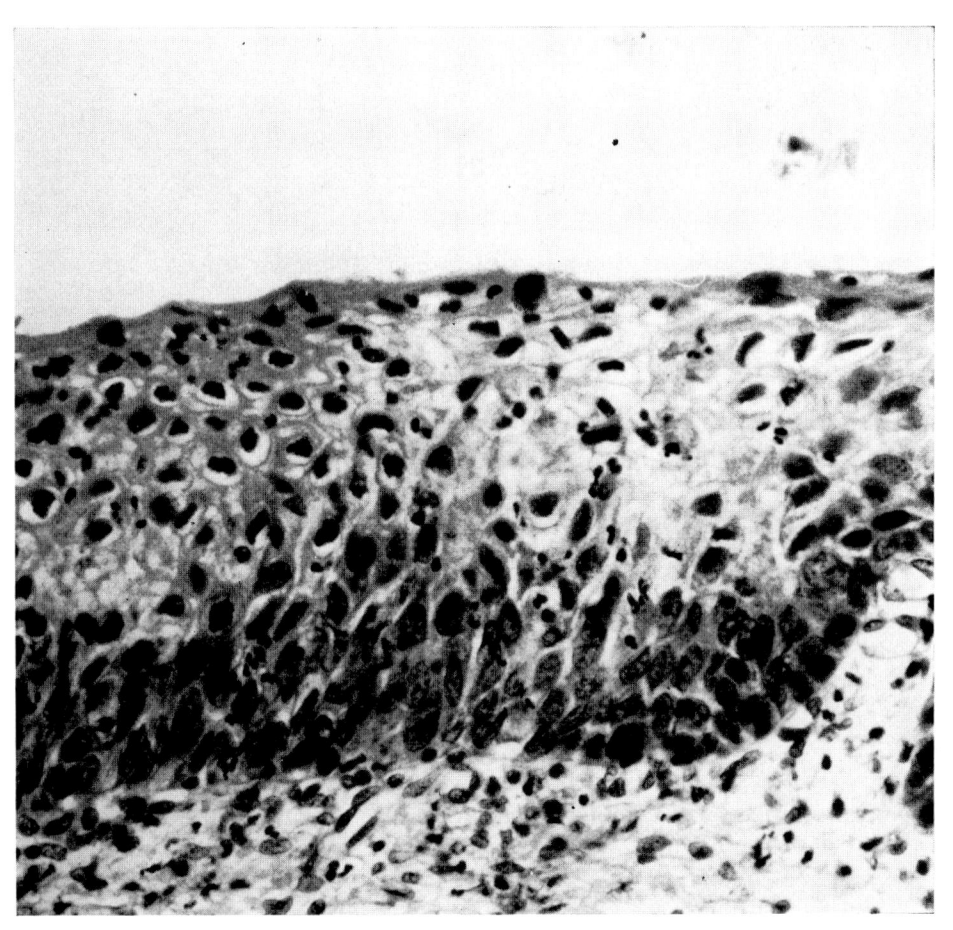

Figure 14. Minor dysplasia. Metaplastic epithelium displaying differentiation in upper layers of the epithelium but increased width of basal layer and minimal changes in nuclear morphology, especially on the right side.

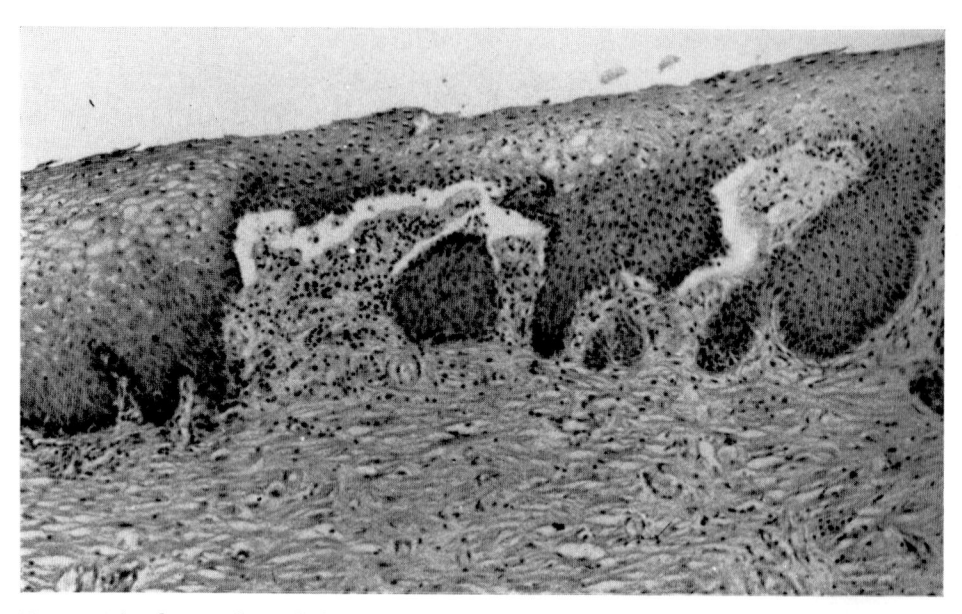

Figure 15. Abnormal epithelium. A variety of metaplastic epithelium displaying differentiation, increased cellularity, and minimal changes in nuclear morphology is seen on the right of the photograph. It adjoins original squamous epithelium on the left.

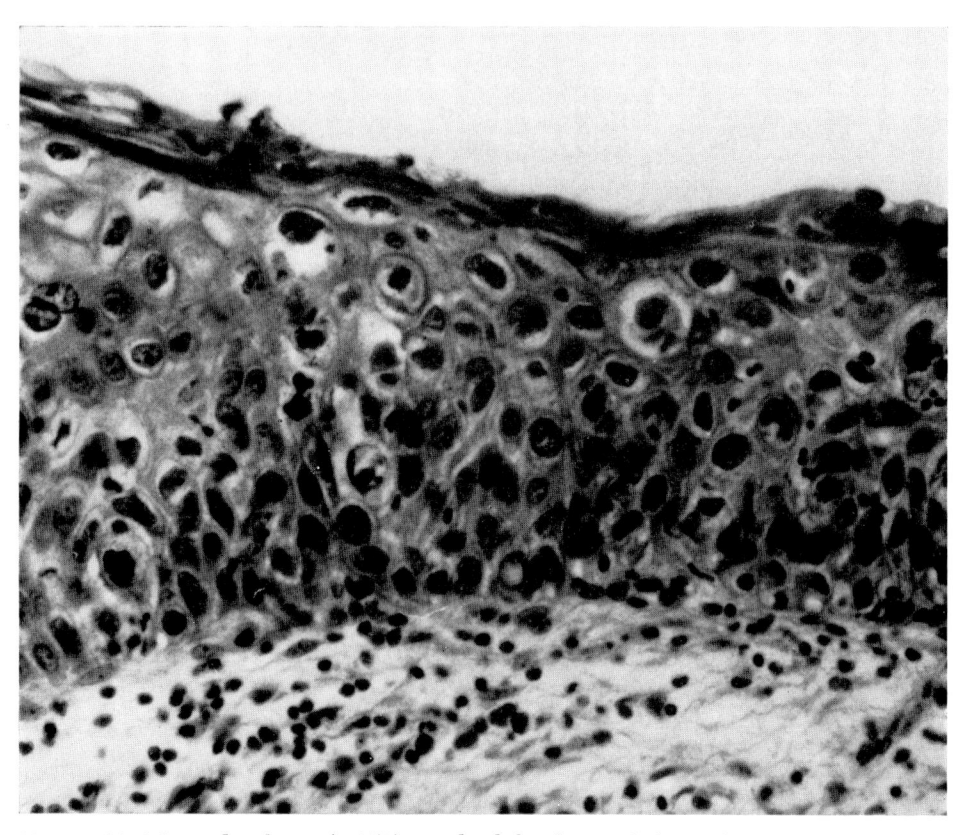

Figure 16. Major dysplasia. (×250) To the left, the epithelium shows major dysplasia with irregularity of structure, pleomorphism, and hyperchromatism amongst its cells. At right, these changes have progressed to a state conventionally termed *borderline carcinoma in situ*.

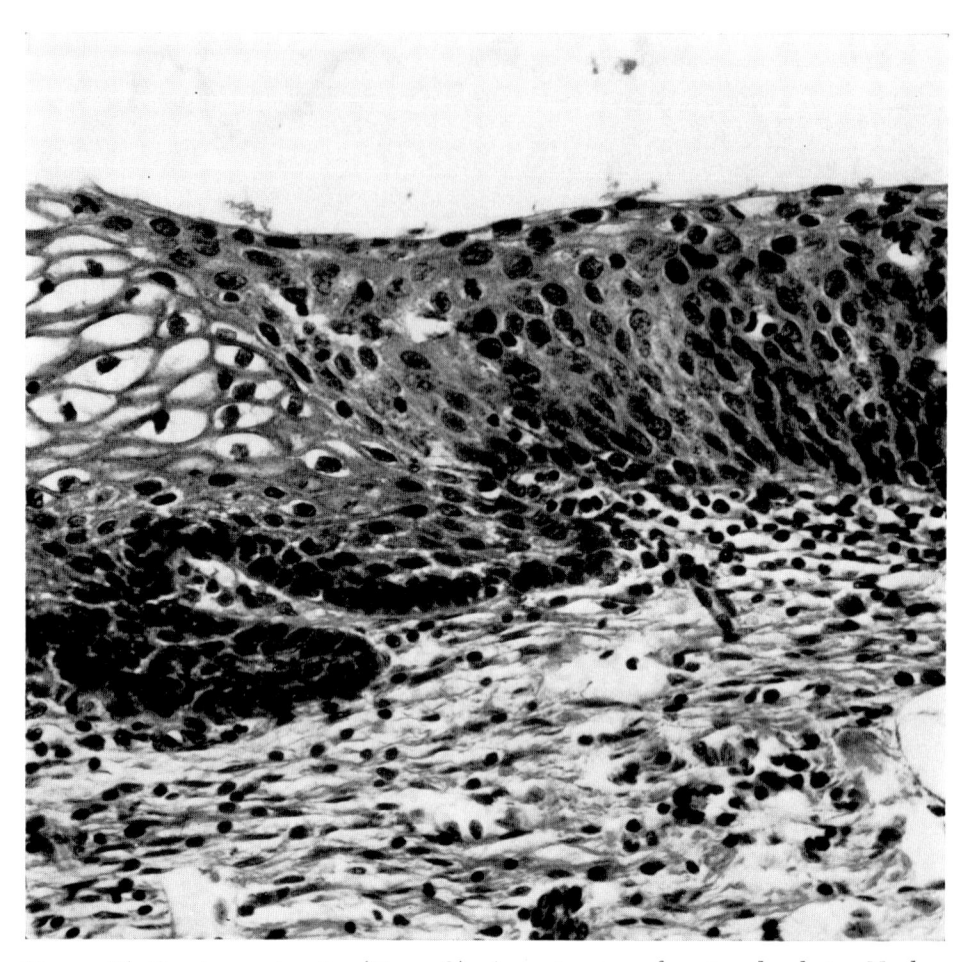

Figure 17. Carcinoma in situ (Stage O). An extension of major dysplasia. Nuclear pleomorphism and hyperchromatism are seen through the full thickness of this undifferentiated epithelium. Towards the left of the photograph, the epithelium shows a characteristic sharp junction with well-differentiated squamous epithelium.

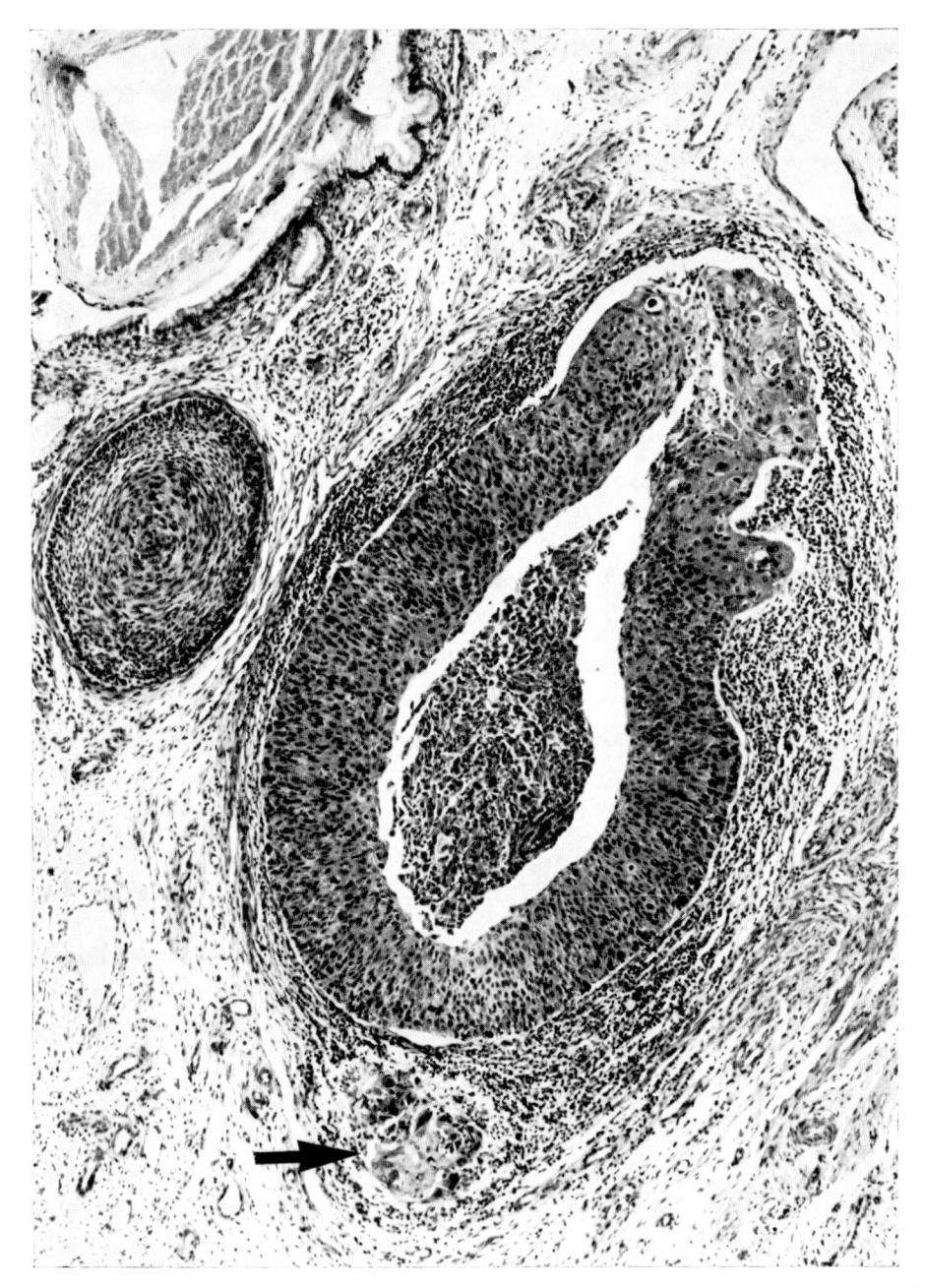

Figure 18. Microinvasive carcinoma. Multifocal microinvasion arising from a gland. Tongues of cells (arrow) extend through the basement membrane from epithelium displaying features of carcinoma in situ.

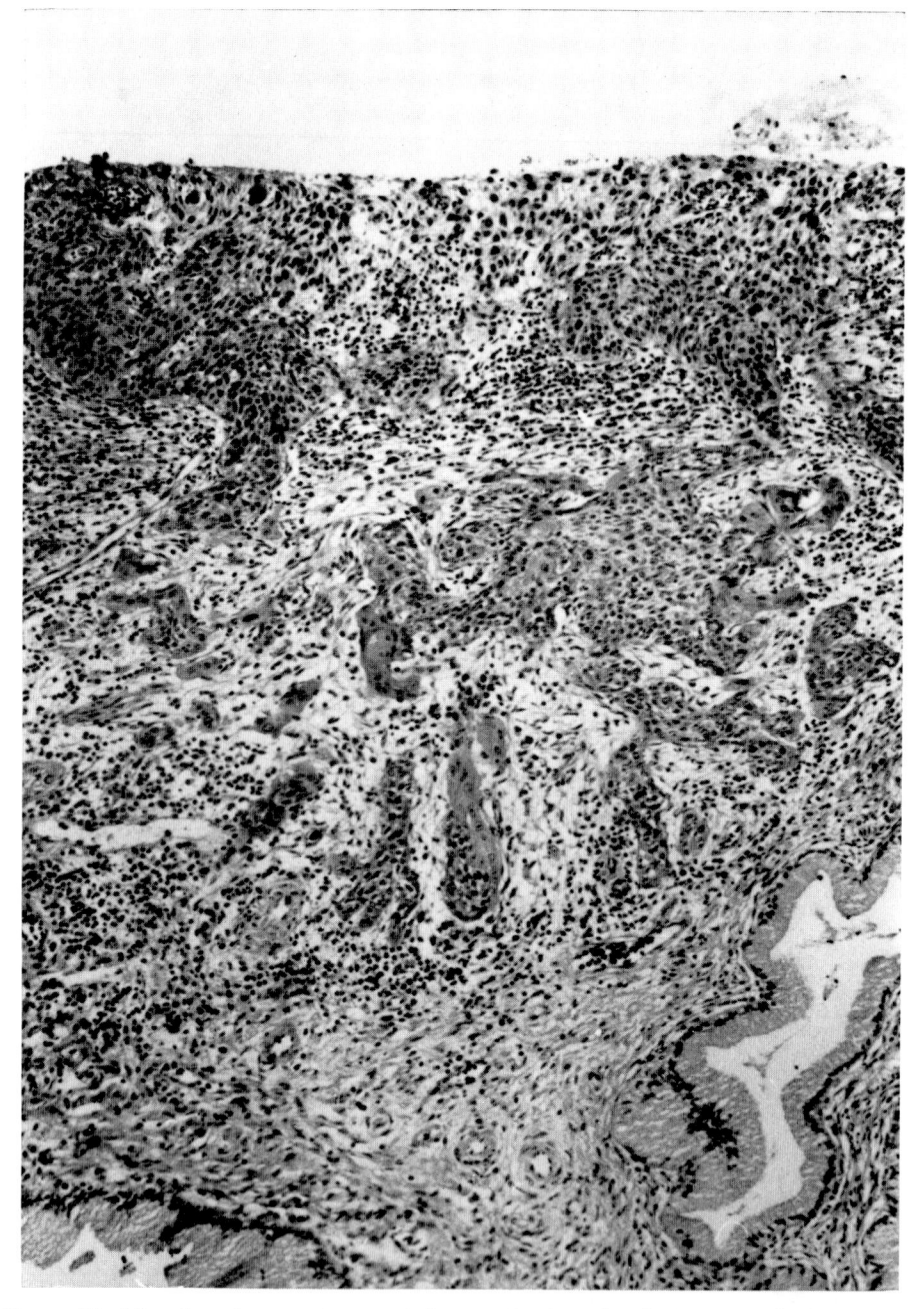

Figure 19. Microinvasive carcinoma. A large microinvasive lesion extends 2 to 3 mm into the stroma. When invasion exceeds 5 mm, the lesion is referred to as an *occult invasive carcinoma*. Differences in the interpretation of this type of lesion are discussed on p. 43.

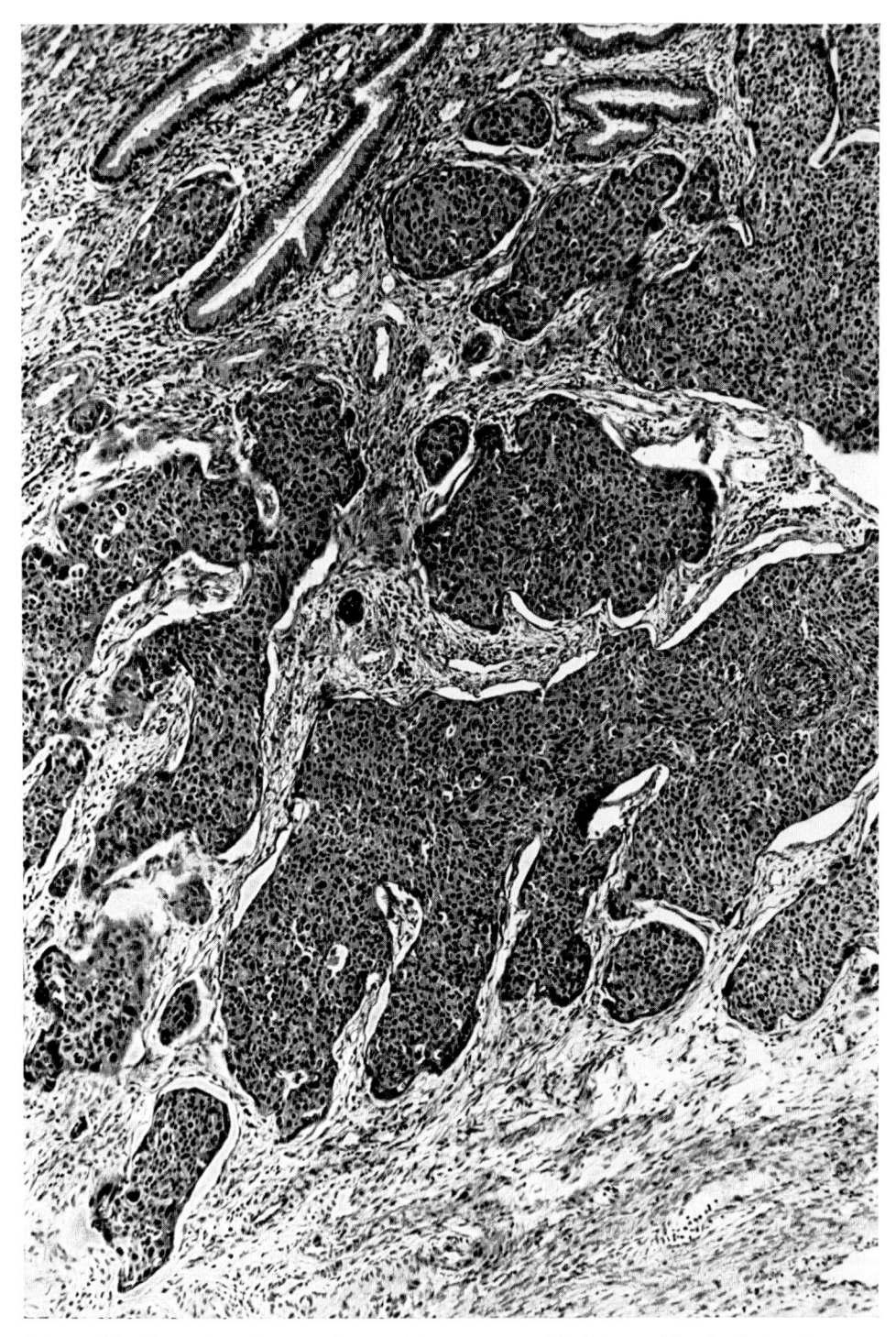

Figure 20. Overt invasive carcinoma. By contrast with Figure 19, the lesion is more extensive in both size and depth of penetration.

To the practising gynaecologist, on traditional grounds, the clinical differentiation of cervix cancer is basic; the lesion is either evident or not evident, clinical or preclinical.

The FIGO classification (International Federation, 1976) is based on "careful clinical examination." However, far more extensive procedures than those traditionally regarded as clinical have been used to produce the definition, and this is the seat of the confusion. For example, the federation's notes to staging state that "conisation or amputation of the cervix should be regarded as a clinical examination." A major component in each of these procedures is the retrospective use of histopathology after the phase of clinical evaluation in cases where there was no gross evidence of cancer. This is no trivial academic point, since diagnosis and therefore all subsequent registration of records has insidiously shifted to the laboratory.

Histological classifications are based on different sets of subjective parameters. Predictably, numerous schemes are offered. Most attempt to subdivide non-clinical invasive cancer into two groups; one where the gynaecologist treats the woman radically (FIGO—occult invasive 1B), the other, where treatment is more conservative (FIGO—microinvasive 1A). The degree of subjectivity in histological diagnosis can be gauged from Table I. The lack of general agreement on features constituting occult invasion is not surprising in view of the absence of consensus on what constitutes microinvasion. The ultimate management of the case by the gynaecologist rests on just this indecision and arbitrariness involved in histological diagnosis. Thus, the World Health Organization (Poulsen et al, 1975), in pointing up the accuracy of pathology, is vague in defining critical parameters concerned, for example, with early invasion. Ill-defined descriptions including "limited to isolated microscopic foci" and lesions which "do not reveal more extensive invasion" abound, calling into serious question conclusions such as "The spread of cancer is more accurately assessed by pathological staging than by clinical staging."

The essence of the problem can be expressed in another way. Every gynaecologist of some experience has encountered unexpected cases of invasive cancer, whether signalled by a positive smear or discovered in a uterus removed for some other indication. Such cases can embrace the full spectrum of histological invasion named in the FIGO and other classifications, from early stromal invasion even to frank invasion. The undoubted fact that the histological appearances of frank cancer can occur in the absence of clinical sign is confusing.

The emergence of the colposcope resolves much of the confusion, since a method for clinical assessment of invasion is at hand. The value of colposcopy in the clinical assessment of preinvasive lesions is now established. We believe it is of equal value in clinical assessment of early in-

TABLE I

STAGE I—CANCER OF CERVIX

INTEGRATION OF TERMS

Clinical	Histological	International Staging (FIGO)
Preclinical invasive cancer*	Microinvasive†	Stage IA
	Invasive‡	Stage 1B (occult)
Clinical cancer	Invasive‡	Stage IB

* Cancer not recognised by traditional methods of examination (including endocervical curettage).

† Great variation in histological definition. Parameters used are arbitrarily determined and include the following:
1. Cutoff points for depth of penetration into stroma; e.g. 1 mm (Nelson, Averette, and Richart, 1975), 3 mm (Mussey, Soule, and Welch, 1969; DiSaia, Townsend, and Morrow, 1975), 5 mm (Ng and Reagan, 1969; Roche and Norris, 1975)
2. Confluency (Boyes, Worth and Fidler, 1970)
3. Permeation of vascular (lymphatic) spaces (Mussey, Soule, and Welch, 1969; Boutselis, Ullery, and Charme, 1971).

‡ Such lesions may be indistinguishable on histological examination. Frank invasion can occur, although lesion is *preclinical*. Such lesions are usually recognisable as *colposcopically suspect overt cancer*.

vasive cancer. By allowing the more precise differentiation of these lesions, a combination of colposcopy and histology becomes paramount in evaluation. The practical result is a more rational management (p. 414). It is to be hoped that nomenclature committees, in future revisions of Stage I of the international classification, will return to the intended "clinical" spirit of staging and introduce the simple subdivision of Stage 1A, *preclinical invasive cancer*, to be subdivided as at present into the two histological entities (microinvasive and occult invasive) and Stage 1B, *clinical invasive cancer* (Table I).

COLPOSCOPIC DEFINITIONS

At this stage, it is necessary to define the main appearances revealed by the colposcope without attempting to describe their range of variation or to explain the tissue basis of these appearances. The theory of colposcopy demands new nomenclature and systems of description. The following colposcopic entities are recognised.

Original Squamous Epithelium

Original squamous epithelium is clearly identified as a smooth, usually featureless covering of the cervix (Fig. 21).

Original Columnar Epithelium

Also with certainty, *original columnar epithelium* is identified as areas exhibiting characteristic multiple villous or grapelike projections (Fig. 22).

Original Transformation Zone

A new term which denotes metaplastic epithelium present in the cervix since the neonatal period, *original transformation zone* (p. 374), is recognisable as a distinct entity in the adult.

Typical Transformation Zone

The area containing metaplastic epithelium of physiological origin is termed *typical transformation zone*. Its characteristic appearances enable the colposcopist to recognise convincingly the histologist's metaplasia (Fig. 23). Just as the early phases of metaplasia are represented on histological examination by undifferentiated or immature metaplastic epithelium, so colposcopic appearances show a similar distinctive counterpart (Fig. 24).

Atypical Transformation Zone

When the metaplastic sheet of epithelium exhibits certain atypical features, specific colposcopic appearances result. It is termed the *atypical transformation zone*. This zone is precisely coextensive with the field of neoplastic potential, which may later be expressed in the development of invasive squamous cancer of the cervix.

Atypical transformation zone exists when one or more of the following specific appearances is encountered, following the application of aqueous acetic acid solution (p. 178). These areas are almost invariably sharply delineated from surrounding areas. Their distal border is always on the cranial side of the original squamocolumnar junction.

WHITE EPITHELIUM: "Geographical" delineated areas of white or whitish grey, opaque epithelium in which vascular structures are either not seen or minimally developed constitute the basic appearance of the atypical transformation zone (Fig. 25).

PUNCTATION: Within areas of white epithelium, intraepithelial capillaries with a punctate or stippled arrangement are frequently seen (Fig. 26).

MOSAIC: Within areas of white epithelium, the intraepithelial capillaries form patterns that are mosaic in arrangement (Fig. 27).

ATYPICAL VESSELS: Within areas of white epithelium, intraepithelial vessels have a bizarre branching pattern (Fig. 28).

KERATOSIS: In the atypical transformation zone, excessive keratin production may result in the appearance of keratosis (Fig. 29). This entity is sometimes evident without colposcopic magnification and may also overlie original squamous epithelium.

"GRADING OF ATYPICAL TRANSFORMATION ZONES": The recognition of variations in quality of the appearances of these areas has necessitated a new form of grading. Three grades are considered significant in histological prediction (p. 156), in assessment of prognosis (p. 403), and in management (p. 397).

Colposcopically Suspect Overt Carcinoma

Colposcopically suspect overt carcinoma is not evident on grounds of clinical examination but revealed at colposcopic examination (Fig. 30). This uncommon but clinically important entity is to be distinguished from overt cancer evident on clinical examination (Fig. 31).

Miscellaneous Findings

A variety of appearances unrelated to metaplasia is encountered. This includes the following.

VAGINOCERVICITIS: This term replaces the classical term *colpitis*, which is etymologically less suitable. Vaginocervicitis refers to appearances due to parasitic and chemical agents (Fig. 32) and not to the condition *chronic cervicitis* used in traditional clinical and histological nomenclature.

ATROPHIC CERVICITIS: Oestrogen-deficient vaginocervicitis: This term is used to denote the characteristic appearances of oestrogen-deprived epithelium (Fig. 33).

TRUE EROSION: An area denuded of epithelium, usually by trauma, is true erosion (Fig. 34).

CONDYLOMA AND PAPILLOMA: Benign, exophytic reactions to a viral agent are condyloma and papilloma (Fig. 35). No distinction is made between the two conditions, and the first term is preferred (p. 286).

CERVICAL ULCER—NON-MALIGNANT: Such lesions are uncommon and usually of inflammatory or traumatic origin (Fig. 36).

INCONSPICUOUS IODINE-NEGATIVE AREAS: Occasionally in the original squamous epithelium, areas inconspicuous on colposcopy become evident as iodine-negative areas after application of Schiller's test. Such areas are frequently due to parakeratosis[*] contained within an original transformation zone and are of no special significance (Fig. 37).

Recommended International Colposcopic Terminology

The classification of colposcopic terminology (Table II) was approved during the Second World Congress for Cervical Pathology and Colposcopy in Graz, Austria, 1975 (Stafl, 1976). This classification, with minor modifi-

---

[*] Parakeratosis = A superficial zone of cornified cells with retained nuclei.

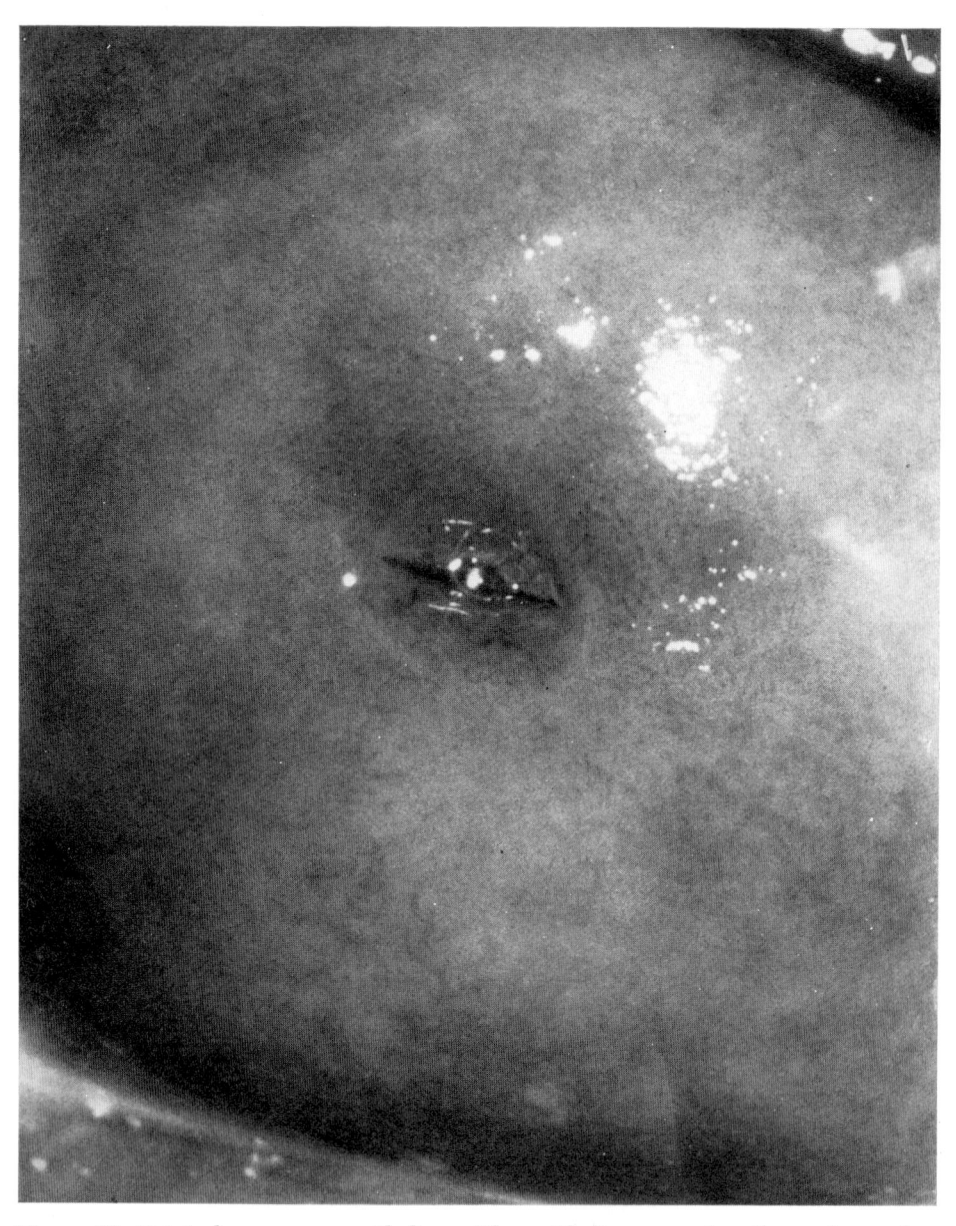

Figure 21. Original squamous epithelium. The epithelium covering the entire surface in this colpophotograph is smooth. There are no pronounced features apart from the presence of some indistinct blood vessels. At the cervical os, a bubble of air with characteristic light reflex lies in the mucus.

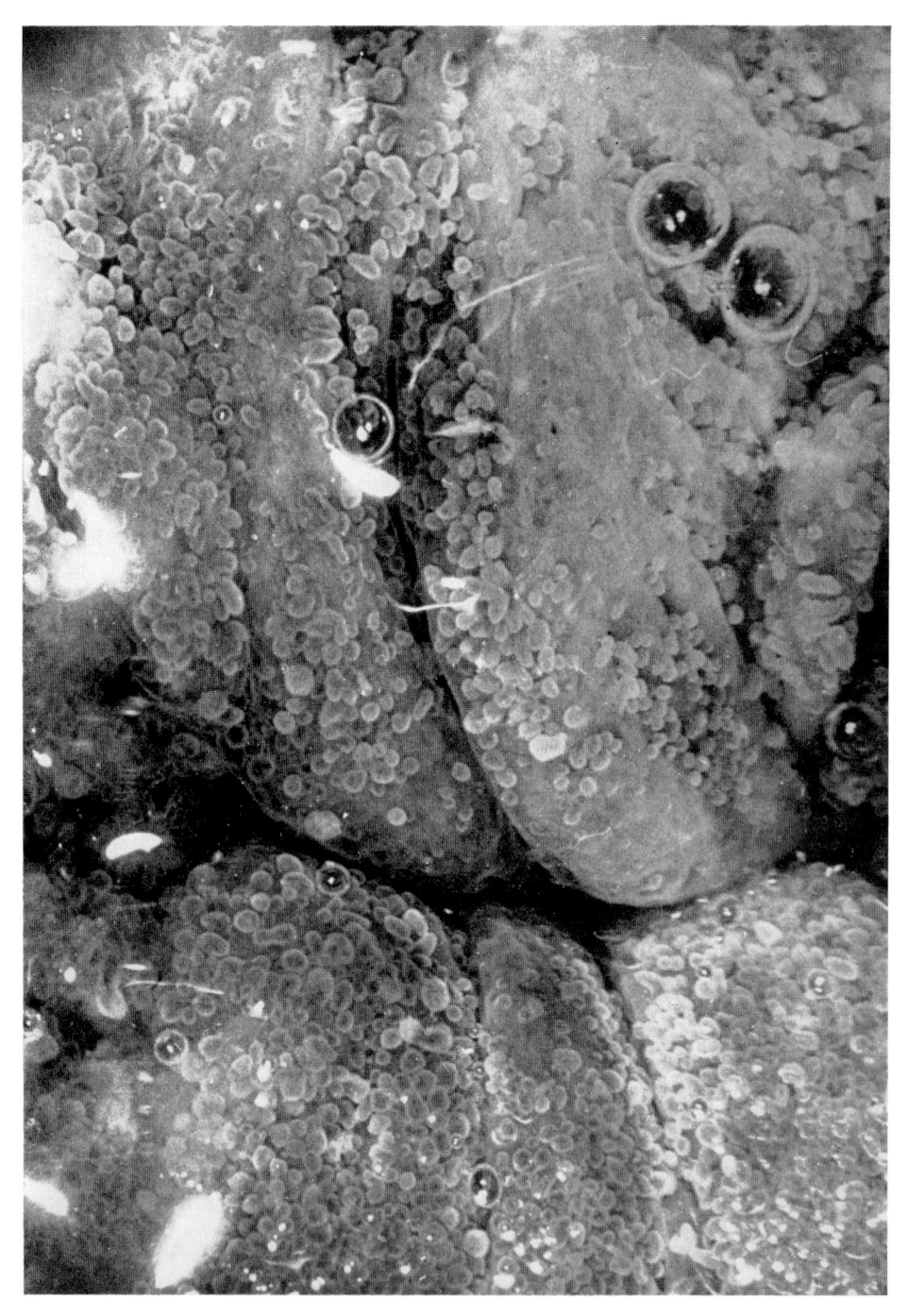

Figure 22. Original columnar epithelium. The whole area depicted in this colpophotograph is columnar in character. Clear mucus is produced in which several air bubbles are trapped. Surface projections like grapes and small fronds are striking. The surface dips into the stroma with deep clefts lying obliquely. Horizontal cleft below centre represents cervical canal.

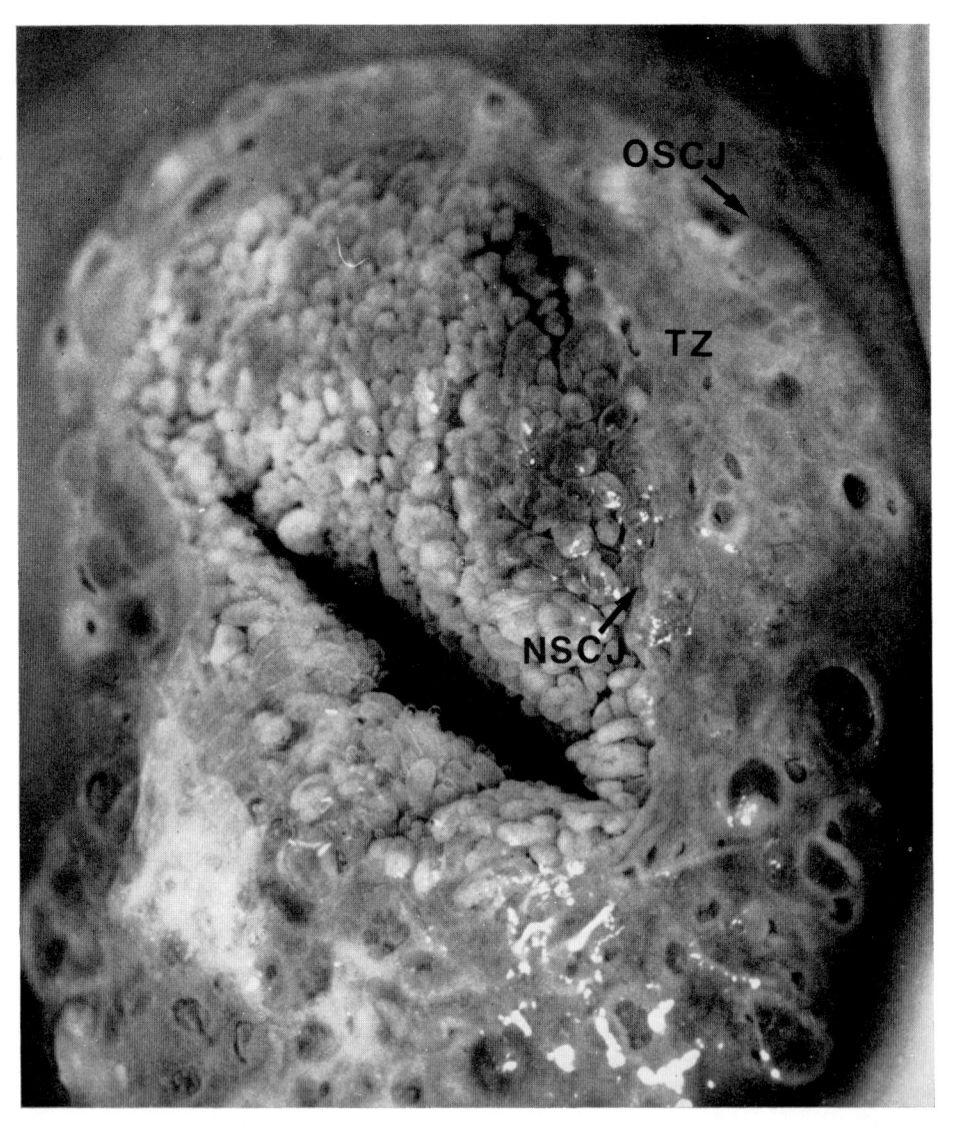

Figure 23. Typical transformation zone. Original squamous and columnar epithelium are seen in this colpophotograph. The original (OSCJ) and new squamocolumnar junction (NSCJ) are evident, and between them lies the transformation zone (TZ). Morphological characteristics are present which distinguish the zone from the other areas. The colour and surface configuration are strikingly different. In particular, openings from the surface to deeper glandular structures are clearly seen.

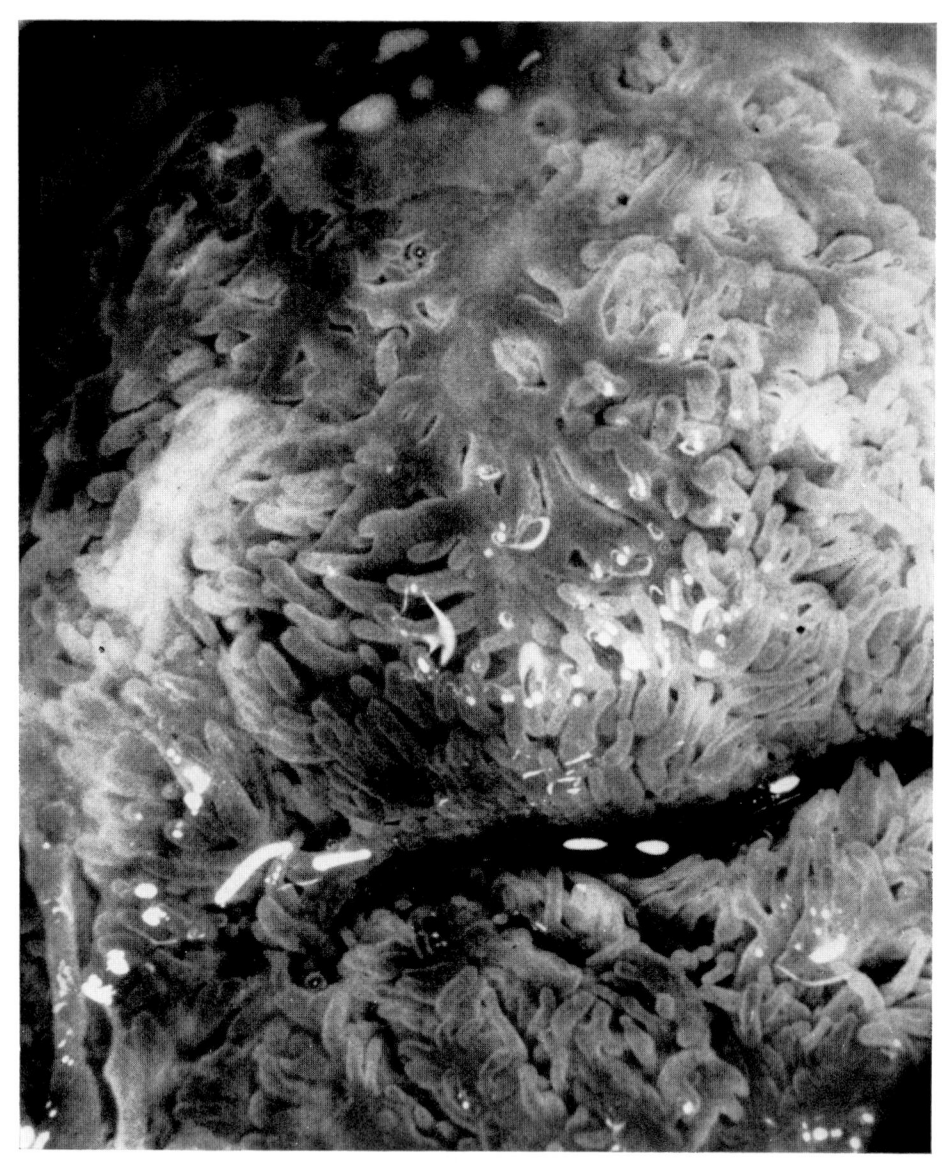

Figure 24. Typical transformation zone (early phase). Observed earlier during its phase of initiation, the metaplastic process may be seen replacing areas of columnar epithelium in the upper portion of the colpophotograph. This early process is represented colposcopically by the fusion of adjacent villi.

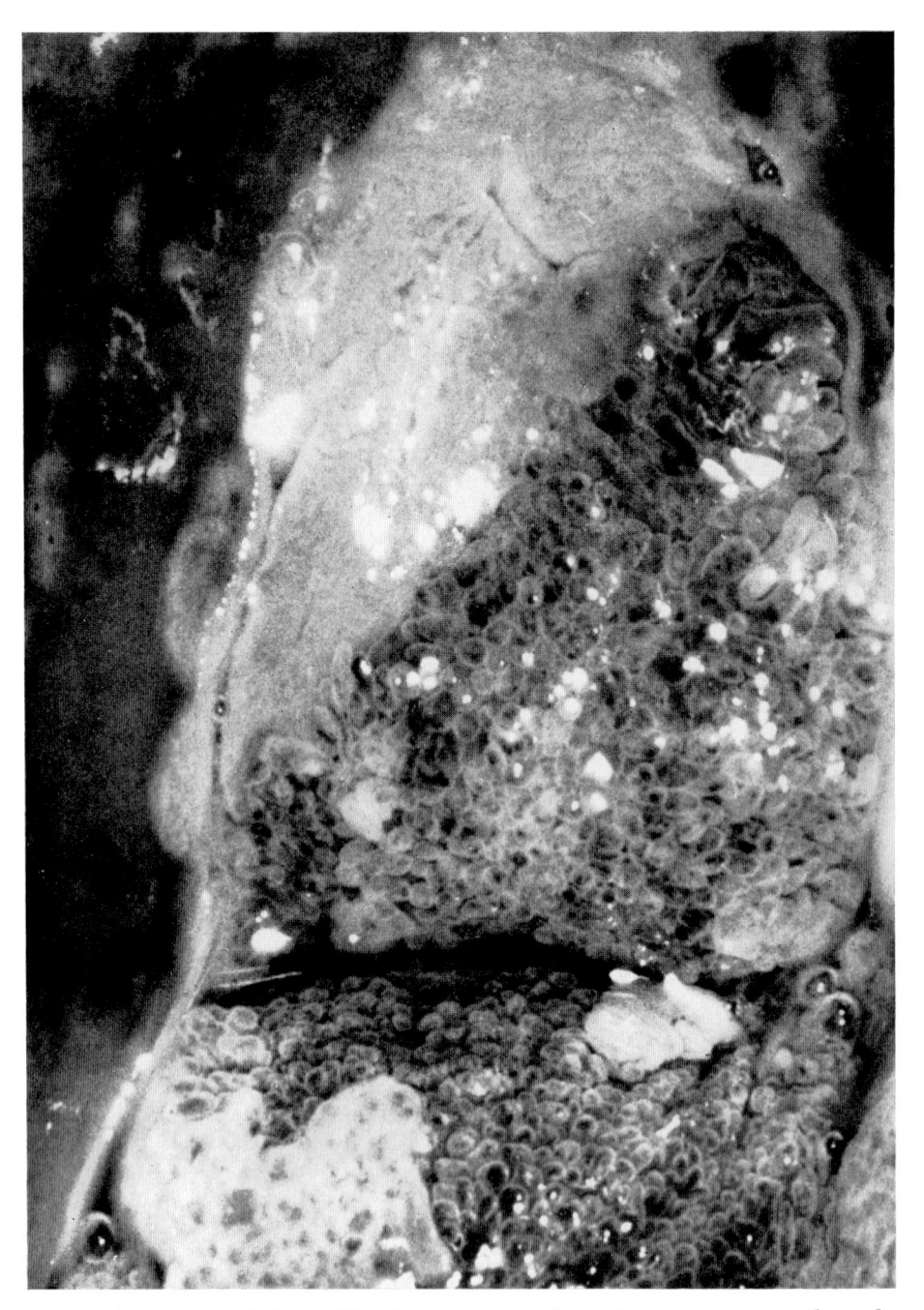

Figure 25. White epithelium. The distinctive transformation zone seen in this colpophotograph differs from those in Figures 23 and 24. It is opaque and white. It lies, however, in the characteristic site, bounded cephalad by the new squamocolumnar junction and caudad by the original squamocolumnar junction.

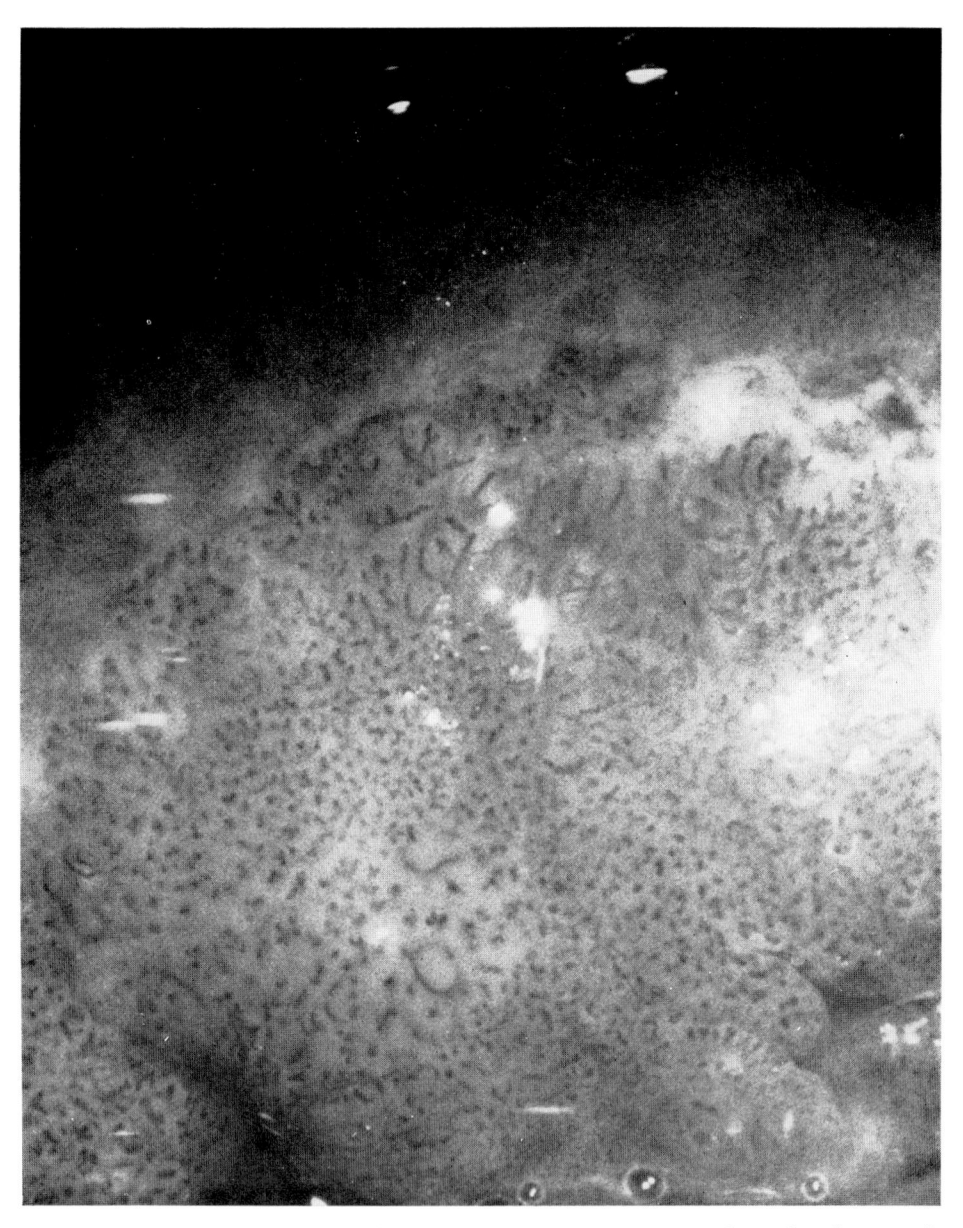

Figure 26. Punctation. The basis for this entity is conspicuous in this colpophotograph. Capillary loops lying within the epithelium are present as dots on a pale surface.

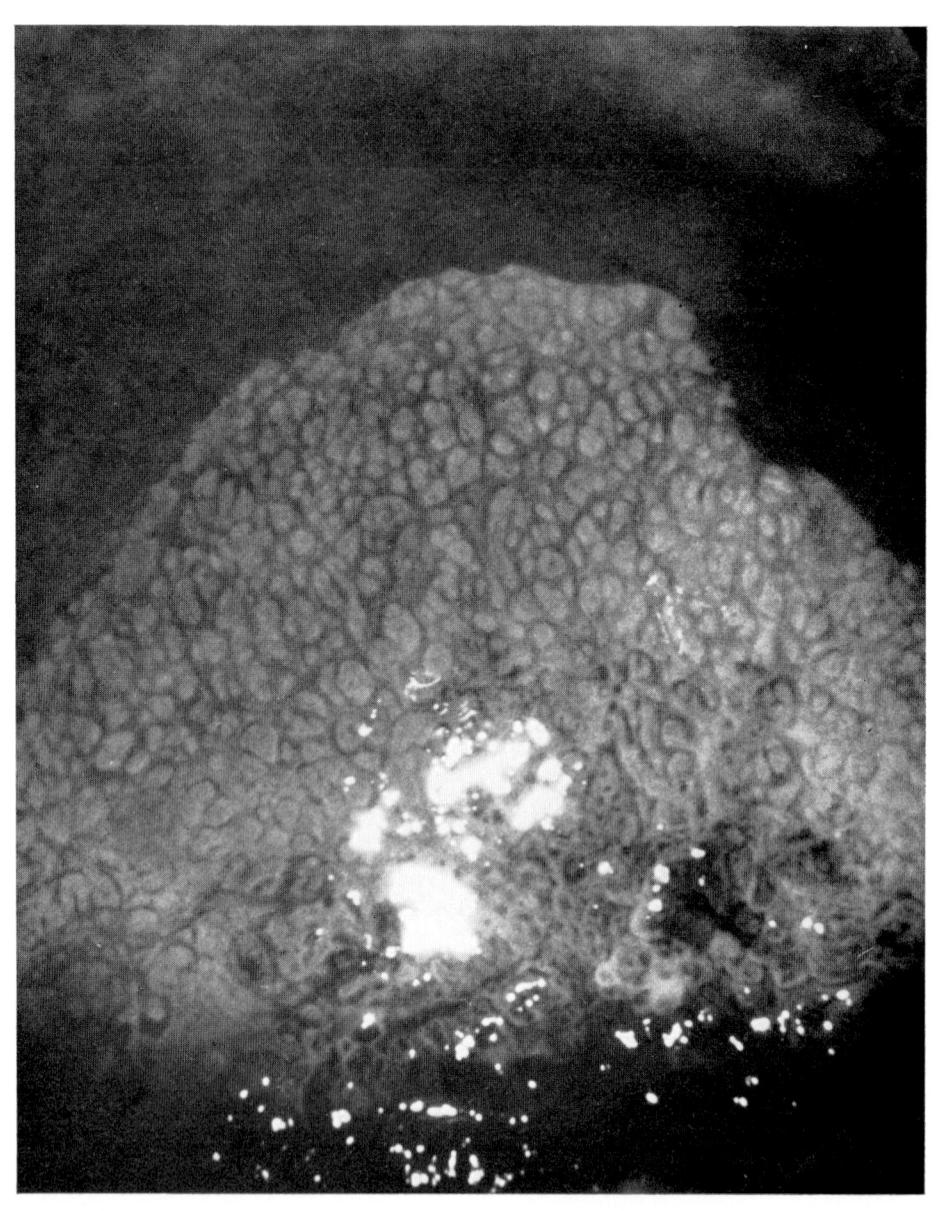

Figure 27. Mosaic. The appearance shown in this colpophotograph is one of the striking aspects of colposcopic morphology. Regular vascular structures of red colour surround pale blocks of epithelial cells to create a surface of mosaic-like appearance.

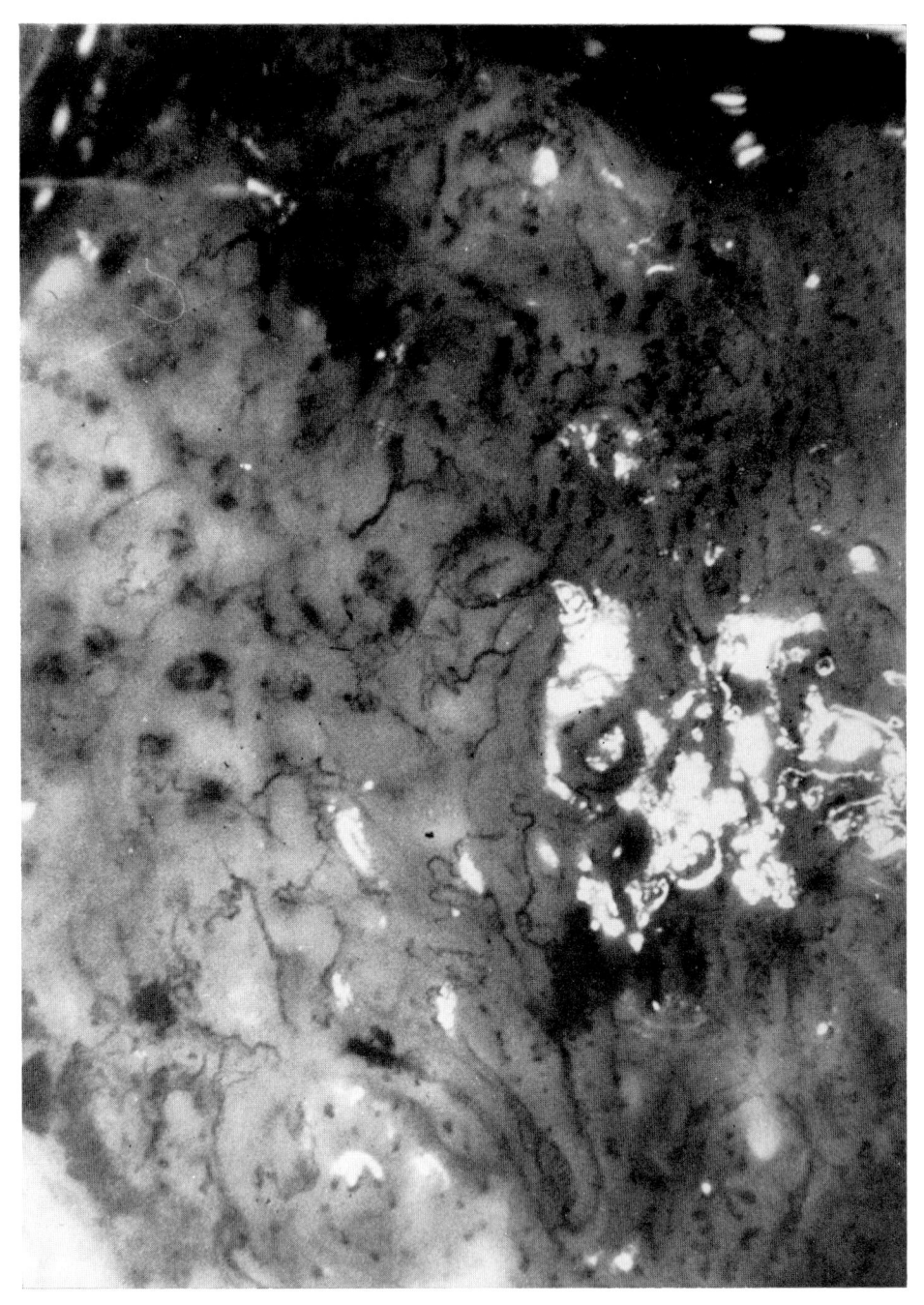

Figure 28. Atypical vessels. This colpophotograph displays blood vessels with bizarre shapes and directions. These vascular arrangements are quite different from the orderly, regular shapes and directions seen in normal structures.

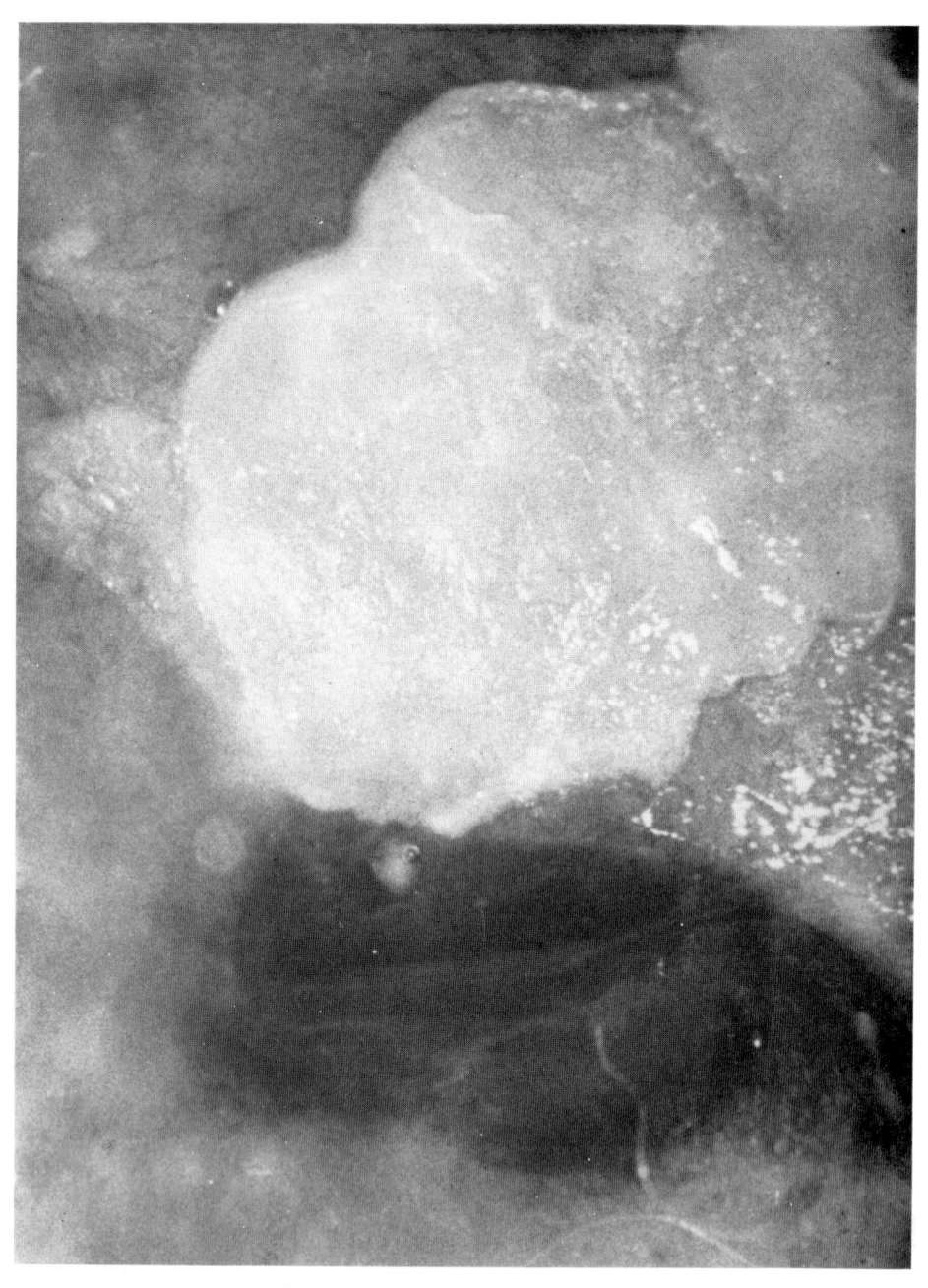

Figure 29. Keratosis. In this colpophotograph, a thick white patch overlies and obscures all features of the epithelium. Such appearances always show on histological section a thick keratin crust. In this case, the keratotic patch was visible with the naked eye.

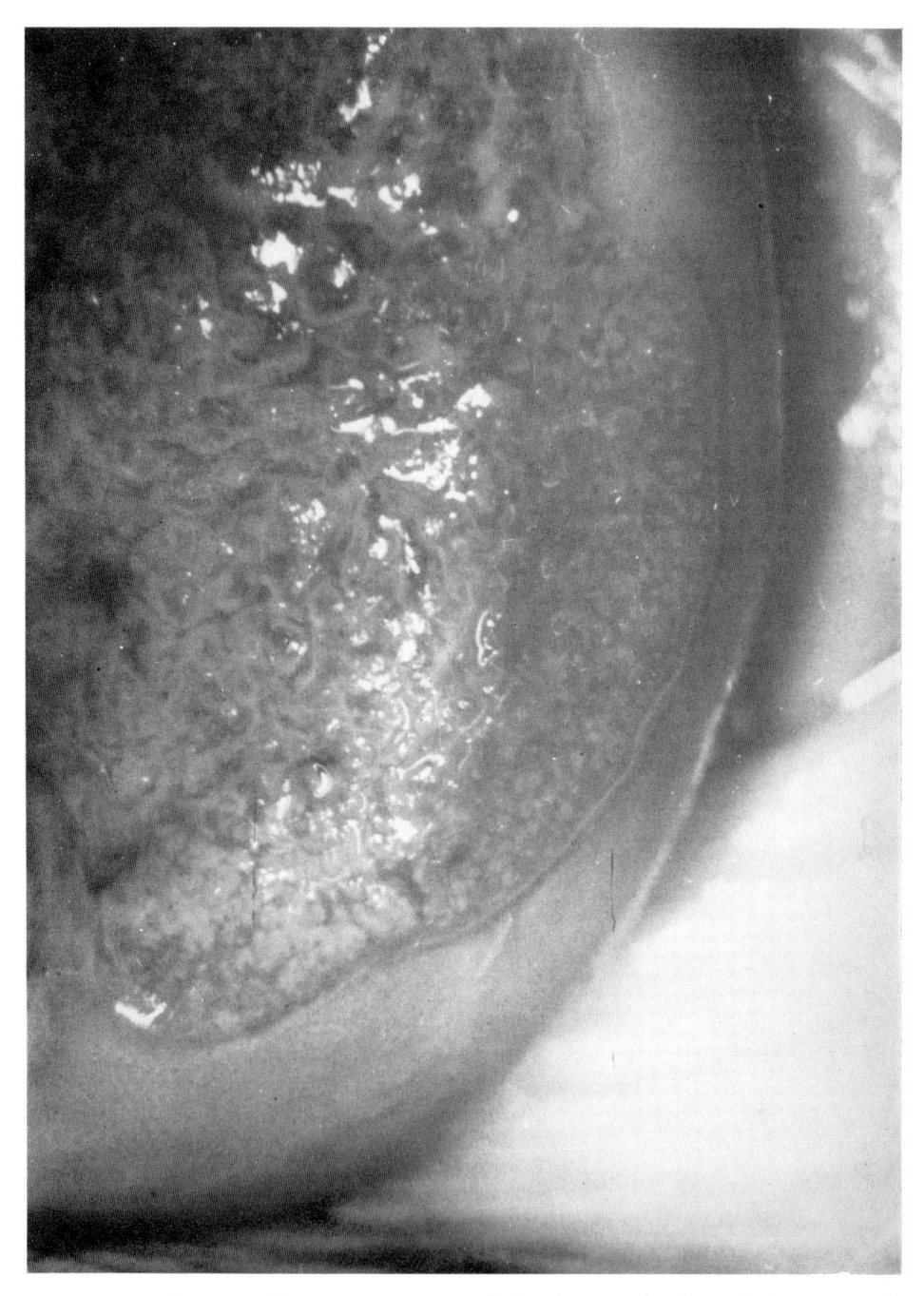

Figure 30. Colposcopically overt carcinoma. Colpophotograph of an obvious, irregular raised papillary growth, the edge of which became sharp and raised following the application of acetic acid. Unsuspected by the naked eye, this invasive carcinoma was discovered on colposcopic examination. This patient was symptom-free with positive cervical smear.

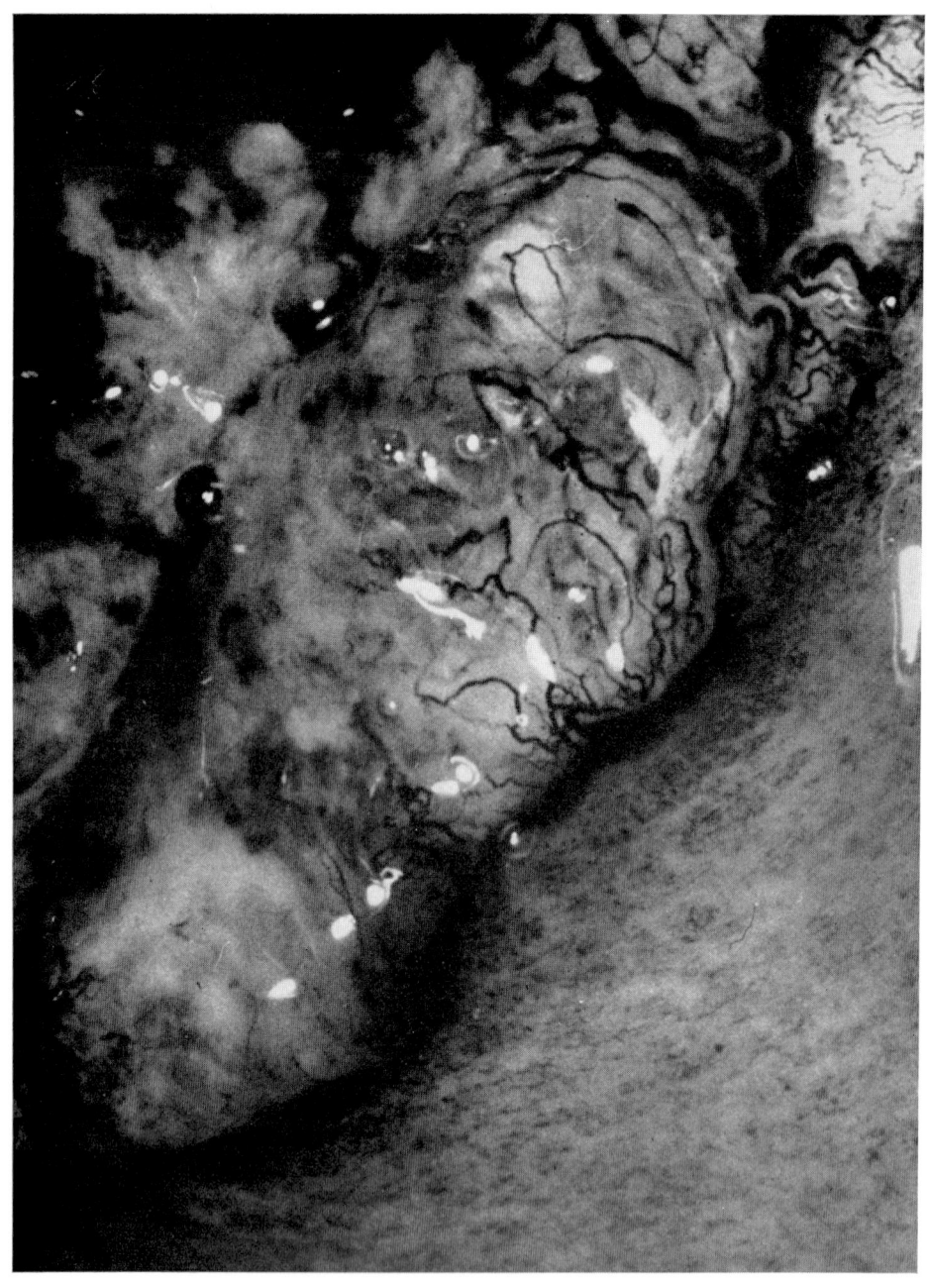

Figure 31. Overt carcinoma. An obvious exophytic carcinoma, raised, highly vascular, and encroaching on the original squamous epithelium towards the right of the colpophotograph.

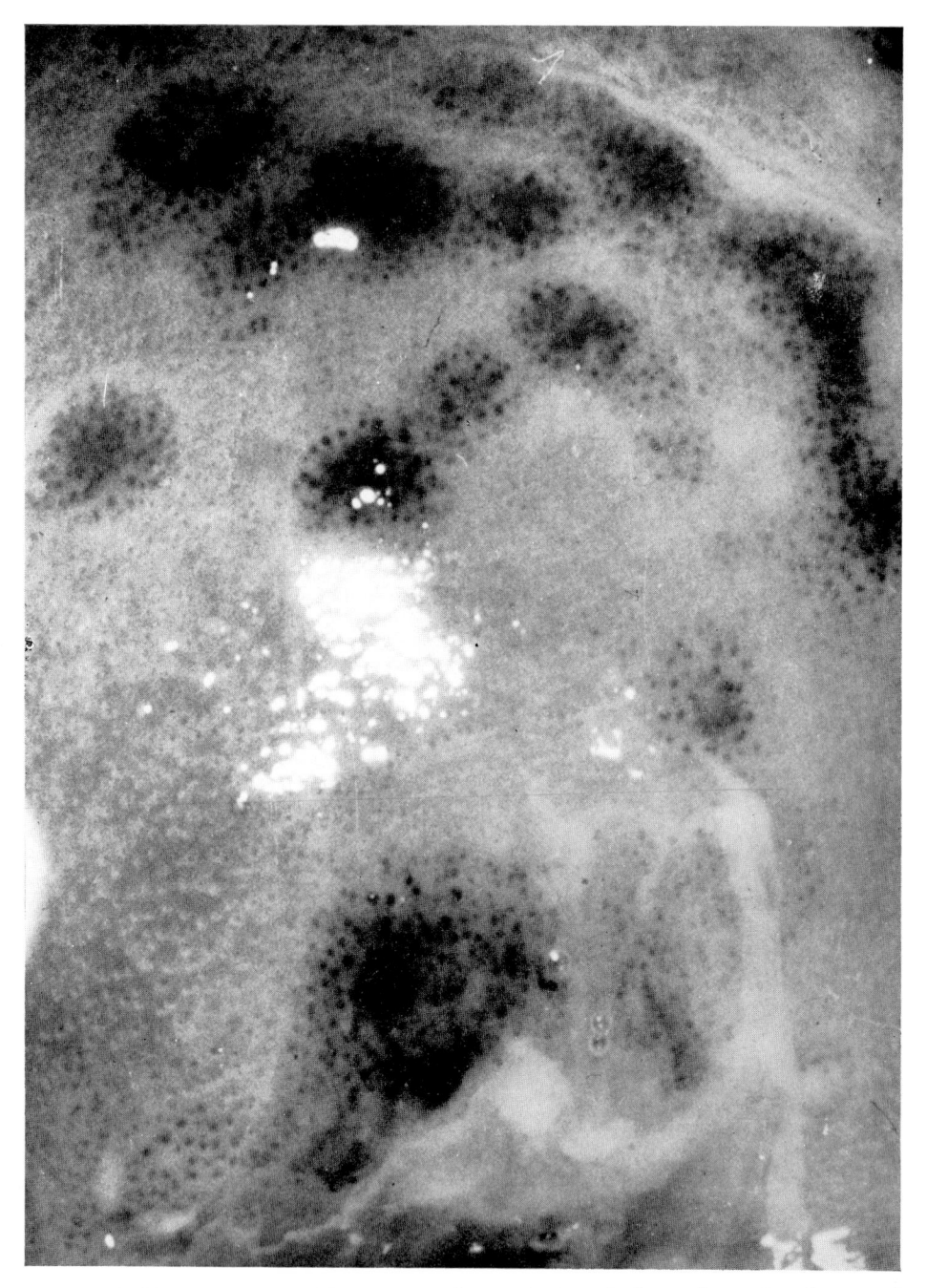

Figure 32. Vaginocervicitis. The increased vascularity which in this colpophotograph is of patchy distribution is characteristic of host response to parasitic infections such as *Trichomonas vaginalis* and *Neisseria gonorrhoeae*. In other cases, the response is more generalized than patchy.

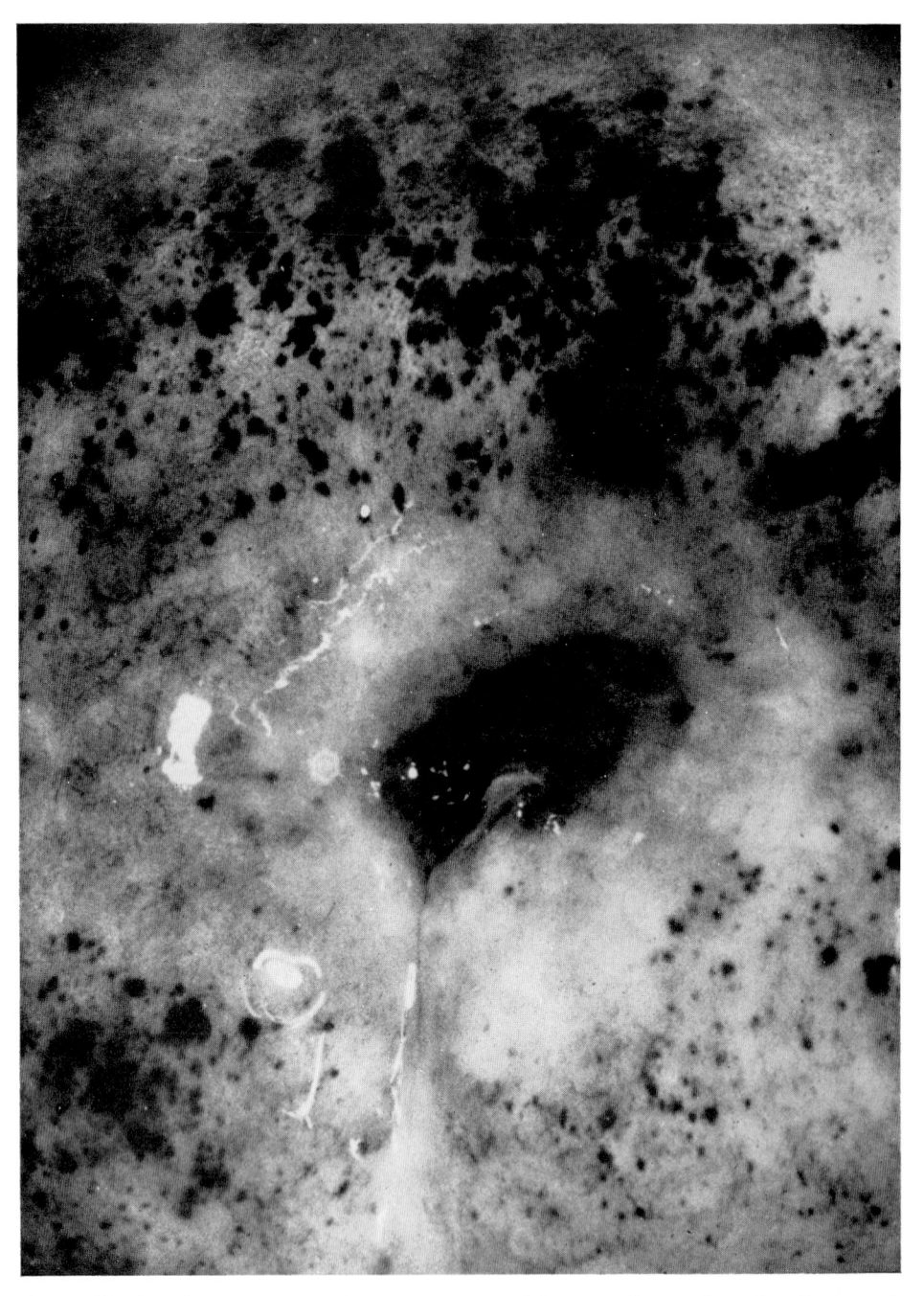

Figure 33. Atrophic cervicitis. The squamous epithelium is thin in the colpophotograph of this postmenopausal cervix, and there are many subepithelial petechiae. The external os is central.

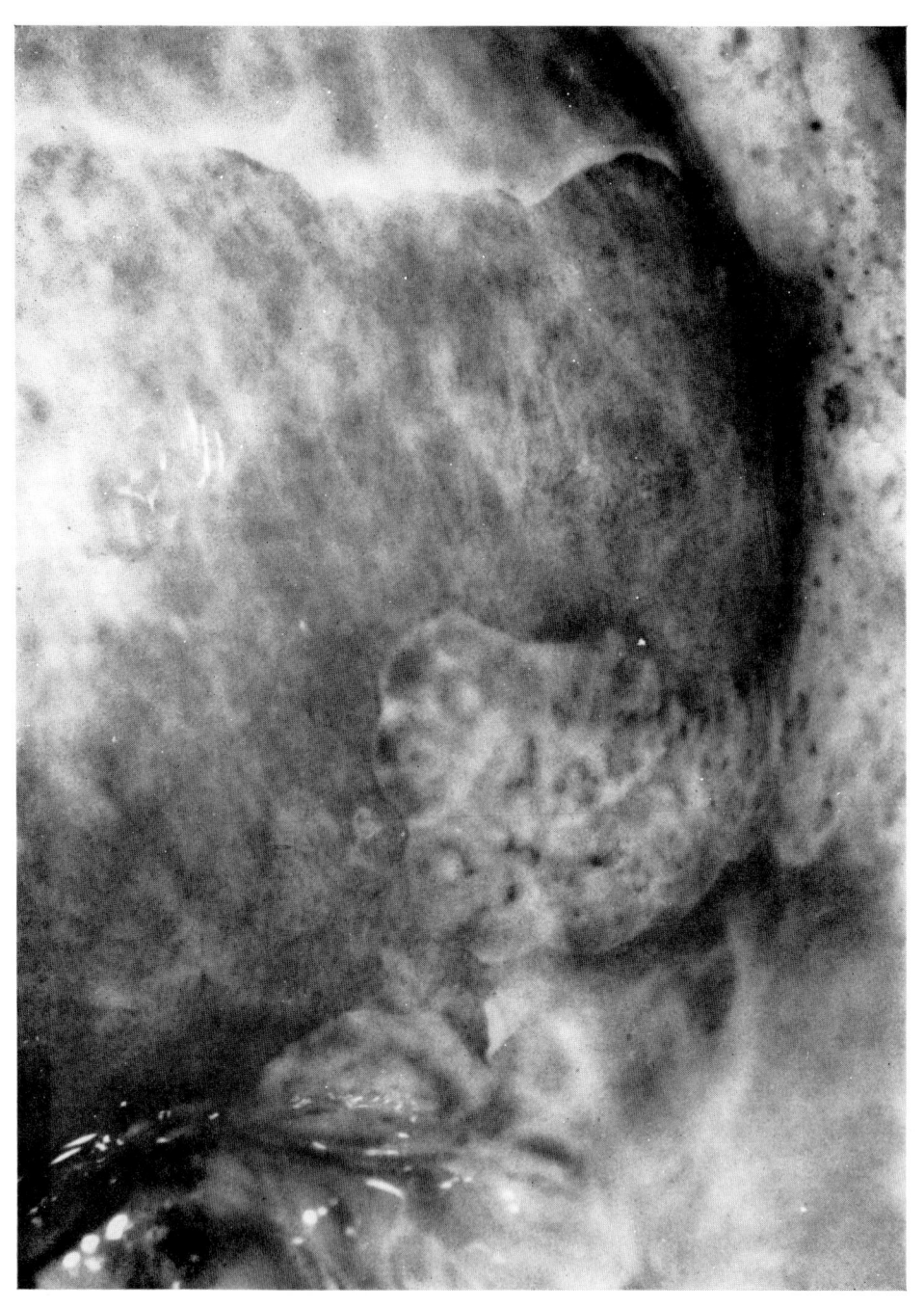

Figure 34. True erosion. A large area devoid of epithelium on the anterior lip of the cervix, occupying most of the left and upper portions of the colpophotograph. This area is below the level of the surrounding epithelium. The external os is at the lower left corner of the photograph.

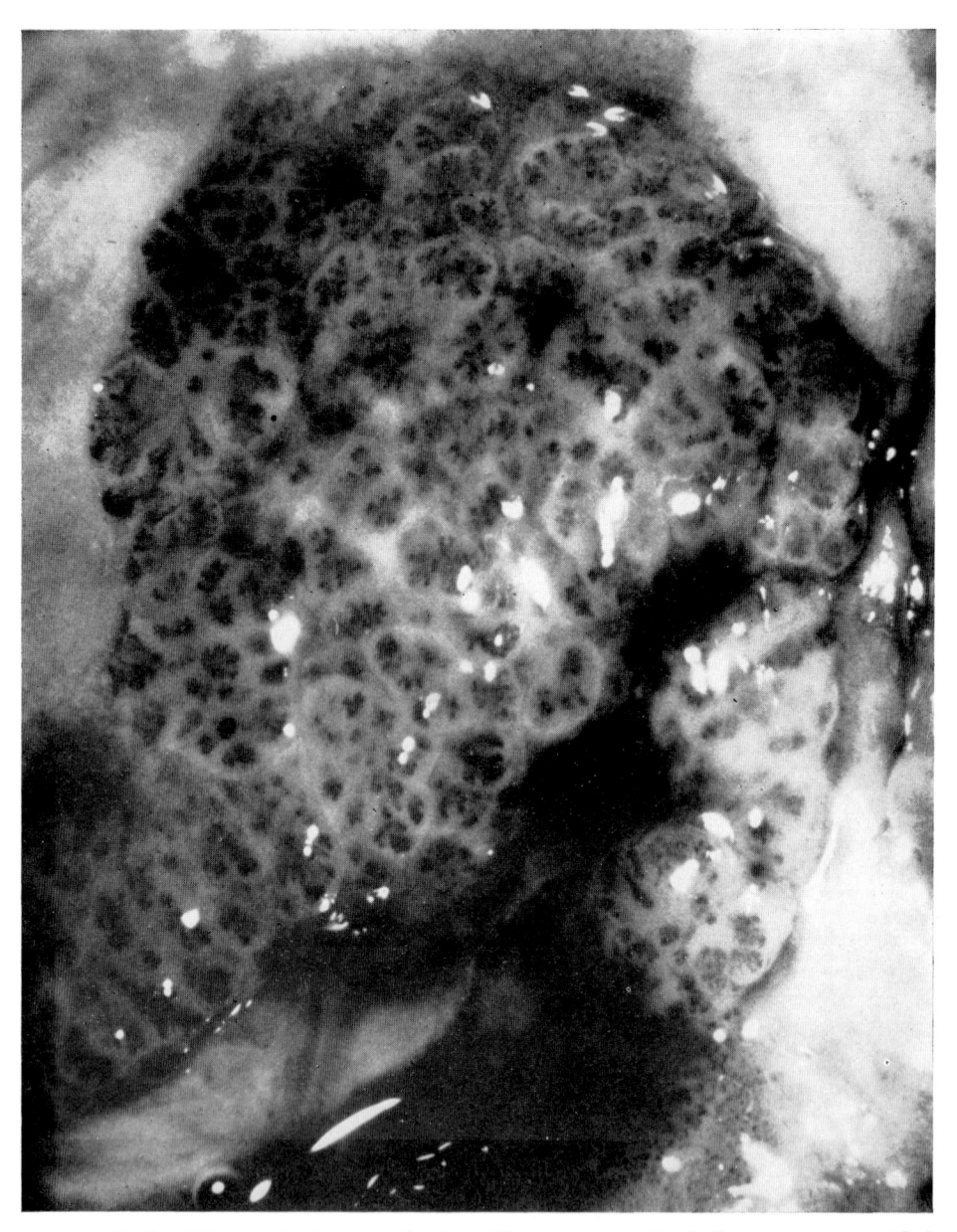

Figure 35. Condyloma. A circumscribed papillary outgrowth of the squamous epithelium with characteristic hyperaemia and regular vessel pattern is seen in this colpophotograph.

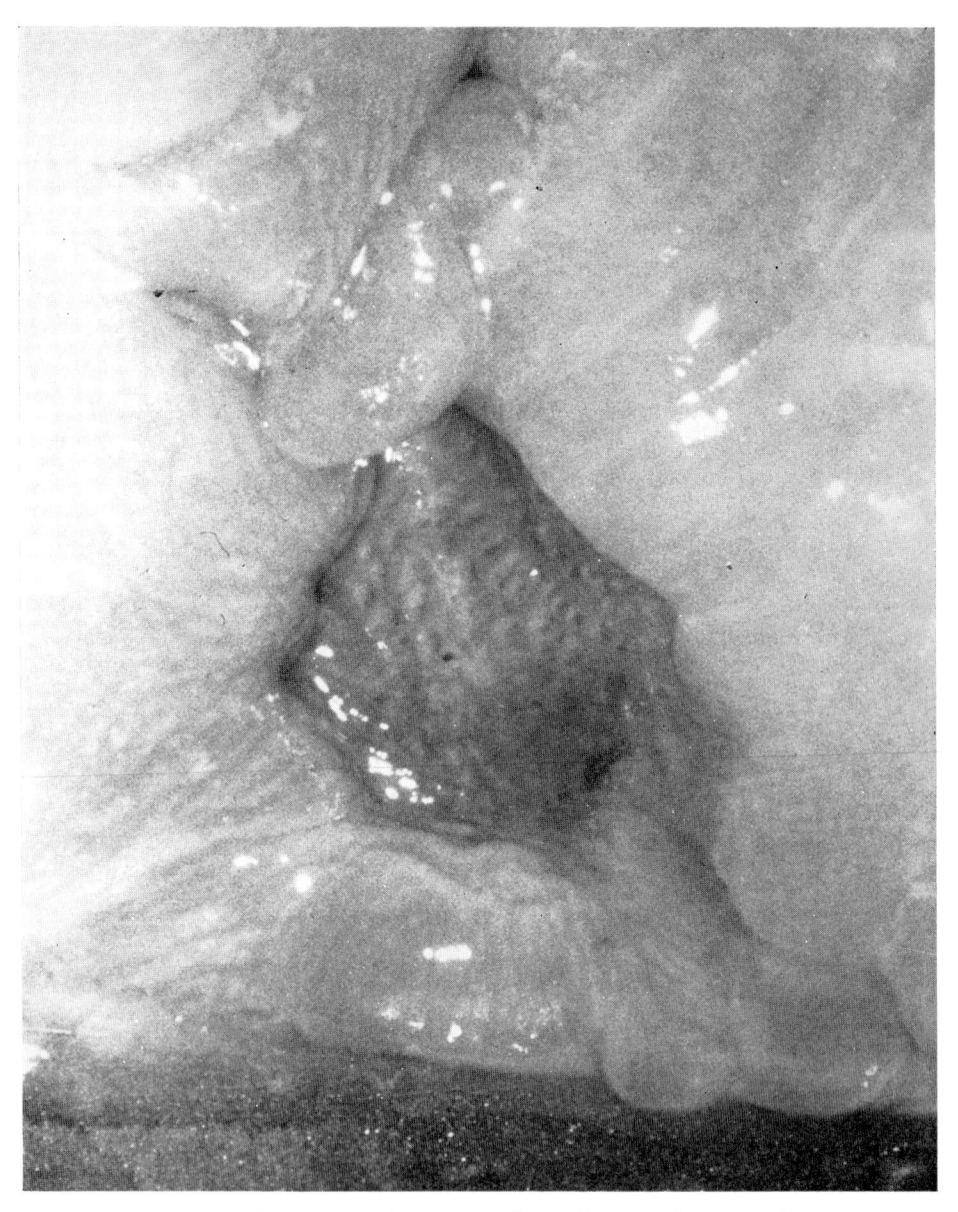

Figure 36. Cervical ulcer; non-malignant. A deep ulcer in the original squamous epithelium is present in the centre of this colpophotograph. The base has been cleansed of necrotic debris and shows the granulating surface of a regenerate process.

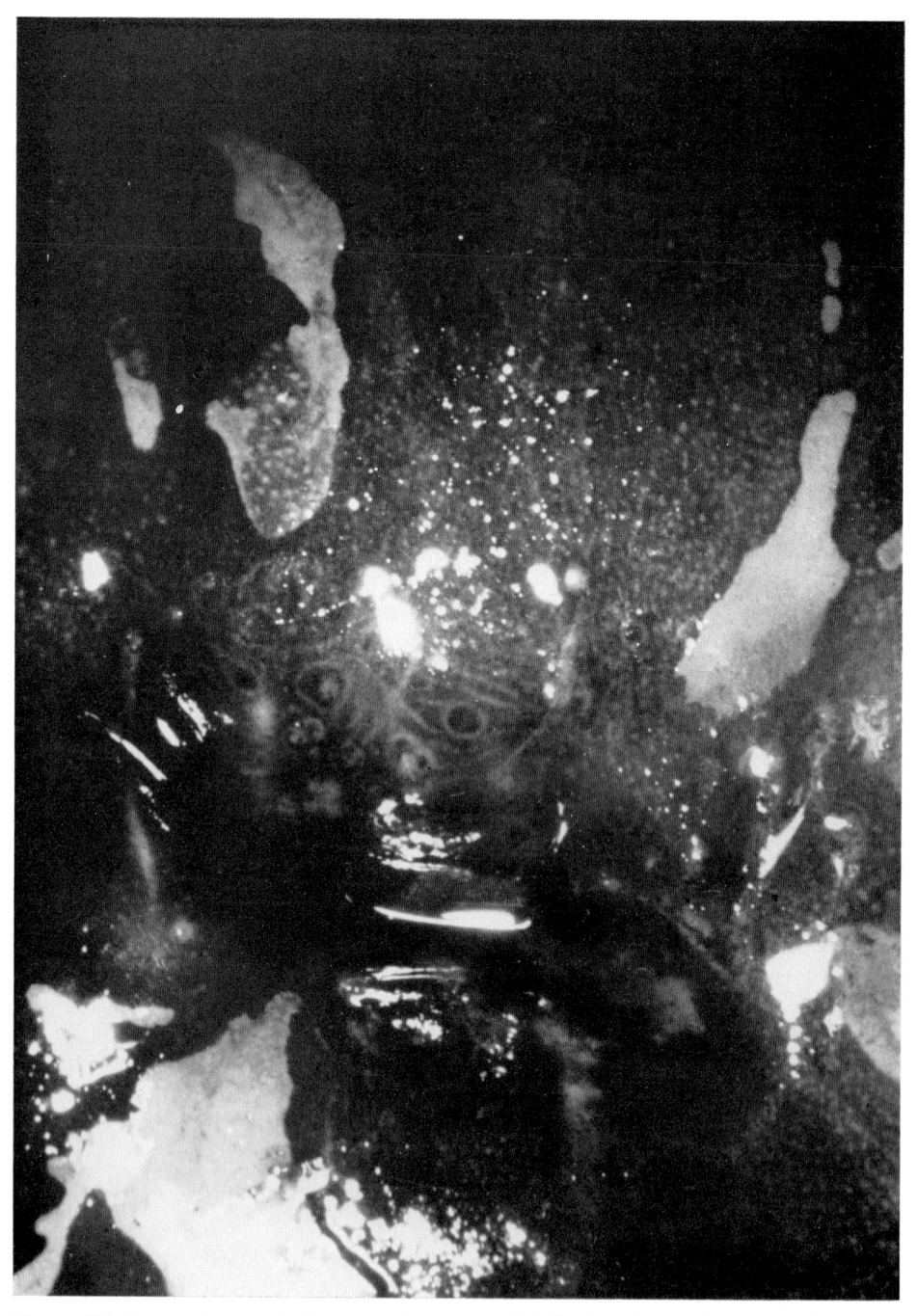

Figure 37. Inconspicuous iodine-negative areas. Schiller's iodine solution has been applied, and the glycogenated original squamous epithelium is dark. Several areas fail to stain. These are thought to be a specific form of non-glycogenated epithelium found within the original transformation zone (p. 374).

cations, resembles an earlier scheme (Coppleson, 1964; Coppleson and Reid, 1967). The modifications are as follows.

Additional Term

Unsatisfactory colposcopic findings is a term used when the new squamocolumnar junction is not visible in the cervical canal, the practical importance of which is discussed later (*see* Chap. 16).

Modified Terms

Punctation has been substituted for ground structure, *keratosis* for leukoplakia, and *atypical vessels* has replaced other atypical vascular structures.

It is evident to the trained colposcopist that the recommended classification differs from the traditional continental conventions. In such schemes, "ground," "mosaic," and "leukoplakia" were thought to arise from "matrix areas" in the original squamous epithelium and were therefore separate from "atypical transformation zone." For such conventions, an integrated concept has been substituted, based on recognition of the origin and development of all atypias as being within the transformation zone and never from the original squamous epithelium. "Ground" (now punctation) and "mosaic" and "leukoplakia" (now keratosis), then take a subsidiary place as examples of the possible range of variations found within the transformation zone.

TABLE II
RECOMMENDED INTERNATIONAL COLPOSCOPIC TERMINOLOGY

I. *Normal Colposcopic Findings*
   A. Original squamous epithelium
   B. Columnar epithelium
   C. Transformation zone
II. *Abnormal Colposcopic Findings*
   A. Atypical transformation zone
     1. Mosaic
     2. Punctation
     3. White epithelium
     4. Keratosis
     5. Atypical vessels
   B. Suspect frank invasive carcinoma
III. *Unsatisfactory Colposcopic Findings*
   (Squamocolumnar junction not visible)[*]
IV. *Miscellaneous Colposcopic Findings*
   A. Inflammatory changes
   B. Atrophic changes
   C. Erosion
   D. Condyloma[†]
   E. Papilloma
   F. Others

[*] The use of the term *squamocolumnar junction* does not distinguish the *original* from the *new* squamocolumnar junction (Figs. 6 and 23).

[†] No distinction is made between condyloma and papilloma in this book. The term *condyloma* is preferred (*see* Chap. 11).

EXFOLIATIVE CYTOLOGICAL DEFINITIONS

There is no doubt that exfoliative cytology is important in mass screening programmes aimed at the detection of women with preclinical cervical carcinoma. In the context of an active colposcopic service, cytology becomes more of an ancillary aid and has been accorded such a place in this book. Thus the only section in this text where exfoliative cytology is relevant is Chapter 16 in which management is discussed. For this reason, it is necessary to define certain terms related to this discipline. The first three terms represent a contraction of systems previously in common use and still used in some clinics.

POSITIVE SMEAR: The report denotes a confident expectation that preclinical carcinoma will be found (Papanicolaou Classes IV and V).

DOUBTFUL SMEAR: In all institutions, a class of smear is recorded in various terms which we have grouped under *doubtful*. Such smears may originate from preclinical cervical carcinoma but also from dysplastic epithelia and occasionally from vaginocervicitis (Papanicolaou Class III).

NEGATIVE SMEAR: Cells desquamated from original and metaplastic epithelia and inflammatory disorders are negative (Papanicolaou Classes I and II).

Some revision of this classification of reporting is now warranted in view of the present practice of incorporating in the report a prediction of the histological findings. This approach is valuable to the clinician and evidently reliable. In the hands of experts with well-prepared material, various grades of dysplasia, carcinoma in situ, and even invasive cancer can be differentiated. At the borders of those grades, the exfoliative cytologist may leave the diagnosis at *abnormal* without qualification by way of histological prediction.

Normal Smear

No evidence of abnormality or presence of a few atypical cells of no probable significance is considered normal. This classification also denotes presence of metaplastic cells (Fig. 38).

Abnormal Smear

An abnormal smear indicates the presence of a lesion including dysplasia, carcinoma in situ, and carcinoma.

PREDICTION OF DYSPLASIA: Large cells with large, often bizarre-shaped nuclei are dysplastic (Fig. 39).

PREDICTION OF CARCINOMA IN SITU: Stigmata of carcinoma in situ include cells, usually in large numbers, of a smaller size than dysplasia with a raised nuclear-cytoplasmic ratio. Nuclei are pleomorphic with prominent chromatin clumps.

PREDICTION OF INVASIVE CARCINOMA: Greater nuclear pleomorphism in the presence of a background of blood, inflammatory cells and cell debris evokes a call of invasive cancer (Fig. 40).

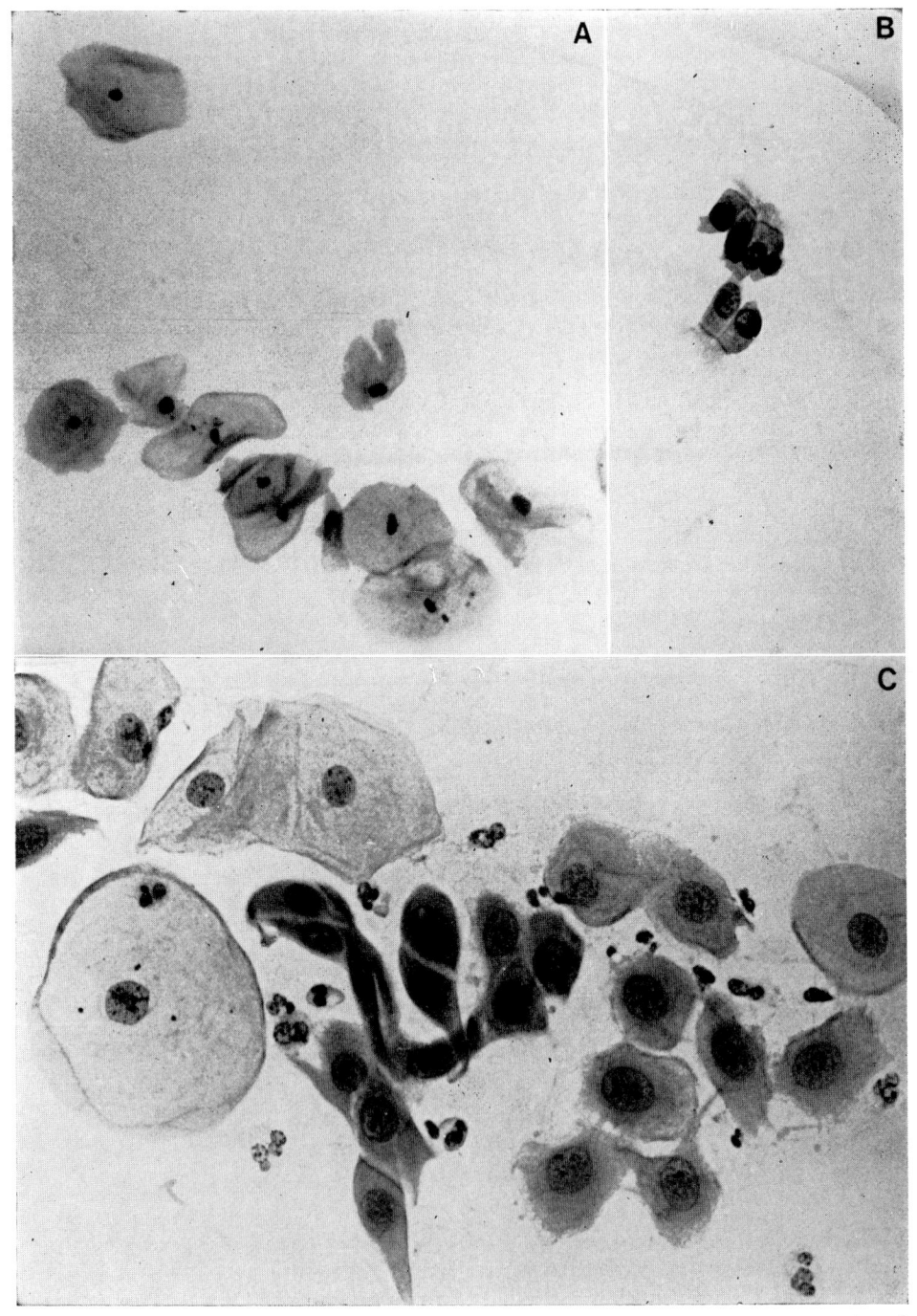

Figure 38. Normal smear. Three common components are illustrated. Cornified and precornified squame cells (A), columnar cells (B), and normal metaplastic cells (C).

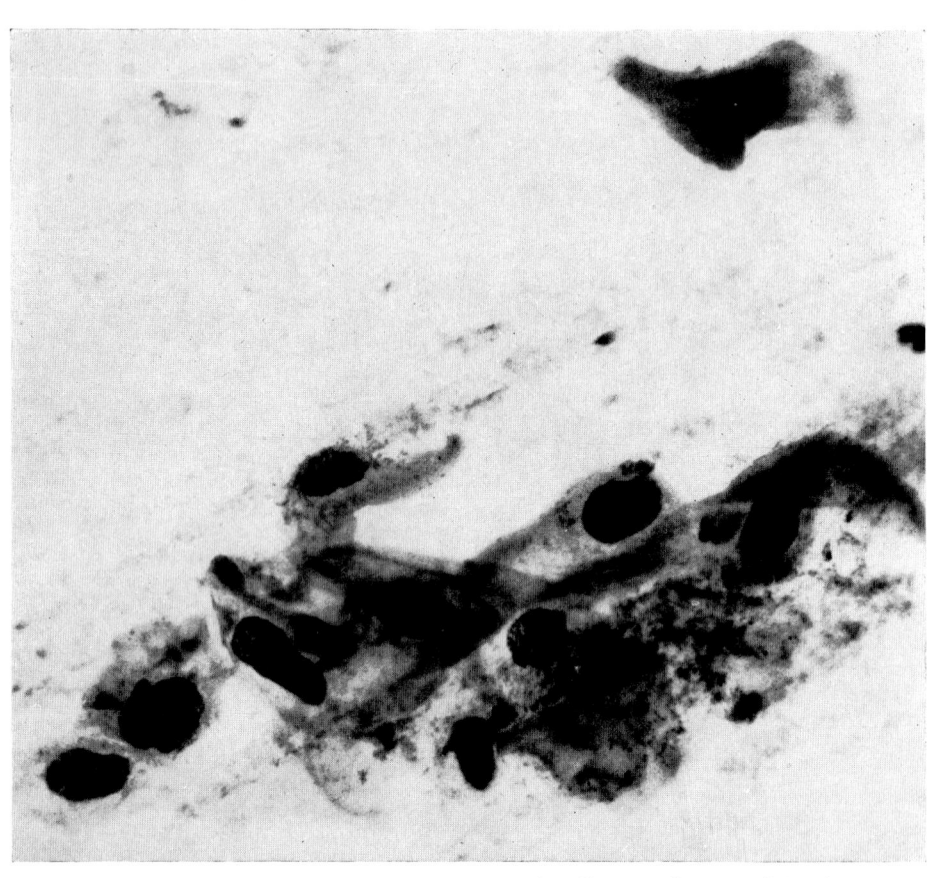

Figure 39. Abnormal smear. Large bizarre nuclei allow prediction of dysplasia.

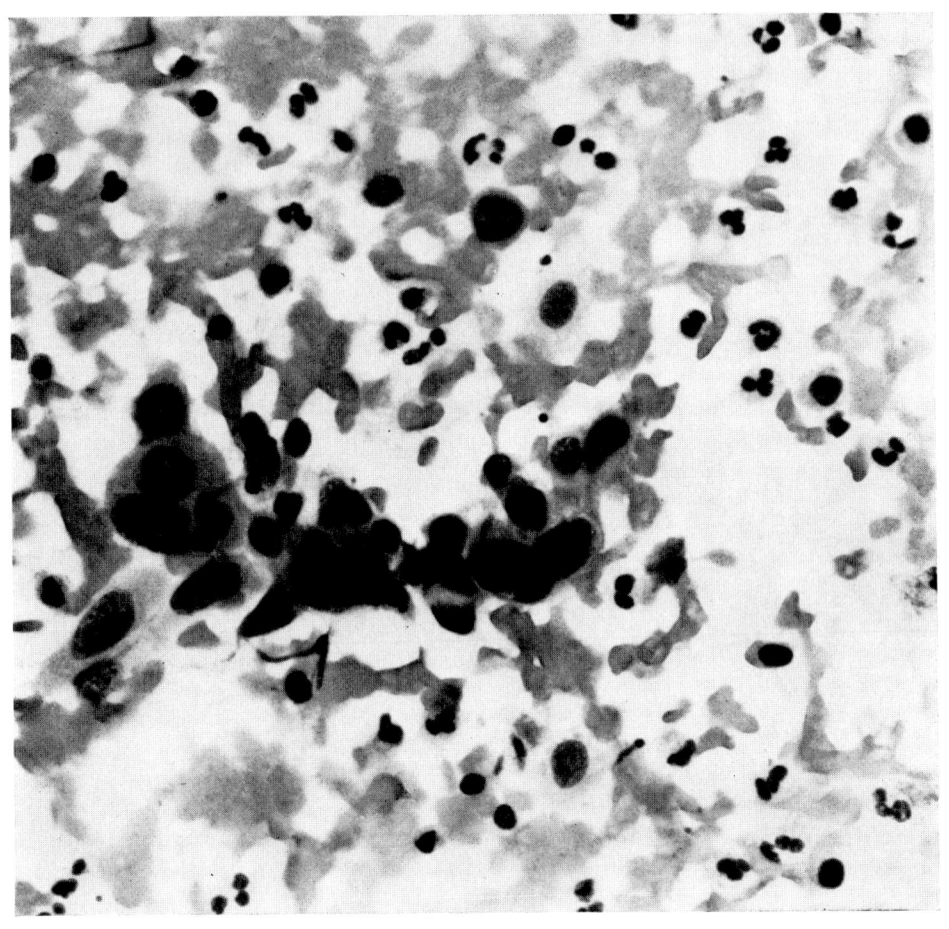

Figure 40. Abnormal smear. Smaller bizarre nuclei with pleomorphism greater than that expected with carcinoma in situ with accompanying inflammatory cells enable prediction of invasive cancer.

Chapter 3

TOPOGRAPHY OF THE CERVICAL EPITHELIA (LOCATION OF PRECLINICAL CERVICAL CARCINOMA AND DYSPLASIA)

THERE IS STILL MUCH DISPUTE in regard to the site of preclinical carcinoma and dysplasia, the relative frequency of an ecto- or endocervical location, and whether in fact dysplasia develops in a different site from that of carcinoma in situ. Appreciation of the topography of the epithelia, normal and abnormal, resolves some of the dissension. The site and extent of abnormal epithelial forms also determine some aspects of investigation and therapy, underlining the important practical advantages that the recognition of topography confers.

Perhaps the most commonly voiced criticism concerning limitations of the colposcopic technique is that histological dysplasia and preclinical squamous carcinoma are frequently found within the endocervical canal and are thus beyond observation. This misconception is partly the result of difficulties encountered in orientation of material provided to the histologist by clinicians, so histologically the exact topographical relationships are not usually evident or frequently misinterpreted (Figs. 41 and 42), and partly to the belief that none of the endocervical canal can be visualised with colposcopy (Figs. 43 and 44).

In fact, in little more than a glance, the whole of the transformation zone, wherein the epithelial disorders lie, can usually be studied during colposcopic examination. The relationships of the cervical epithelial forms to each other and to important anatomical reference points of the lower genital tract become strikingly evident and, in particular, the metaplastic epithelium and its atypical forms, dysplasia and preclinical carcinoma, are readily identified in terms of site and extent.

With the awareness of the many opinions concerning the site of dysplasia and carcinoma in situ, an attempt to define accurately topographical relationships was made. The topographical identity of physiological squamous metaplasia, dysplasias, and carcinoma in situ was clear when characteristics such as site and distribution were compared. The range of variations in these characteristics observed in physiological metaplasia then defines the range within which these abnormal forms are observed.

Combined colpophotographic and histological methods have been used in examination of a series of female subjects, including foetuses, pre-

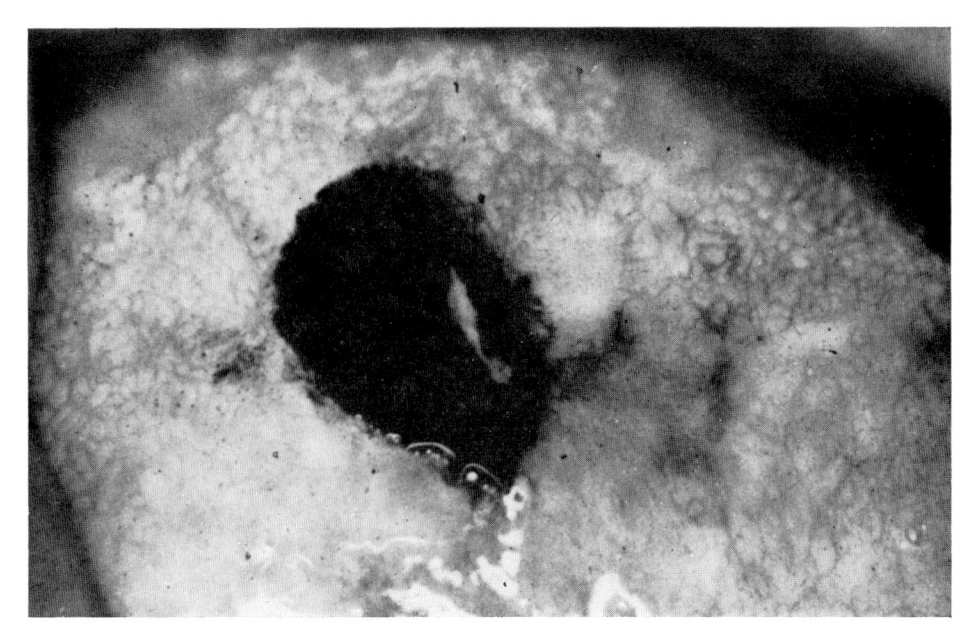

Figure 41. Colpophotograph of atypical transformation zone with white epithelium and mosaic. The punch biopsy site is easily seen, and histological examination of this tissue showed carcinoma in situ. The appearance is real and not apparent (p. 17), indicating a truly ectocervical site. Note the carcinoma in situ has developed inside the line at the top of the photograph which marks the original squamocolumnar junction.

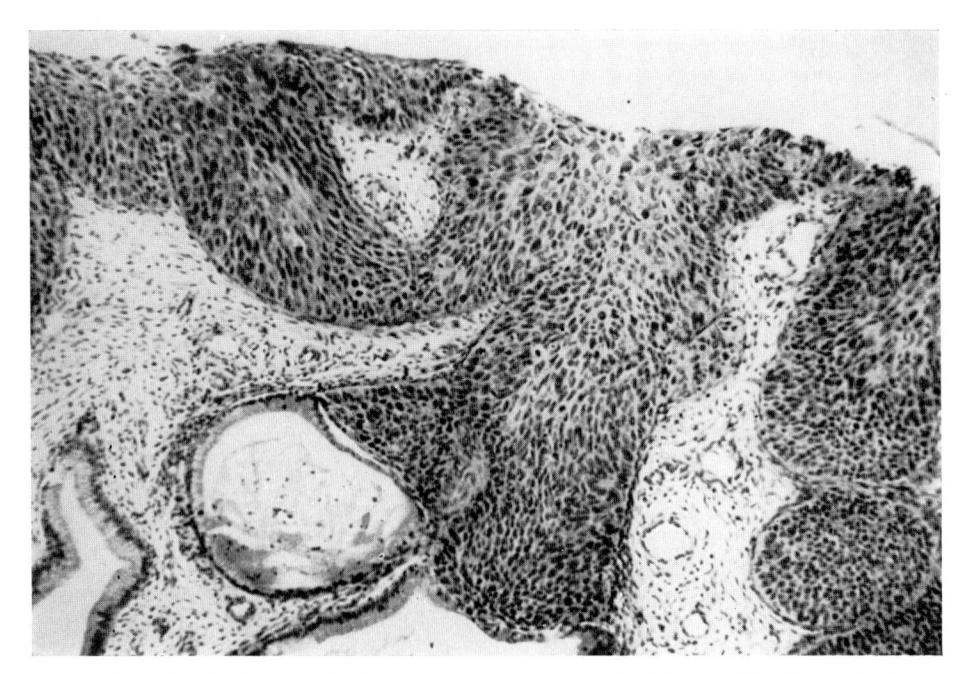

Figure 42. Histological study from biopsy site seen in Figure 41. Cervical glands, usually presumed to be endocervical in site are seen, yet this lesion was ectocervical.

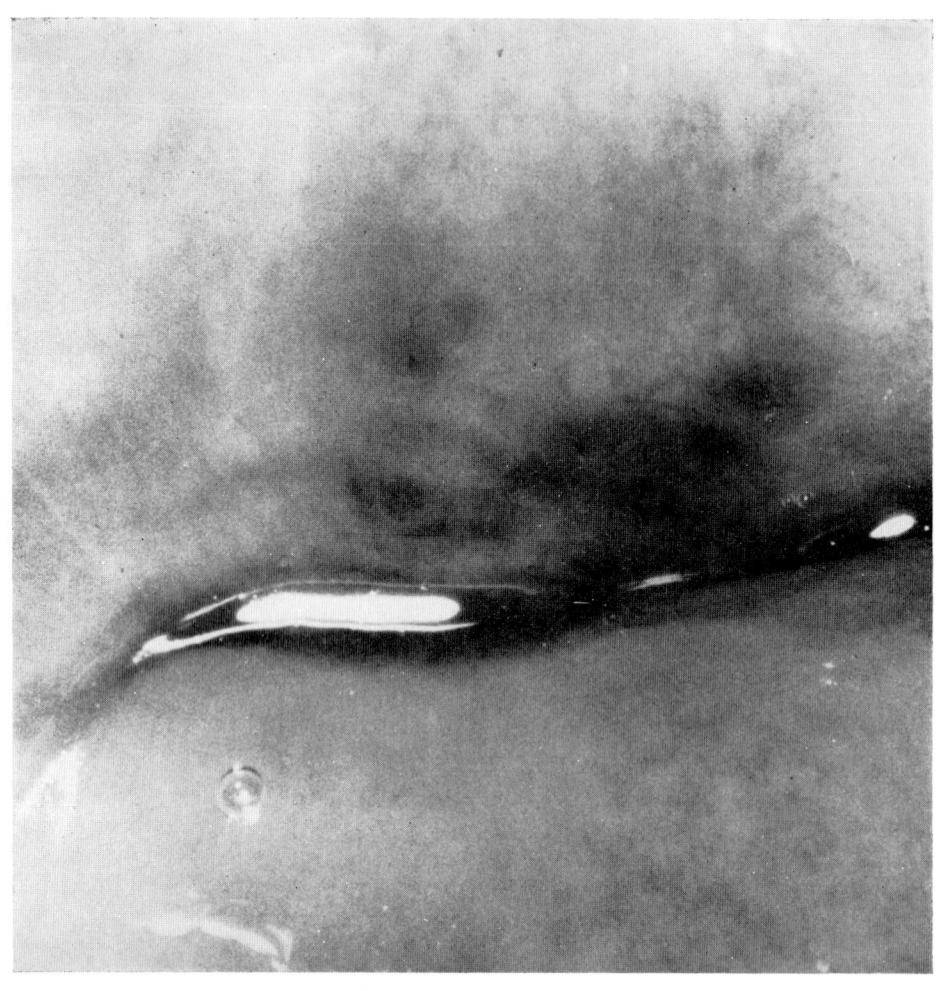

Figure 43. *Real view* of cervix (compare with Figure 44) in subject whose cervical smear was positive. When speculum blades are closed, original squamous epithelium is identified to the external os.

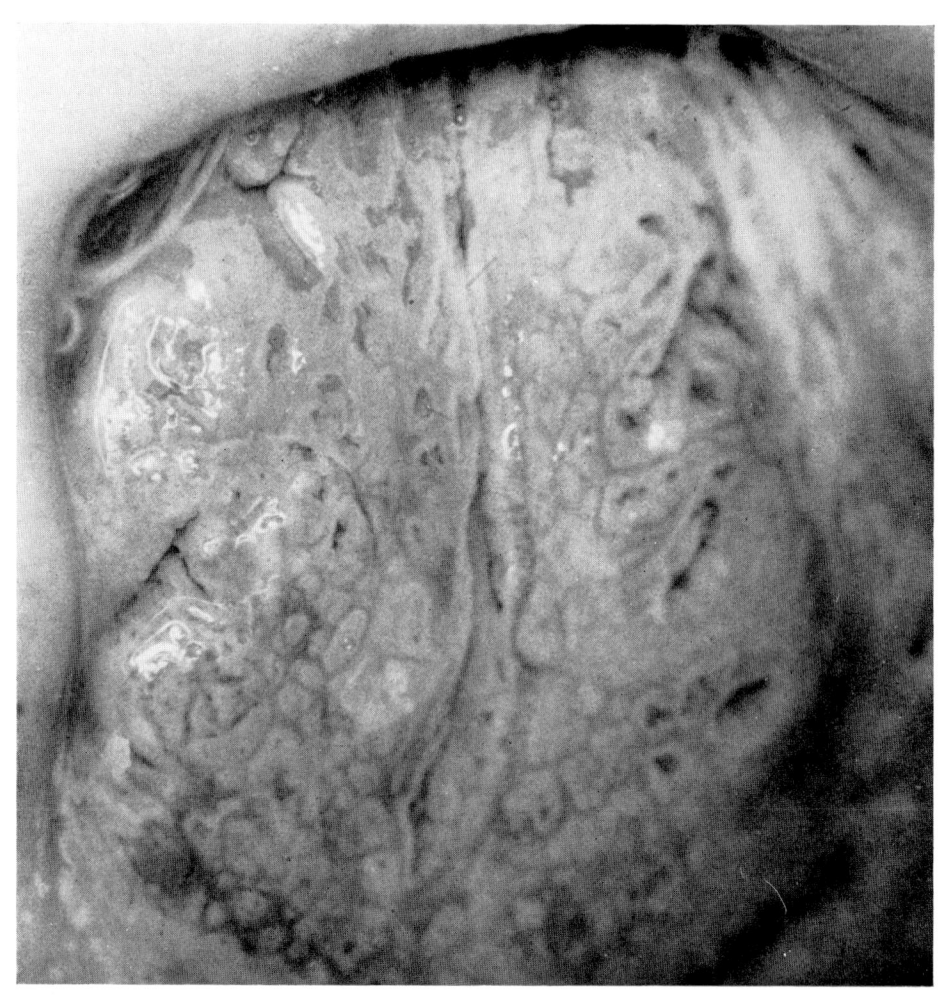

Figure 44. Same subject as Figure 43, *apparent view*. Eversion of the canal with the blades of the vaginal speculum open displays a surprising extent of the posterior aspect of cervical canal in which atypical transformation zone is present. Biopsy showed carcinoma in situ.

72   Colposcopy

pubertal and adolescent females, and women seen during pregnancy, the reproductive years, and following the menopause. By colposcopic examination, the extent and relationship of the epithelia to such anatomical reference points as the vaginal fornix and external os were studied. By histological examination of blocks taken from regions of known orientation within preserved specimens, such relationships were confirmed, and in addition, traced within the endocervical canal and into the depths of glandular structures.

The findings in this study show the variations to be observed in the distribution of the various forms of epithelium present in the cervical region of the genital tract.

The systematised findings are presented in schematic drawings of the cervix and adjacent vagina. This device is required, because techniques of macrophotography do not allow the whole extent and distribution to be displayed in living subjects. Topographical aspects are, however, evident in the colpophotographic illustrations used throughout the book.

TOPOGRAPHICAL VARIATIONS

For purposes of description, three epithelial arrangements are recognised.

1. The original squamocolumnar junction lies at or cephalad to the external os. Original squamous epithelium covers the entire ectocervix and

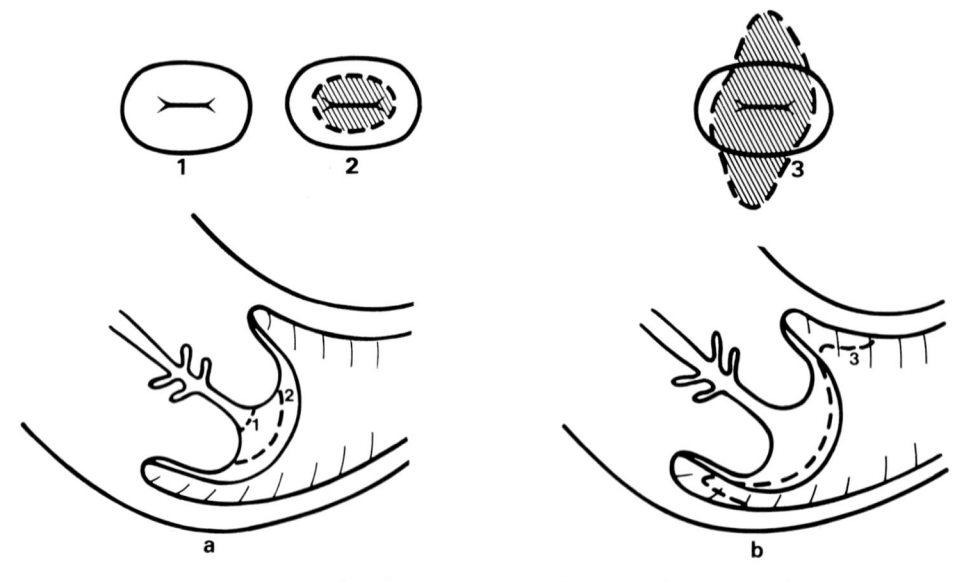

Figure 45. (a1) In both sagittal and surface views the original squamocolumnar junction coincides with the external os. (a2) The original squamocolumnar junction is caudad to the external os and encloses an elliptical area of columnar and metaplastic epithelia (shaded in the surface view). (b3) An extensive area is enclosed by the original squamocolumnar junction, which continues from the cervix onto the vagina (shaded in the surface view).

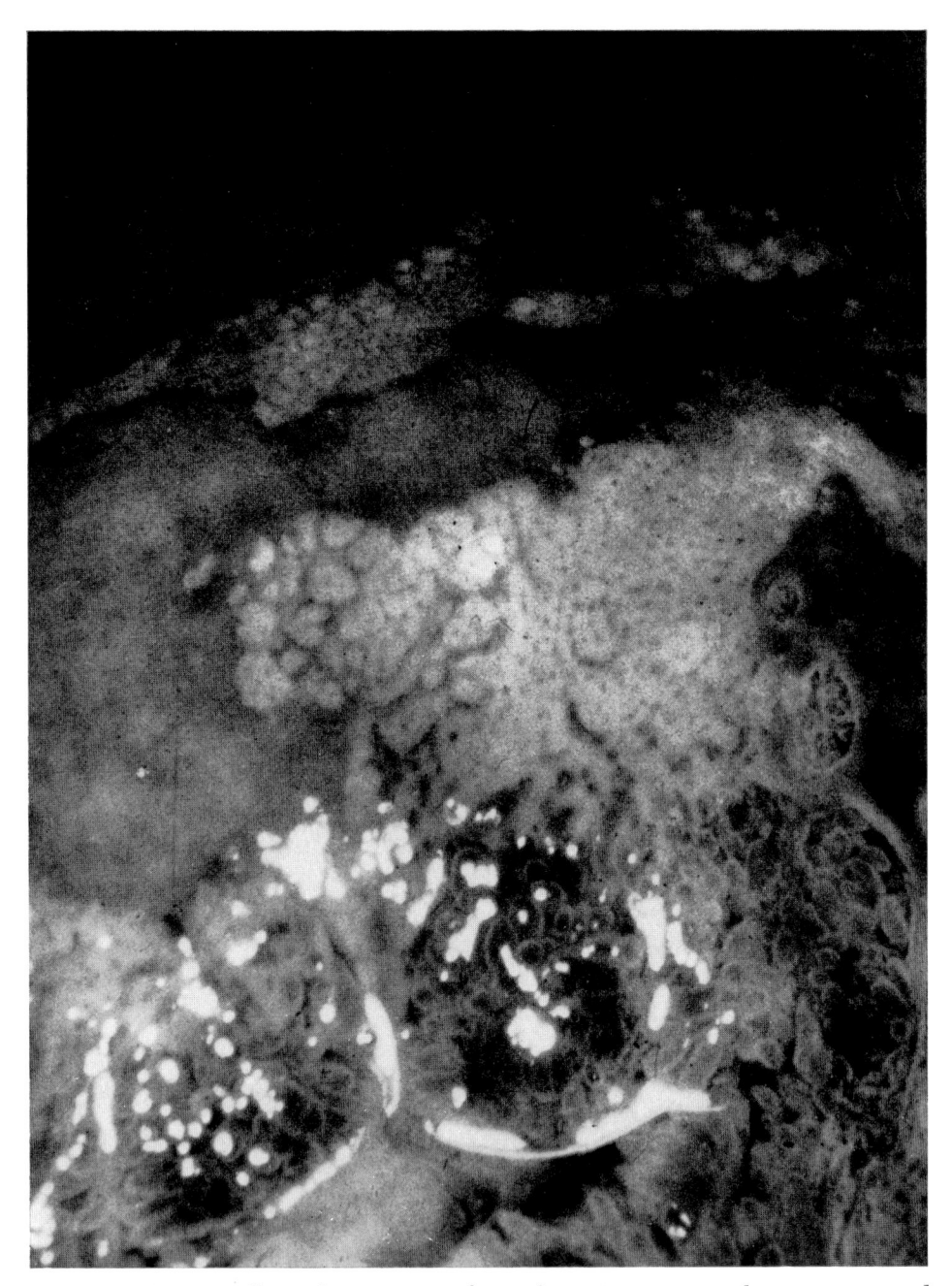

Figure 46. Occasionally, a discrete area of transformation zone can be seen separated from the main zone, apparently lying within original squamous epithelium. In this colpophotograph, the transformation zone is atypical and displays punctation and mosaic.

may line a portion of the lower endocervical canal. The transformation zone, when present, lies entirely within the canal. The clinician recognises this as the "normal" cervix of classical description (Fig. 45-1).

2. More commonly, the original squamocolumnar junction lies on the ectocervix. It usually circumscribes an elliptical area of variable size, within which the columnar and metaplastic epithelia display a highly variable admixture (Fig. 45-2). This arrangement is the morphological basis of what is so frequently and erroneously termed erosion, eversion, or ectopy.

3. Seldom, the original squamocolumnar junction can be traced onto portion of the vaginal epithelium. This arrangement, seen in 4 per cent of subjects, results in portion of the upper vagina as well as the cervix being covered with columnar and metaplastic epithelia (Fig. 45-3).

Most of the arrangements described above are regular and mainly symmetrical. Occasionally, the original squamocolumnar junction is haphazard and small isolated areas of transformation zone lie separate from the main zone (Fig. 46).

COLPOSCOPIC COUNTERPART OF THE VARIATIONS

It is evident that wide variations in site and extent of metaplasia can be observed. These are of significance for both the conduct of the colposcopic examination and the practical management of clinical problems.

The undoubted existence of metaplasia within the cervical canal may seem to offer a problem to the colposcopist. However, equally undoubted is the observation that when the vaginal speculum is introduced and its blades separated, in most instances, the cervical lips part to cause an apparent eversion of canal epithelia to be examined (see Figs. 43 and 44). Even without eversion, a valid comment may usually be made on the nature of the cervical epithelia within the lower portion of the canal (Fig. 47).

It is possible simply to define the topographical variations of the metaplastic epithelium as follows:

In one quarter of the material, metaplastic epithelium (typical and/or atypical) is entirely within the canal and is, in most instances, seen through the canal or can be everted for inspection.

In the remainder, the metaplastic epithelium (typical and/or atypical) occupies variable portions of the ectocervix and endocervical canal in continuity. The endocervical portion is usually everted by speculum examination as described (p. 17), and the new squamocolumnar junction can usually be identified, thus rendering obvious the whole of the area.

The large majority of atypical metaplasia, the histologist's dysplasia, and preclinical carcinoma share the features applying to physiological metaplasia discussed in this chapter and so are visible. Almost invariably, therefore, the precursors of squamous cancer are examinable by the experienced colposcopist.

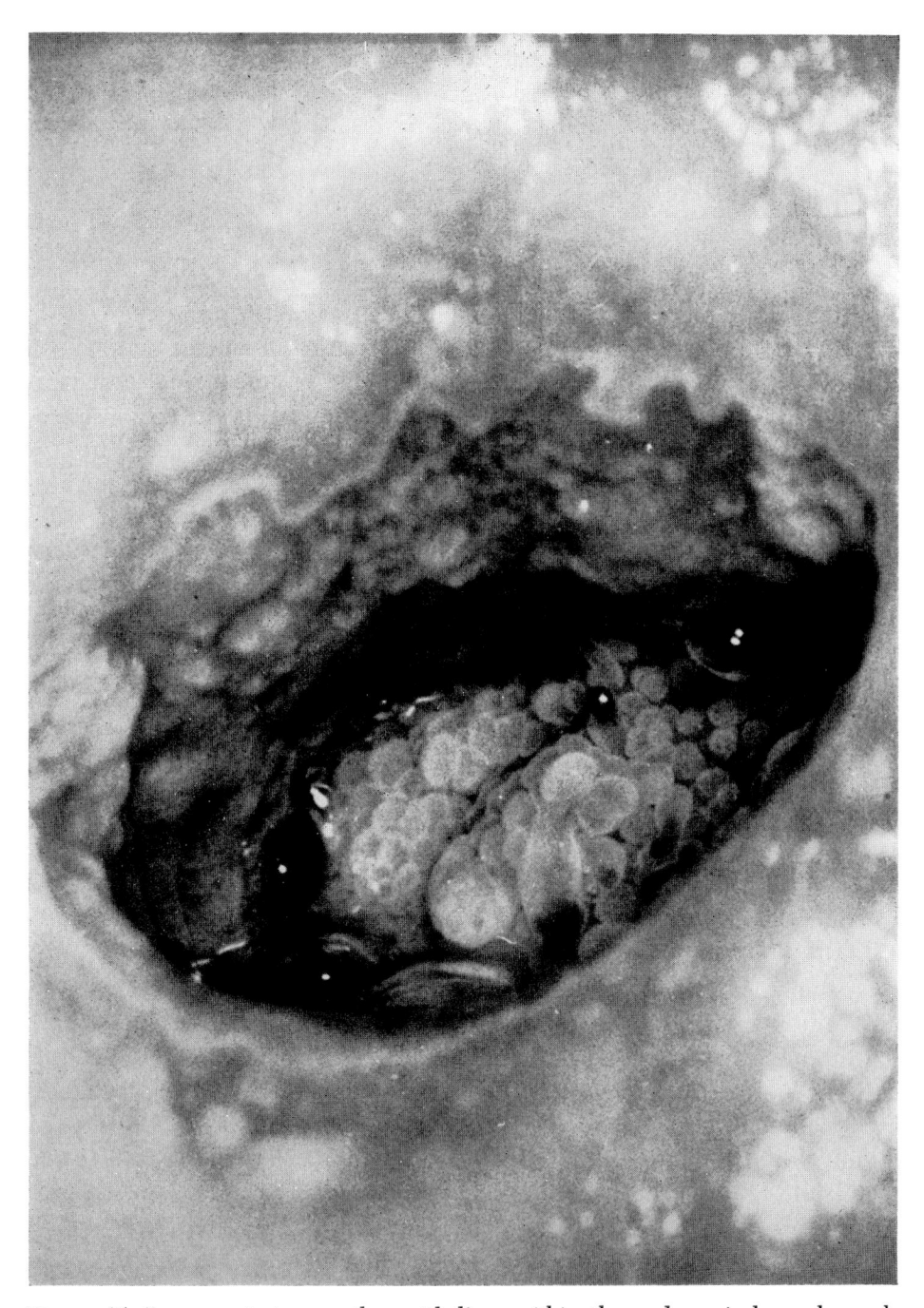

Figure 47. In many instances, the epithelium within the endocervical canal can be identified by colposcopy without eversion by the vaginal speculum. In this colpophotograph, columnar epithelium is seen in the cervical canal well above the external os.

Chapter 4

NATURAL HISTORY OF SQUAMOUS METAPLASIA AND THE TRANSFORMATION ZONE

THE ORIGIN AND DEVELOPMENT OF THE TISSUE AT RISK

THE PRINCIPAL FOCUS of enquiry in colposcopic examination is the transformation zone. This area requires precise understanding as a prelude to training in the techniques of the method, for it is here that preclinical squamous cancer of the organ and other epithelial dysplasias develop. The concept of the transformation zone is of such central importance to the method of colposcopy that an exhaustive textual and pictorial treatment of the area forms the basis for this book.

The areas where metaplastic epithelium (physiological and atypical) is identified constitute the transformation zone. Various aspects already described, such as site and extent, are readily appreciated during colposcopic examination. Their comprehension effectively eliminates the confusion existing in the minds of clinicians and histologists concerning this important area of the cervix.

The caudal limit of the transformation zone is readily defined by a line separating two squamous epithelia of differing origin and morphology: the original and the metaplastic. This line marks the site of the original squamocolumnar junction (Fig. 48). The cephalic limit of the zone lies at the junction of the metaplastic and columnar epithelia, the new squamocolumnar junction.

Most significantly, this process of metaplastic transformation seems to be a common physiological activity which in certain cases proceeds at or after initiation in an abnormal direction. It is evident from both histological and colposcopic study that in the majority of subjects, metaplastic activity results in the development of new squamous epithelium which is at first immature (p. 80). This normal transformation process, forming a *typical transformation zone* (Fig. 48), having reached maturity, does not seem subject to the development of squamous cancer. On the other hand, there is much evidence to show that some phases of the initial process are vulnerable to the equivalent of a genetic change, resulting in the emergence of a new squamous epithelium whose whole cell population has somehow acquired neoplastic potential. Such epithelia exhibit morphological characteristics that constitute the *atypical transformation zone* and define the precursors of squamous cancer of the cervix (Fig. 49).

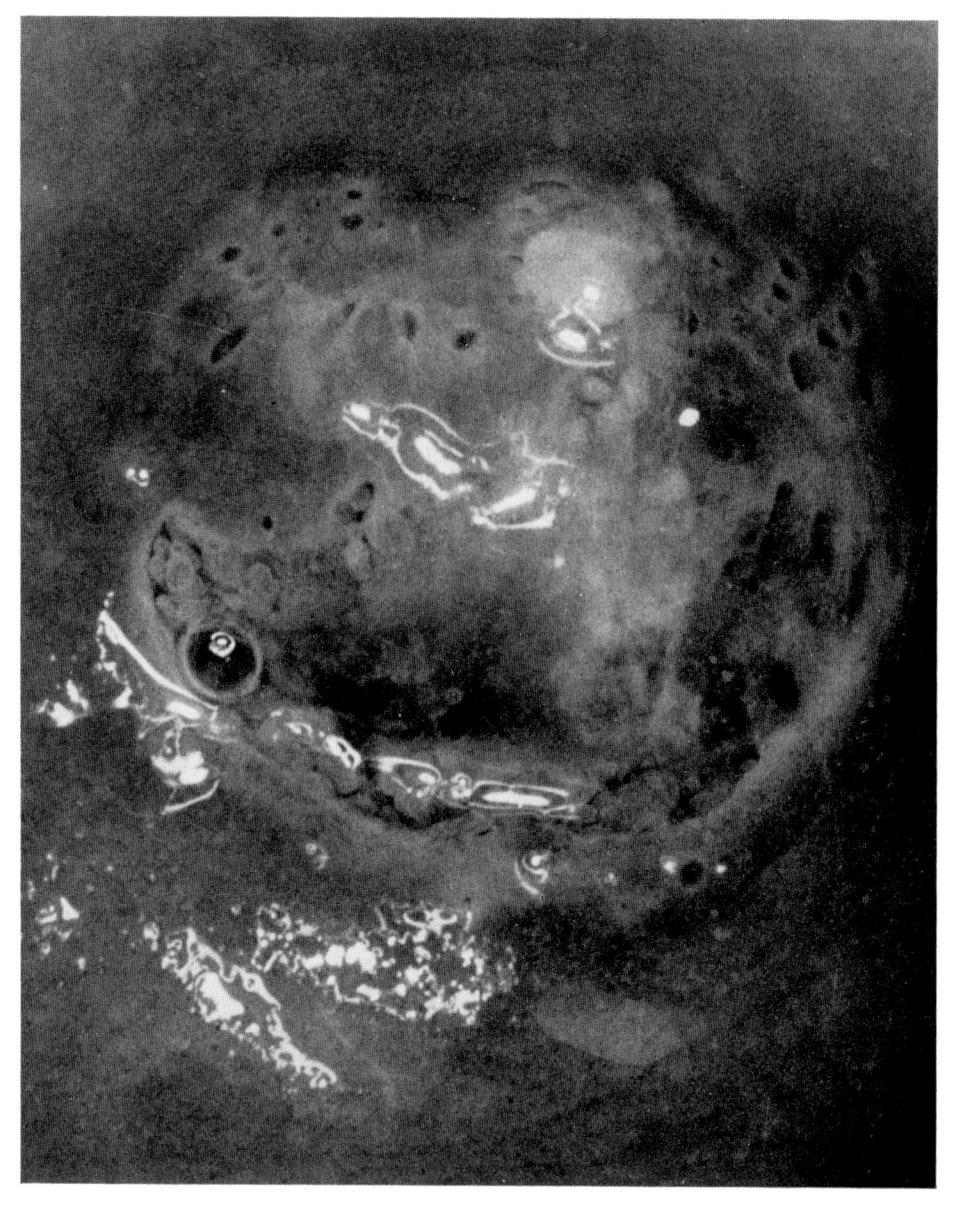

Figure 48. The product of physiological squamous metaplasia-typical transformation zone. The zone is demarcated peripherally from the original squamous epithelium at the original squamocolumnar junction, and its origin from preceding columnar epithelium is apparent from the presence of gland openings. Such a zone has no neoplastic potential.

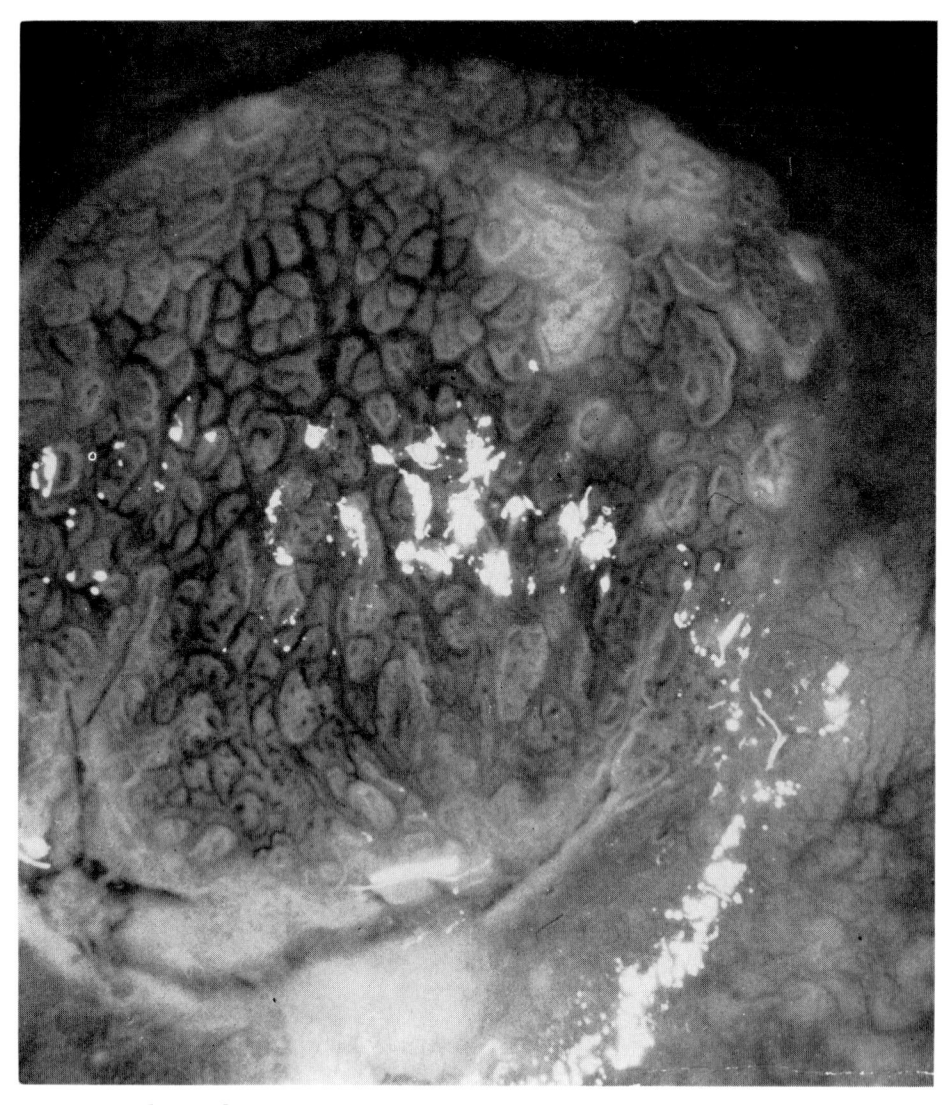

Figure 49. The product of atypical squamous metaplasia-atypical transformation zone. The zone is demarcated peripherally from the original squamous epithelium at the original squamocolumnar junction. Cancer may develop in this area; this is the *field of neoplastic potential*.

The interrelationships between the various epithelial forms which arise during physiological and pathological behaviour are amplified in Figures 50 and 51.

Atypical transformation zone denoted colposcopically by its white epithelium with or without punctation, mosaic, atypical vessels, and keratosis (Fig. 49), is almost invariably found in areas where dysplastic epithelia or

HISTOLOGY

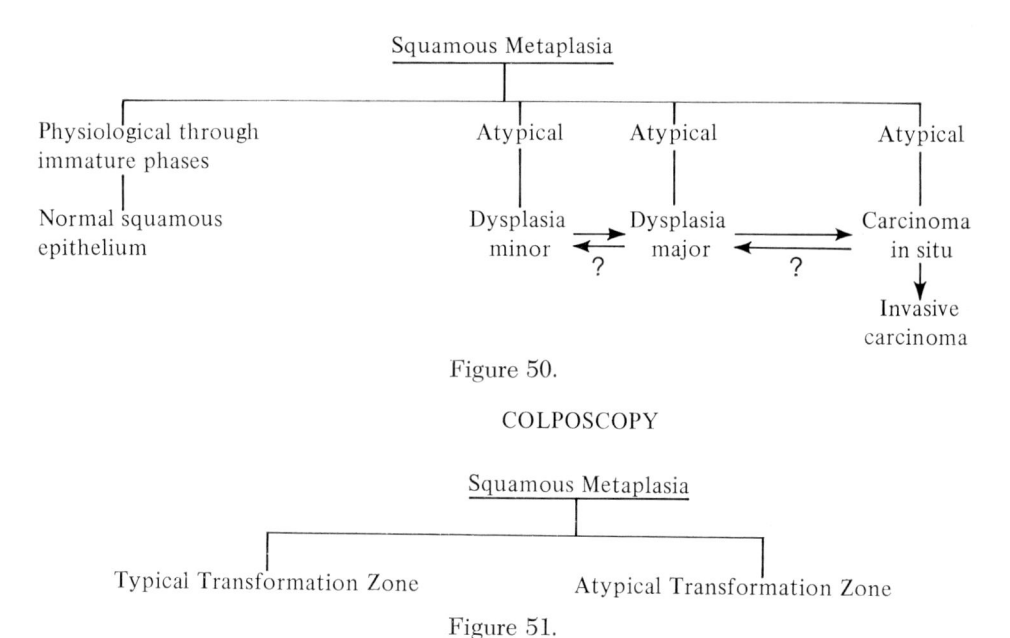

```
                        Squamous Metaplasia
         ┌───────────────────┬──────────┬──────────┐
Physiological through     Atypical   Atypical   Atypical
immature phases              │          │          │
     │                    Dysplasia  Dysplasia  Carcinoma
Normal squamous            minor ⇌    major  ⇌   in situ
epithelium                      ?           ?       │
                                                 Invasive
                                                 carcinoma
```

Figure 50.

COLPOSCOPY

```
                 Squamous Metaplasia
         ┌──────────────────┴──────────────────┐
  Typical Transformation Zone        Atypical Transformation Zone
```

Figure 51.

preclinical carcinoma are diagnosed histologically. Our interpretation of the atypical transformation zone includes a grading of the colposcopic appearances and, with its attempt to identify the more significant lesions, forms an integral part of our approach to the diagnosis and management of patients (p. 396).

Atypical transformation zones, especially the minor grades, may also be present in areas where histological examination reveals an epithelium containing minimal disorders of nuclear morphology and even normal metaplastic epithelium. This paradox referred to later (Chaps. 5, 9, and 15) forms one of the disappointments experienced by clinicians during their early use of the colposcope. The paradox is partly resolved when the reasons underlying the colposcopic morphology are understood.

BEHAVIORAL ASPECTS OF METAPLASIA

The behaviour of squamous metaplasia holds the key to the understanding of oncogenesis in this area and affords the opportunity for the development of neoplastic potential. Thus, the study of the life history and behaviour of metaplasia may well reveal factors important in carcinogenesis here and elsewhere. Particular aspects of behaviour which would seem to be important are its initiation and progress.

The onset of the metaplastic process can be recognised during sequential colposcopic examination. This we have termed the *dynamic phase* of metaplasia. During this phase emerges a new *immature metaplastic epithelium*. Subsequently, the new epithelium undergoes changes recognisable as *maturation*. It should be noted that these three phenomena apply to the origin and development of both physiological and atypical metaplasia. Indeed, the development of the two types of metaplasia, especially in their earlier phases, is so interrelated as to demand a detailed consideration of the former for any basic appreciation or understanding of the latter.

The chronological aspects of metaplasia may be appreciated only by methods that allow a continuous process to be observed from time to time and highlight the contribution of the colposcopic method to the study of squamous metaplasia. Isolated histological studies give only a picture of an arrested instant of the continuous process.

The colposcope has proved of great value in allowing sequential observation of the metaplastic process with time and when physiological episodes such as pregnancy, parturition, and the menopause occur. Two methods of study have been used to explore behavioural characteristics of the metaplastic epithelia. In one, the findings in groups of females categorised by age and reproductive status have been compared. In the other, individuals have been observed over several years and the findings recorded photographically.

DYNAMIC ASPECTS OF METAPLASIA

Although the initiating phase of metaplasia precedes a physiological outcome in most cases, it is also possibly the period of activity when neoplastic potential is acquired. The possibility highlights the need for close study of when and how an area of metaplasia comes into existence. It is unlikely that such behavioural characteristics can be adequately studied using histological methods. When such techniques are used, a major deficiency arises in that the bulk of material examined comes from age-groups when gynaecological disorders are common, resulting in inadvertent selection of material, mainly from the middle decades of life. Material from subjects in the early decades is scarce. Our studies suggested that new metaplastic activity is low during the middle decades and that already by this time extensive metaplasia has occurred and reached a mature stage. This assessment applies equally well to atypical epithelium.

Seeking the earlier and perhaps more significant phases in the life history of metaplasia, interest was initially focused on changes to be seen in pregnant women. Serial colpophotographic observations were made during and immediately after pregnancy in multiparous women supported by histological correlations, but a similar static picture emerged. On the other hand, when primigravidas were examined, it became evident that active metaplasia involving rapid replacement of columnar epithelium could be observed in some women, especially during the middle months of pregnancy. This activity refers to the *dynamic phase*, the initial process by which metaplastic epithelium succeeds columnar. During the dynamic phase, a well-defined zone of metaplasia, physiological or atypical, comes rapidly into existence.

The process observed during pregnancy cannot, however, explain the existence of some degree of transformation zone observed so frequently amongst most nulliparous women. The existence of this degree of metaplasia led us to examine the extent of the phenomenon in earlier age groups. Two other dynamic phases when metaplasia was active became apparent. These were during foetal life (p. 92) and in early adolescence (p. 100), especially if the latter was associated with the onset of sexual activity. Thus, it is our belief that this process of epithelial succession, from columnar to metaplastic during the life of the individual, results mainly from one or more of three possible episodic dynamic phases of metaplasia. The process at other times is minimal.

Our synthesis of the dynamics of metaplasia has been fashioned after many colpophotographic and histological correlations and describes the essential changes of an apparently short-lived dynamic phase. The appearance of several adjacent villi of cervical epithelium may be used to illustrate and explain this process. Demonstrated are the means by which the complicated villiform convoluted surface of the columnar epithelium is rendered smooth by metaplastic transformation. Three stages characterise the earliest phases of squamous metaplasia.

Prior to metaplasia, the villus is seen with its stromal core and terminal vascular structures covered by a single layer of mucus-secreting cells of the columnar epithelium. The earliest detectable colposcopic change of metaplasia, *Stage I*, is a loss of translucency of the tip of the villus, the vascular structures becoming distinct (Fig. 52a). Histological examination of the area demonstrates a reduction in the mucus content of the epithelial cells, which become flattened and cuboidal. The stromal cells lose their quiescent appearance of a dark nucleus with scant cytoplasm and develop a less densely staining nucleus and increased cytoplasm, which is drawn out into long processes (Fig. 53). These appearances are referred to as *activated stromal cells*. We believe that these stromal cells together with the altered columnar cells transform directly to an epithelium (Fig. 54). Similar cells above the basement membrane are usually described as the *columnar reserve cells*.

The changes are a prelude to the appearance of a multilayered undifferentiated sheet of epithelial cells by rapid division of the activated stromal cells capping the villus and extending into the cleft between two adjacent villi.

Stage II is observed in adjacent, more mature areas where individual

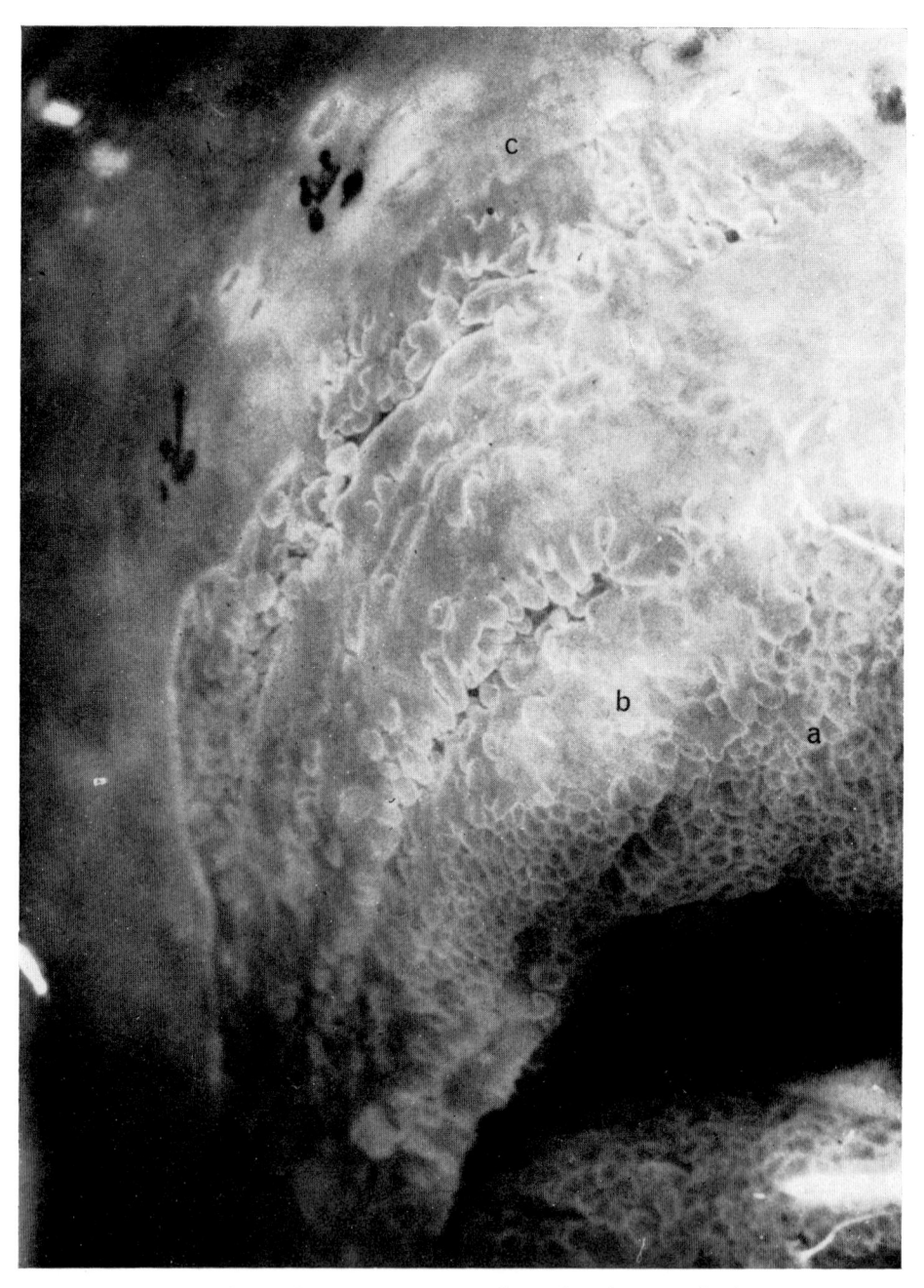

Figure 52. Portion of transformation zone in this colpophotograph shows various appearances characterising the transition from columnar to metaplastic squamous epithelium during the dynamic phase of metaplasia. (a) Within the endocervical canal and nearby, the columnar villi are unaffected. (b) Adjacent to (a) villi become indistinct or glazed (Stage I) and then undergo fusion (Stage II). (c) In other areas, all semblance of the original structure is lost, and the smooth surface characteristic of squamous epithelium is evident (Stage III).

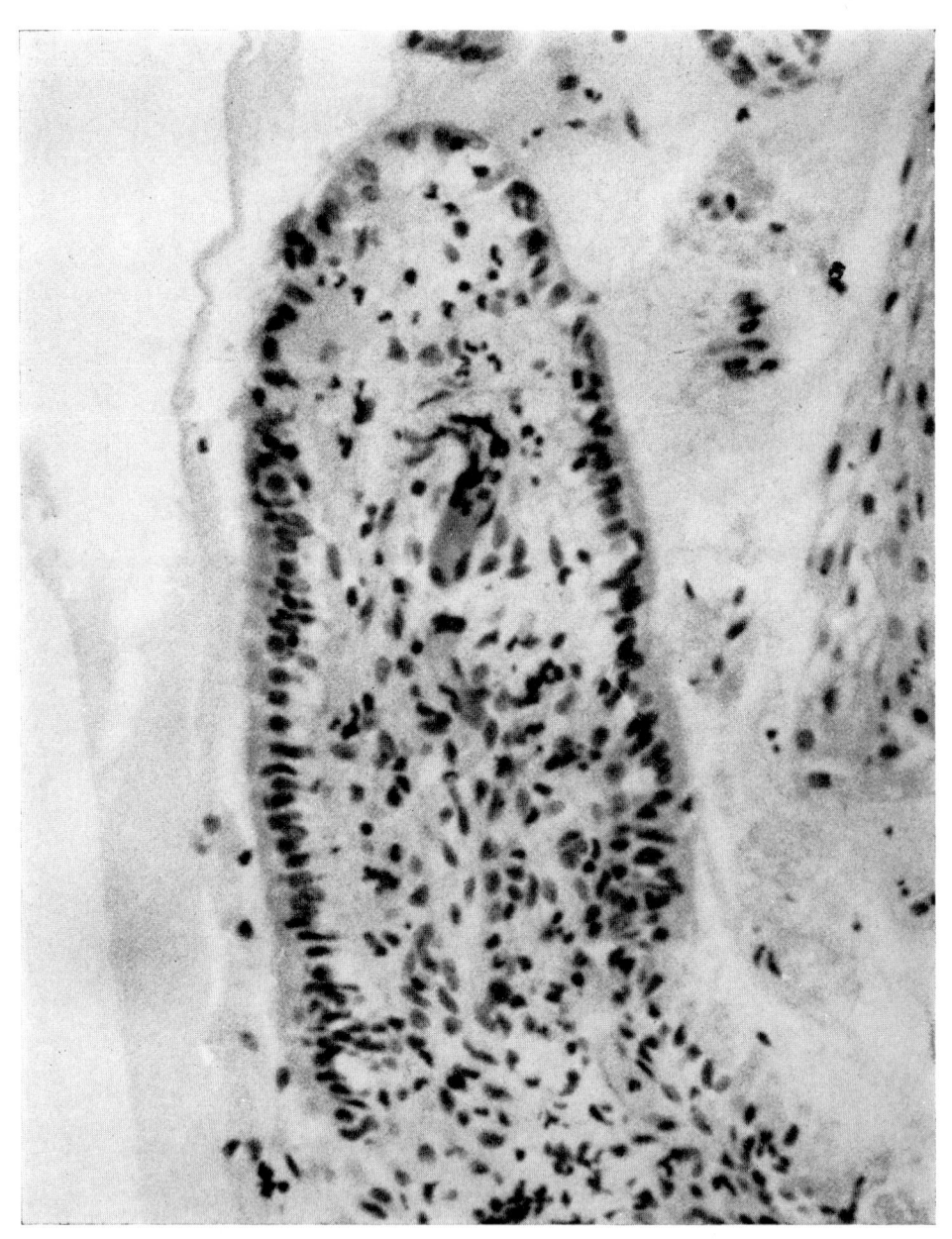

Figure 53. Metaplasia. Stage I. Histological section of a single columnar cell covered villus. Towards the tip of the villus, the tall columnar cells are replaced by low cuboidal cells.

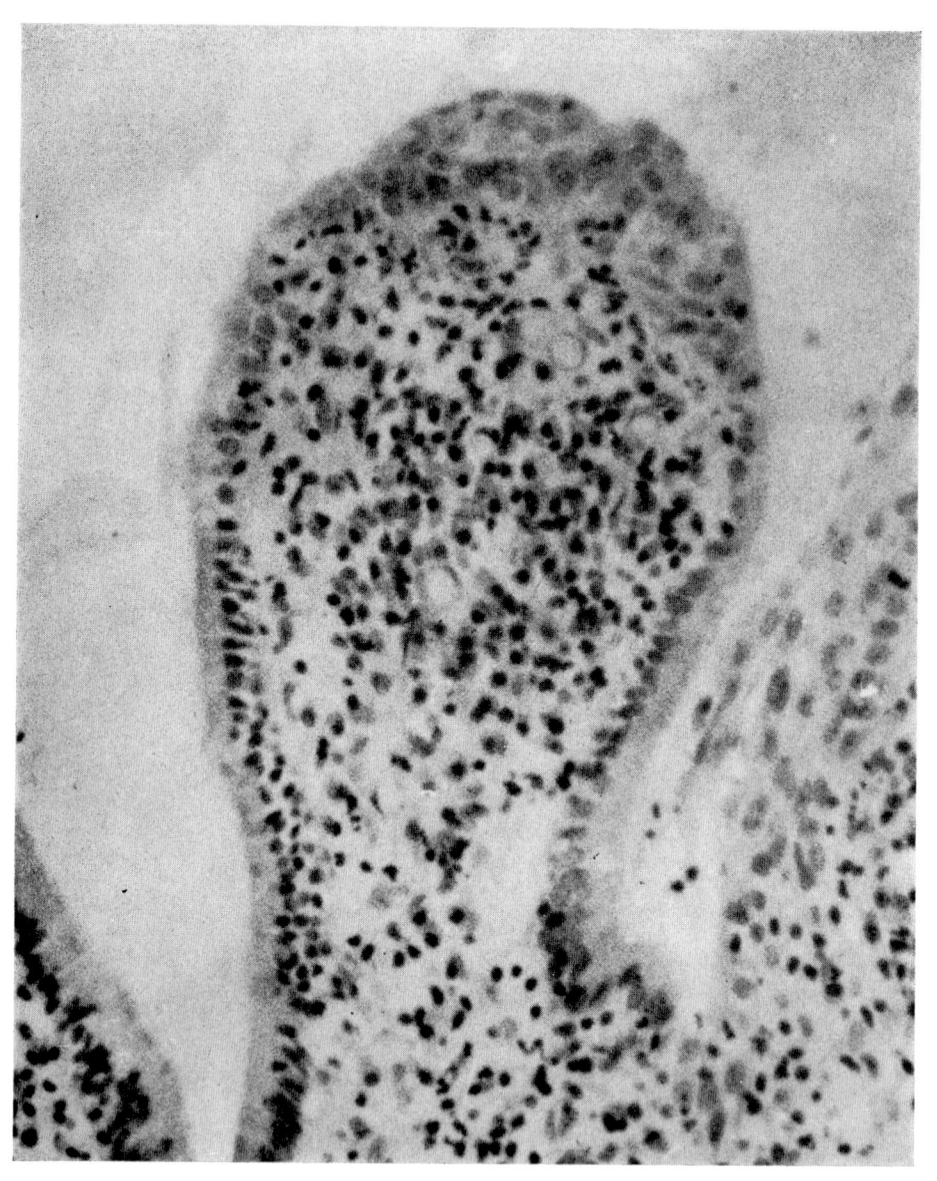

Figure 54. Early metaplasia. Histological section of villus at a later stage. The epithelium is now multilayered, and the stroma is packed with small round cells.

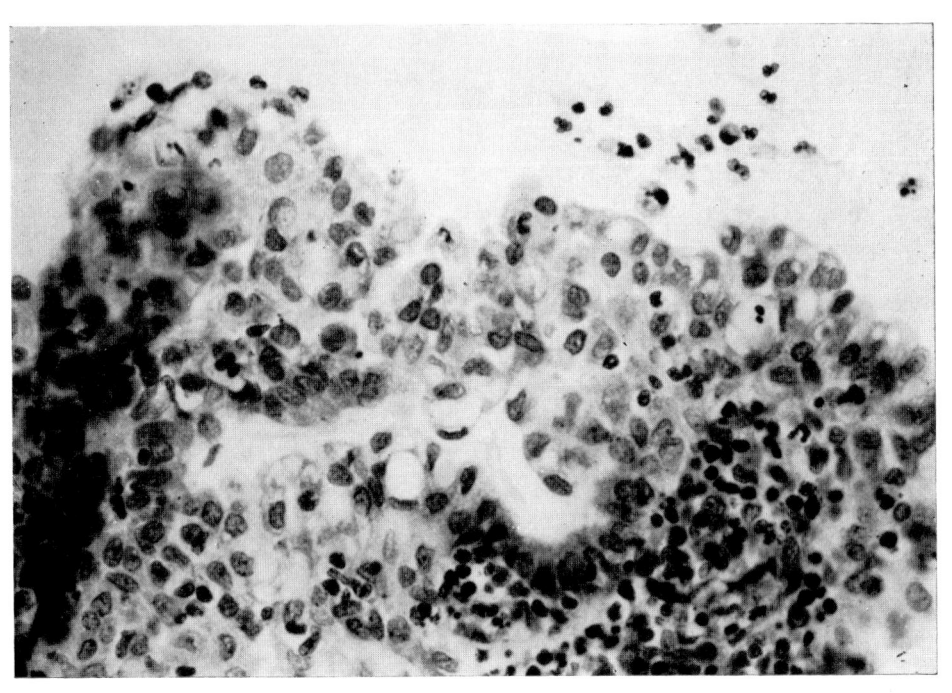

Figure 55. Metaplasia; Stage II. Histological section shows the epithelium of two adjacent villi which has fused. The original villous surface configuration is still evident. The new epithelium is now six to ten cells thick.

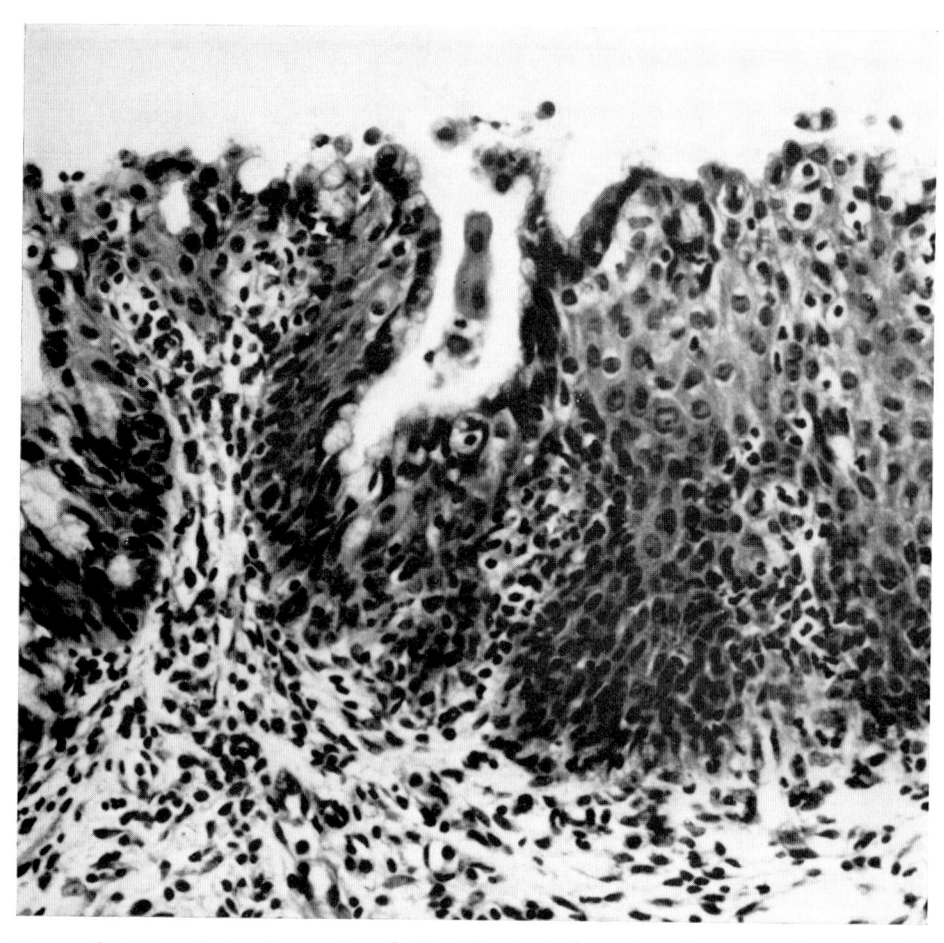

Figure 56. Metaplasia; Stages I and III. Histological section shows, on the right, the stratified epithelium of two adjacent villi has fused and now forms a new smooth surface to the area (Stage III). The two stromal cores of the original villi are incorporated as intraepithelial papillae. On the left is a villus in late Stage I.

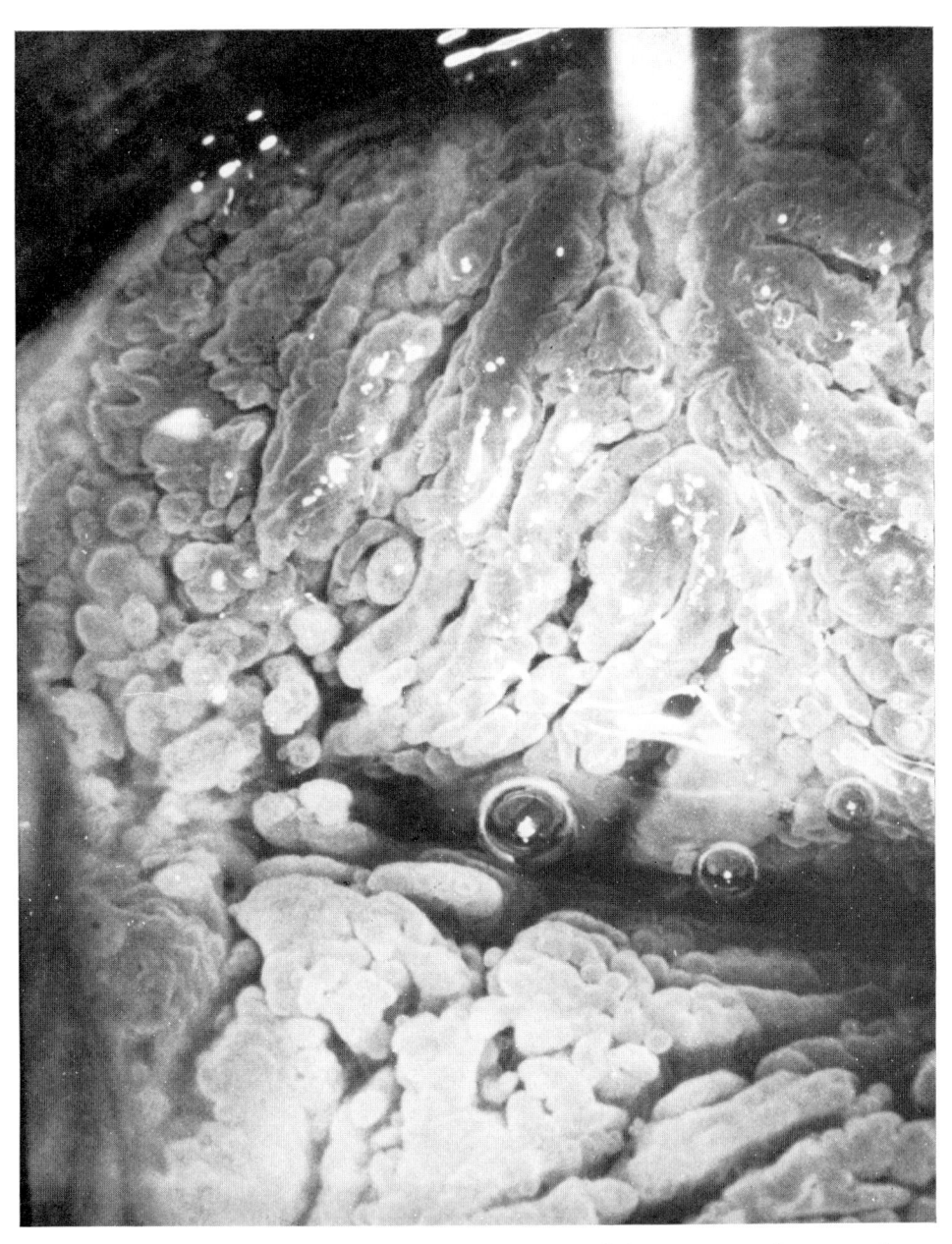

Figure 57. Evolution of metaplasia. The columnar epithelium in several areas is being modified. Villi are becoming glazed and confluent as the early phases of metaplasia modify the surface pattern. Single villi are still demonstrable in the deeper clefts. The metaplastic areas just above the canal on the right of the colpophotograph are discrete and clearly indicate an origin by *in situ* transition rather than ingrowth.

opaque villi appear fused but in which the origin of the new surface is still apparent. Minute humps are present, representing the tips of the old villi (Fig. 52b). Histologically, the clefts have been obliterated by extension downwards of the multilayered epithelium and fusion of their opposed surfaces. The stromal core persists as a structure now seen to be intraepithelial (Figs. 55 and 56).

Stage III is the near obliteration of the original structure, producing a smooth surface (Fig. 52c) of multilayered, undifferentiated epithelium, into which has been incorporated the original vascular structures proper to the stromal cores of the now effaced villi (Fig. 56).

There are three other features worthy of mention in discussing the replacement of columnar by squamous epithelium. First, the process starts at the tips of villi, suggesting that the stimulus for the change is to be found in the external environment provided by the vagina (Fig. 57). There is much evidence to indicate that the acid pH of the vagina is a major factor. Second, the essential process is believed to be in situ, so that the new epithelium emerges from beneath and is not an ingrowth from the original squamous epithelium (Fig. 57). Third, the process proceeds from patches representing fused villi interspersed with unchanged columnar epithelium. The final cover of the transformation zone, despite a superficial homogeneity, is thus an assembly of patches.

MATURITY OF METAPLASIA

The new metaplastic squamous epithelium emerges from the dynamic phase as a six- to ten-cell thickness of undifferentiated surface cells (*see* Fig. 11). The subsequent fate of the undifferentiated metaplastic epithelium is a gradual process of maturation. That these stages may be confused with other undifferentiated epithelia such as carcinoma in situ and dysplasia is of practical importance (Fig. 58). The many and various forms of this immature epithelium are observed in histological literature in various terms (p. 25) which do not often recognise its nature. Generally, the immature forms of metaplasia have their colposcopic counterparts in the immature transformation zones (*see* Fig. 24). Similar confusion is possible in attempts to colposcopically distinguish immature metaplastic epithelium of the physiological and atypical varieties (p. 227).

The ultimate maturity of this functionally and structurally immature epithelium is its development to a fully differentiated squamous epithelium, distinguishable with difficulty from the original squamous variety (Fig. 59). However, it is apparent that any episode of metaplasia may be arrested at any intermediate stage, either to persist in an immature state throughout life or to await further stimuli before tending again towards further maturity. The mature state may be reached relatively early and

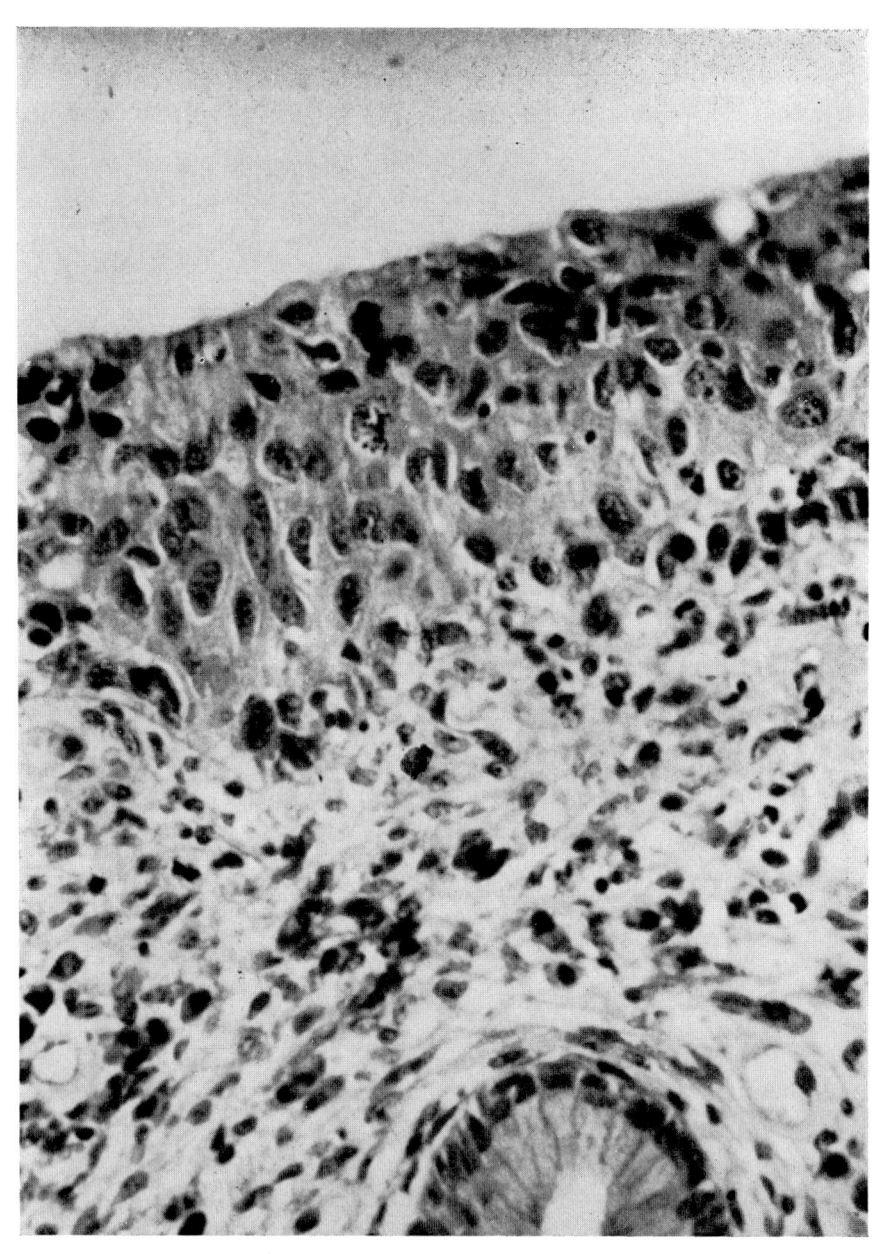

Figure 58. Photomicrograph of undifferentiated cervical epithelium demonstrating the difficulty of differentiating immature metaplastic epithelium from cervical intraepithelial neoplasia.

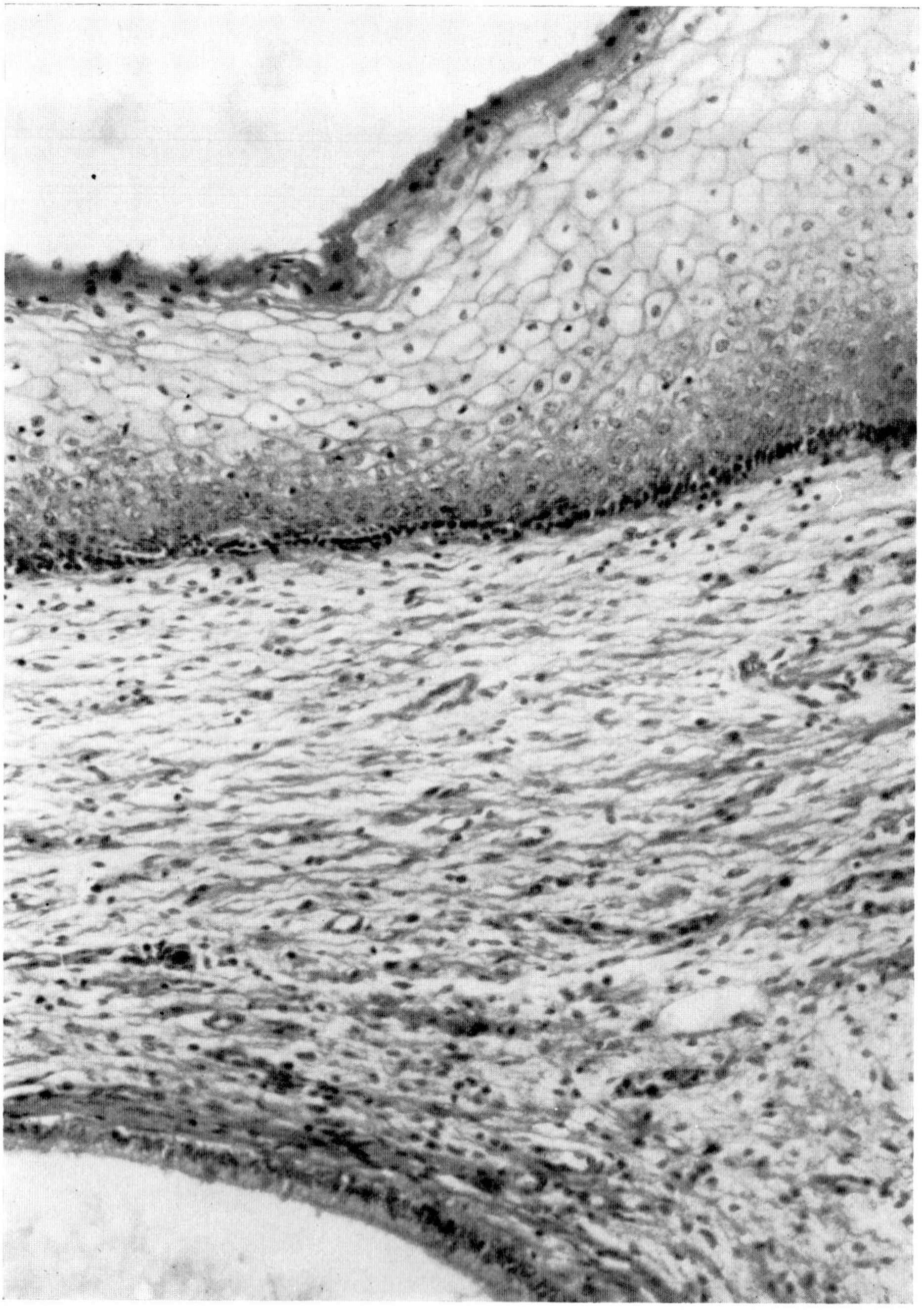

Figure 59. Maturation. After initiation, metaplastic epithelium matures eventually, and in time its histological appearance may closely resemble that of the original variety. Associated columnar structures as seen in the lower left corner of this photomicrograph usually assist in identifying it.

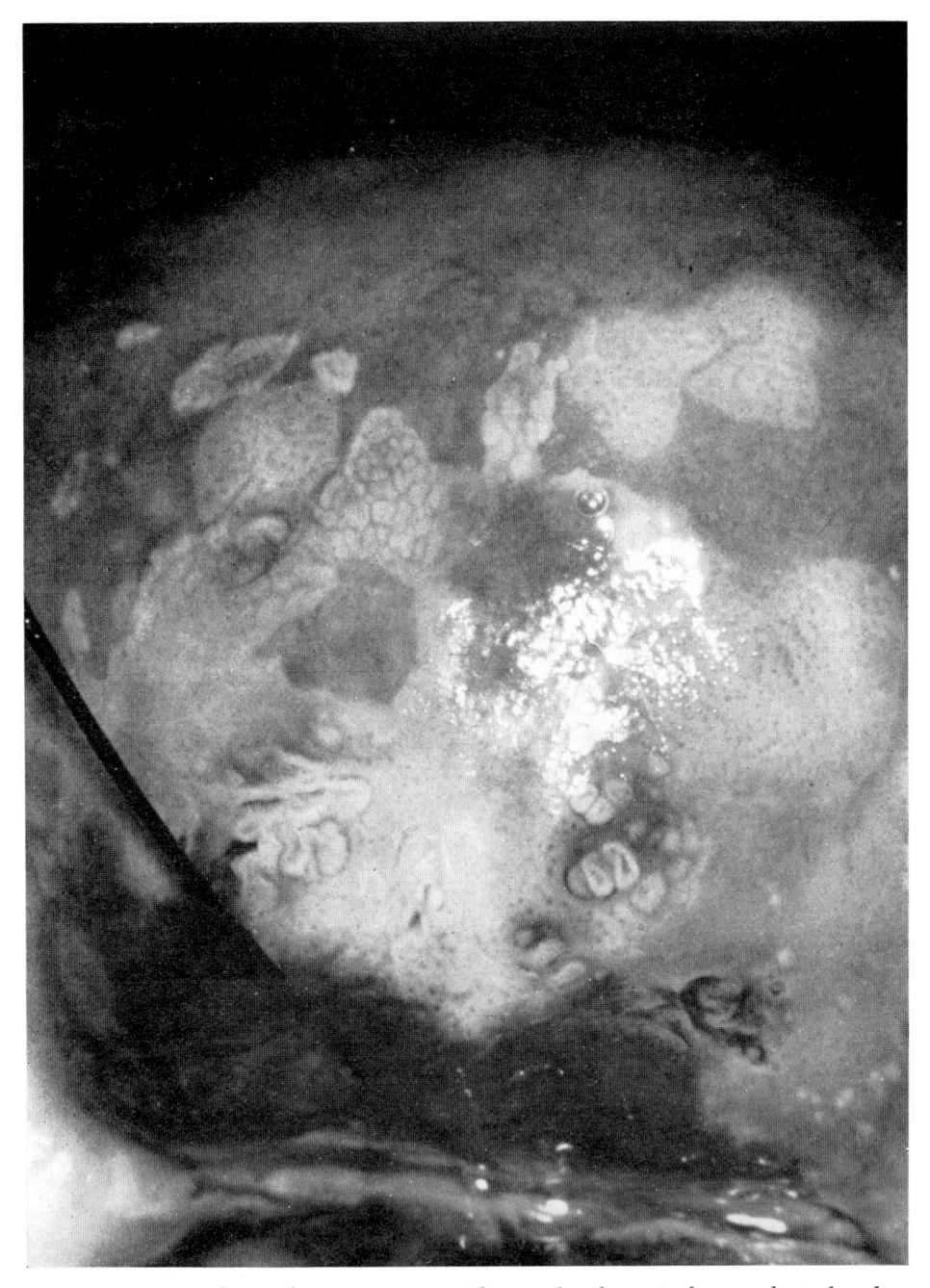

Figure 60. Atypical transformation zone. The result of atypical metaplasia has here been patchy and is thus multifocal. Two patches of normal metaplasia are also seen as islands within the transformation zone.

has even been seen in some foetuses. On the other hand, immature forms are identified in postmenopausal women. It is apparent that the tendency towards maturity is characterised by great variability.

Atypical metaplasia may take origin subtly during a dynamic phase in the way discussed for physiological metaplasia. The patchy nature of the origins of physiological metaplasia applies equally to atypical epithelium, with the result that the origin of the disease is frequently multifocal (Fig. 60). The role of atypical metaplastic epithelium as the tissue at risk cannot be overemphasised. The analogy with physiological metaplasia continues with arrest or progression with varying degrees of loss of differentiation or maturity. Intermediate stages are common and present to the histologist as varying degrees of dysplasia and carcinoma in situ. The end point of the process, definitive expression as frank cancer, is uncommon.

METAPLASIA IN VARIOUS AGE-GROUPS

It is evident that the complete understanding of the natural history of squamous metaplasia can only be approached by study of the process from its origin onwards throughout life. A pattern emerges from examination of the cervix in groups of females ranging from the foetus through senility. A short presentation of the colposcopic appearances of these age groups follows.

The Foetal Cervix

It has not been possible to establish any understanding of events prior to about twenty-four weeks gestation, but from then on, many of the typical epithelia become evident.

Our experience of the foetal cervix has been gained through colpophotographic study of preserved specimens supported by histological examination of blocks taken from known sites. In this fashion, the topography, colposcopic appearance, and histological variations encountered in over 300 subjects have been analysed. The following description is based upon analysis of specimens of gestational ages of twenty-four weeks onwards to one month of age.

In the foetal to one-month-old group, the original squamous epithelium of the cervix and vagina are often identical displaying over the whole extent a rugose character (Fig. 61). In formalin-preserved specimens, it is usually easy to identify the extent and distribution of various epithelial forms, although the usual colour variation and vascular structures are destroyed by lengthy immersion in preserving fluids.

The columnar epithelium is poorly developed in specimens of less than twenty-eight weeks gestation. It is usually present only within the endocervical canal as a simple flat sheet with a few shallow clefts. By thirty-two weeks, the results of advancing organogenesis are seen in the increas-

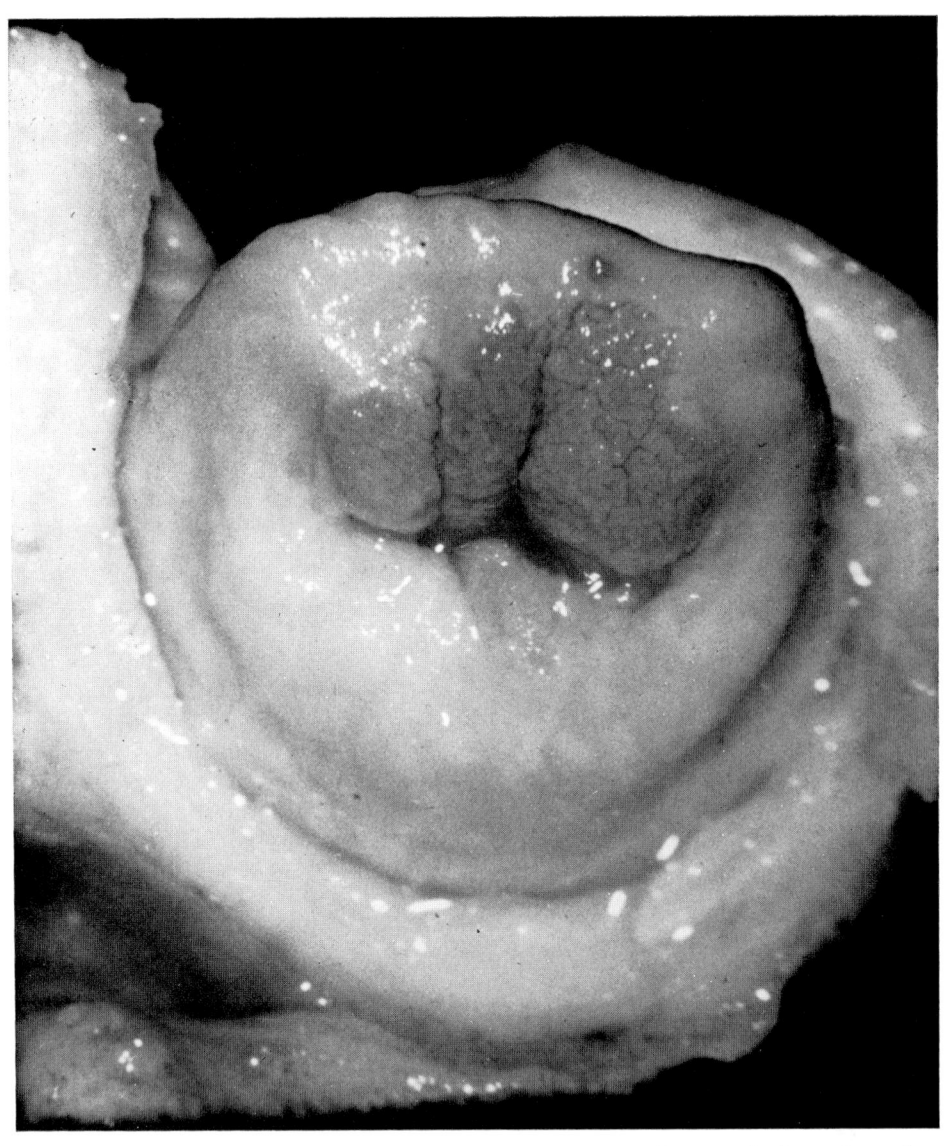

Figure 61. Cervix of neonate. Original epithelia can be distinguished in the colpophotograph, despite fixation in formalin. The original squamous epithelium is rugose like the vagina. Villi and clefts of the columnar epithelium are seen.

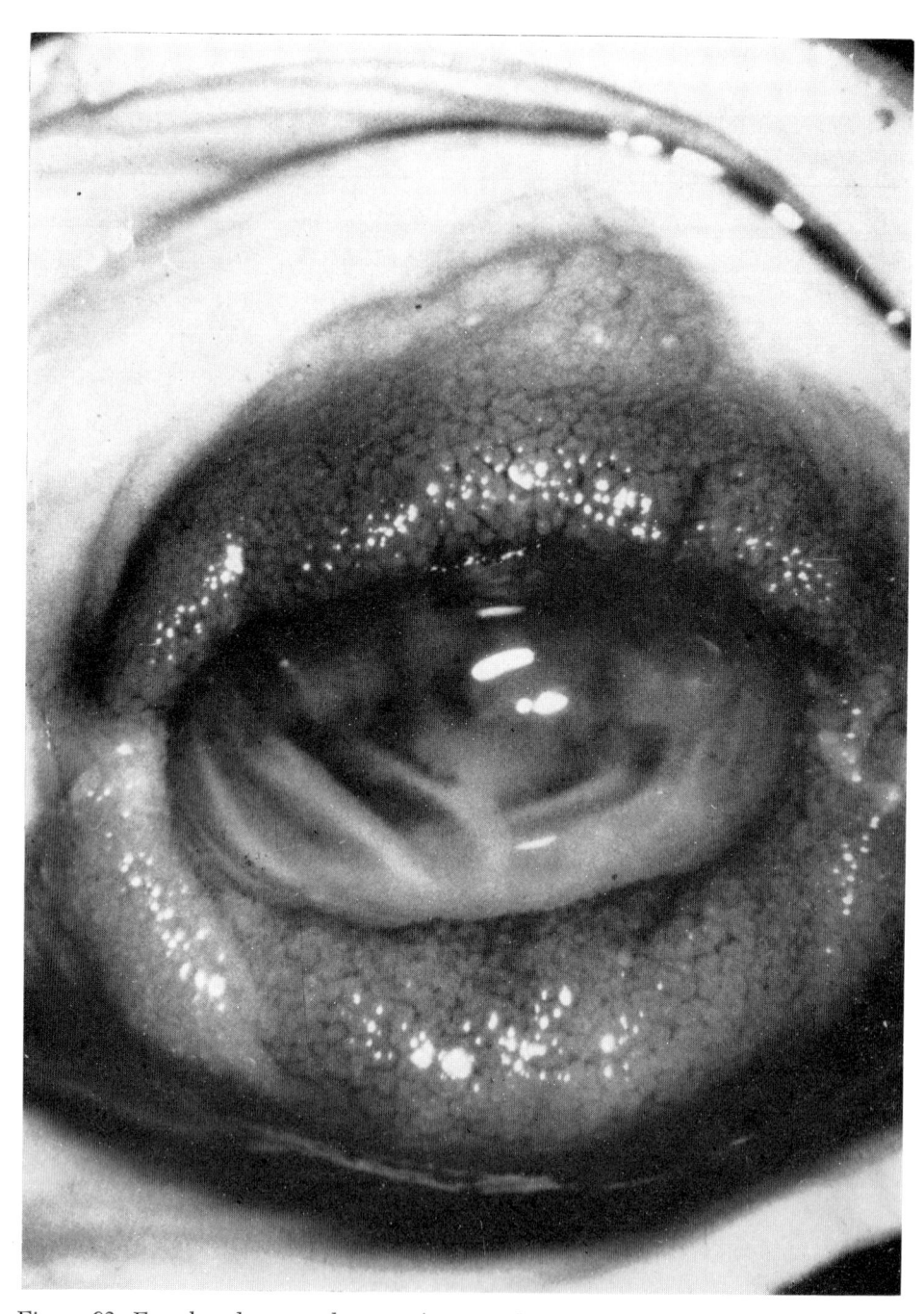

Figure 62. Foetal and neonatal cervix (preserved specimen). In this colpophotograph, columnar epithelium is seen on the ectocervix adjoined by an area of metaplastic epithelium at twelve o'clock. The arbor vitae uteri may be seen developing within the cervical canal.

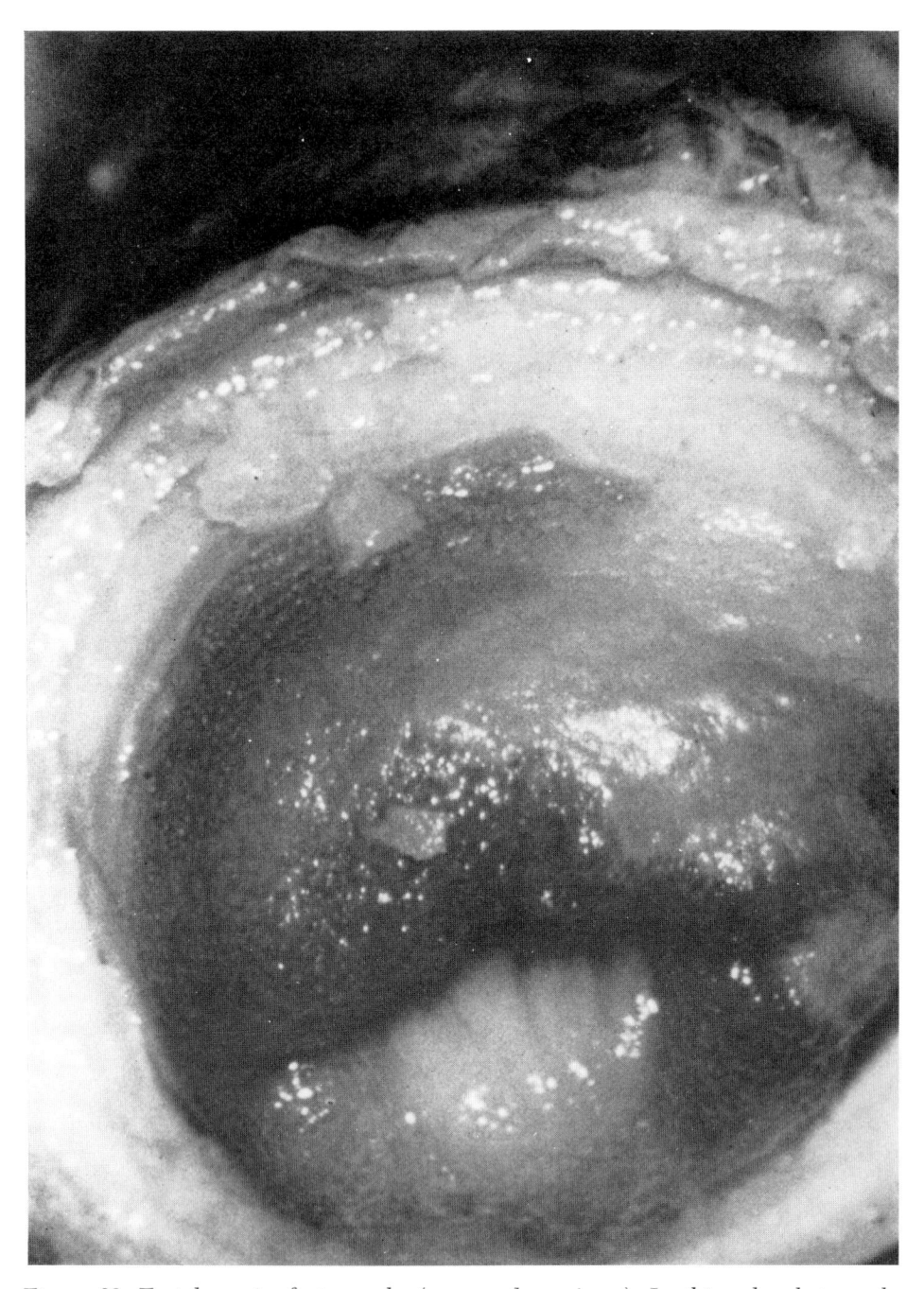

Figure 63. Foetal cervix; forty weeks (preserved specimen). In this colpophotograph, columnar epithelium and metaplastic epithelium form the main covering of the ecto-cervix. The transformation zone has the distribution commonly seen in the adult.

A

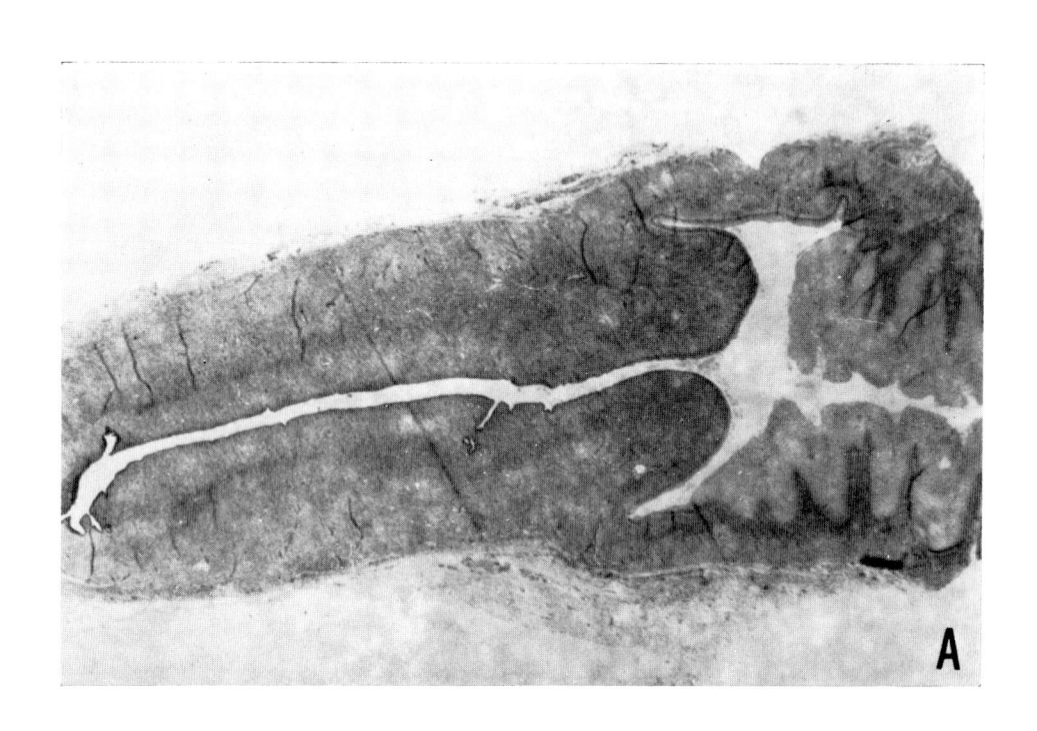

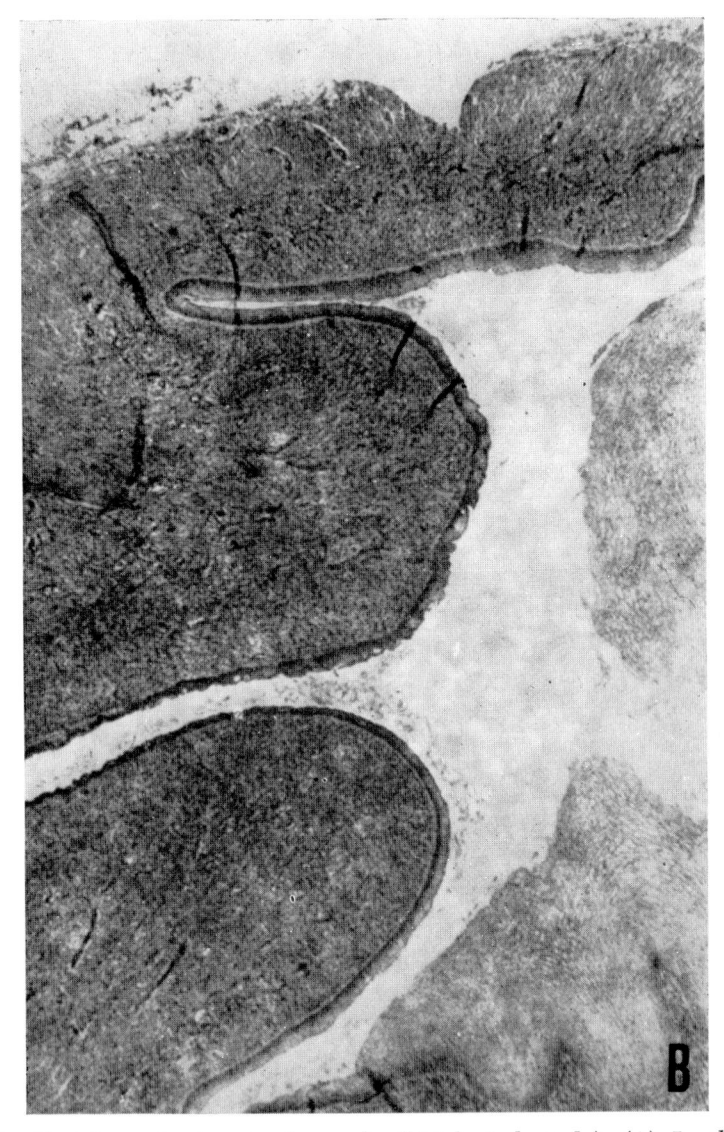

Figure 64. Foetal cervix; twenty-six weeks (histological study). (A) In the sagittal plane demonstrated, metaplastic epithelium is seen to extend from the upper vagina over the ectocervix into the canal. (B) Higher magnification of this area.

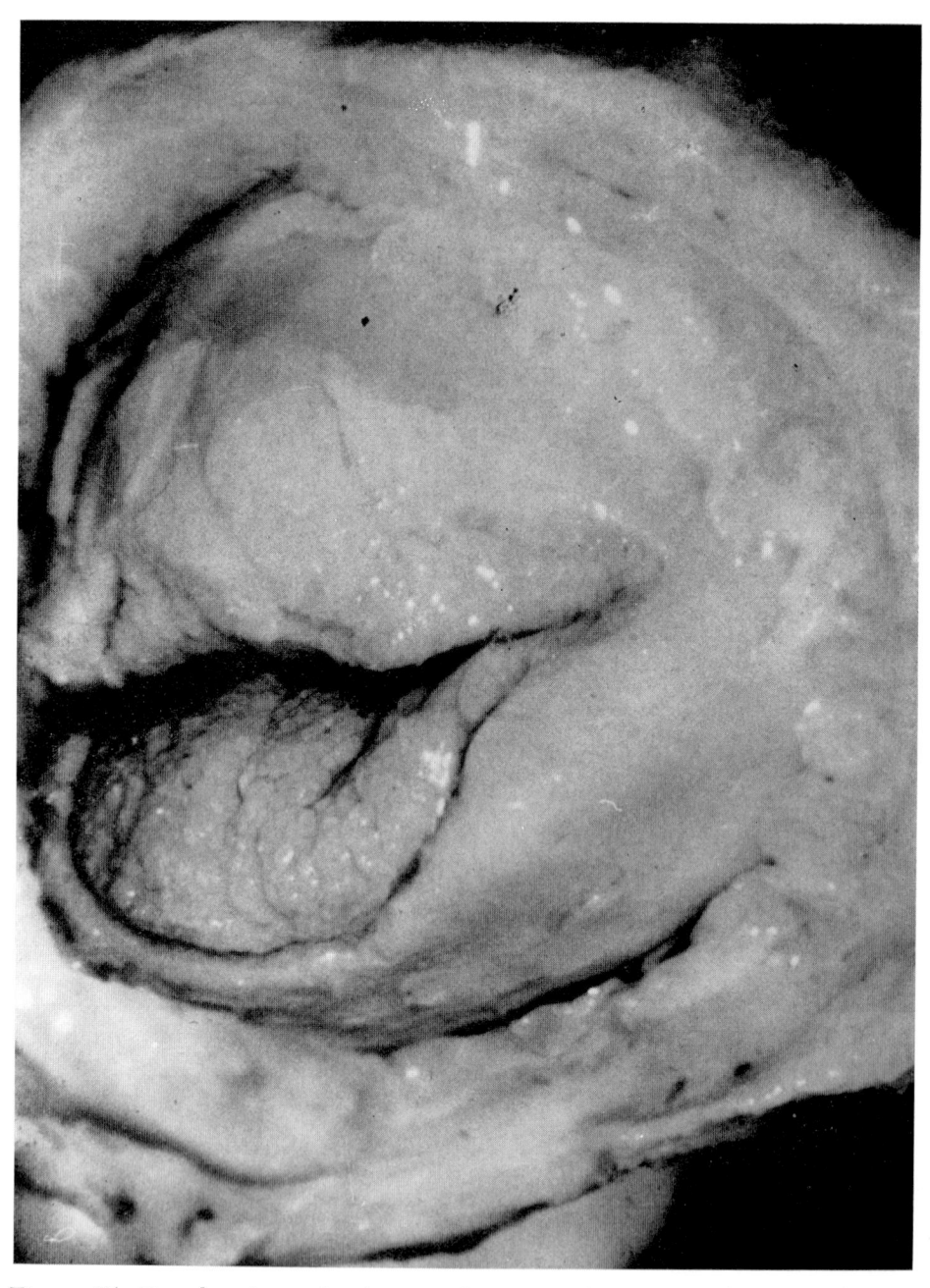

Figure 65. Prepubertal cervix (preserved specimen). In this three-year-old girl, columnar epithelium-covered villi, less obvious than in colpophotographs of living cervices, form part of the ectocervical covering. Laterally, the transverse external os ends in a slit resembling a laceration. The original squamocolumnar junction is seen.

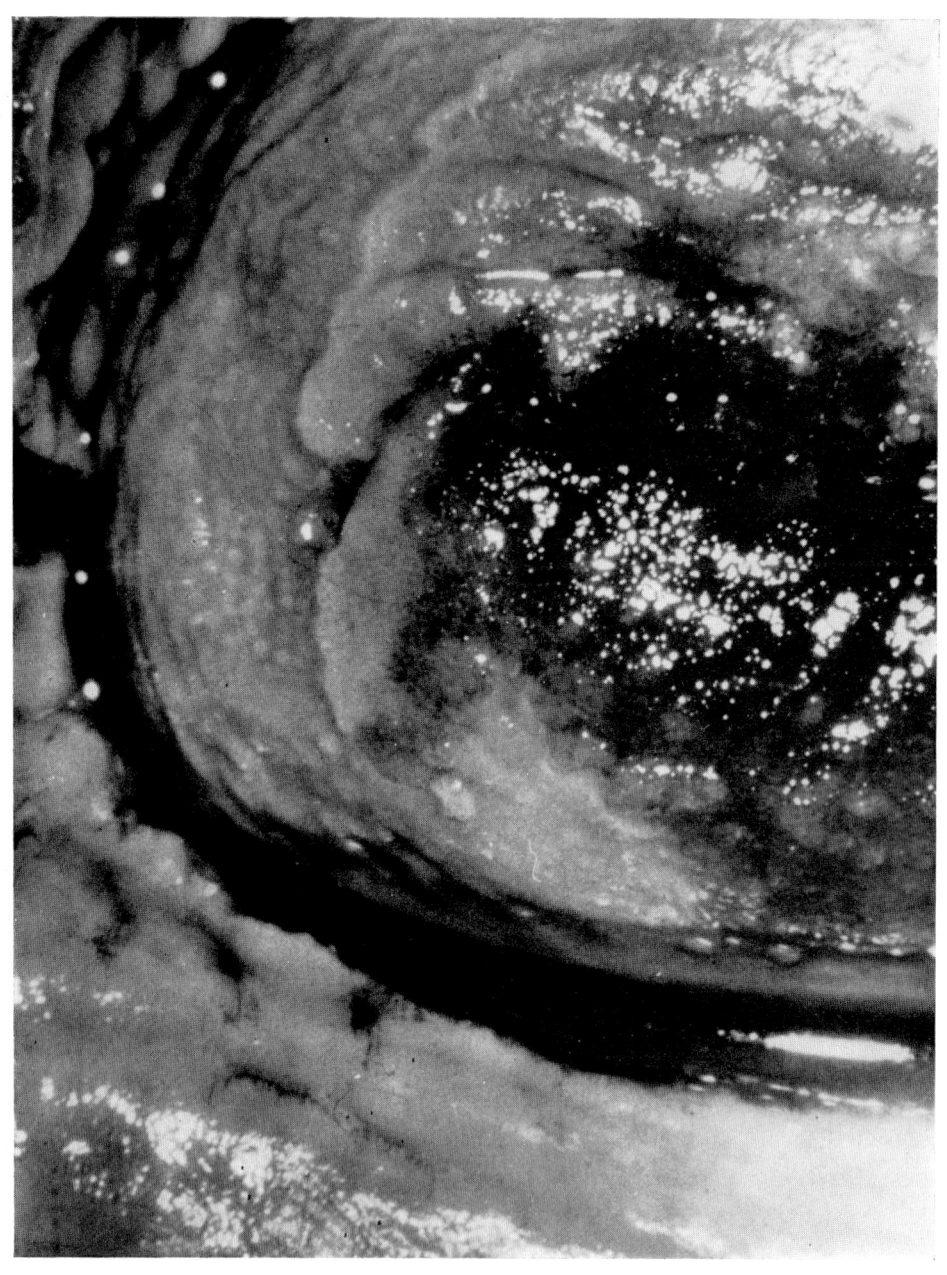

Figure 66. Prepubertal cervix (preserved specimen). Colpophotograph of cervix of a twelve-year-old girl. Between the crescentic area of original epithelium on the ectocervix on the left of the photograph and the bloodstained area on the right is an irregular crescent of white epithelium.

ing surface convolutions and subsurface structures now also found frequently on the ectocervix. Apparently, the original squamocolumnar junction is displaced caudad as the extent and complication of the columnar epithelium is increased. At birth, the epithelial structures and their topography closely parallel those seen in the adult (Fig. 62).

Physiological metaplasia is common (Fig. 63). In histological examination of single sagittal sections from each subject, it was found in 66 per cent of cases. It was extensive in 39 percent of instances, surprisingly so in the occasional case (Fig. 64A and B). Its principal distribution is in the distal or caudal zone of the original columnar area, its caudal boundary is the original squamocolumnar junction, and its cranial margin is the site at which further episodes of metaplasia may later be initiated. The real entity is appropriately termed *original transformation zone* and is discussed at length in Chapter 15.

Prepubertal Years

Available accounts of the structure and development of the cervix in this era have suggested that epithelial structures present at birth revert into the endocervical canal until puberty. Our studies of a large number of necropsy specimens have not confirmed this. The morphology of the original epithelia is substantially unchanged by physiological influences of the first decade of extrauterine existence.

The contribution of organogenesis to the morphology of the adult cervix is reflected in various appearances of the external cervical os. In most subjects, it is seen in the form of a transverse slit. This may extend laterally, creating the appearance of a traumatic laceration (Fig. 65). Persistence into adult life of such structures may make it difficult to distinguish their origin as congenital or acquired.

Atypical transformation has been identified rarely in the prepubertal group (Fig. 66) and is presumably the form which is described later as *original transformation zone* (p. 374).

The Cervix in Adolescent Nulliparae

The epidemiologist has called attention to early sexual activity and multiple coital partners as central factors in the aetiology of cervical carcinoma. This makes the study of metaplasia in the sexually active adolescent one of the principal current requirements of those interested in aetiology. Control studies in non-promiscuous and virginal groups need to be included.

Several hundred cervices in the second decade of existence have now been examined. Some observations have been made on preserved specimens and include histological examination of sections from sagittal planes. Advantage has been taken, during gynaecological examination under anaesthesia, of the opportunity to examine and photograph as many virgin cervices as possible. Changing sexual mores have facilitated the examination of sexually active teenage girls. It has also been possible to examine girls with known higher levels of activity. Detained promiscuous girls under legal compulsion to submit to bacteriological examination of the vagina have been available. Opportunity has been taken during these examinations for colpophotographic studies, and in some cases, permission has been obtained for biopsy and histological study (p. 366).

The years after puberty, with the onset of menstruation and possibly of coital activity, is the first opportunity for environmental factors to influence local activity in the cervix, especially during the vulnerable phases of metaplasia.

Knowledge of topography determined in prepubertal females is useful in anticipating the overall variations in epithelial distribution likely to be found in early adolescence. The majority of females progress to early adulthood with the cervix displaying the prepubertal ectocervical areas of columnar epithelium in which some metaplasia has usually occurred. This metaplasia may still be in immature phases, susceptible to further dynamic change, as is the still-present columnar epithelium. The traditional *virginal cervix* covered by squamous epithelium is uncommon.

Virgins

Almost all morphological variations have been observed in the virgin group. Extensive areas of columnar and metaplastic epithelium are present on the ectocervix in 75 per cent of subjects (Fig. 67). Typical transformation is present, often immature in early adolescence, and either represents persistence of prepubertal and foetal metaplasia or is of recent origin. Our impression is that the extent of metaplasia is less than that observed in sexually active groups.

Atypical transformation zone is present in a proportion of undoubted virgins (Fig. 68). Two explanations are now tenable. First, recent insight indicates that atypical transformation zone originating in intrauterine existence may present in adult life to explain the anomaly. This entity, the original transformation zone, is discussed later (p. 374). Second, immature metaplasia during adolescence can produce the same picture.

Sexually Active Adolescents

Examination of the sexually active group shows atypical transformation with striking frequency (Figs. 69-71). Typical transformation is also seen in this group (Fig. 72). Dynamic phases of the transformation process are prominent. There seems little doubt that in some of this group, the initial

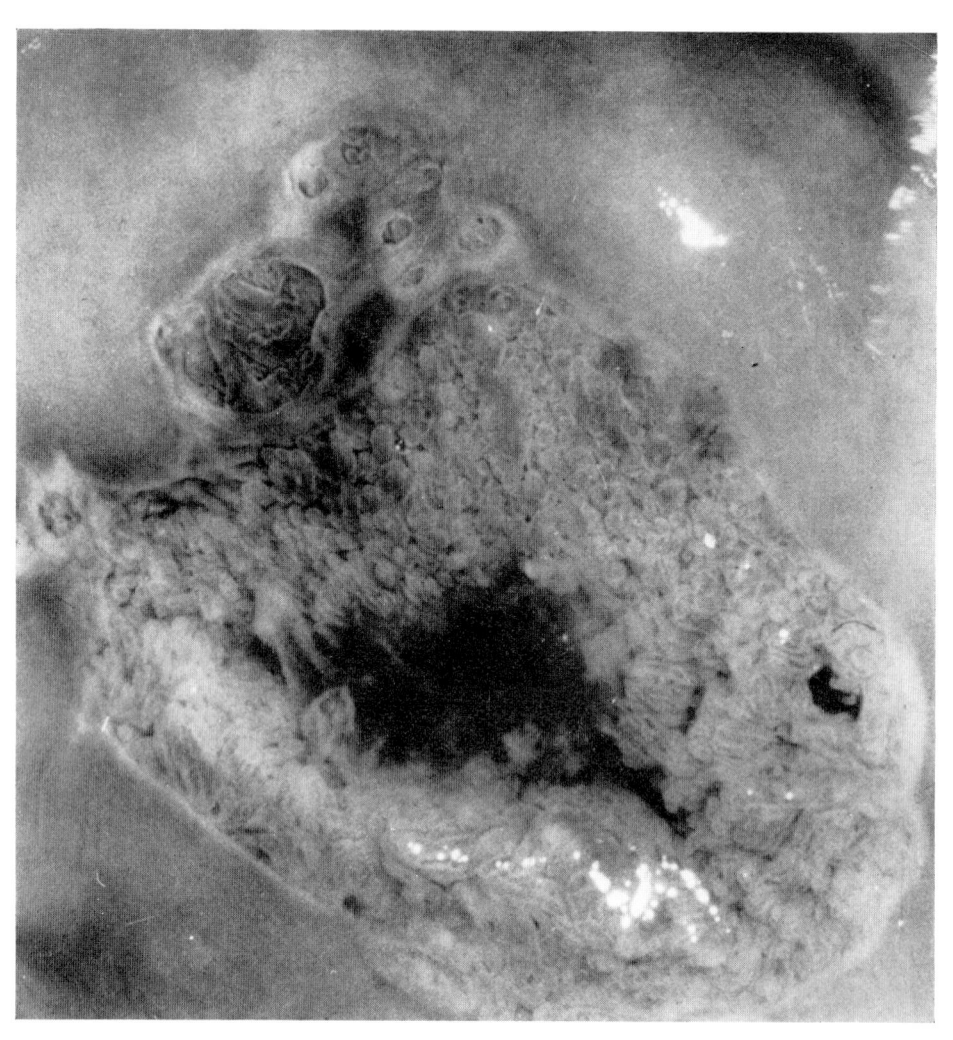

Figure 67. Adolescent cervix: virgin. Typical transformation zone showing varying grades of maturity of metaplastic squamous epithelium. These appearances, frequently seen, resemble cervices of other groups of females and are more common than the traditional virgin cervix of the literature. Adjoining the original epithelium at eleven o'clock is mature metaplastic epithelium, probably congenital in nature. Elsewhere are varying stages of fused villi indicating metaplasia of more recent origin and villi covered by columnar epithelium.

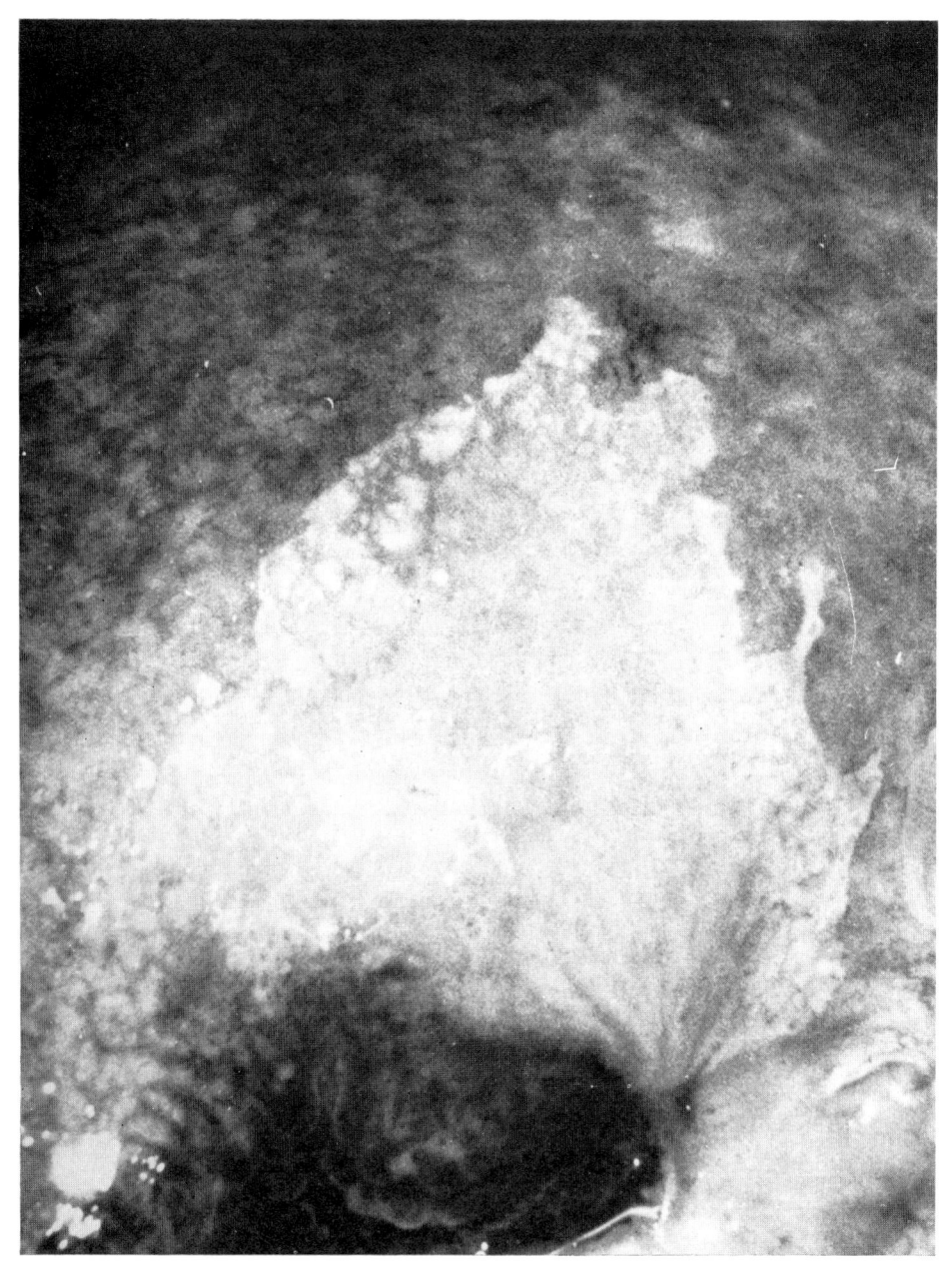

Figure 68. Adolescent cervix: virginal. Atypical transformation zone is present as a triangular area on the anterior lip mainly in the form of white epithelium. This is probably the original form of transformation zone (p. 374).

moment of the complicated sequence leading to the development of squamous carcinoma of the cervix is being observed. Some of the sexually active adolescent girls exhibiting atypical transformation zones must harbour an epithelial aberration, which in time develops to a stage recognizable histologically as one of the range of potentially neoplastic disorders. Subsequent observations on this group suggest that in others, as in the virginal group, the atypical appearances represent either special varieties of immature metaplastic epithelium preceding the development into mature physiological metaplastic epithelium or original transformation zone (p. 374).

Pregnancy

The importance of the first pregnancy, in which eversion may result in dynamic metaplasia, has already been stressed. Pregnancy is the event that may materially alter the embryologically determined epithelial relationships. The first pregnancy is the phase other than adolescence when dynamic change and environmental factors coincide and is thereby of aetiological importance.

The principal change in many women is the occurrence of eversion. Successive photographs of a woman observed throughout pregnancy demonstrate progressive eversion of the lower canal epithelium to an ectocervical site. The everted epithelium may be subject to a striking dynamic phase of metaplasia (Figs. 73-76), usually of a physiological character but occasionally atypical. The dynamic phase of metaplasia seems mainly restricted to the first pregnancy, resulting in the production of an area which persists and is returned, partly or completely, to the canal in the puerperium. In second and subsequent pregnancies, the now pre-existent area of metaplasia may again be everted, but these pregnancies exhibit minimal, if any, further dynamic phases of metaplasia.

Observations of other women in first and subsequent pregnancies have not revealed evidence of either eversion or dynamic metaplasia (Fig. 77).

In nearly all subjects, the cervix increases in its dimensions in varying proportions, with associated remodelling of surface contours. There is also a general increase in vascularity.

Birth trauma in the form of lacerations and true erosions, more common in the primigravida, is also productive of epithelial regeneration. This phase also produces a further opportunity for the installation of atypical epithelium.

The Reproductive Years

A large group of females has been observed over a number of years in order to determine the changes with time. Three major observations have been made. First, when areas photographed on several successive occasions were compared, the appearances most often were closely similar or indicat-

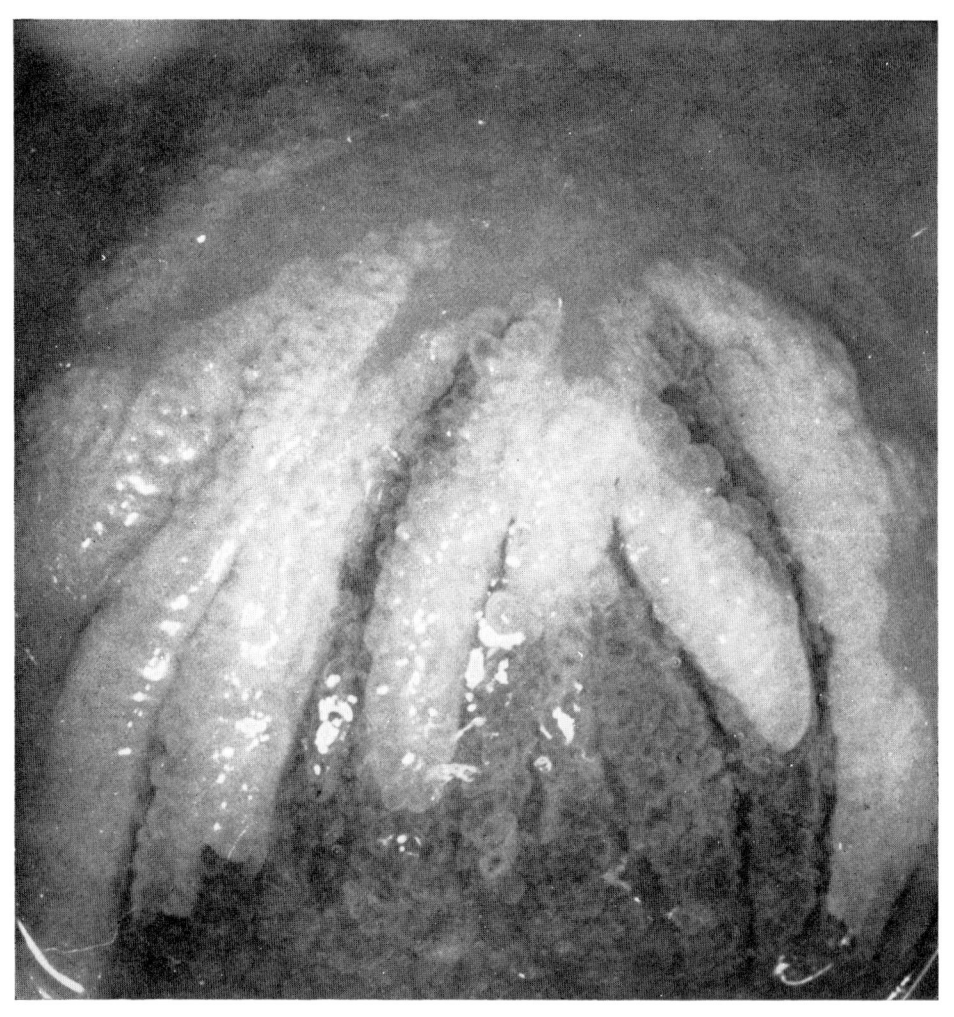

Figure 69. Adolescent cervix: promiscuous. The cervix of a fifteen-year-old girl displaying atypical transformation zone. The original villous structures can be seen to have fused, and the new surface emerges as a thick white epithelium.

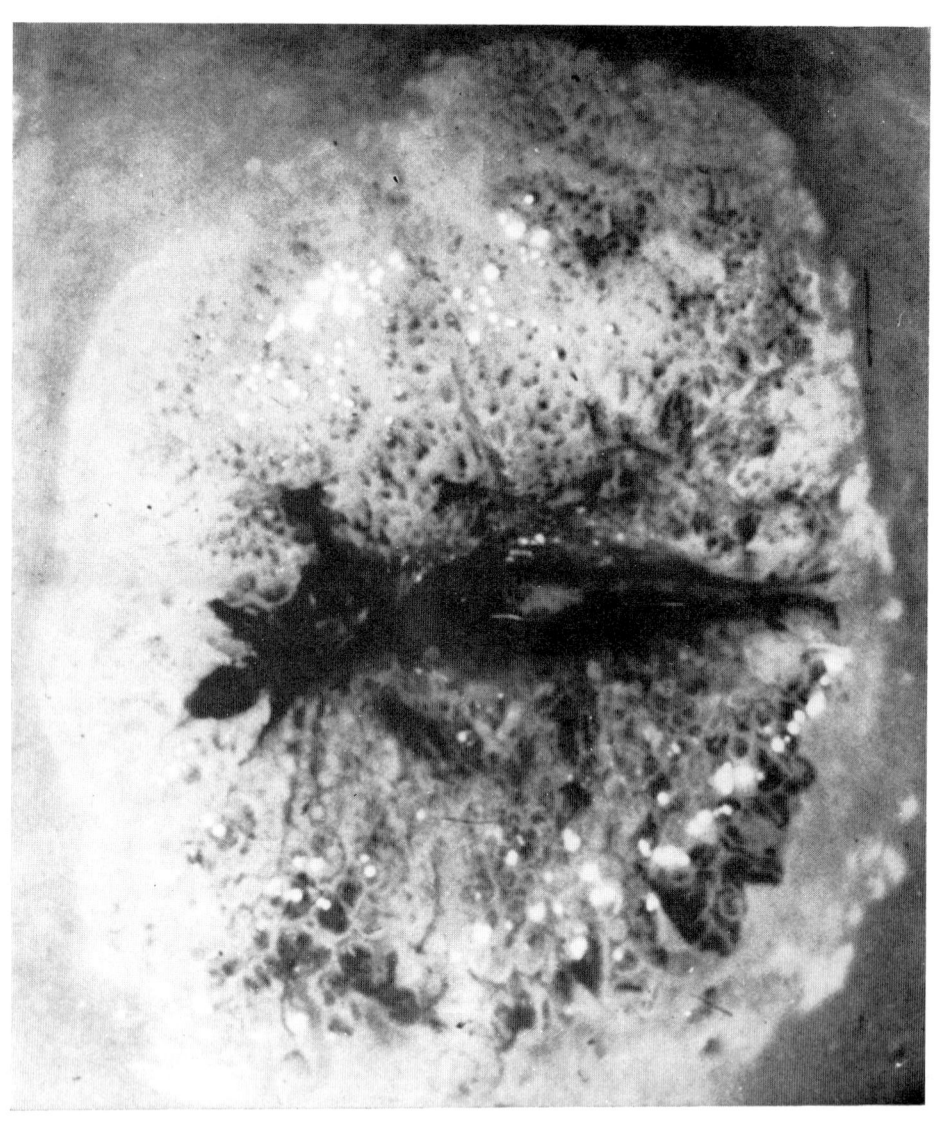

Figure 70. Adolescent cervix: promiscuous. Within a sharply demarcated original squamocolumnar junction, atypical transformation zone displaying white epithelium and punctation has formed. The subject is fourteen years old.

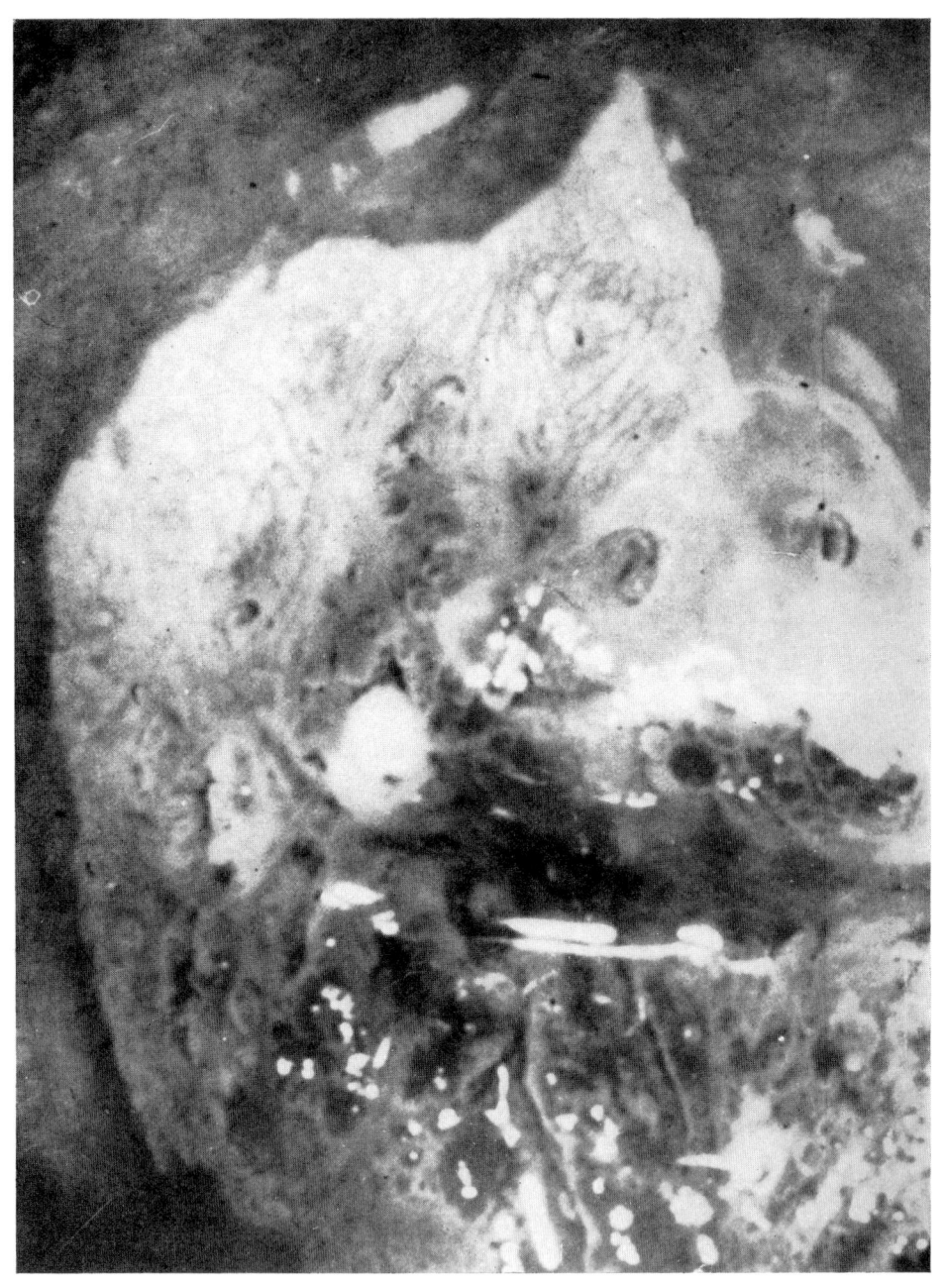

Figure 71. Adolescent cervix: promiscuous. A mature atypical transformation zone with white epithelium and faint vascular markings is present over a large portion of the anterior lip of the cervix. The cervical canal is below the centre of the colpophotograph.

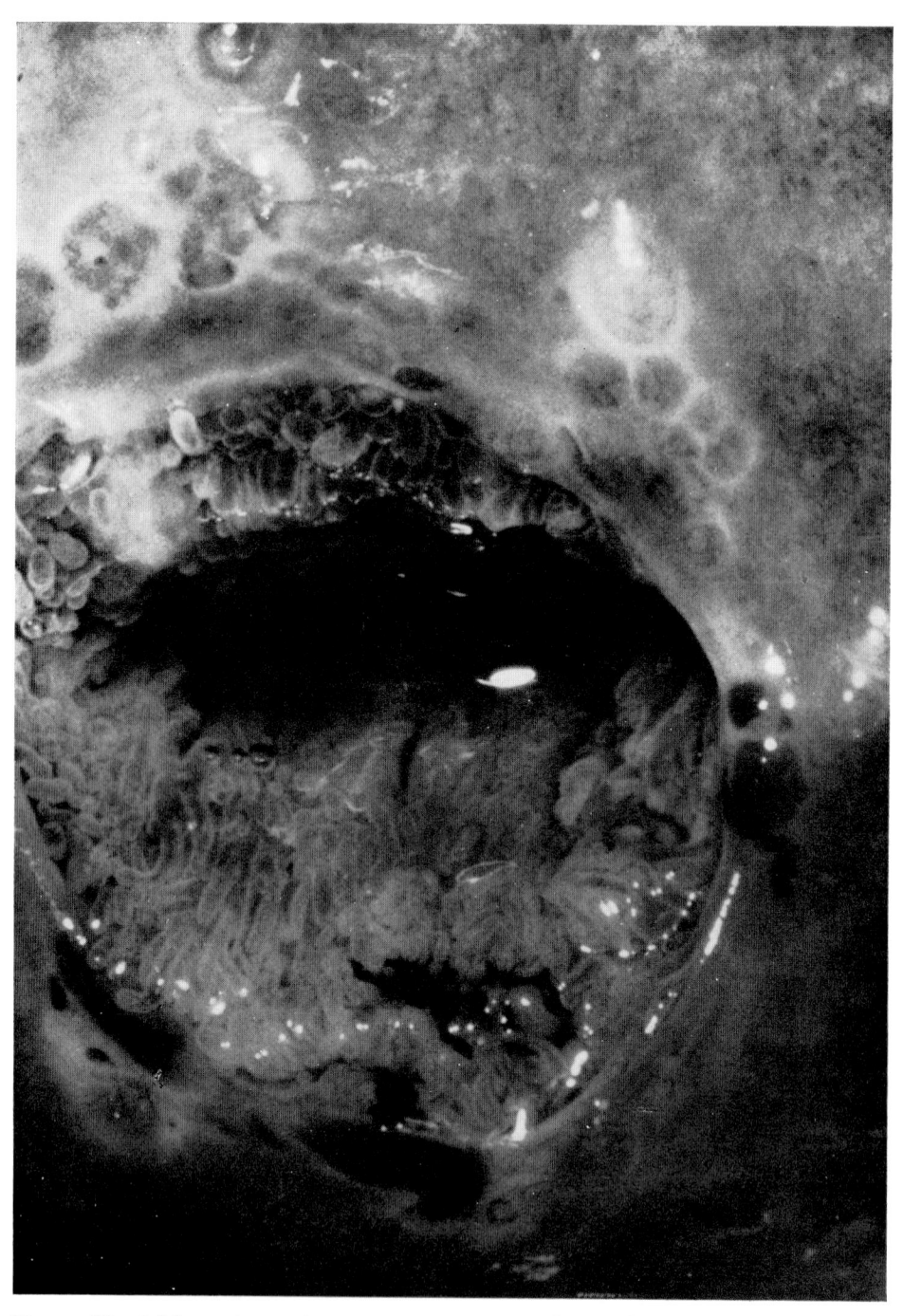

Figure 72. Adolescent cervix: promiscuous. Typical transformation zone, showing mainly mature metaplastic epithelium with gland openings at the periphery of columnar epithelium seen within the cervical canal. This colpophotograph is representative of those girls in the promiscuous group whose cervices are not atypical. The appearances are similar to those of physiological metaplasia in other groups.

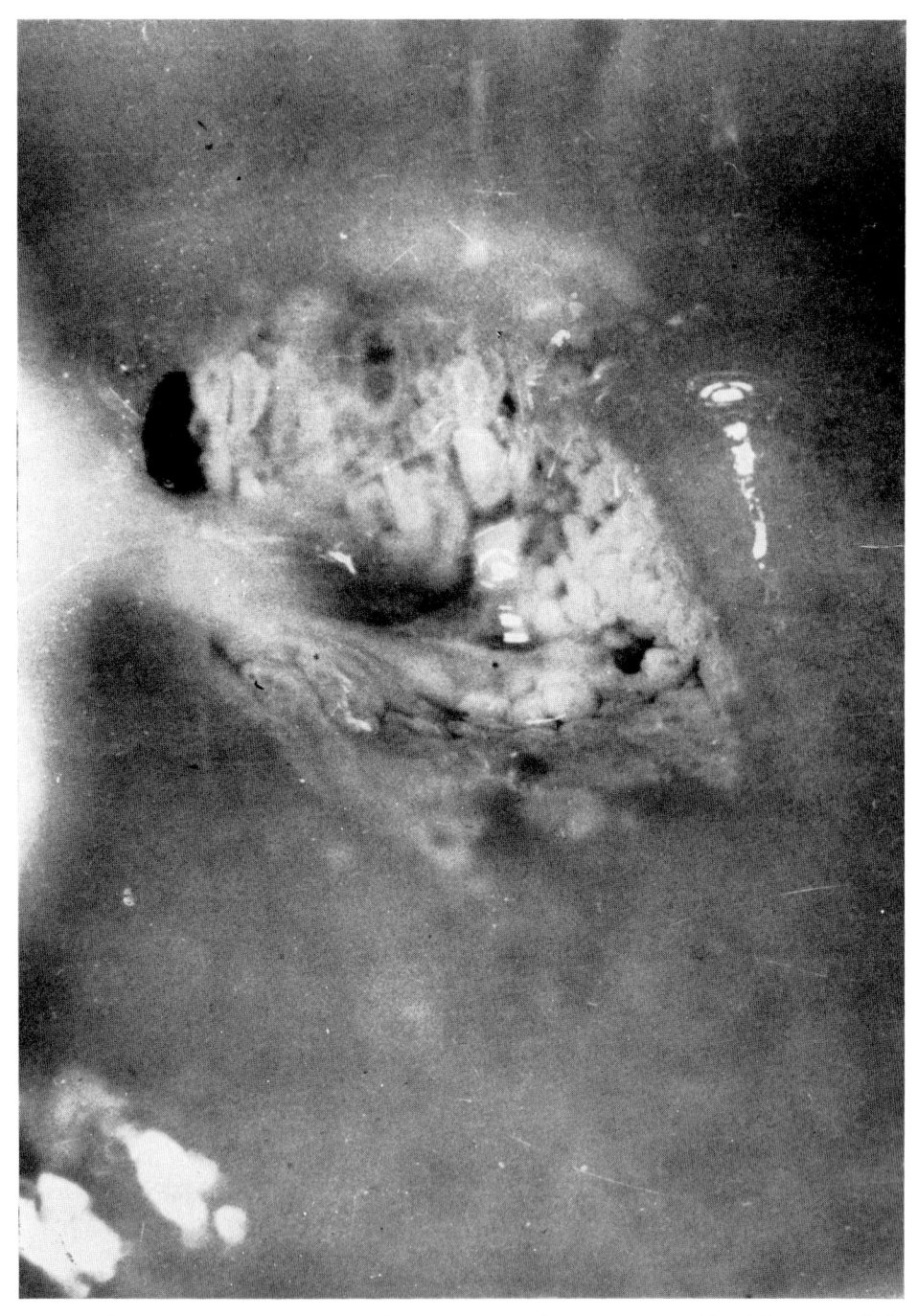

Figure 73. Cervix at sixteen weeks pregnancy in a primigravida. There is slight eversion, and villi representing the columnar epithelium are readily seen on the ectocervix.

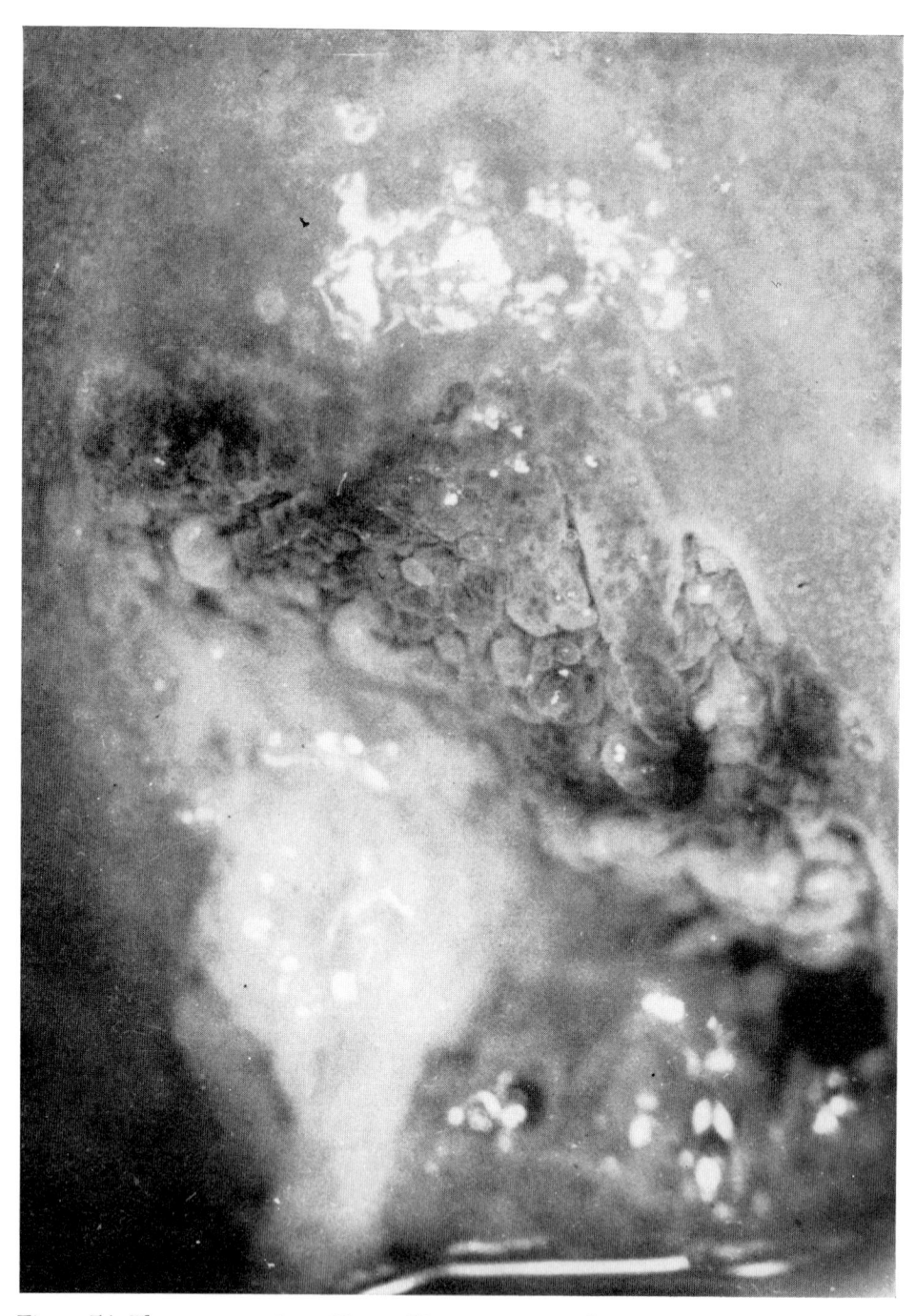

Figure 74. The same cervix as Figure 73 at twenty weeks pregnancy. There is further eversion. Early metaplasia has started on the anterior lip proximal to the original squamocolumnar junction and is best seen in the centre of the picture. Much white mucus is present to the left side of the cervical os.

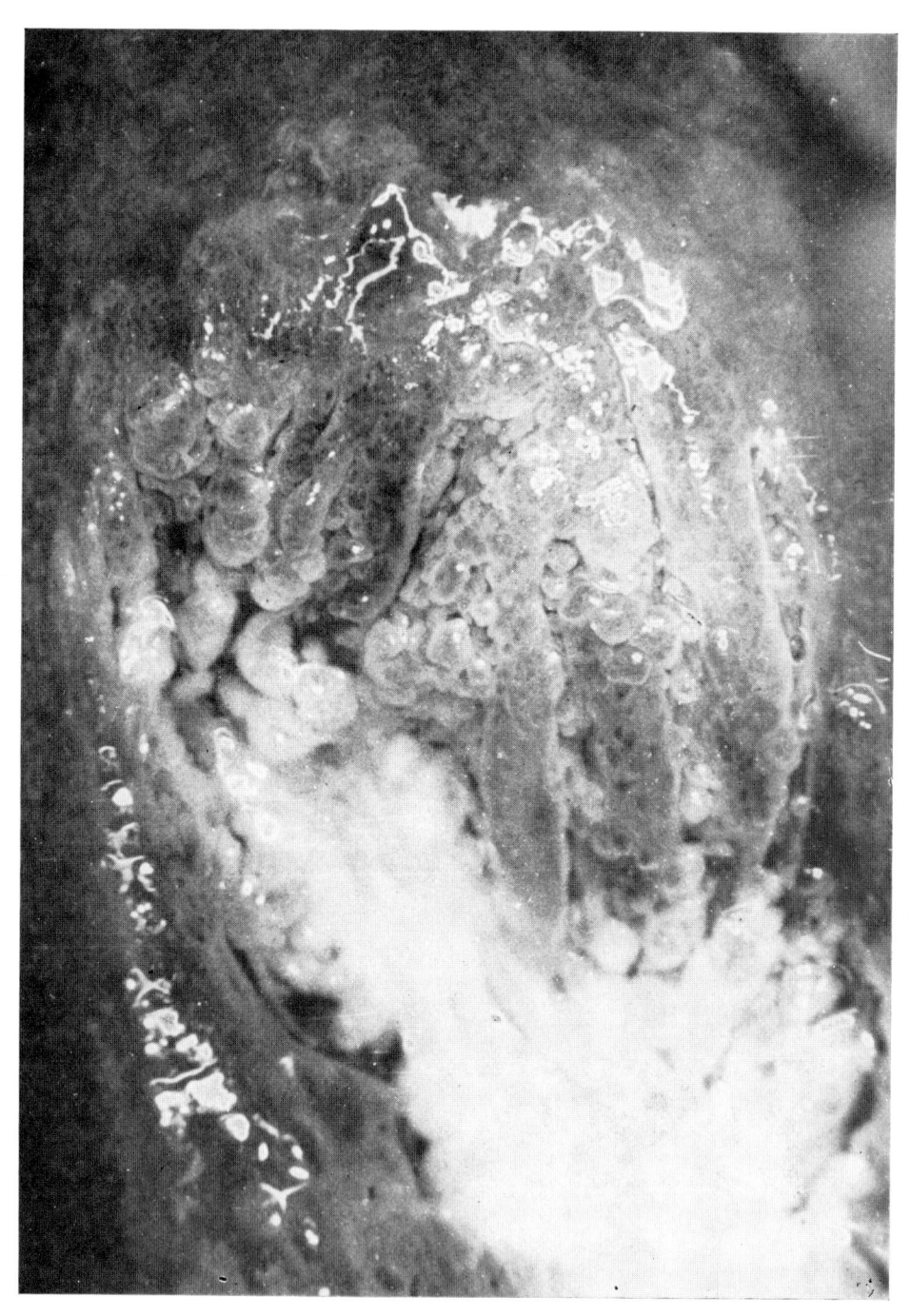

Figure 75. The same cervix as Figures 73 and 74 at twenty-four weeks pregnancy. Further eversion of canal epithelium has occurred. Several ridges of fused villi can now be seen to be covered by smoother metaplastic squamous epithelium. Columnar epithelium can be seen elsewhere.

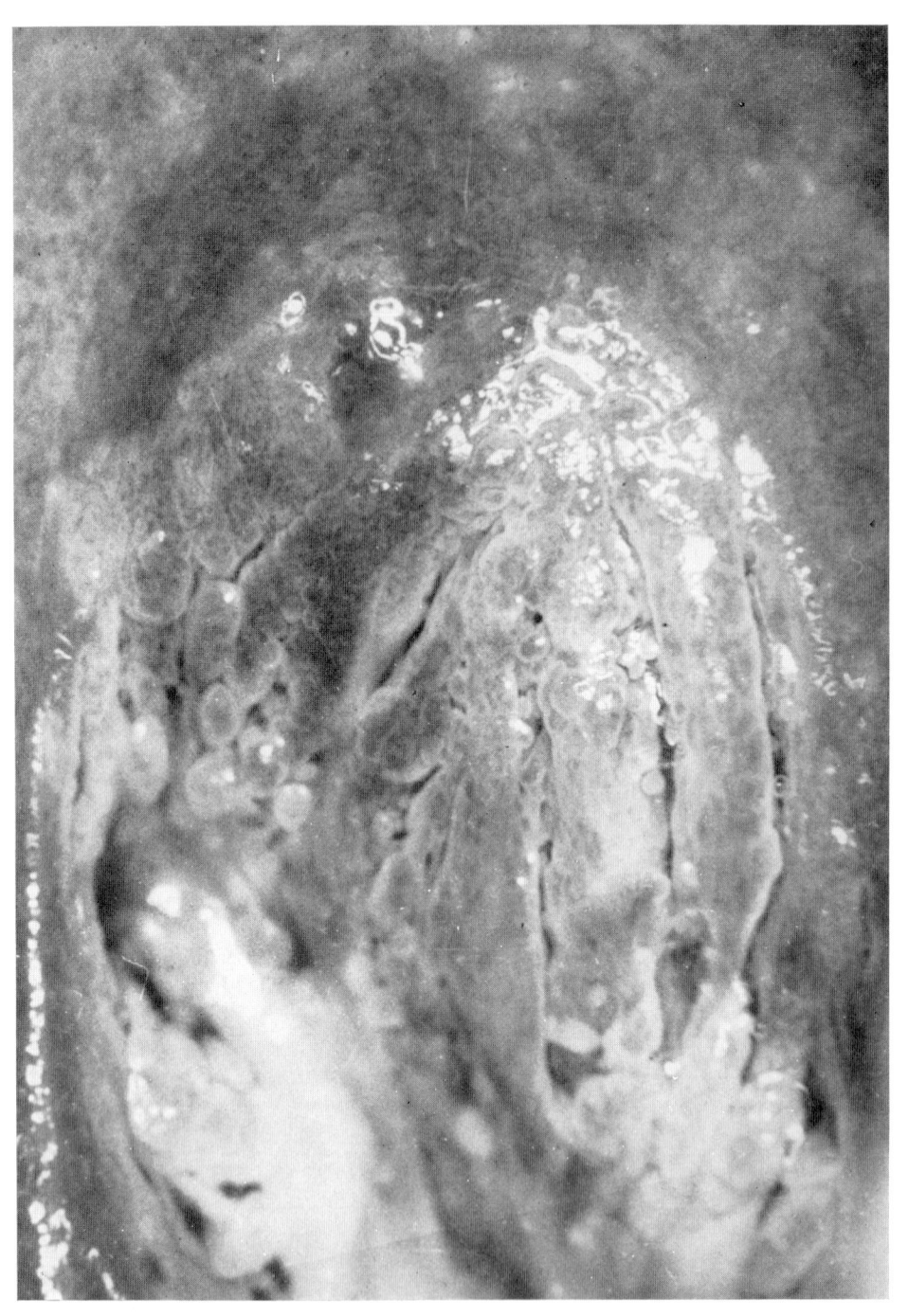

Figure 76. The same cervix as Figures 73 to 75 at thirty-nine weeks pregnancy. There is no further eversion but greater maturity of the metaplastic squamous epithelium as shown by the increasing opacity covering the ridges.

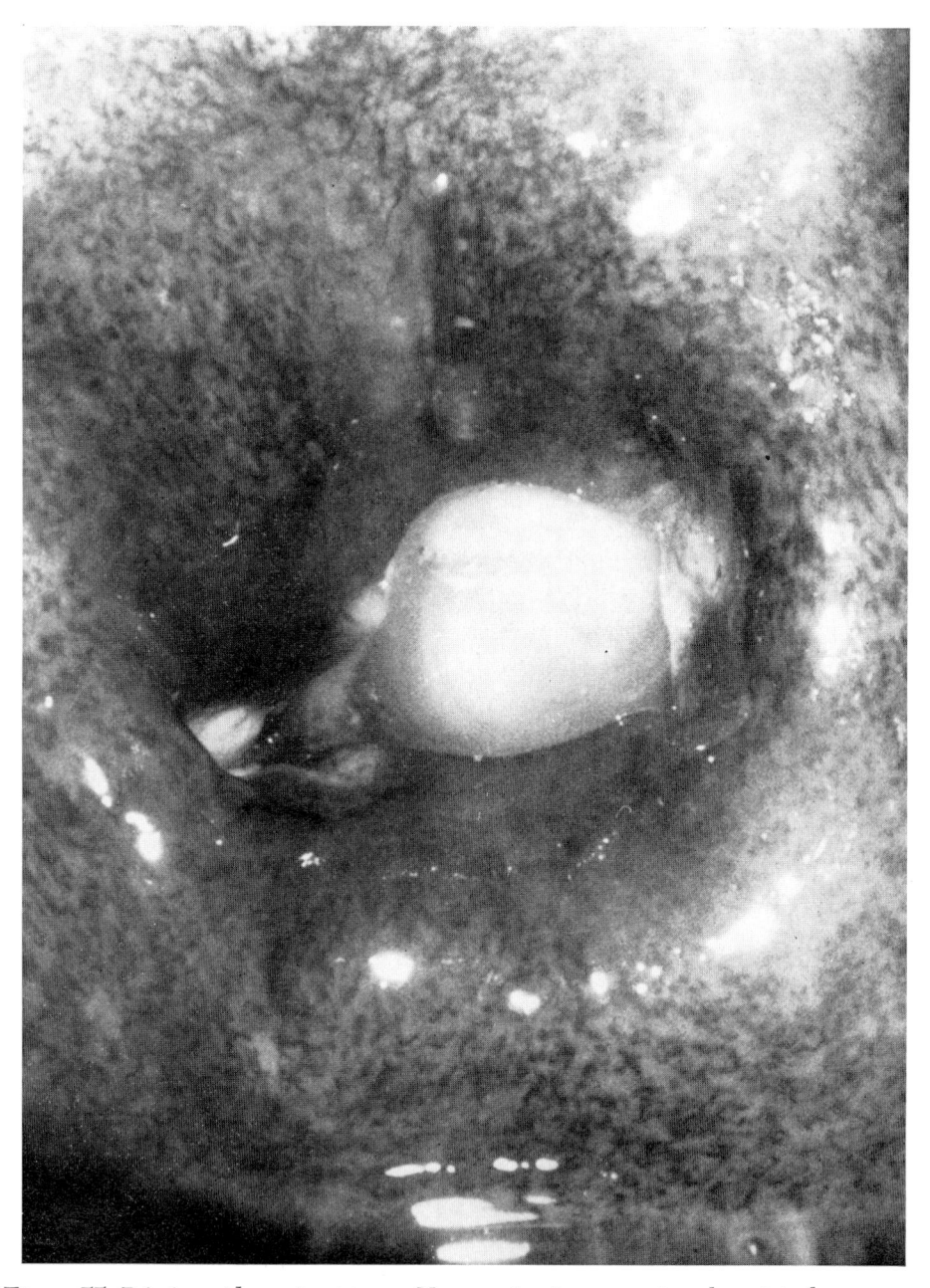

Figure 77. Primigravid cervix at term. No eversion is apparent, only original squamous epithelium being seen. A plug of mucus obscures the canal.

ed a slow succession of metaplastic change. During this change usually involving only increasing maturity, the appearance gradually tends towards the type of mature typical transformation zone seen in the middle and later decades of life (p. 209). Likewise, many atypical appearances beginning at an earlier stage share this inactivity (p. 432). Second, no case of dynamic phase was seen during this era, except during pregnancy. Third, in no subject was there evidence of the "to-and-fro" movement of the epithelial types, columnar and squamous, a concept which still figures prominently in traditional literature. This now historic view is disproven and should be discarded. There is no reason to believe that metaplasia is other than a permanent change.

The Postmenopausal Years

Widely held views that after the menopause the transformation zone undergoes reversion into the endocervical canal have not been confirmed in the studies. Many subjects exhibited ectocervical columnar and metaplastic epithelia, the presence of which casts doubt on this traditional view. However, it may well be that a degree of postmenopausal reversion occurs in some cases. Until adequate numbers of women are followed through and after the menopause, the frequency of reversion will remain undetermined. We have formed an impression that time and metaplasia cause a gradual decrement in the extent of the original columnar epithelium. There results an apparent contraction of the epithelial elements most evident when the atrophy of the menopause accelerates the change.

After the menopause, the colposcopic picture becomes lacklustre, surface features are reduced in size, and the terminal vasculature is virtually closed down. To confuse the picture further, the thin squamous epithelia are subject to trauma and frequently display petechial haemorrhages of traumatic origin or a background of bacterial vaginocervicitis, which makes identification of specific epithelia difficult (Fig. 33).

An additional problem encountered in the postmenopausal group is the gradual reduction in size and lack of elasticity which renders examination of the canal difficult. This reason may underlie the undoubted difficulty of a comprehensive colposcopic survey and subsequent interpretation in many women in this age group. The number of unsatisfactory colposcopic findings (p. 179) increases significantly.

Oestrogen administration restores the colposcopic appearances to much the same prominence as occurred premenopausally (Fig. 78). It then becomes apparent that the cervical epithelia display well into the sixth, seventh, and even eighth decades of life characteristics that have been merely subdued by hormone deprivation.

In the case of atypical metaplasia, this possible reversion has practical implications, in that the tissue at risk may be lost from colposcopic vision.

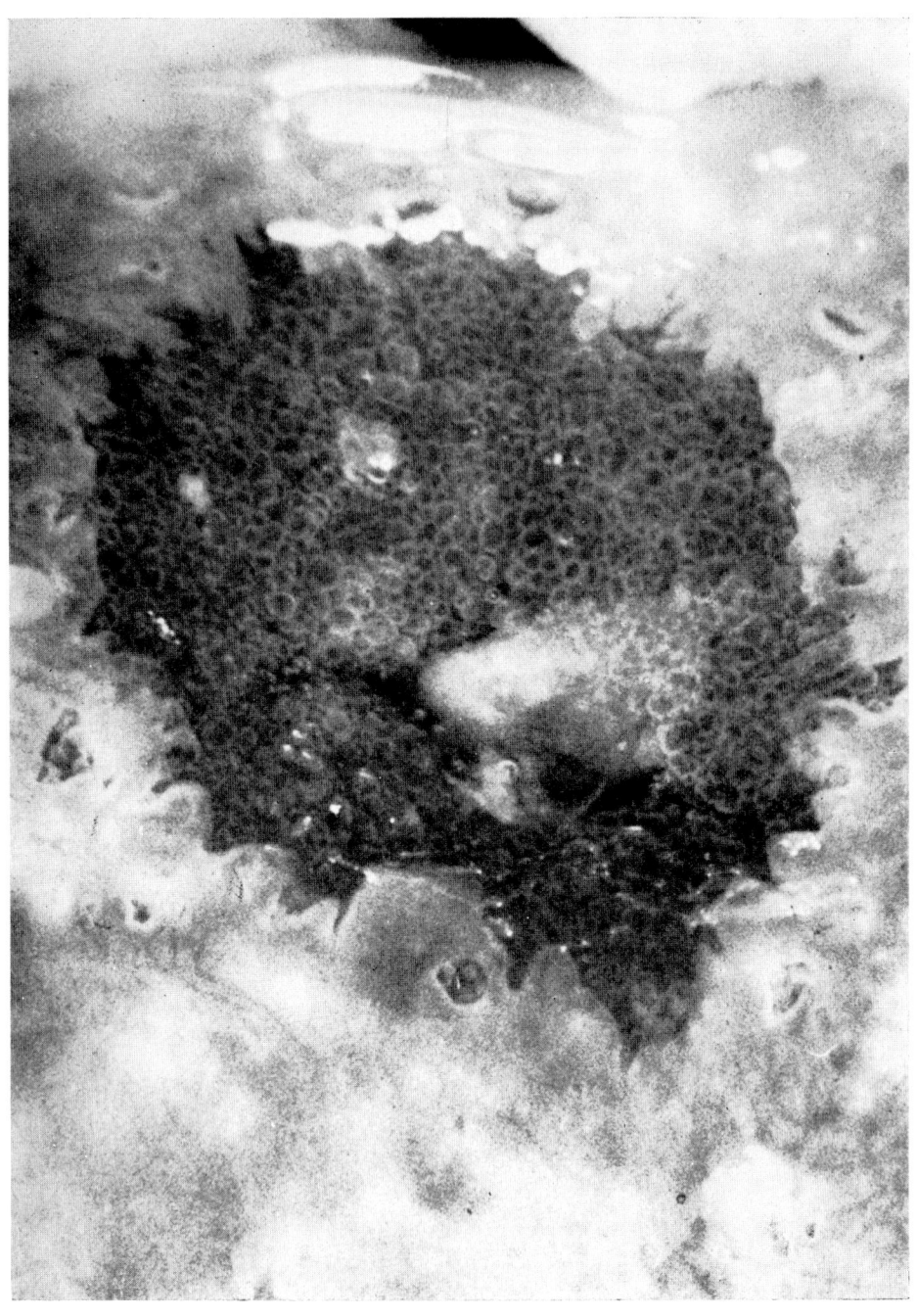

Figure 78. Cervix of nullipara, aged sixty years. Vaginal oestrogen administered for two weeks. The lacklustre, small size, and obliteration of the terminal vasculature, features of the postmenopausal cervix, have been replaced by premenopausal appearances. Such a restoration indicates that basic patterns of cervical epithelia do not necessarily disappear by recession into the cervical canal.

THE CONTRACEPTIVE PILL AND METAPLASIA

It has been suggested that ingestion of oral contraceptives might significantly evoke dynamic metaplasia and influence the natural history of squamous metaplasia. Several authors have suggested that specific alteration in the morphology of the cervix can be attributed to the effects of the oral contraceptive pill, especially the development of the so-called erosion.

We have not specifically investigated the proposition but have nevertheless observed many subjects using oral contraception for the first time and over lengthy periods and have had the opportunity frequently to record the appearances before and after the start of medication. Our comments are based on a comparison of the appearances with subjects who have not used the preparation. The extreme variability of cervical morphology makes valid comparison difficult.

It is our impression that the use of sequential preparations providing a high dose of oestrogen results in a secretory response, causing hypertrophy of the cervix and its glandular structures (Fig. 79). It is possible that some eversion of the lower endocervical canal occurs in some of these subjects, especially in those whose columnar epithelium is extensive and complicated. A degree of metaplasia might then result. No impression has been gained that the combined oral contraceptive preparations significantly alter the morphological and dynamic characteristics of the epithelia other than to increase the production of mucus. Some preparations seem to induce the shade of blue in the original squamous epithelium that is seen in some patients in early pregnancy. No characteristic of metaplasia is apparently affected by use of these preparations.

There is no evidence of an increased incidence of atypical metaplasia in women using oral contraception.

METAPLASIA AND CARCINOGENESIS

The natural history of cervical squamous cancer is summarised in Figure 80. The simplicity of the scheme testifies to the value of previous colposcopic research in permitting a clear overall concept of events of obvious clinical value. At the same time, the scheme is of great academic moment for its heuristic value in elucidating further study of carcinogenesis. Our teaching experience dictates that some amplification of such a scheme is often sought by clinicians in assuaging a thirst for more knowledge on the vexatious problem of carcinogenesis both on the cervix and elsewhere. Parallels do exist with the well-known subdivisions of carcinogenesis in experimental animals into *initiation* and *promotion*.

Initiation represents the hit by the carcinogens on its target cells, in this case, those of early metaplasia. In this clinic, the role of sperm has been under active investigations for fifteen years, particularly its deoxyribo-

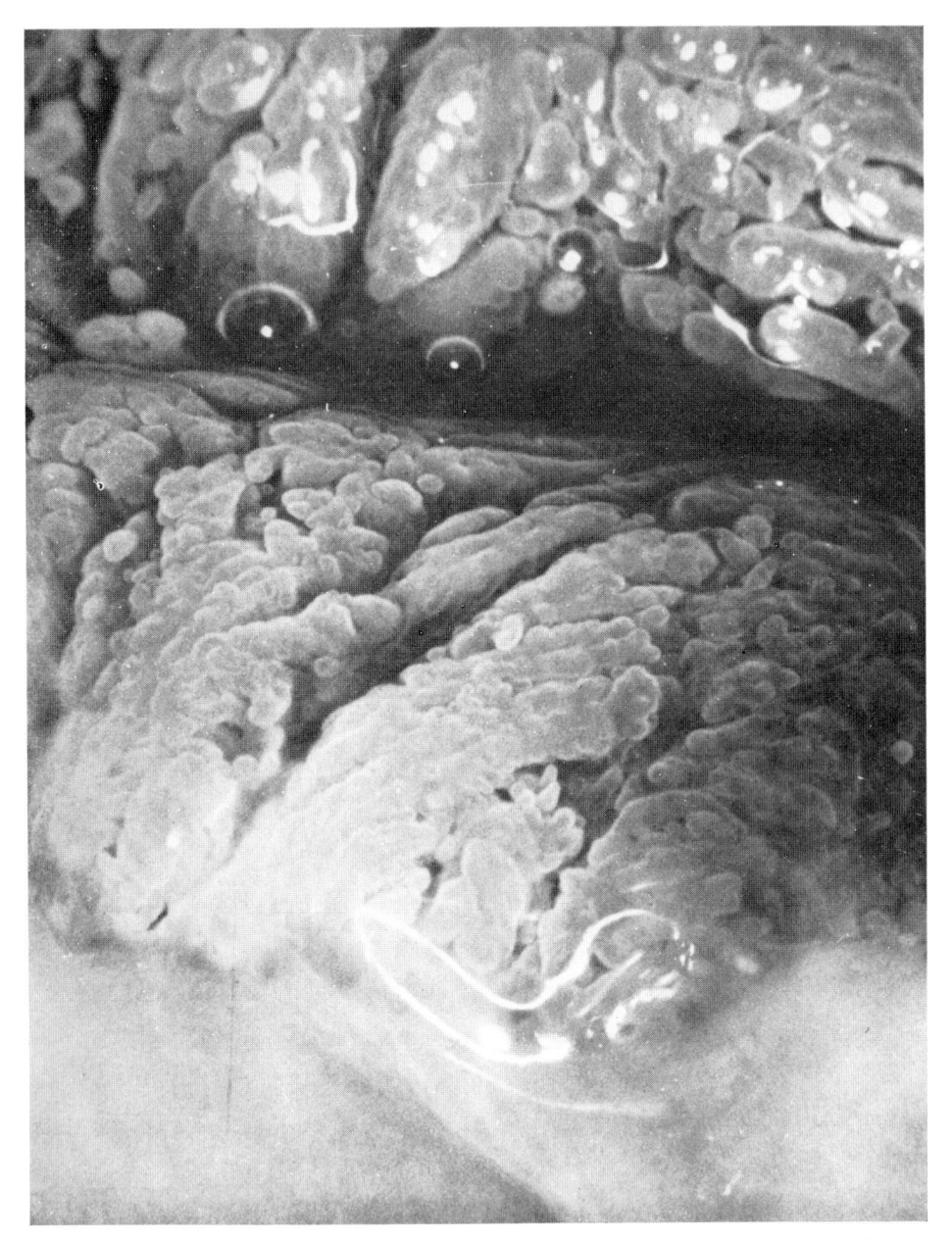

Figure 79. Cervix, effect of sequential contraceptive pill. Hypertrophy of the columnar epithelium is seen, with the deep clefts being filled and distended by clear mucus.

nucleic acid (DNA) component. Recently, we had more compelling reasons for an interest in a protein connected with the DNA content, sperm histones (Coppleson and Reid, 1975, Reid and Coppleson, 1976). A recent school in the United States has, however, rekindled an interest in the DNA

NATURAL HISTORY OF SQUAMOUS CARCINOMA OF CERVIX

*INITIATION**

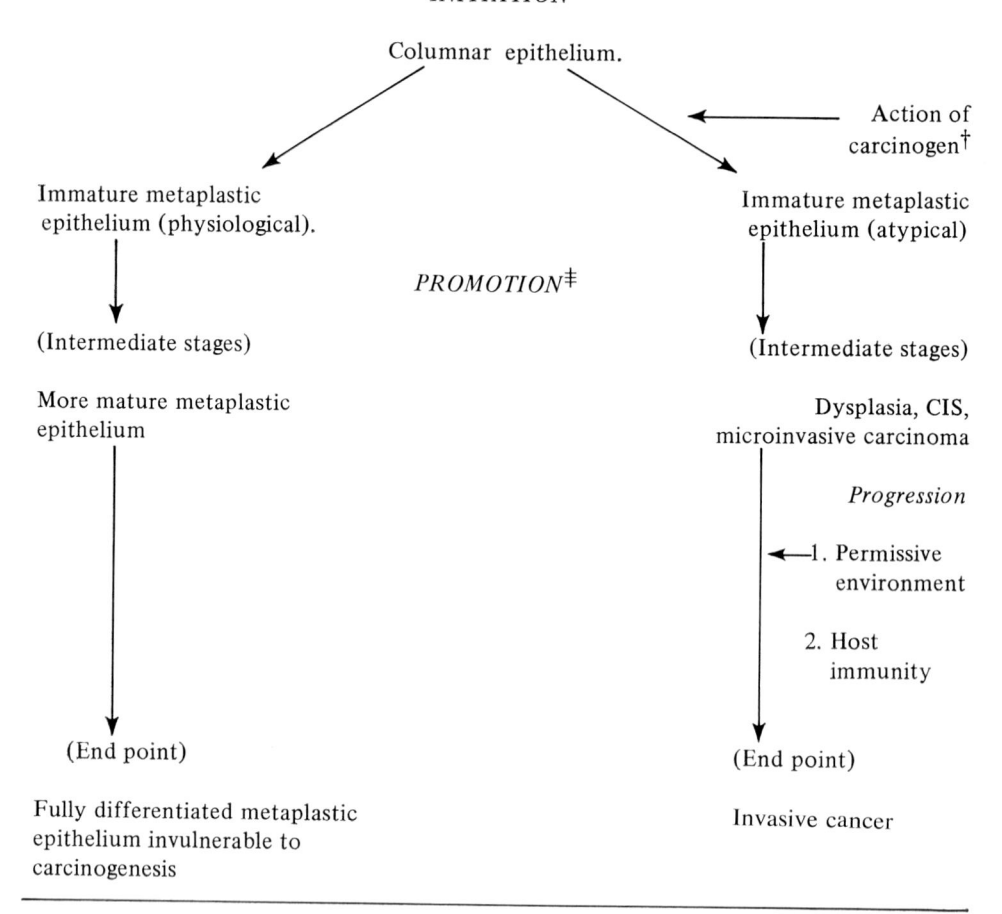

Columnar epithelium.

Action of carcinogen[†]

Immature metaplastic epithelium (physiological).

Immature metaplastic epithelium (atypical)

PROMOTION[‡]

(Intermediate stages)

(Intermediate stages)

More mature metaplastic epithelium

Dysplasia, CIS, microinvasive carcinoma

Progression

1. Permissive environment

2. Host immunity

(End point)

(End point)

Fully differentiated metaplastic epithelium invulnerable to carcinogenesis

Invasive cancer

---

*Initiation. The "hit" by the carcinogen.
[†]The carcinogen is transmitted by coitus.
[‡]Arrest may occur at any of the early or intermediate (physiological or atypical) stages, for months, years, or a lifetime.

Figure 80

content by highly refined biological research (Bendich, Borenfreund, and Sternberg, 1974). Other very active research groups in the United States promote the virus of herpes genitalis in the same role. In any event, the onset of the disease is universally regarded as venereal.

Initiation in the metaplastic cell is followed by a promotion phase in which intermediate stages occur. These are recognisable histologically as dysplasia, carcinoma in situ, and so forth and may be the site in the life history of its arrest for variable periods up to a lifetime. For presently obscure reasons, equally obscure promoting agents may carry the initiated cell through its various intermediates to the stage of clinically invasive cancer. Under active study at present are the promotional roles of steroids, blood and nerve supply, pH, and the status of immune mechanisms. Whatever our present ignorance, progress in the elimination of these manifest obscurities will be both quickened and enlightened by the labours of the colposcopist working in conjunction with the basic sciences team.

Chapter 5

THE TISSUE BASIS OF COLPOSCOPIC APPEARANCES: INTERRELATIONSHIP WITH HISTOLOGY

GENERAL CONSIDERATIONS

THE HISTOLOGIST is conventionally the final arbiter on questions concerning the nature of epithelial changes: benign, premalignant, and malignant. However, certain information concerning such changes is not available to him in the majority of circumstances. It is this information, including topographical characteristics of epithelial surfaces and minute features of the surface morphology in the living state, which is uniquely obvious to the colposcopist. This additional information, considered with that derived from histology and other sources, allows a far more precise understanding of the origin, nature, and behaviour of the tissue than is possible by the use of histology alone.

Each specific characteristic especially obvious on colposcopic examination reflects a particular aspect of the tissue pattern. These characteristics are termed *prime morphological features* and provide the basis of a scheme utilised in subsequent descriptive chapters on colposcopic appearances. These features are (1) topography (*see* Chap. 3), (2) colour, (3) surface configuration, and (4) angioarchitecture. In the sections relating to abnormal tissues, a further characteristic is added; (5) grading.

Extensive variations observed in the prime morphological features are so numerous they produce in the colposcopic appearances of each cervix a fingerprintlike individuality. Despite this, the various forms of epithelia, normal and abnormal, have appearances almost as characteristic as those seen on histological examination. The fundamental considerations involved in the colposcopic method are illustrated in synoptic form in Figure 81.

Colour

Some characteristics of the epithelium modify the colour arising from the stromal blood vessels. Specific properties such as epithelial height, cell density, cellular differentiation, and keratin production alter the optical response, which is evident in variations of the colour and opacity of the epithelium.

Surface Configuration

The epithelial growth characteristics are displayed not only by colour and vascularity but by a further structural aspect, surface configuration.

Variations in configuration generally reflect embryonic and physiological variations of columnar or original squamous epithelium. Highly significant variations encountered in the major grades of atypical transformation zone reflect growth disorders of the epithelium, especially those accompanying potential neoplastic activity. Ultimately, just as the gross clinically overt cancer may exhibit exophytia, clinically unsuspected degrees of exophytia become overt at magnification.

Angioarchitecture

The principal colposcopic feature almost indiscernible in standard histological sections is the spatial arrangement and specific structure of the surface and subepithelial vascular tree. Generally speaking, the terminal capillary network and to a lesser extent the terminal vessels of the venous tree are clearly visualised. Looped and network capillaries form the basic pattern stemming from deeper, usually branching terminal vessels. Vessels may be sub- or intraepithelial. If they are intraepithelial, a thin stromal coat always persists as the stromal papilla.

Subsequently, the original vascular structures may be modified by the following:
1. Trauma, resulting in destruction of the pattern and replacement with regenerate vascular patterns
2. Metaplasia, which may obliterate original structures or modify them, resulting in the appearance of punctation and mosaic
3. Neoplasia, wherein angiogenesis creates new and bizarre structures, the atypical vessels
4. Alteration resulting from changes related to age or to infection by micro-organisms, both of which are usually reversible.

Important differences occur in the size, shape, calibre, arrangement, course, number, and general disposition of the vasculature. Conspicuous variations in these vascular patterns allows distinction between physiological and pathological areas of cervical epithelium.

Grading

In the systematic description of the atypical transformation zone another feature of the atypical lesion is described, that of grading. This attribute, though subjective, is held by us to be of the utmost importance in practice. Grading refers to degrees of difference which can be observed in the prime morphological features; variations range from minimal to maximal and often demonstrate a relationship with both histological grading and potential for neoplastic progression. We believe that gradings determined colposcopically, while often correlating with histology, are independent of it and that they contribute substantially to the authority of colposcopy asserted elsewhere.

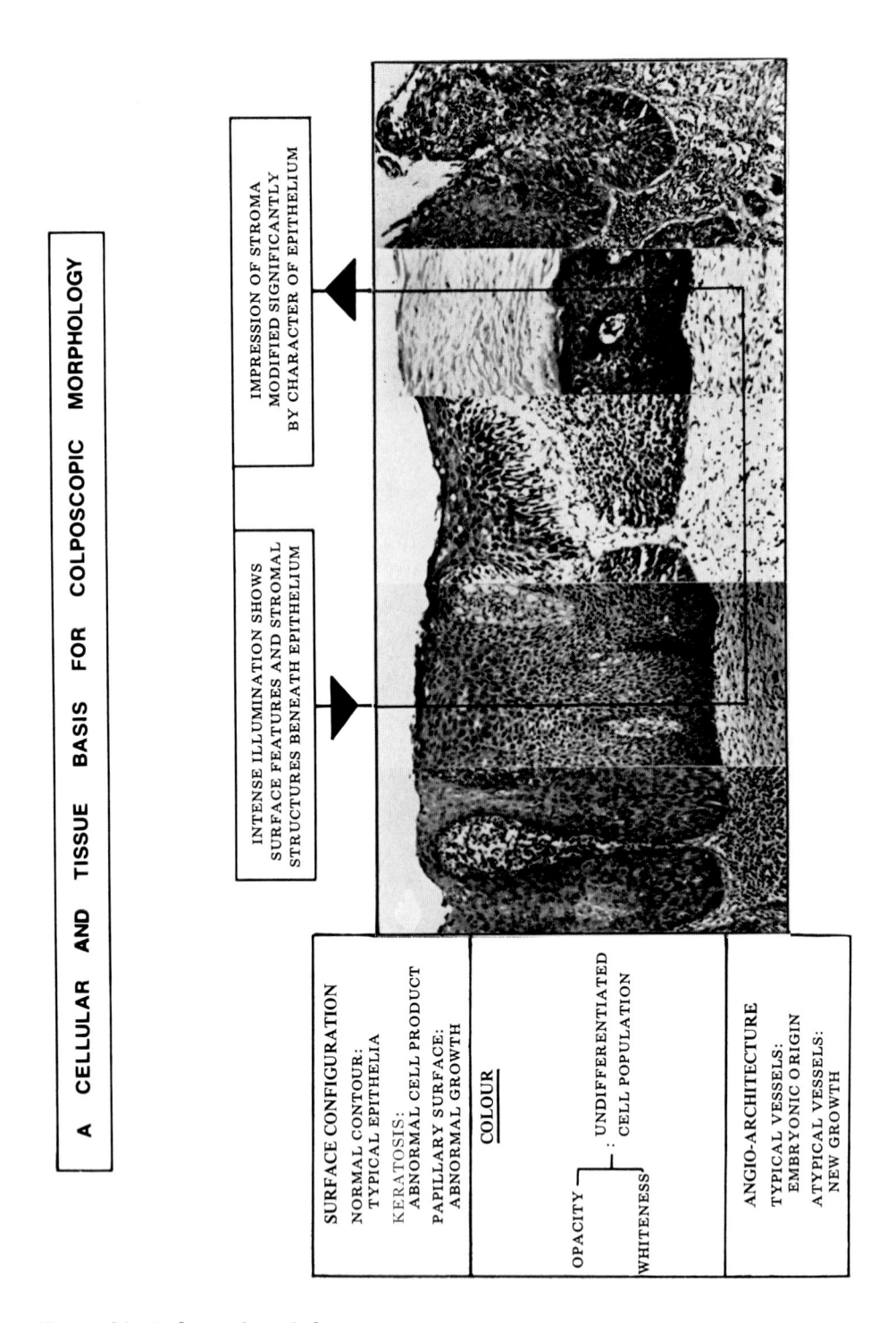

Figure 81. A sheet of epithelium intervenes between the light source and the underlying stroma. The stroma exhibits a diffuse colour whose origins are probably vascular. This colour, observed through the epithelium, is further modified by the cellular character of the epithelium. Opacity is an important reflection of the cell density of the epithelium. Variations in surface configuration are manifest, especially when stereoscopic apparatus is employed. Cellular products such as keratin and mucus may overlie all appearances.

BASIC COLPOSCOPIC AND HISTOLOGICAL CORRELATIONS

Each colposcopic image is the counterpart of a particular tissue pattern. For adequate comprehension of this relationship, certain basic considerations are necessary.

The two principal aspects of the tissue pattern are the epithelium and the terminal vascular arrangements (angioarchitecture) of the related stroma. With most colposcopic prime morphological appearances, satisfactory correlations have followed comparison of colpophotographs with material obtained either from target biopsy or the extirpated cervix and submitted to standard histological preparation. With angioarchitecture, on the other hand, more elaborate methods are required, modifications of the standard tissue preparation. At times, a more refined colpophotographic technique is used.

The impetus of our own angioarchitectural studies has been greatly accelerated by using Kos's (1960, 1962) and Stafl's (1962) alkaline phosphatase technique as a stain for capillaries and viewing these preparations through thick, cleared sections. This enhances the appearance of the various stromal blood vessels, especially capillaries. The convoluted capillary course in the various papillae is especially apparent and provides histological confirmation for the dominating influence of these blood vessels in the colposcopic image. The outlines of blood vessels with this technique are more striking with atypical epithelia than with physiological epithelia. The special technique of colpophotography of Koller (1963) and Kolstad (1964) has also done much to define the importance of the minute structure of terminal blood vessels. An instructive correlation of the Kos-Stafl technique with the special technique for colpophotography appears in an atlas on the subject (Kolstad and Stafl, 1977). Our descriptions are mainly in accord with the original work of these authors, whose elegant pictures provide the most comprehensive study of this basic aspect presently available.

Original Squamous Epithelium

The appearance of original squamous epithelium shows little variation from subject to subject either colposcopically or histologically. The pink, translucent epithelium seen through the colposcope (*see* Fig. 21) is the counterpart of the characteristic fifteen to twenty layers in this stratified and differentiated squamous epithelium (*see* Fig. 8).

Special colposcopic pictures are usually necessary to show looped capillaries (Fig. 82), a network capillary system (Fig. 83), or a combination of both. With alkaline phosphatase studies, the stromal arrangement within which the terminal vasculature ramifies is seen in similar form. It exists either as a flat sheet upon which the epithelium rests, or from it, finger-like papillae project in varying numbers into the epithelium (Fig. 84). In

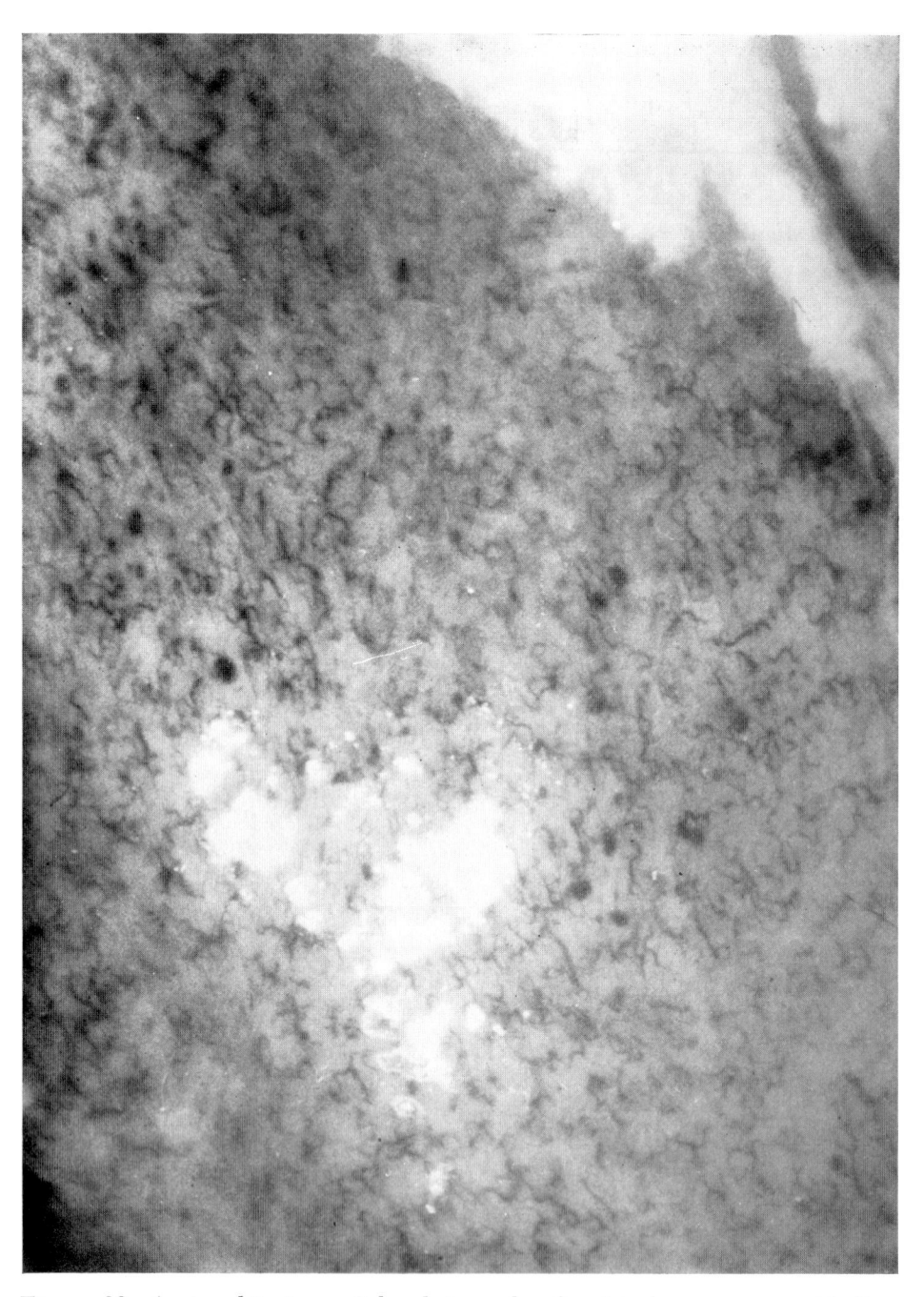

Figure 82. Angioarchitecture. Colpophotograph of original squamous epithelium. Terminal looped capillaries lying within the original squamous epithelium, course mainly tangential to the surface.

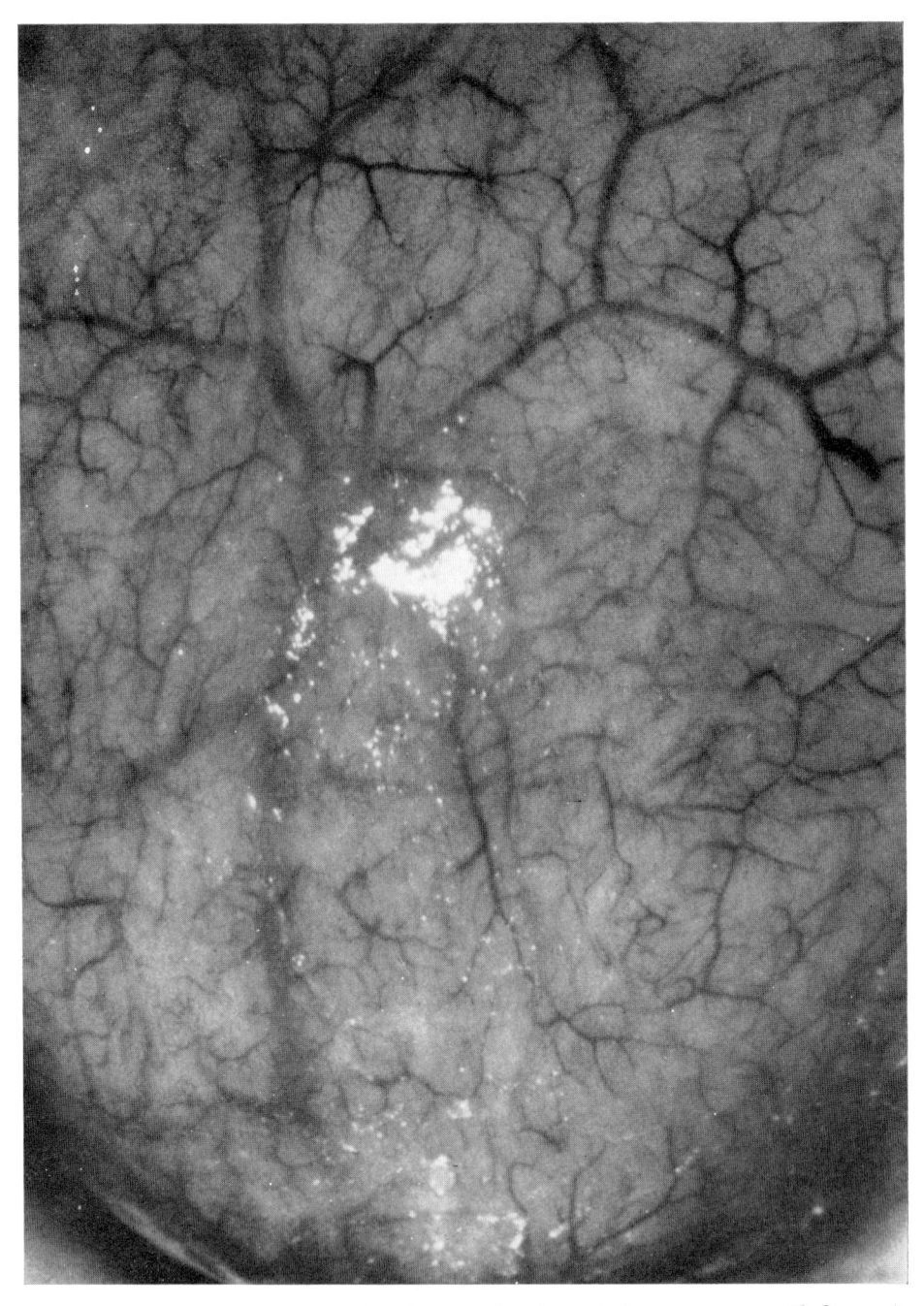

Figure 83. Angioarchitecture. Colpophotograph of original squamous epithelium. An inclusion cyst from within the cervical canal has enlarged sufficiently to underlie the original squamous epithelium, displaying the terminal vessels in usual detail. Large veins within the stroma show orderly branching, and between the finest branches an epithelial capillary network pattern is evident. This network differs from the terminal looped intraepithelial arrangement seen in Figure 82.

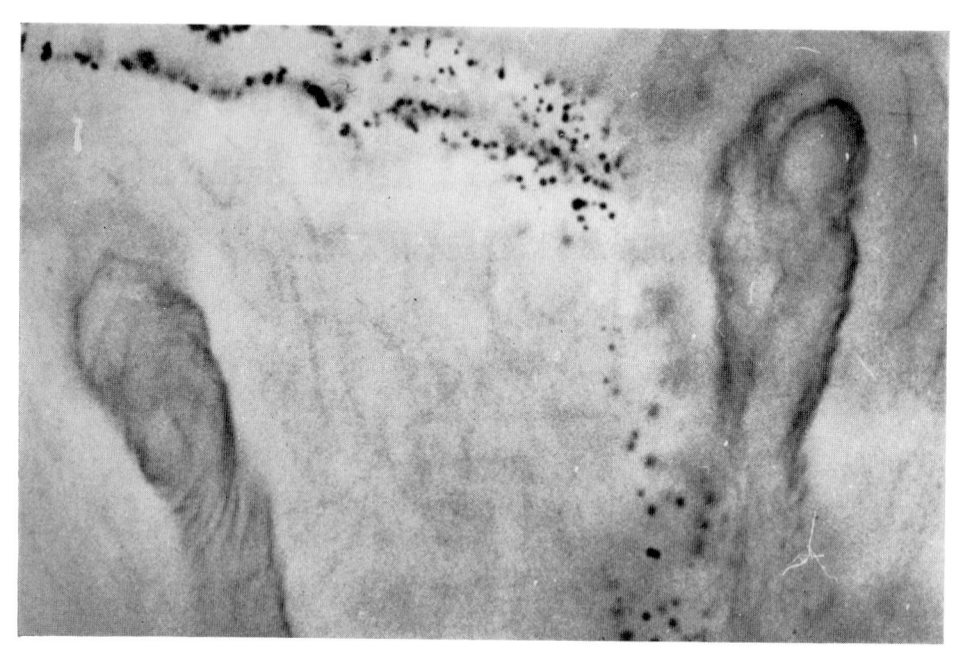

Figure 84. Angioarchitecture. Photomicrograph of original squamous epithelium (angiography using alkaline phosphatase, 125 μ section). Two papillae are shown within the original squamous epithelium containing looped capillaries. The papillae arise from the stroma, which is not visible in the photograph. In the absence of such papillae, the vessels are distributed as a network beneath the epithelium.

the former, a subepithelial network capillary system forms parallel to the surface, whereas in the latter, looped capillaries, usually single, extend for a variable distance towards the surface.

Cervical Columnar Epithelium

The characteristic grapelike appearances of the columnar epithelium seen on colposcopy represent variations in surface contour, which is the essential characteristic of this mucus-secreting component of the cervical epithelia (Fig. 85). This surface configuration of variable pattern is distinctive and allows immediate identification of the epithelium. In histological sections, papillary and villiform excrescences form the counterpart of the surface configuration seen in colposcopy (Fig. 86). A smooth single-layer columnar epithelium overlies the stroma, which produces the surface contours.

Within the subjacent stroma of the columnar epithelium, the vascular arrangements are variable. Beneath the common villous structure, branching vessels can sometimes be seen (Fig. 87). Within the villus itself, looped capillaries of degrees of complexity usually constitute the main vessel structure (Fig. 88). The counterpart of the deep branching vessels and the looped vessels of the villus core are well shown by alkaline phosphatase study (Fig. 89).

When viewed either through the colposcope or with the unaided eye, the rich vascular bed and single-layer transparent epithelium combine to give the tissue its intense red hue.

Typical Transformation Zone

The colposcopic counterpart of the phases and extent of physiological metaplastic epithelium is treated fully in Chapter 8. There are, however, several important tissue arrangements characteristic of the more mature phases of metaplasia which are basic features of the transformation zone and which have colposcopic appearances relevant at this stage. A detailed description of the histological correlation with colposcopic appearances of the dynamic phases of metaplasia has already been given (p. 81).

Within the area bounded by the original squamocolumnar junction, the colour of the metaplastic epithelium is usually different from the original squamous areas (Fig. 90). Histologically, these colour differences in the metaplastic epithelium may be correlated with lesser degrees of differentiation, the appearances of the basal layer of cells, and often the presence of glandular elements of columnar epithelium. In the best circumstances, an oblique line is seen to separate two squamous epithelia of undoubtedly different, though normal appearance (Fig. 91). This is the histological evi-

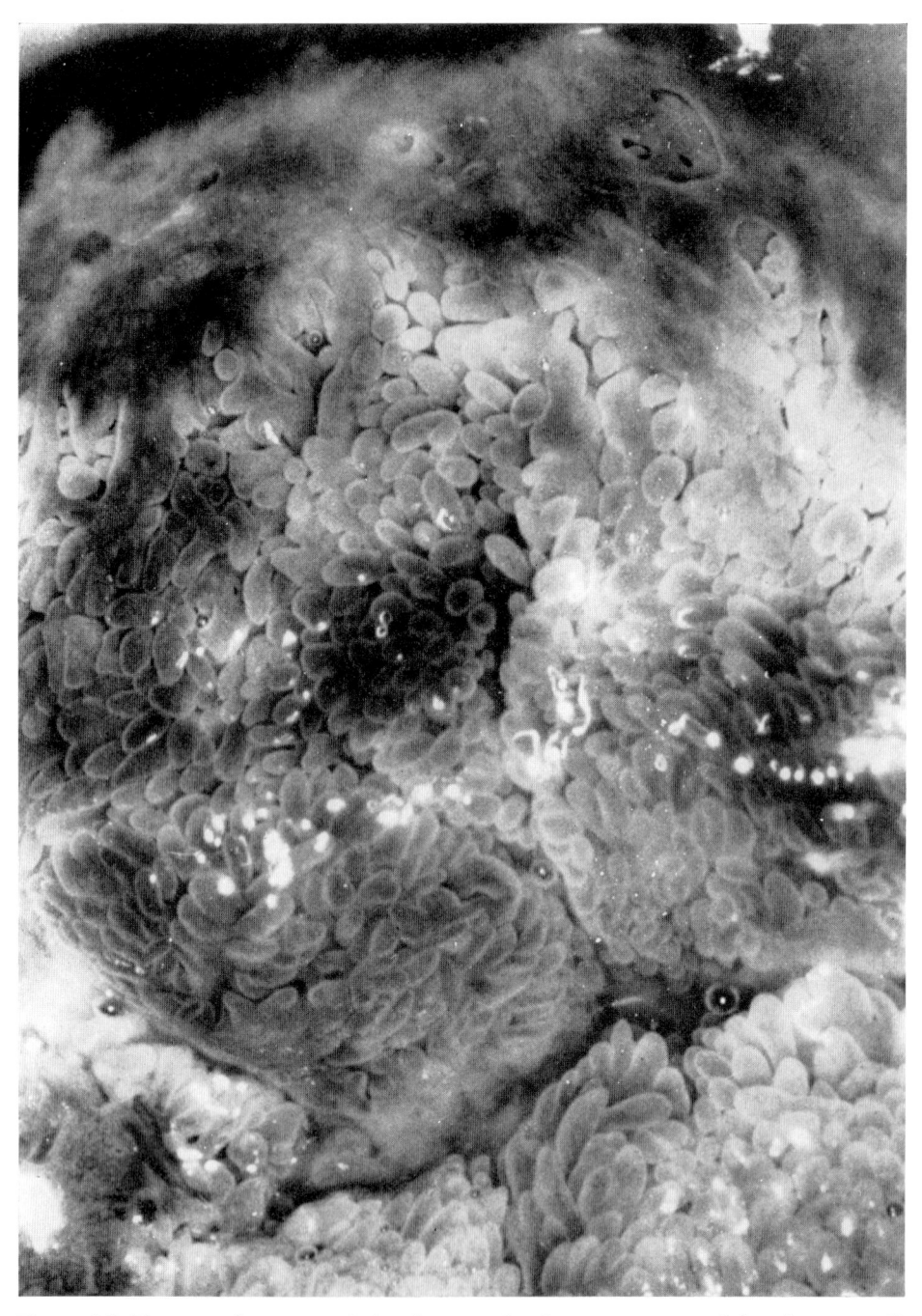

Figure 85. Tissue architecture. Colpophotograph of anterior cervical lip showing villi of varying dimensions. These are always covered by columnar epithelium.

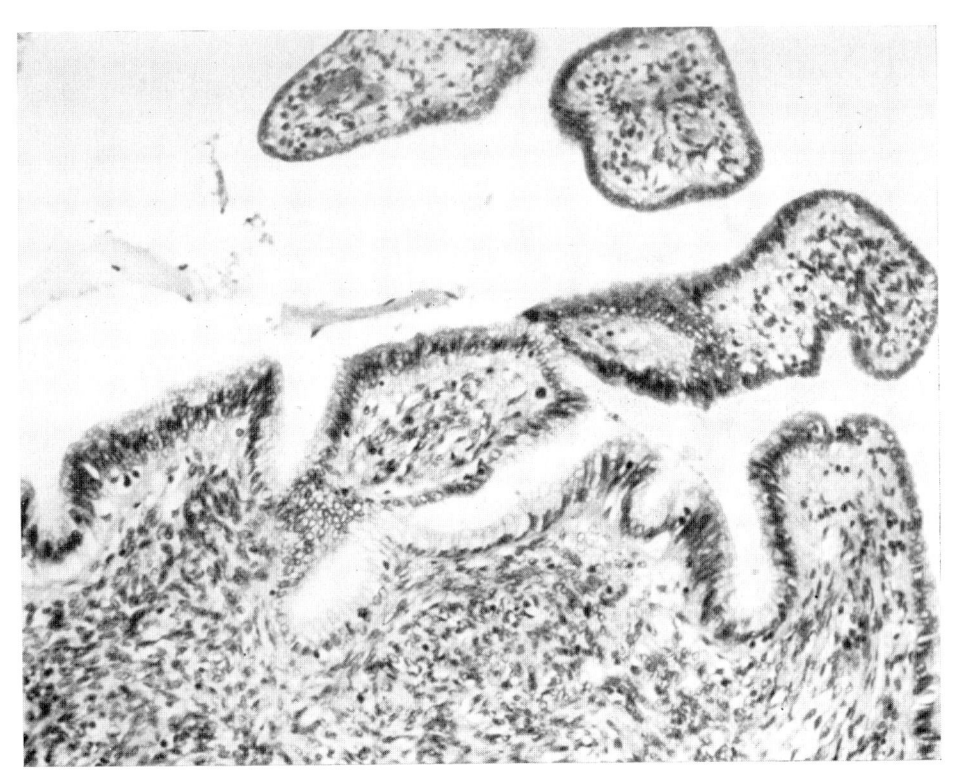

Figure 86. Tissue architecture. Photomicrograph of cervical columnar epithelium. Histological study from area similar to Figure 85. The columnar epithelium is disposed in various forms, including villi and papillae. The elongated nature of the villi is indicated by the three cross sections lying above the surface.

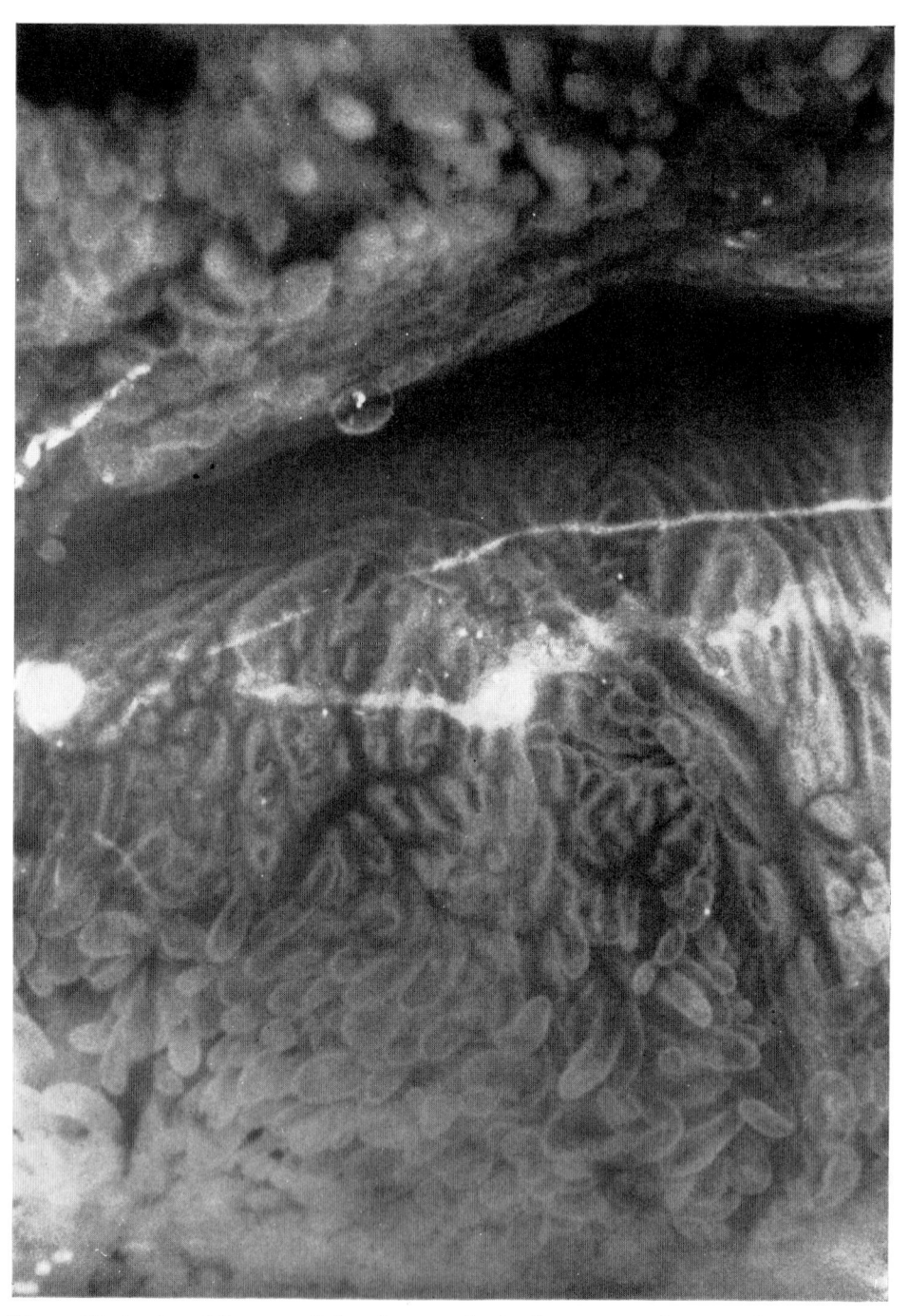

Figure 87. Angioarchitecture. Colpophotograph of villous area indicative of the presence of columnar epithelium at external os. Large branching vessels are visible deep to the epithelium.

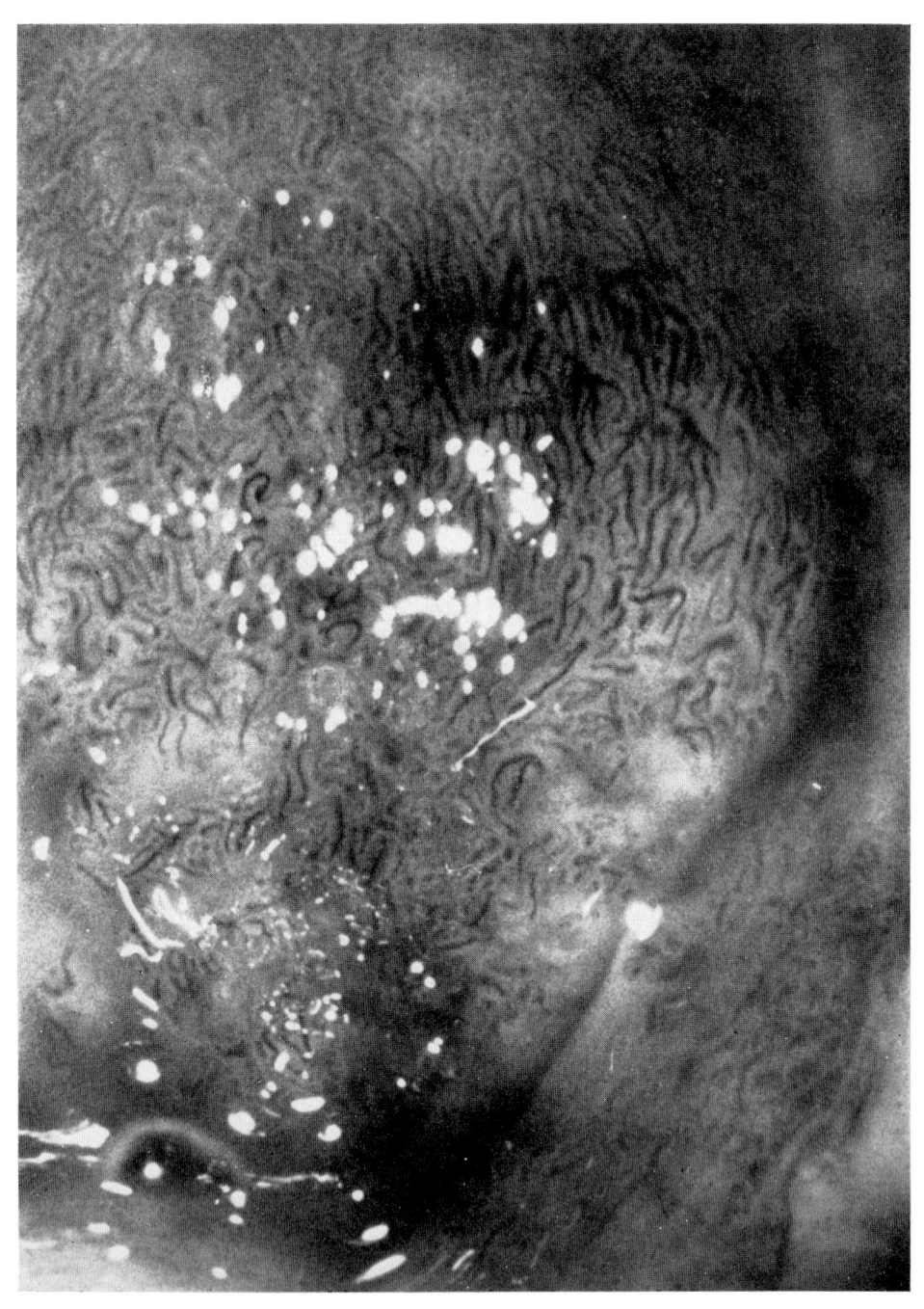

Figure 88. Angioarchitecture. Colpophotograph of an area of villous columnar epithelium. Looped terminal vessels are seen in the stromal cores of the villi, which have arisen from similar branching vessels seen in Figure 87.

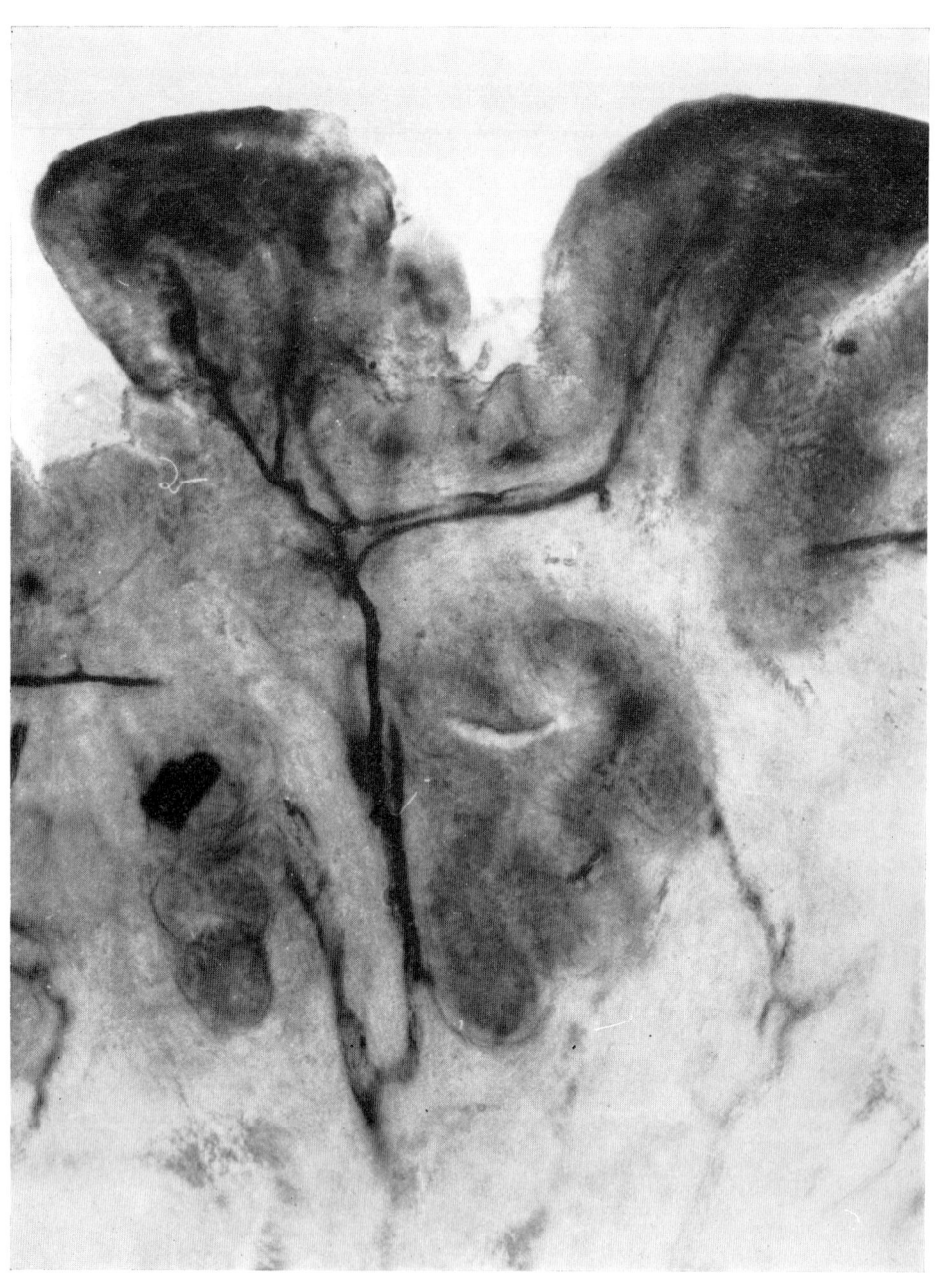

Figure 89. Angioarchitecture. Photomicrograph of cervical columnar epithelium (angiography using alkaline phosphatase, 125 μ section). Two villi contain capillary loops arising from subepithelial branching vessels.

dence of the original squamocolumnar junction, seen so readily on colposcopy. In some specimens, the two epithelia are so nearly identical they are indistinguishable on morphological grounds, except by the presence of associated glandular structures. These glandular structures are readily identified on both colposcopic and histological examination as clefts and cystic structures lying deep to the metaplastic epithelium (Figs. 90 and 92).

The angioarchitecture of the typical transformation zone is one of its more distinctive characteristics. As observed at colposcopy, it represents the persisting arrangement from the original columnar structure, modified by remodelling processes during metaplasia, including compression and sloughing.

The vascular patterns observed are variable and systematized with difficulty. The basic structure is the branching vessel of the subepithelium sometimes seen emerging in newly formed transformation zone (Fig. 93). Its arborization is highly characteristic. In many zones, the pattern is distorted by inclusion cysts (Fig. 94), and the subepithelial vessels are best seen when stretched over large inclusion cysts (Fig. 95). In some women, the typical branching vessels remain as the only reminder of metaplastic activity (Fig. 96).

Atypical Transformation Zone

White Epithelium

In general, an epithelium with increased cellular and nuclear density produces colposcopic appearances of opacity and paleness. This important quality makes whiteness and opacity the distinctive characteristic of both preclinical carcinoma and dysplasia. However, degrees of paleness and opacity may be exhibited by physiological undifferentiated metaplastic epithelia, and thus may be seen by some to be a source of confusion (see Chaps. 9 and 15).

Surface changes do not become apparent until the growth characteristics of the cell populations disturb the usual contour and produce irregularities.

The nature of the terminal vascularization of atypical transformation zone is important, as within it, reactive changes apparently concurrent with the growth disorder can be seen.

Although it is clear that the terminal vasculature of the original columnar epithelium is in some way incorporated into the new atypical squamous epithelium, the precise nature of the process by which these original structures may be modified or how the different vascular patterns in atypical transformation zone develop is not fully understood.

In areas where white epithelium only is seen, a characteristic angio-

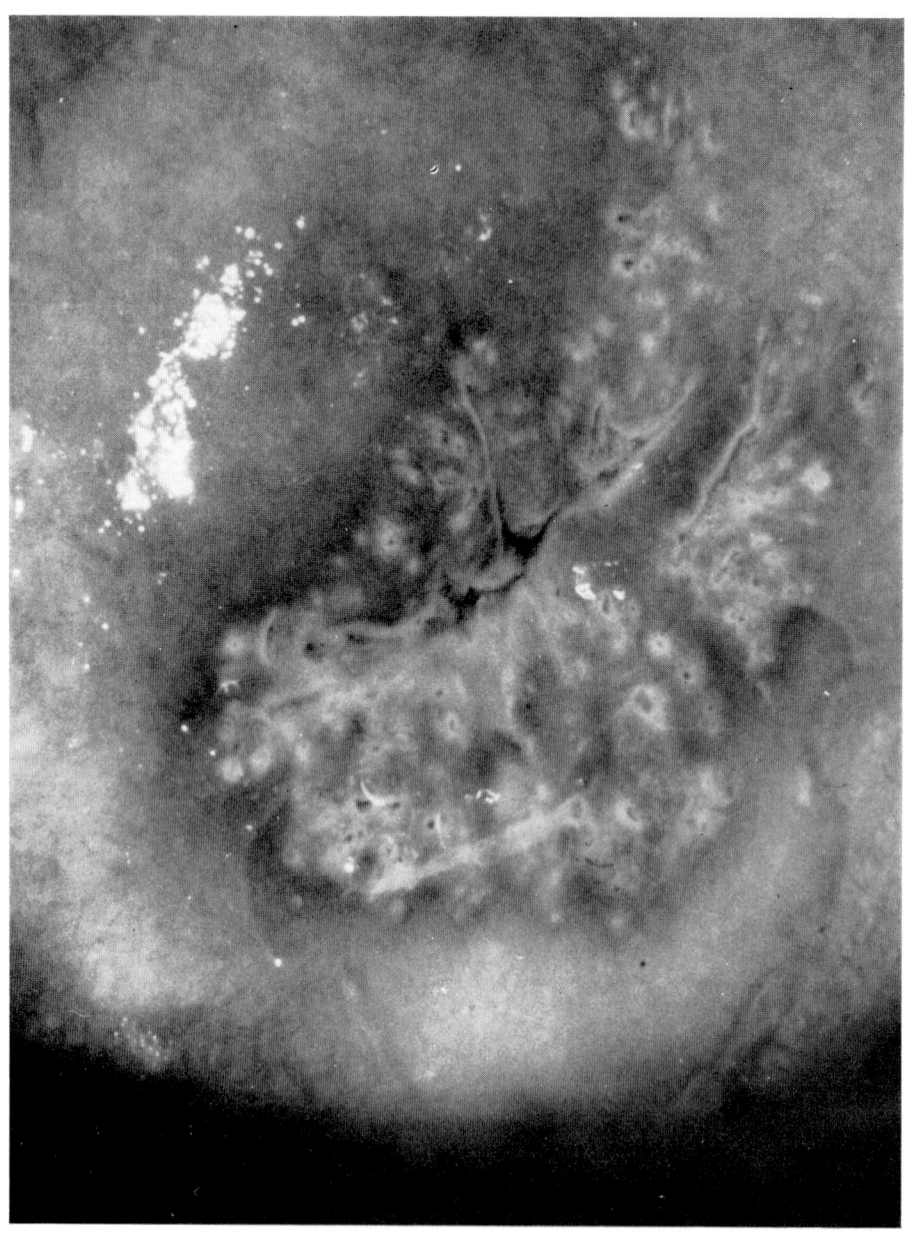

Figure 90. Angioarchitecture. Colpophotograph of typical transformation zone. Within the designated area, the metaplastic and columnar structures may be darker, except where white rings surround gland openings.

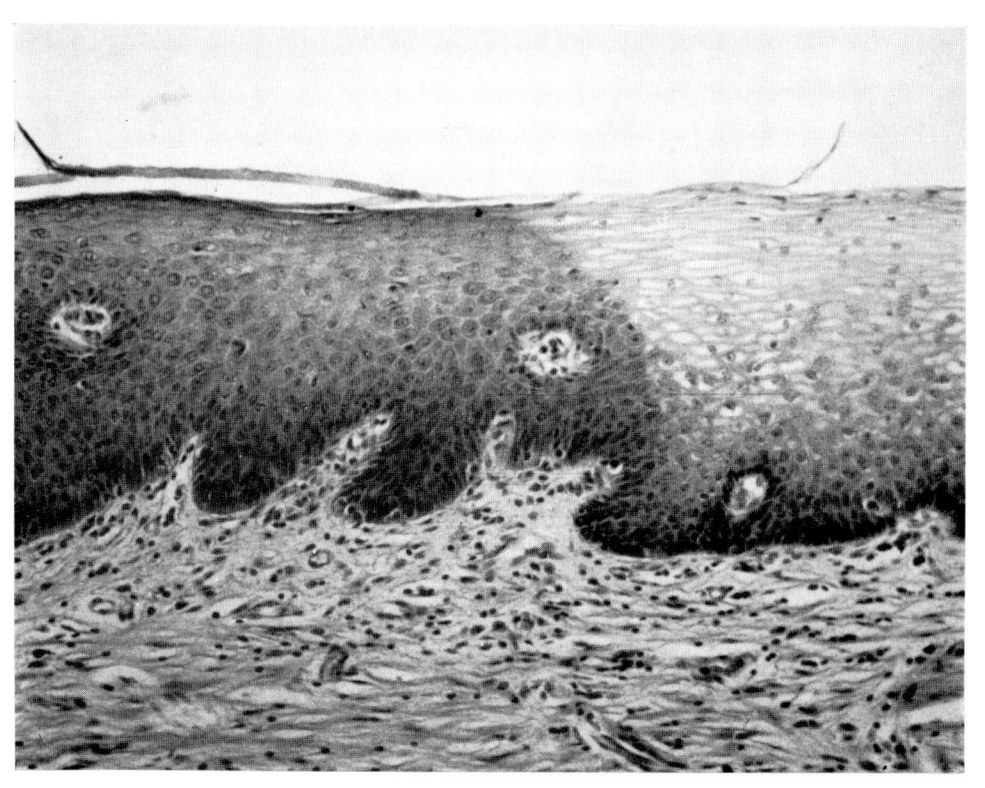

Figure 91. Tissue architecture. Photomicrograph of metaplastic epithelium. Histological section showing oblique line separating two epithelia: original squamous epithelium on the right and metaplastic epithelium on the left.

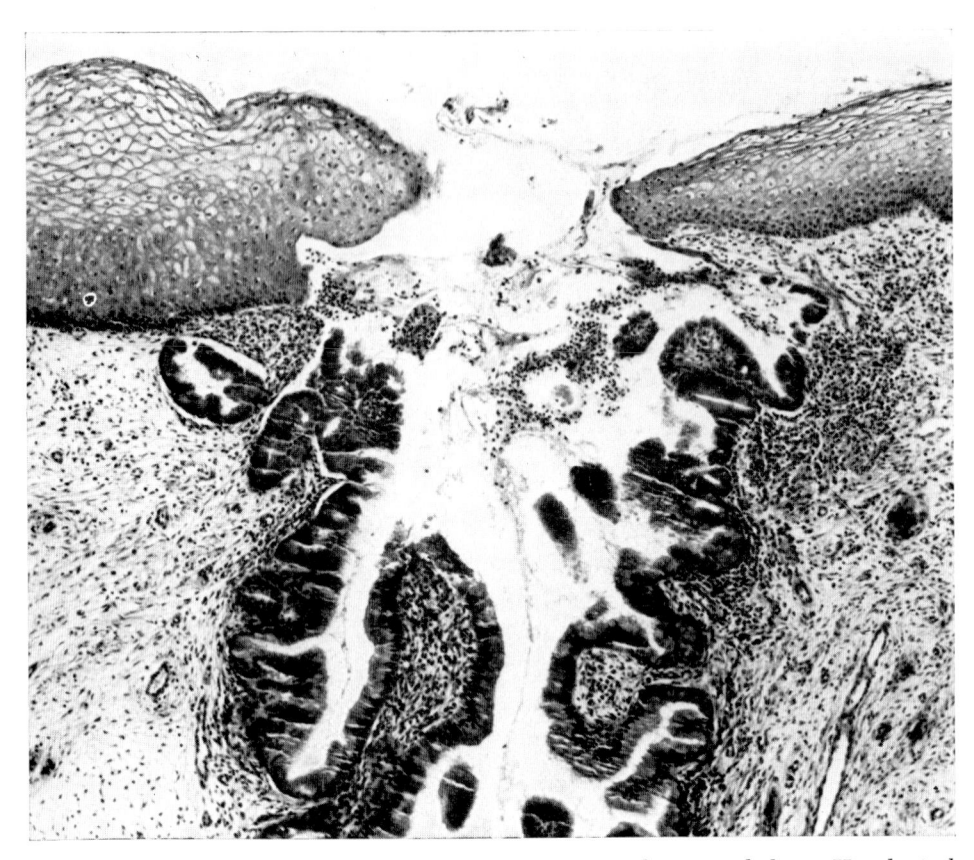

Figure 92. Tissue architecture. Photomicrograph of metaplastic epithelium. Histological section displaying metaplastic epithelium with underlying glandular structures indicating its origin from columnar epithelium.

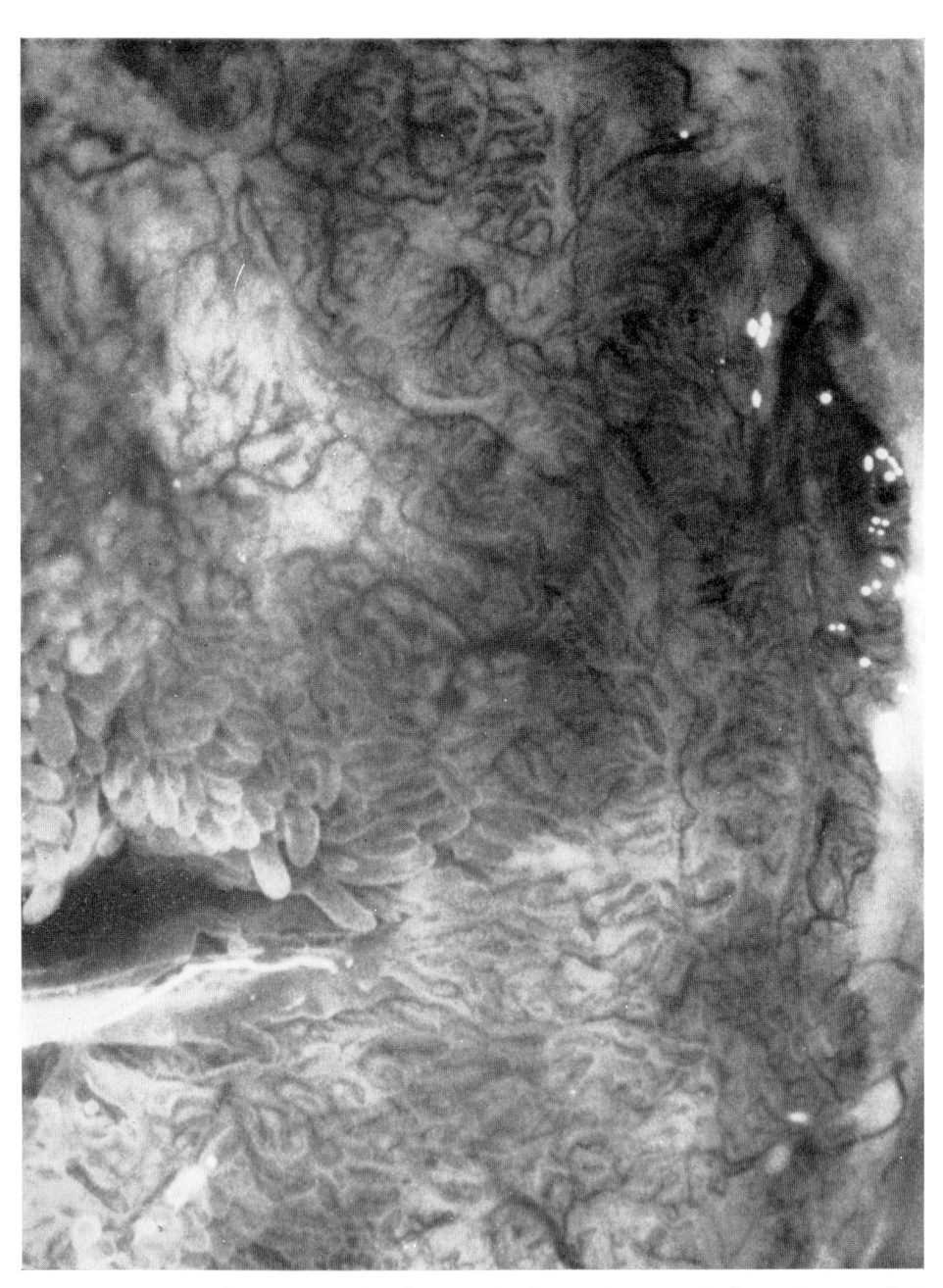

Figure 93. Angioarchitecture. Colpophotograph of metaplastic epithelium. As metaplasia transforms the distal areas of columnar epithelium, the original branching vessels deep to the columnar epithelium become visible in the emerging typical transformation zone.

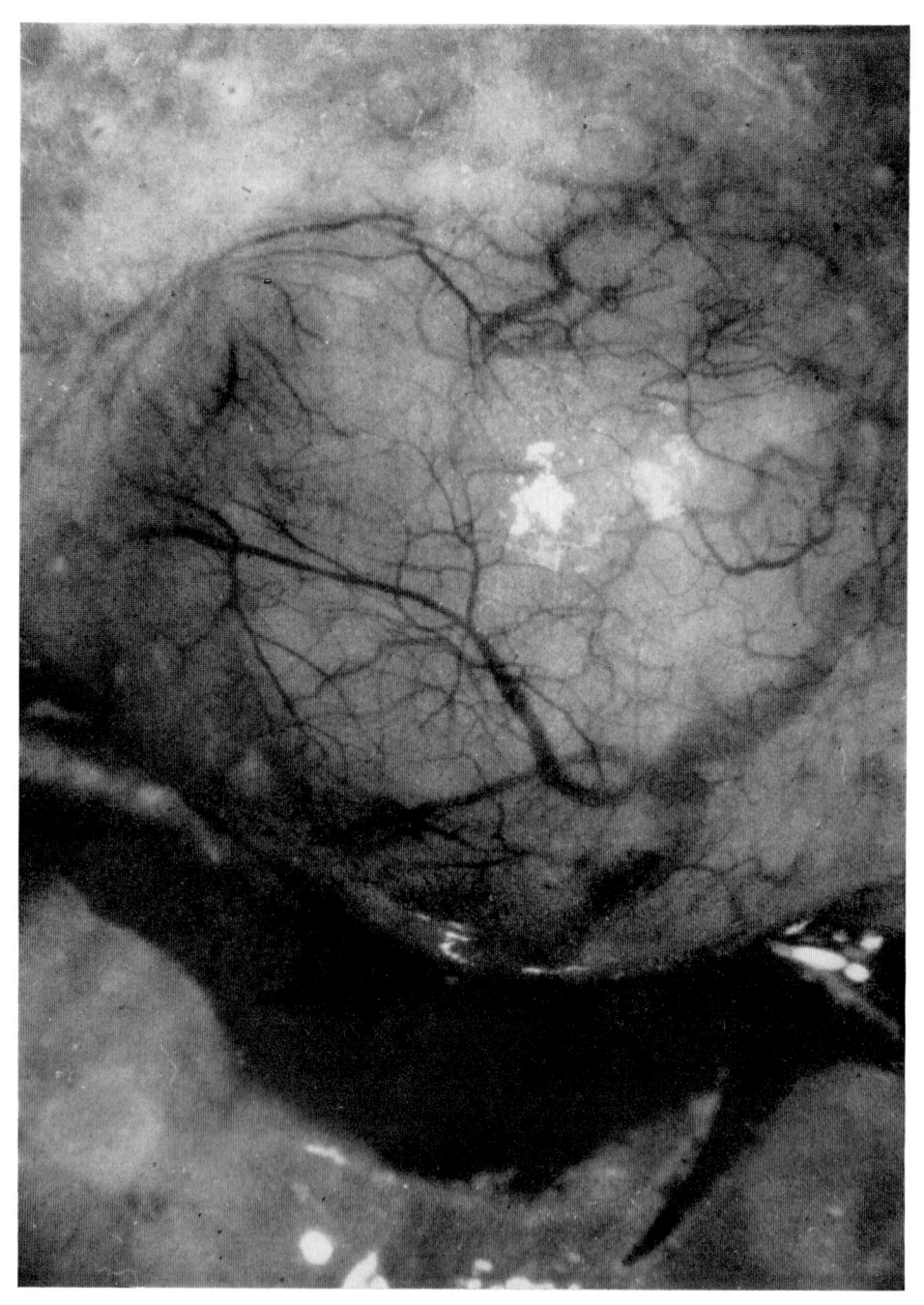

Figure 94. Angioarchitecture. Colpophotograph of metaplastic epithelium. Subepithelial vessels form a complicated branching network over a large nabothian cyst.

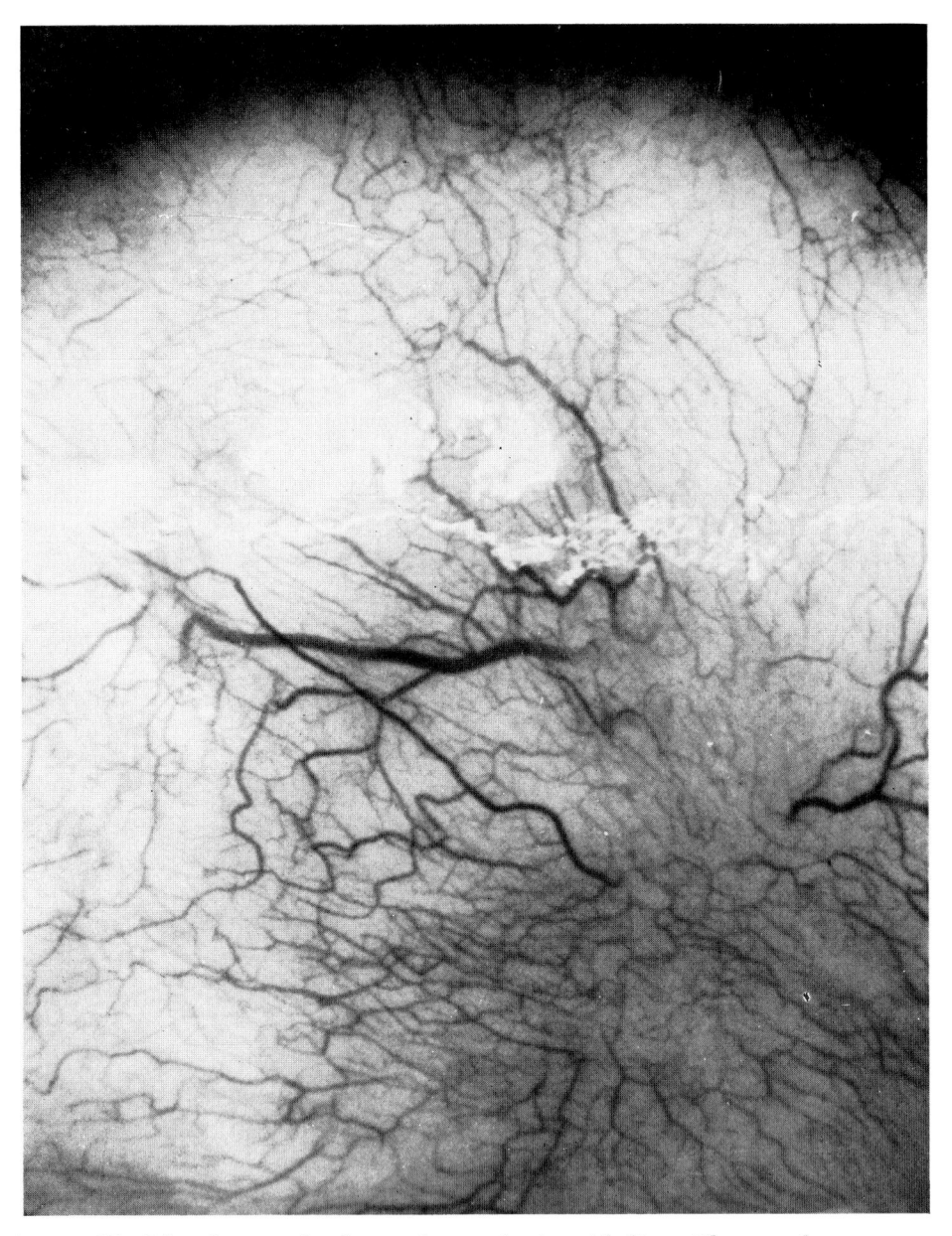

Figure 95. Colpophotograph of normal metaplastic epithelium. The vascular structures are displaced towards the surface and compressed by a cystic formation. The vessels branch regularly and diminish in calibre as they eventually terminate in the capillary network.

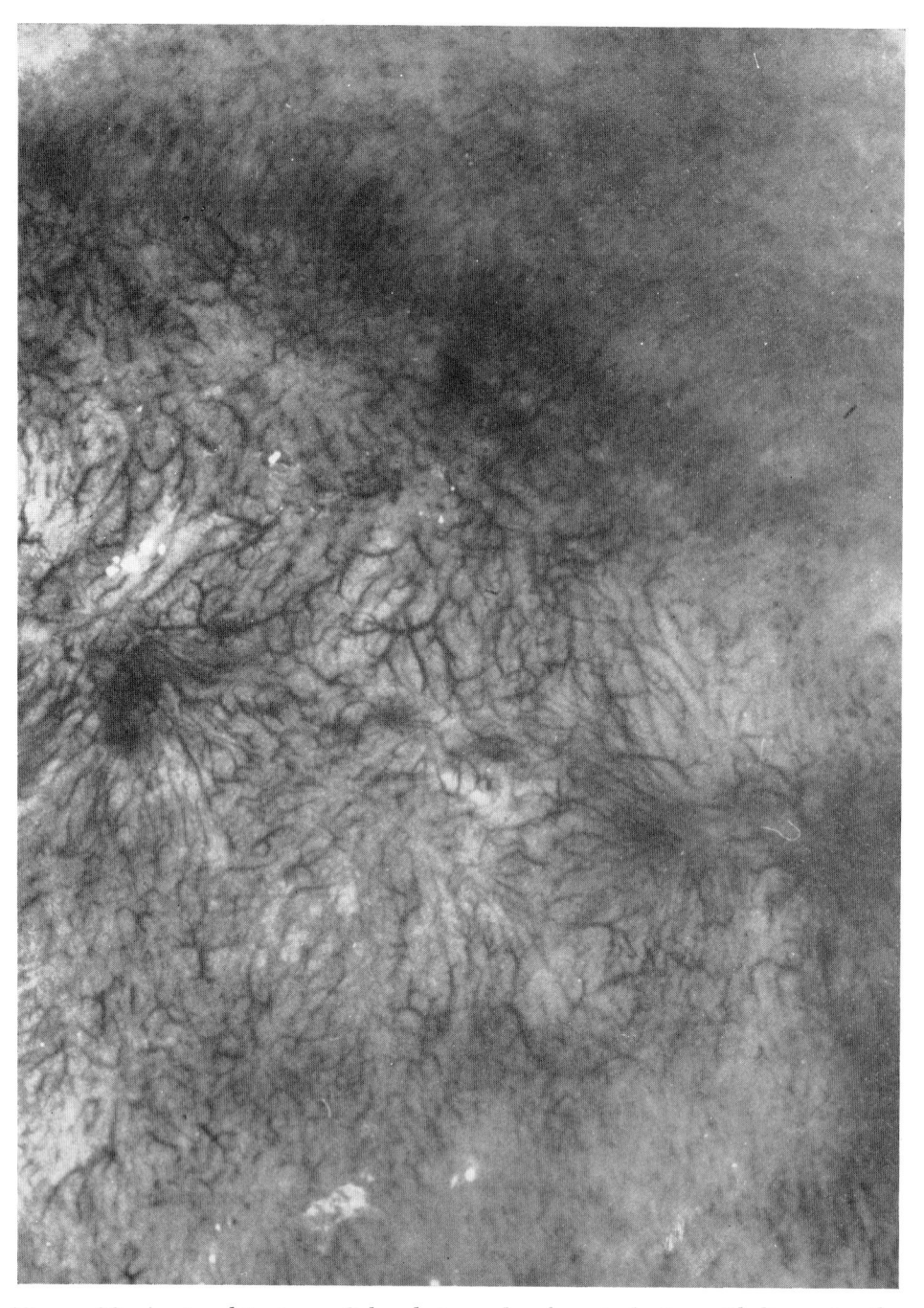

Figure 96. Angioarchitecture. Colpophotograph of metaplastic epithelium. In the fully developed transformation zone, branching vessels are the main distinguishing feature. They form a network capillary system. The original squamous epithelium is seen in the upper right corner.

architectural pattern emerges (Figs. 97 and 98). The epithelium is devoid of intraepithelial stromal papillae and thus of terminal vessels. Due to the opacity of the epithelium, the stromal vascular bed is not seen, so that the observer sees the tissue as white.

In other areas, the colposcopic features concerning either intraepithelial capillaries or a keratin covering are imposed on the background of white epithelium and modify the appearance. These are described.

Punctation

The essential colposcopic appearance in punctation is a series of fine red dots in a whitish background (Fig. 99). More marked degrees show dilatation of the dots and their replacement by a coiled or twisted appearance (Fig. 100). In such areas, the basic tissue arrangement is that of an epithelium into which the fingerlike stromal papillae containing the terminal vascular structures protrude. Alkaline phosphatase studies of tissue representative of the various atypical colposcopic grades show that the basic arrangement of vessels can be similar in each grade. Single, looped, coiled capillaries course perpendicularly or obliquely towards the surface (Figs. 101 and 102). The coarse, coiled structure is only evident colposcopically on occasion. Whether this striking alteration in vessel pattern is predominantly due to hyperaemia or to a more basic alteration in the structure of the capillary wall contingent on the increased demands of the active epithelium or to both are topics for future research.

Mosaic

Mosaic structure is a common basic tissue arrangement (Figs. 103 and 104). Like punctation, the distribution of the capillaries is within the epithelium, but instead of being fingerlike, the stroma is disposed as a wall or ridge circumscribing blocks of epithelium. Adjacent ridges meet in a honeycomb-like disposition (Fig. 105). The ridges are continuous and interconnected, so that when viewed from the surface, their vascular arrangements are seen as red mosaic lines and dots delineating white or pale blocks of epithelium. As in punctation and presumably from the same cause, variations occur in the calibre of these vessels.

Atypical Vessels

Atypical branching intraepithelial vessels, striking in their aberration and consisting of the most bizarre loops and networks, present with sudden variations in calibre and direction (Fig. 106). They represent the ultimate stage of a series starting with fine punctation and/or mosaic. This abnormal arrangement is probably caused by compression of the expanding epithelium on the stromal papillae, so that the sole outlet for any expansion of the system is at the surface.

Keratosis

The colposcopic white areas of thickened surface layer termed *keratosis* have their microscopic equivalent in considerable thickening of the squamous layer of the epithelium (Fig. 107). Up to fifty layers of thin, keratinous squames overlie an epithelium (Fig. 108) which is not necessarily histologically atypical (p. 233). The opacity so caused produces a thick, white keratin crust through which the subepithelial tissue can only be seen by the mechanical removal of the layer. Intraepithelial papillae of the fingerlike or laminar form may be present, representative respectively of punctation and mosaic.

Colposcopically Suspect Overt Carcinoma

The ultimate development of abnormal appearances occurs in invasive cancer, where there is a gross exaggeration of all the abnormal features of colour tone, surface contour, and blood vessel pattern already described. The magnification and ample lighting of the colposcope have allowed the clear discernment of the colposcopically suspect overt cancer denied the naked eye (Fig. 109).

CORRELATION BETWEEN COLPOSCOPIC AND HISTOLOGICAL DIAGNOSIS

The final appeal of the usefulness of colposcopy to the clinician is judged on its ability to render satisfactory correlations with histological diagnosis. In fact, the colposcopic appearances usually show predictable histological correlations. These are described.

Original Cervical Epithelia

The unremarkable qualities of original squamous epithelium and the characteristic appearance of original columnar epithelium require no further comment. They are unmistakable colposcopically.

Typical Transformation Zone

When the colposcopic appearances of typical transformation zone are clearly evident, one can be sure that this epithelium, if biopsied, will not show preclinical carcinoma.

The typical transformation zone with its many and varied colposcopic appearances (*see* Chap. 8) shows squamous metaplasia of varying degrees of maturity. Thus, there may be islands of columnar epithelium in gland crypts; immature squamous epithelium and mature squamous epithelium distributed in adjoining areas in patchwork fashion. Beneath the meta-

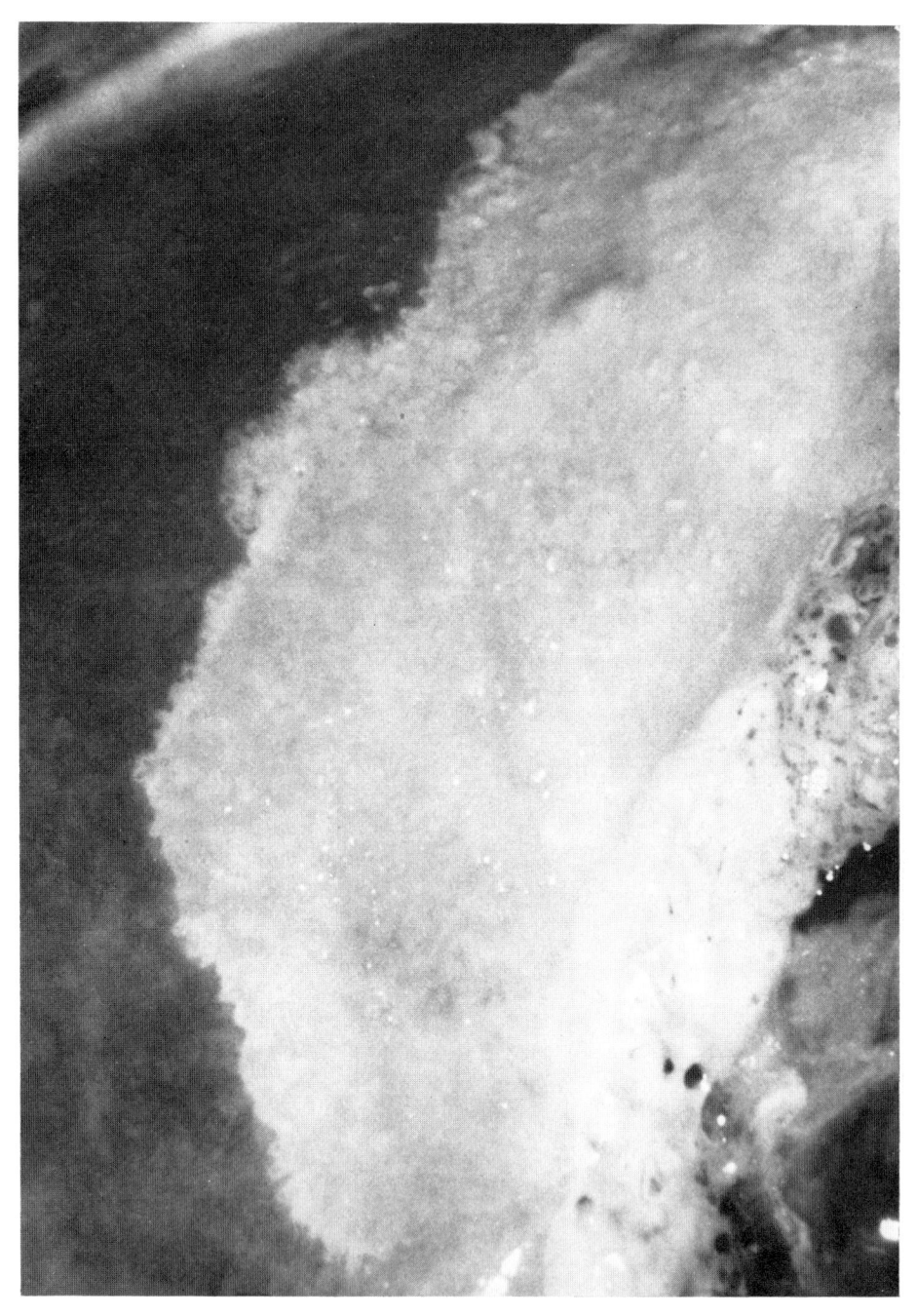

Figure 97. Colpophotograph of lateral cervical lip where the transformation zone shows white epithelium. In most of this area, no terminal vascular structures are seen.

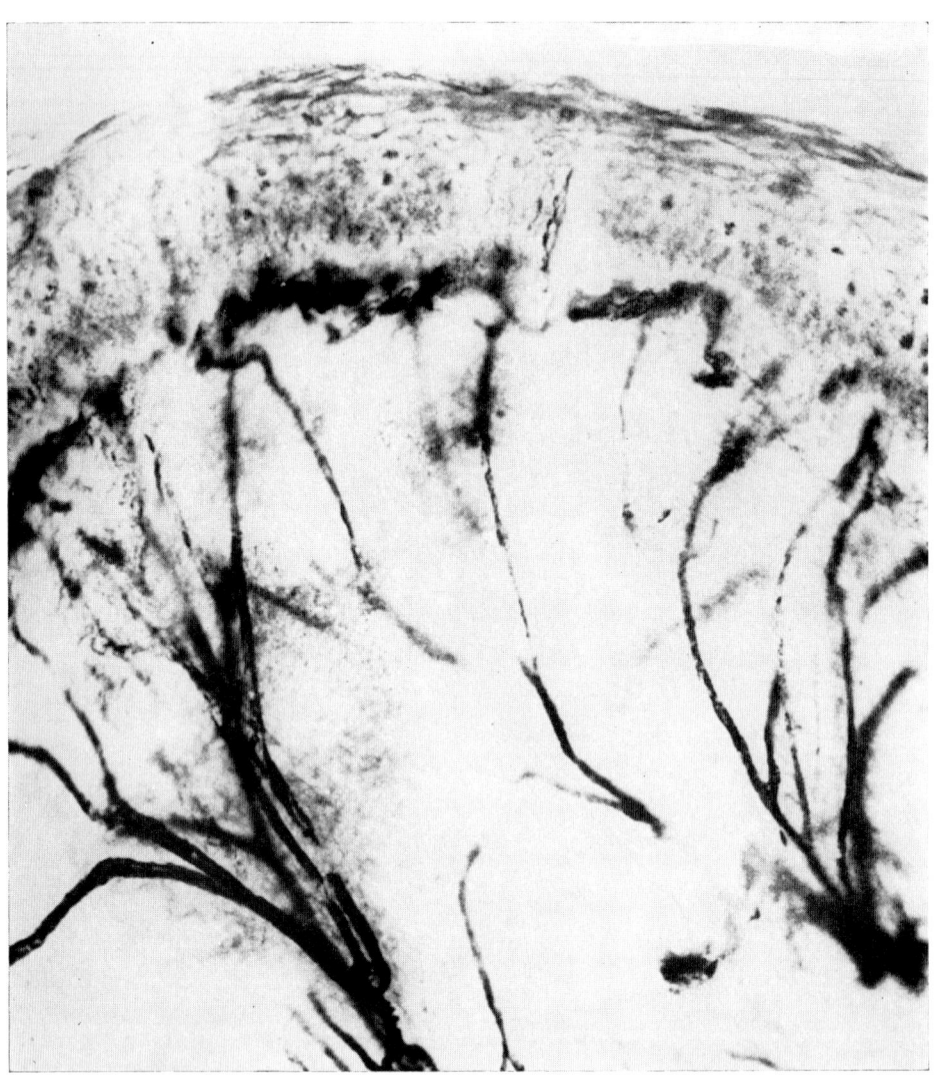

Figure 98. Angioarchitecture. Photomicrograph of biopsy of atypical transformation zone (angiography using alkaline phosphatase, 125 μ section). The atypical transformation zone displaying white epithelium only (Fig. 97) has numerous subepithelial vessels ending in a capillary net beneath the epithelium. There is an absence of intraepithelial vessels.

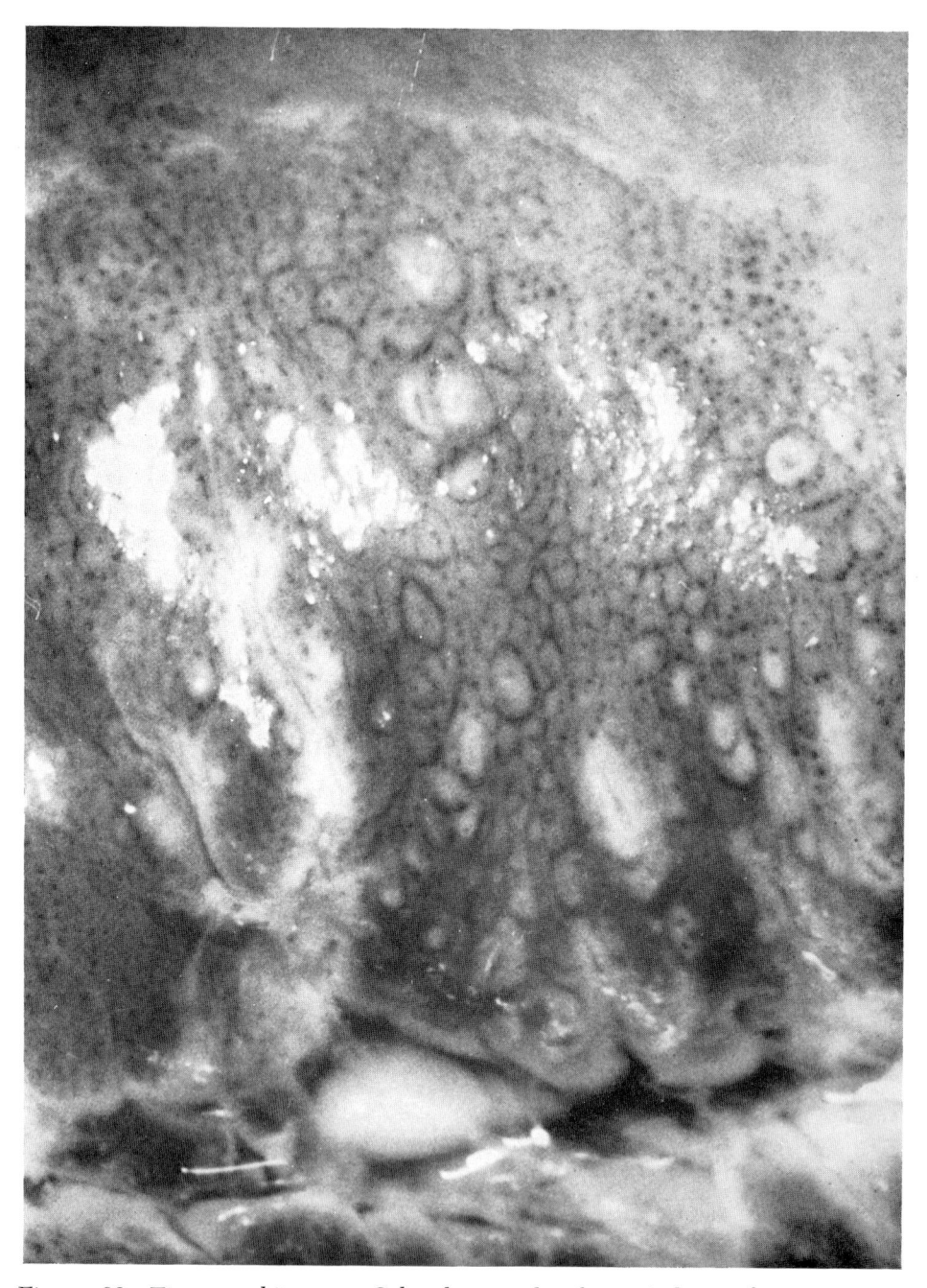

Figure 99. Tissue architecture. Colpophotograph of atypical transformation zone showing both punctation with noncoiled capillaries and mosaic.

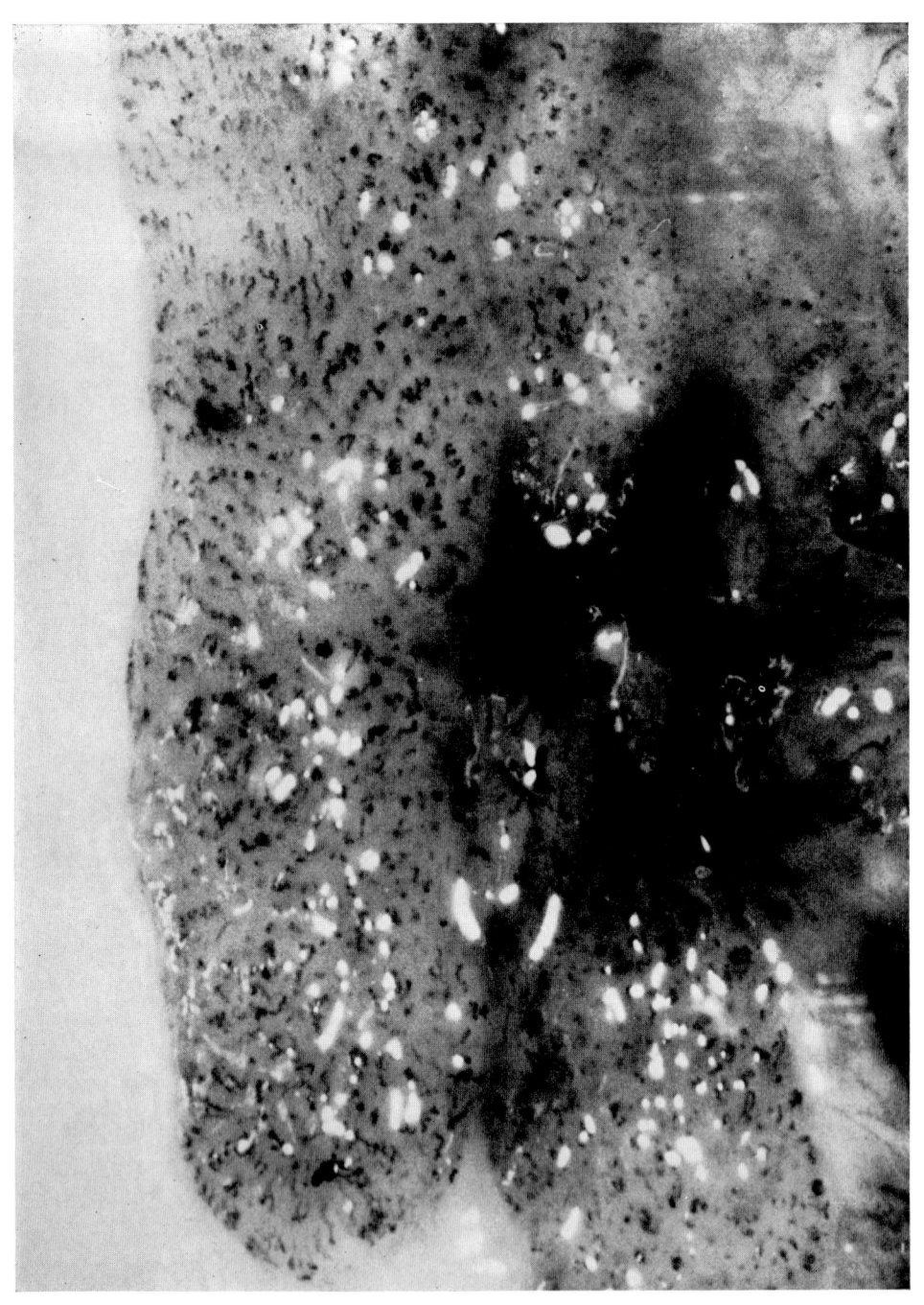

Figure 100. Tissue architecture. Colpophotograph of atypical transformation zone. In contrast to Figure 99, the white atypical transformation zone displays coiled and widely separated vessels in the punctation.

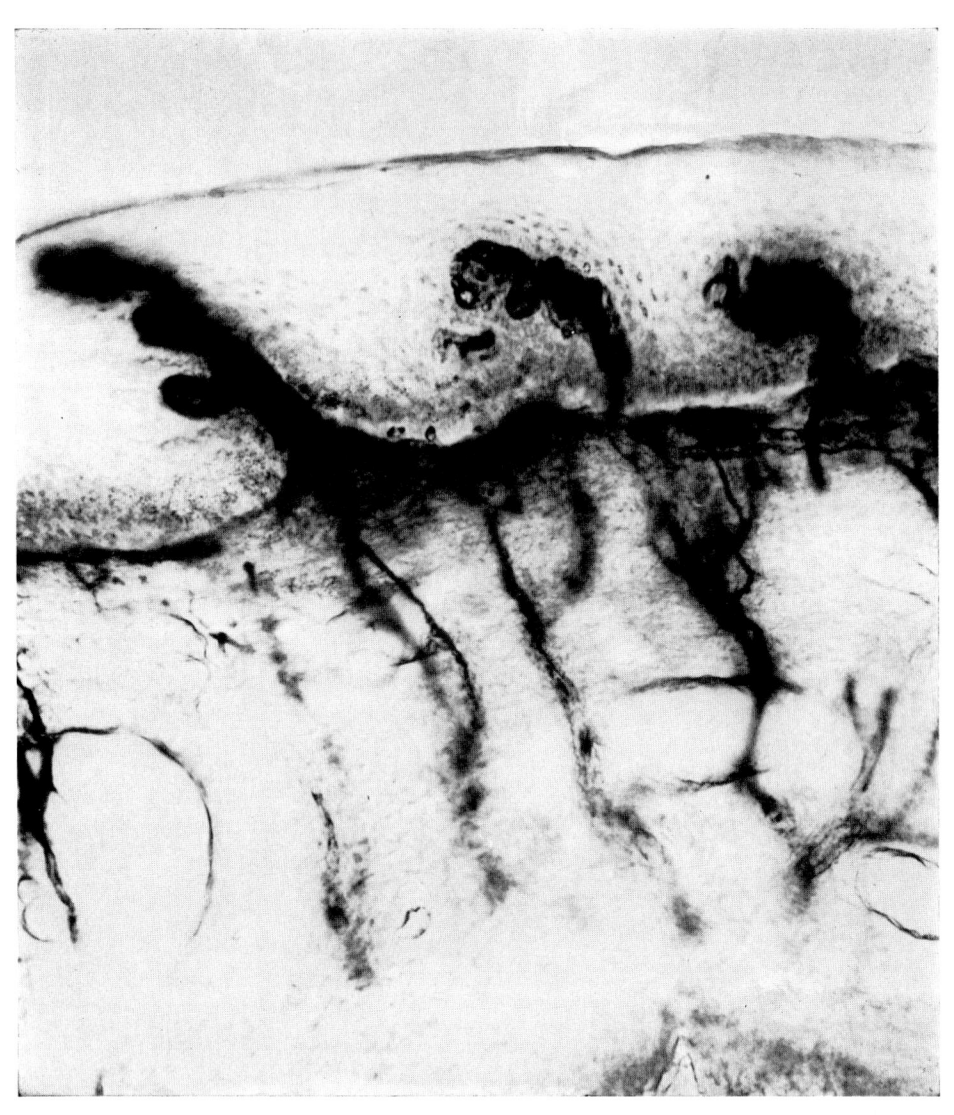

Figure 101. Angioarchitecture. Photomicrograph of biopsy of atypical transformation zone (angiography using alkaline phosphatase, 125 μ section). Tissue from an area of punctation shows coiled intraepithelial capillaries, one of which reaches almost to the surface.

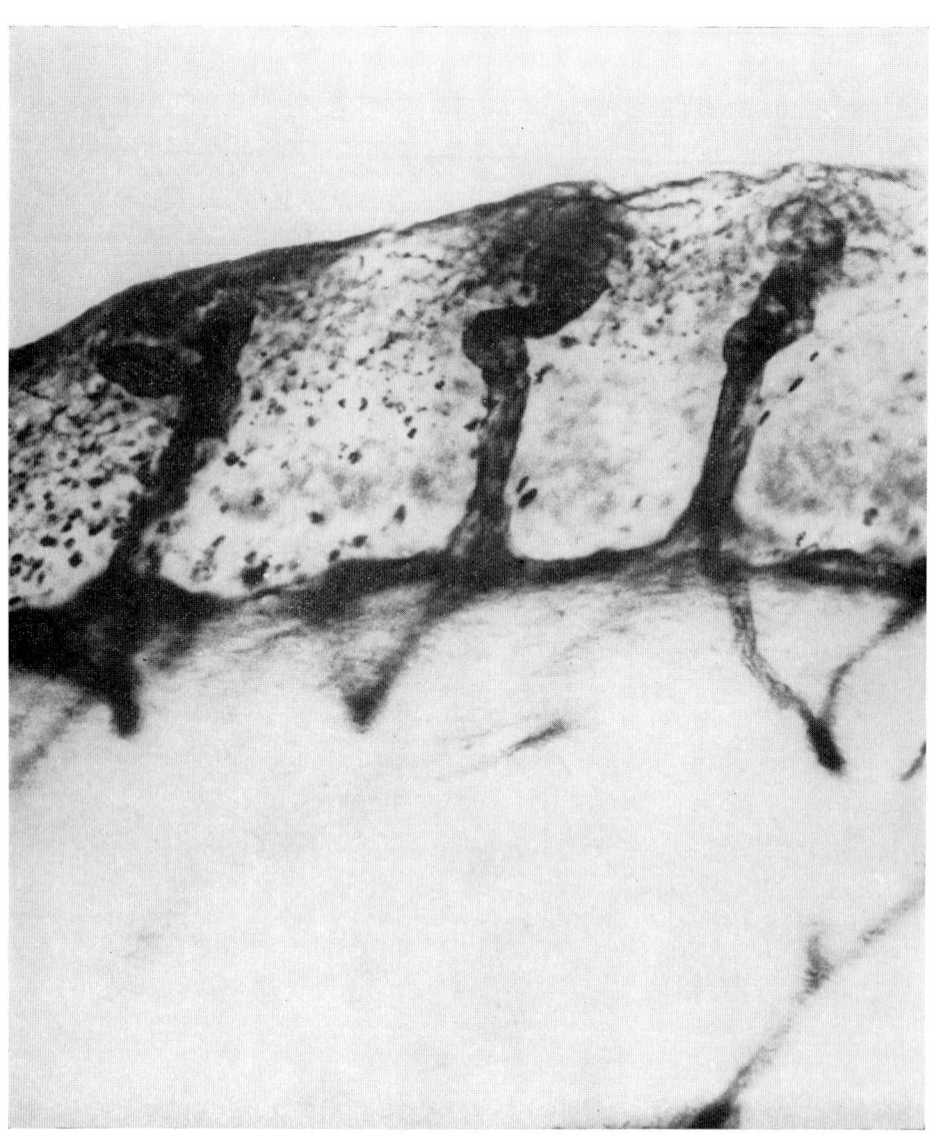

Figure 102. Angioarchitecture. Photomicrograph of biopsy of atypical transformation zone (angiography using alkaline phosphatase, 125 μ section). Tissue from an area of punctation displays intraepithelial capillaries with an oblique, twisted course. The twisted structure here and in Figure 101 is usually not evident colposcopically (Fig. 99). On the other hand, it is usually evident in alkaline phosphatase studies. This suggests that the difference is due to an increased blood flow rate associated with major epithelial atypias.

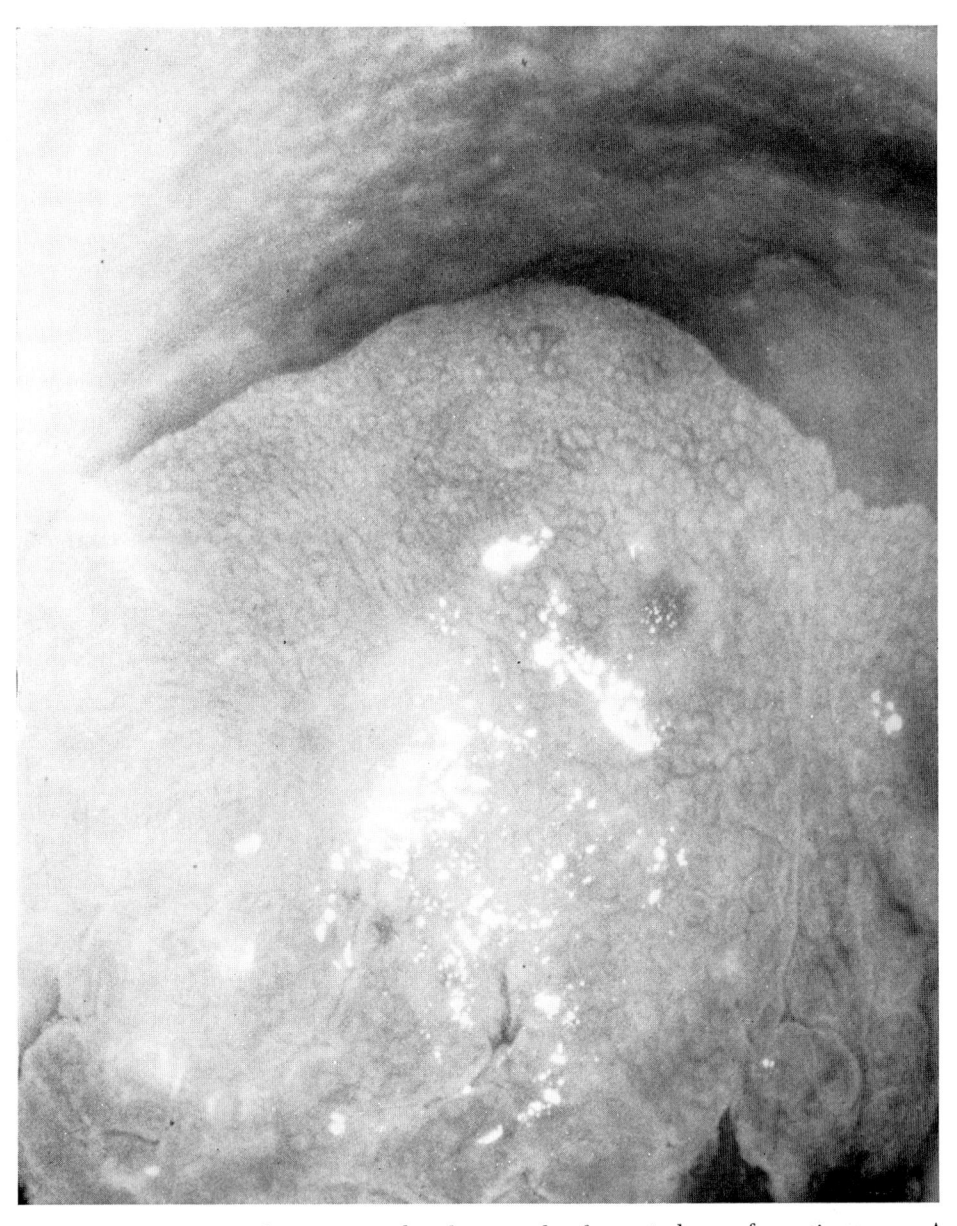

Figure 103. Tissue architecture. Colpophotograph of atypical transformation zone. A regular arrangement of fine blood vessels etches a mosaic pattern in the white epithelium on the anterior cervical lip.

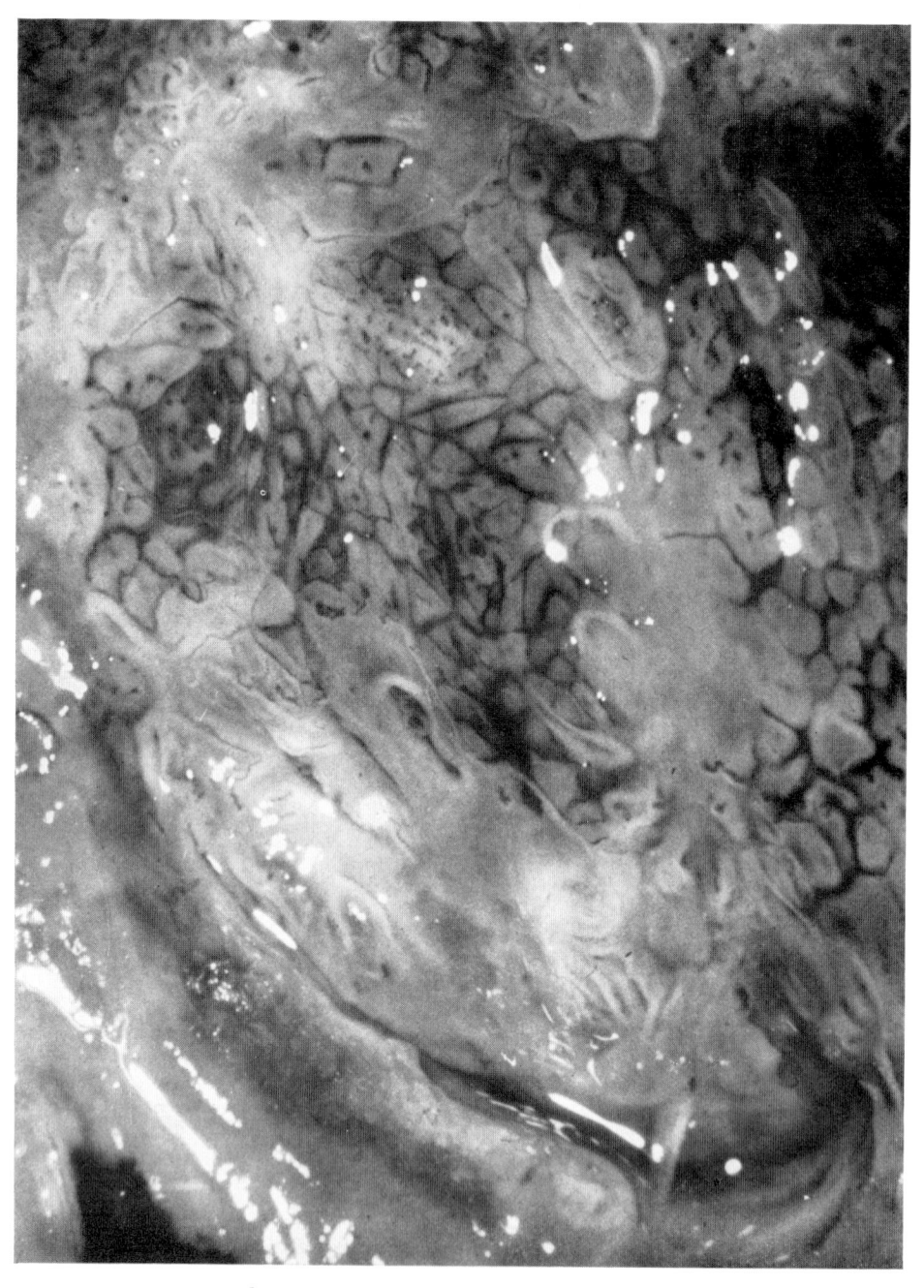

Figure 104. Tissue architecture. Colpophotograph of an atypical transformation zone which exhibits a coarse mosaic structure showing wide variations in area of the blocks and increased dilatation of the vessels, compared to Figure 103.

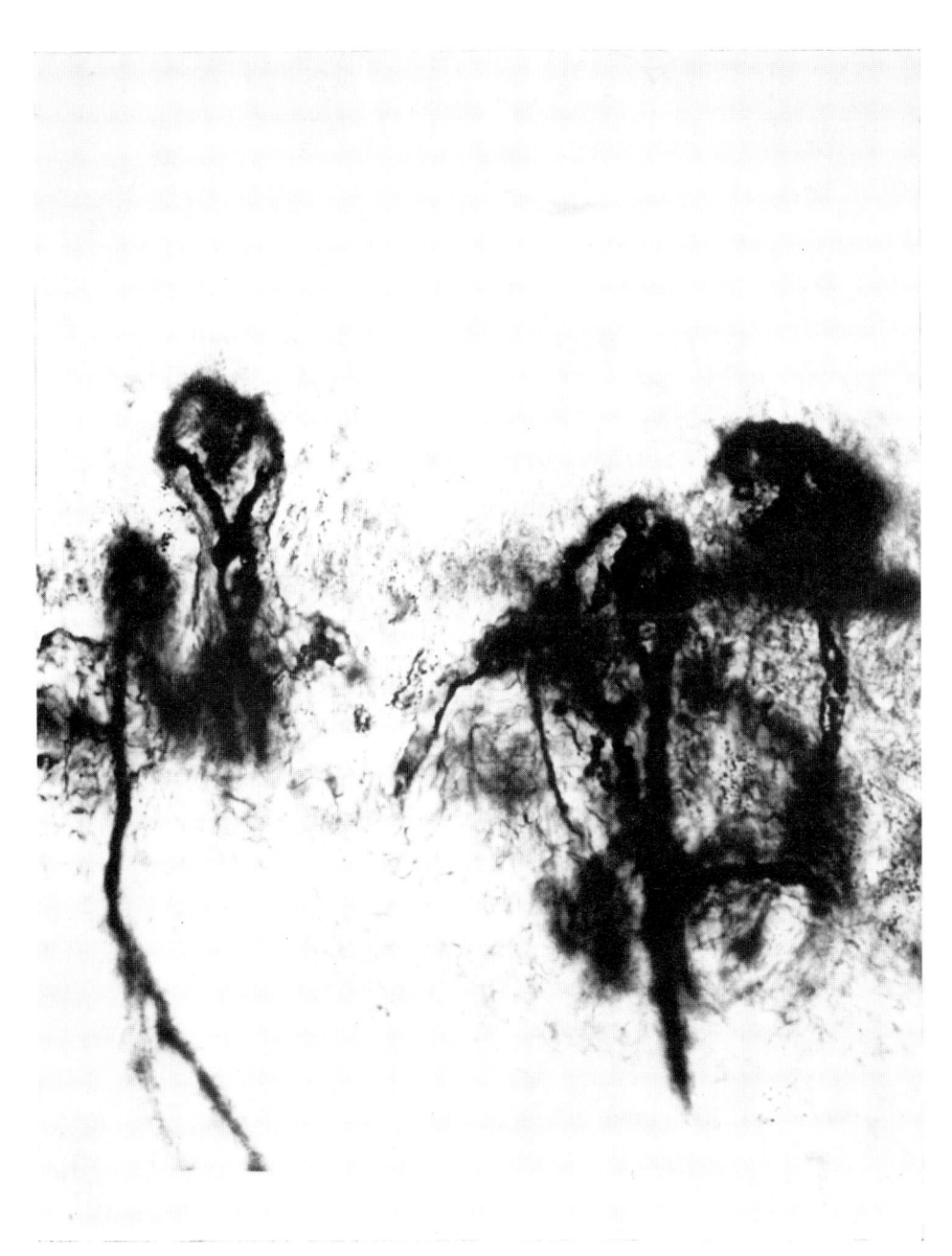

Figure 105. Angioarchitecture. Photomicrograph of biopsy of atypical transformation zone (angiography using alkaline phosphatase, 125 μ section). Tissue from an area of mosaic showing coiled intraepithelial capillaries which appear to lie in tissue ridges vertical to the surface and also to form capillary loops within the ridges. The papillae associated with mosaic are wider than those seen with punctation and in a surface view would link up to form the characteristic pattern. The more obvious vessel dilatation in Figure 104, when compared to Figure 103 is due to vascular hyperaemia.

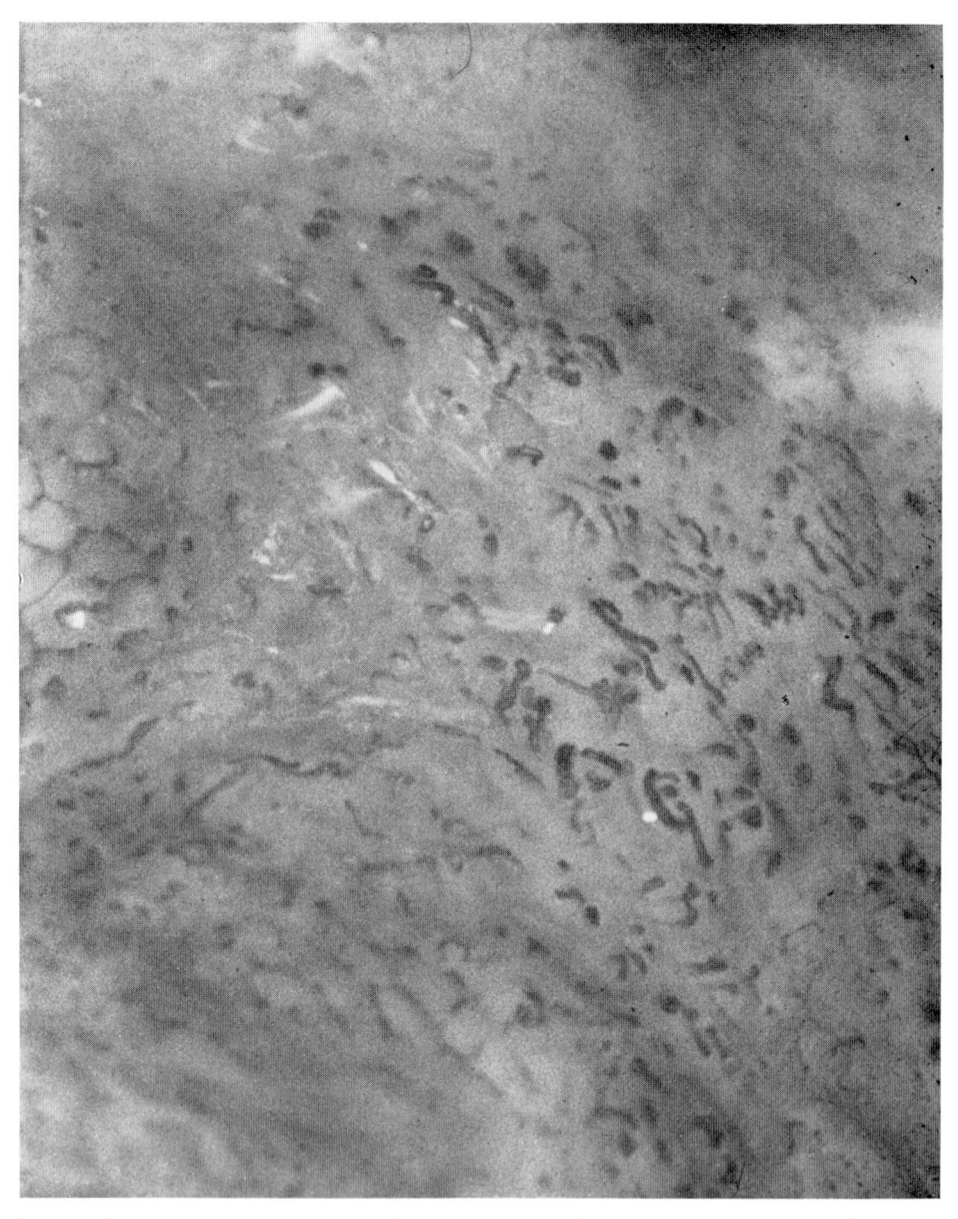

Figure 106. Angioarchitecture. Colpophotograph of part of atypical transformation zone showing atypical vessels. Towards the left margin of the study, mosaic and punctation patterns are evident. Elsewhere terminal capillaries are grossly dilated, bizarre in their shape, and irregular in their course in the epithelium.

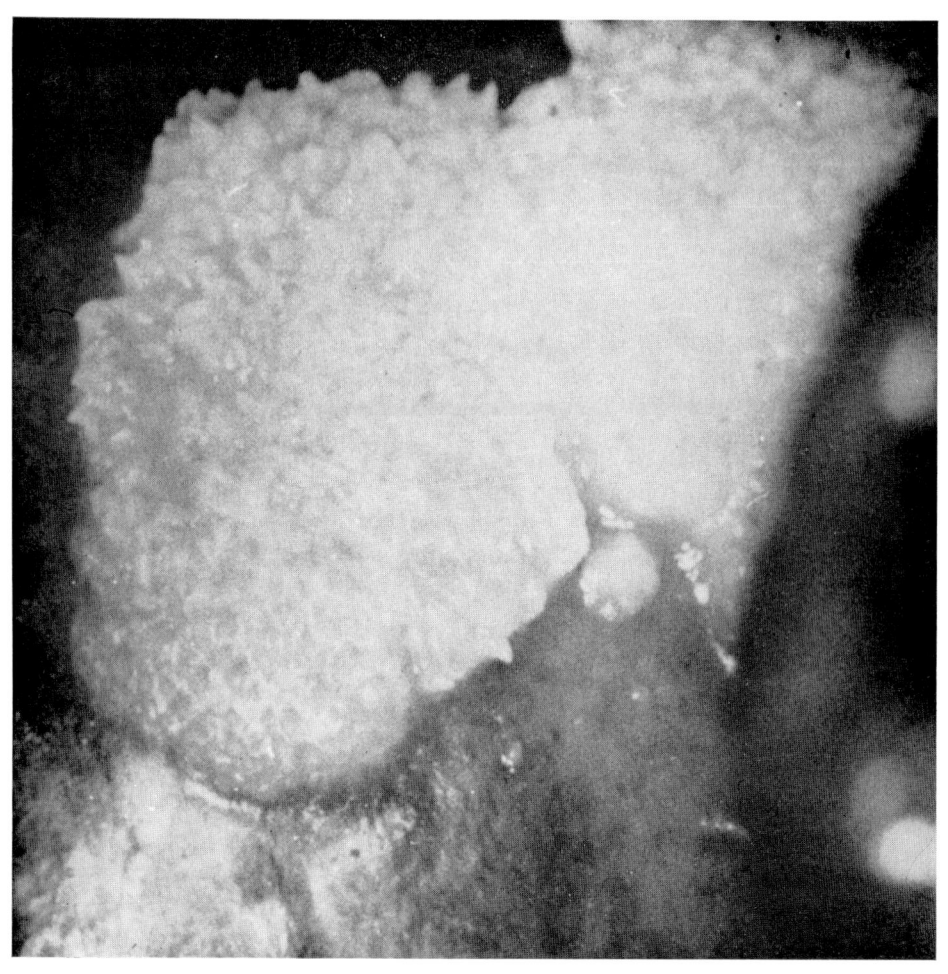

Figure 107. Tissue architecture. Colpophotograph of atypical transformation zone (keratosis). The epithelium is covered by a thick white patch of keratin that is raised above the general surface level.

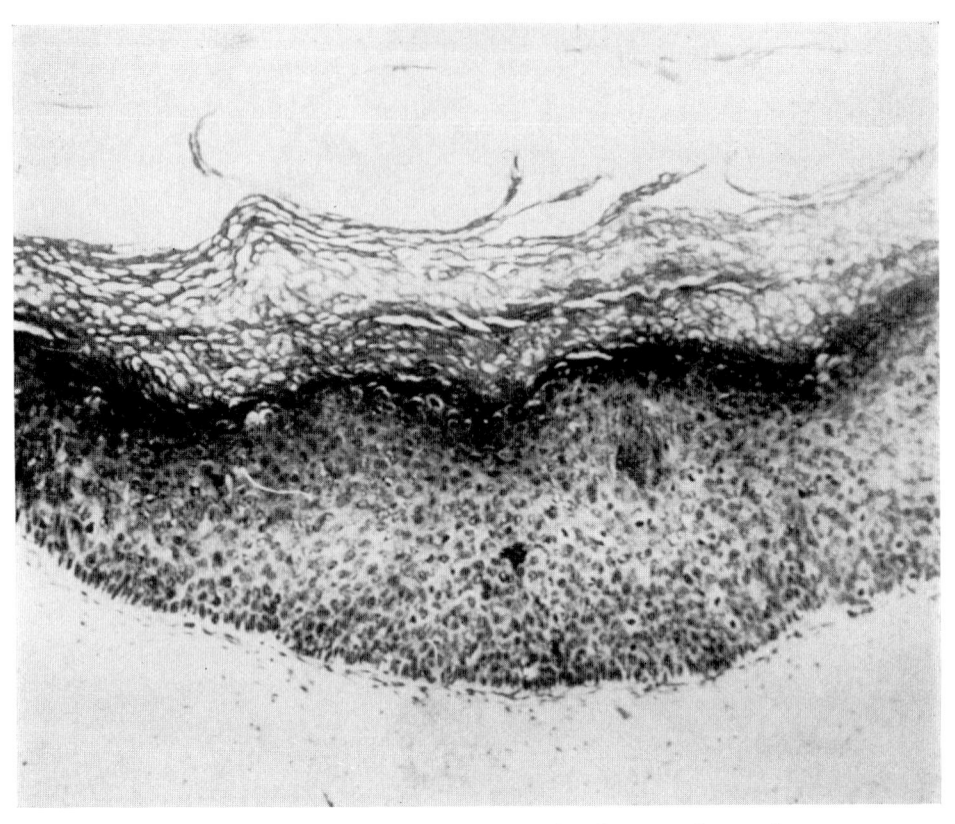

Figure 108. Tissue architecture. Photomicrograph of atypical transformation zone. Overlying the surface epithelium, which shows appearances of major dysplasia, many layers of keratin material have formed.

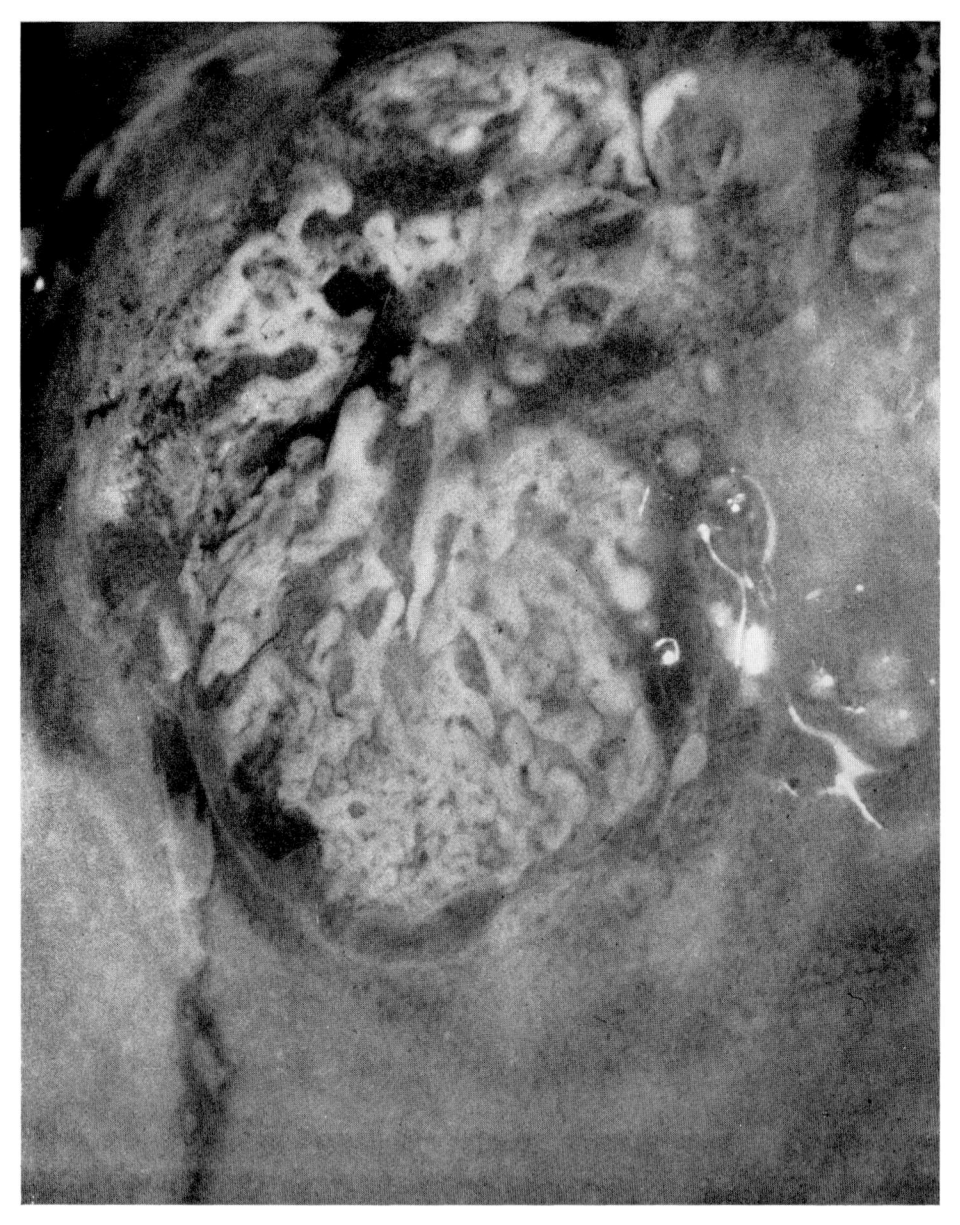

Figure 109. Colpophotograph showing colposcopically overt cancer. An area in the transformation zone displays a sharp edge, bleeds slightly, and contains atypical vessels, features discerned only by colposcopic examination.

plastic epithelium, entrapped columnar epithelium may be present as inclusions or as functional clefts opening onto the surface. The openings are recognisable colposcopic features (see Fig. 90). In general, the most mature squamous epithelium adjoins the vaginal limit of the transformation zone, where its histology approaches closely that of the original squamous epithelium. The distinction between the two types of squamous epithelium may, in the absence of glandular structures, be possible only on colposcopic grounds by virtue of subtle variations in the angioarchitecture.

The histological assessment of immature metaplastic epithelium is often difficult. The characteristic colposcopic appearance of the early stages of typical transformation assists the diagnosis.

Atypical Transformation Zone

Three grades (Grade I, Grade II, and Grade III) of the atypical transformation zone are recognised. In general, the greater the histological abnormality, the more pronounced are the colposcopic changes. The colposcopic characteristics of each grade and the importance of grading in management are discussed later (see Chaps. 9 and 16).

The grading of colposcopic lesions depends on the following:
1. The degree of "whiteness" of the epithelium (after acetic acid application)
2. The nature of the surface contour, whether flat or irregular
3. The fineness or coarseness (dilation) of the calibre of epithelial blood vessels and the regularity or irregularity of vessel shape
4. The presence of a regular or irregular pattern of punctation or mosaic
5. The presence or absence of atypical vessels
6. The intercapillary distance

Not surprisingly, the range of features introduces a large subjective element into the evaluation. Attendant errors, both in the one observer at different times and between different observers, are a natural consequence. Because of this inherent subjectivity, we consider it unwise in grading to attempt a system confined by rigorous correlation with histology. Our leaning has been towards a very simple and practical subdivision into appearances which are *insignificant* (Grade I), *significant* (Grade II), and *highly significant* (Grade III). This has involved a minor revision of the grading originally proposed in the first edition of this book. Experience from continuing correlative studies of histology and colposcopy has shown that the revised scheme has more practical application.

Grade I

Atypical colposcopic appearances of minor significance compatible with an overlapping histological series from normal metaplastic epithelium to minor dysplasia are considered Grade I (Figs. 110 and 111).

Grade II

Atypical colposcopic appearances of significance compatible with a major dysplasia or carcinoma in situ are Grade II (Figs. 112 and 113). In general, the epithelium is whiter and the terminal vascular structures more dilated and irregular than in Grade I.

Grade III

Atypical colposcopic appearances of high significance compatible with carcinoma in situ or preclinical invasive cancer are Grade III (Figs. 114 and 115). Extreme variations in calibre, course, and intercapillary distance are seen in this grade. Atypical vessels and minute papillary exophytia observable only on stereoscopic viewing indicates the probable presence of invasive cancer.

Colposcopically Suspect Overt Carcinoma

The ultimate in abnormality of preclinical colposcopic appearances that indicates the presence of invasive cancer is *colposcopically suspect overt carcinoma* (*see* Fig. 109).

DISCREPANCY BETWEEN COLPOSCOPIC AND HISTOLOGICAL DIAGNOSIS

In most cases, the correlations are as described in the previous section. Within this range and histological overlap described, minor discrepancies are acceptable. The recognition that one-step differences in the histological report, e.g. severe dysplasia or carcinoma in situ, are generally unimportant in management render these minor discrepancies unimportant.

Major discrepancies also occur. Thus, colposcopic appearances consistent with a minor Grade I classification turn out, on histological examination, to show full-thickness loss of differentiation and thus attract the histopathological label of carcinoma in situ. Grade II colposcopic appearances may be associated with minor dysplasia or apparently insignificant epithelial changes or, on the other hand, may be associated with preclinical invasive carcinoma. Major discrepancies with Grade III colposcopic appearances are rare. Such discrepancies have, of course, salutory and chastening effects but in no way minimise the general efficiency of the technique of colposcopy. In this sense, they are to be expected and call for more research to establish reasons for the discrepancy rather than comment as to the "worthlessness" of the technique. They serve as a continuing reminder that no single technique can hope to correlate even substantially with a process as complicated and unpredictable as carcinogenesis.

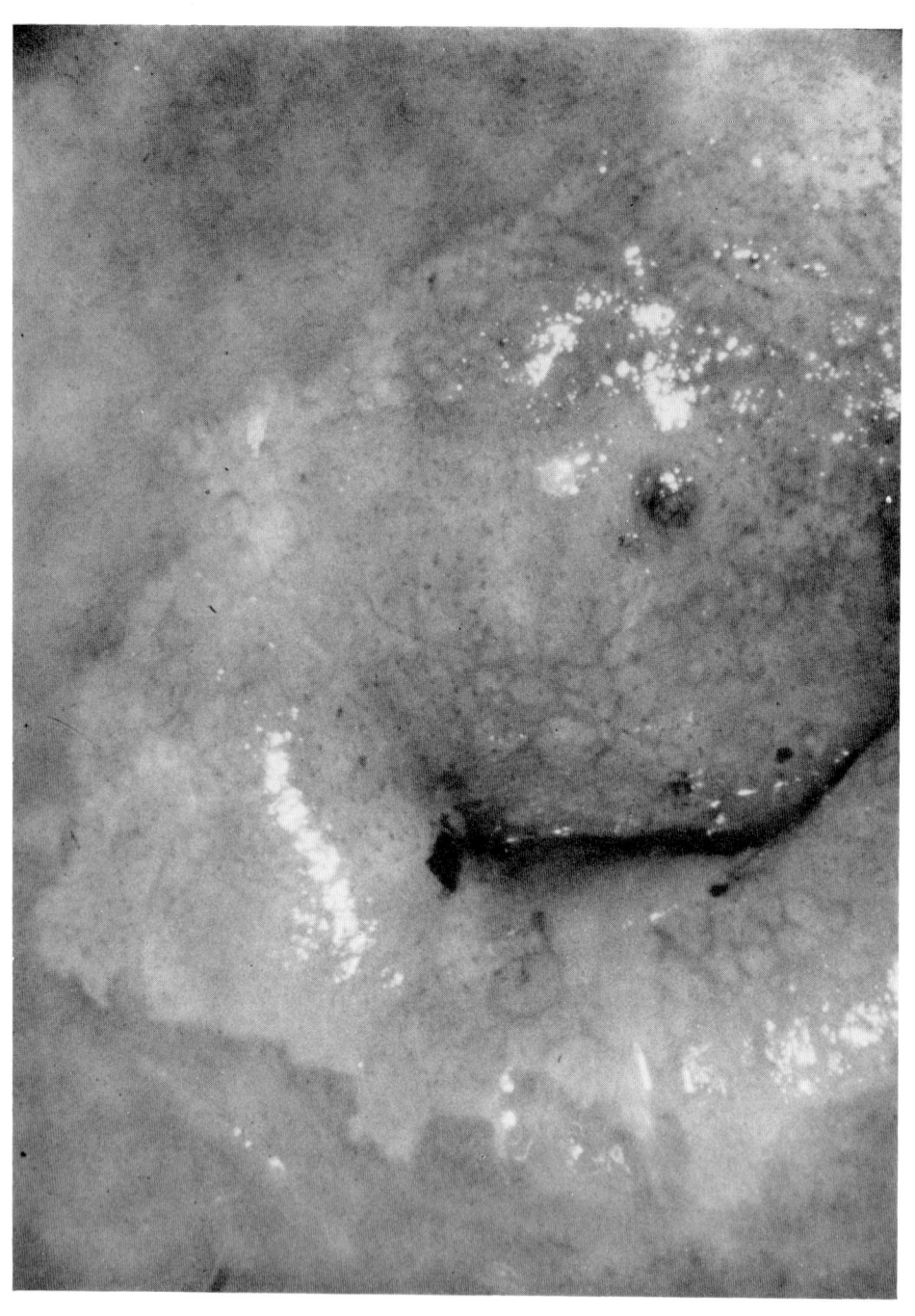

Figure 110. Colpophotograph of atypical transformation zone (Grade I lesion) displaying white epithelium with inconspicuous punctation and mosaic. Histological examination showed minor dysplasia, the presumptive diagnosis with Grade I atypical colposcopic lesions.

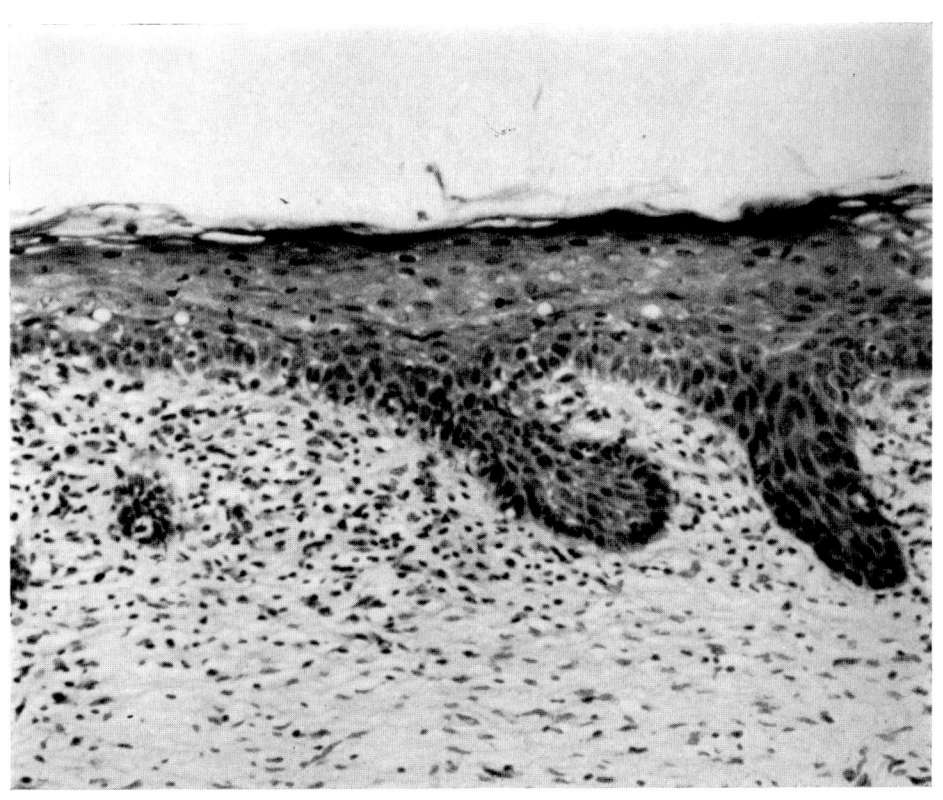

Figure 111. Photomicrograph of biopsy of atypical transformation zone (Grade I lesion). This minimal disorder of epithelial pattern, termed *abnormal epithelium*, is a common histological finding with Grade I atypical colposcopic appearances.

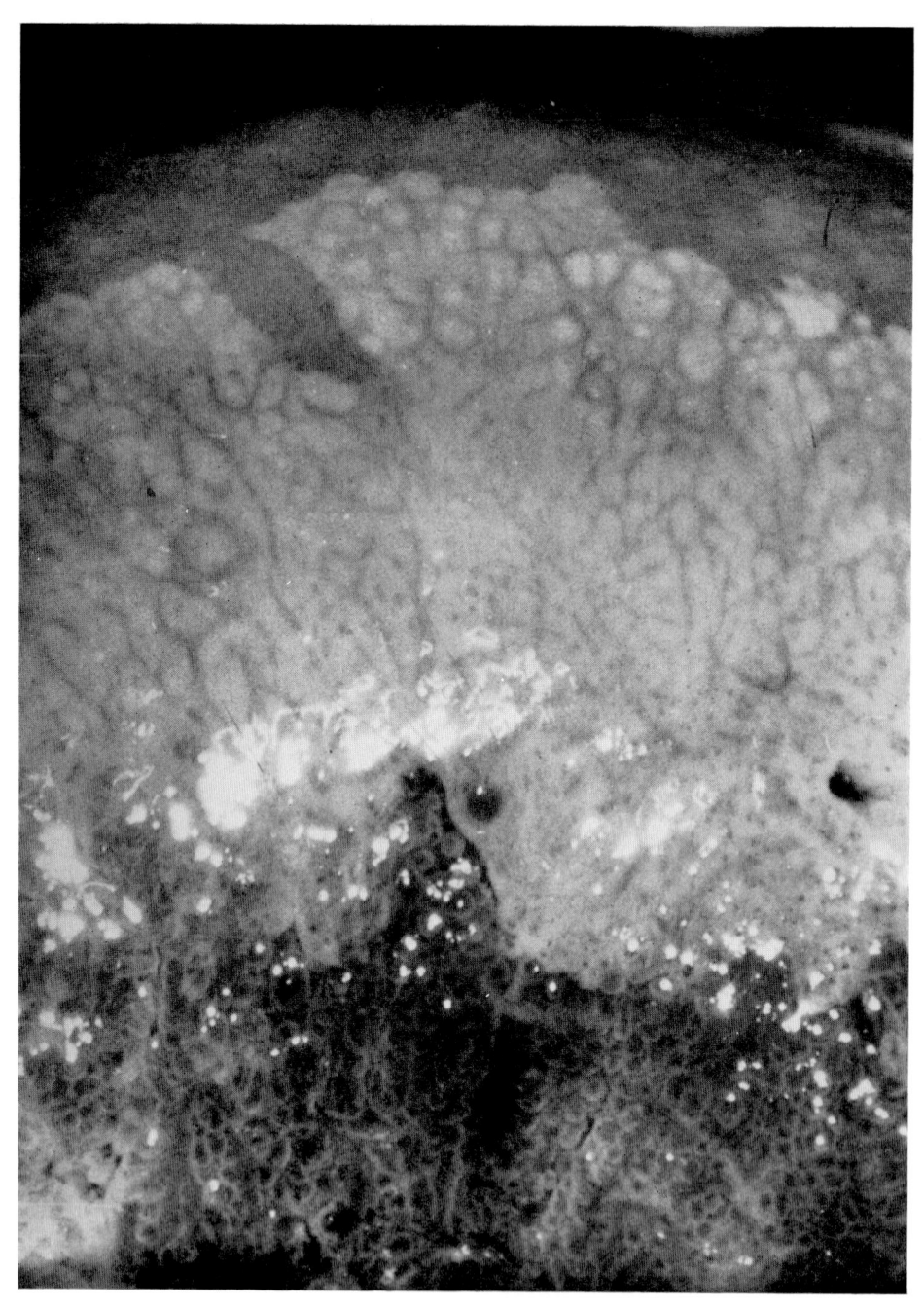

Figure 112. Colpophotograph of atypical transformation zone (Grade II lesion). The white epithelium contains vascular structures arranged mainly to form mosaic patterns. In several areas, especially near the junction with columnar epithelium, an associated punctation is also evident.

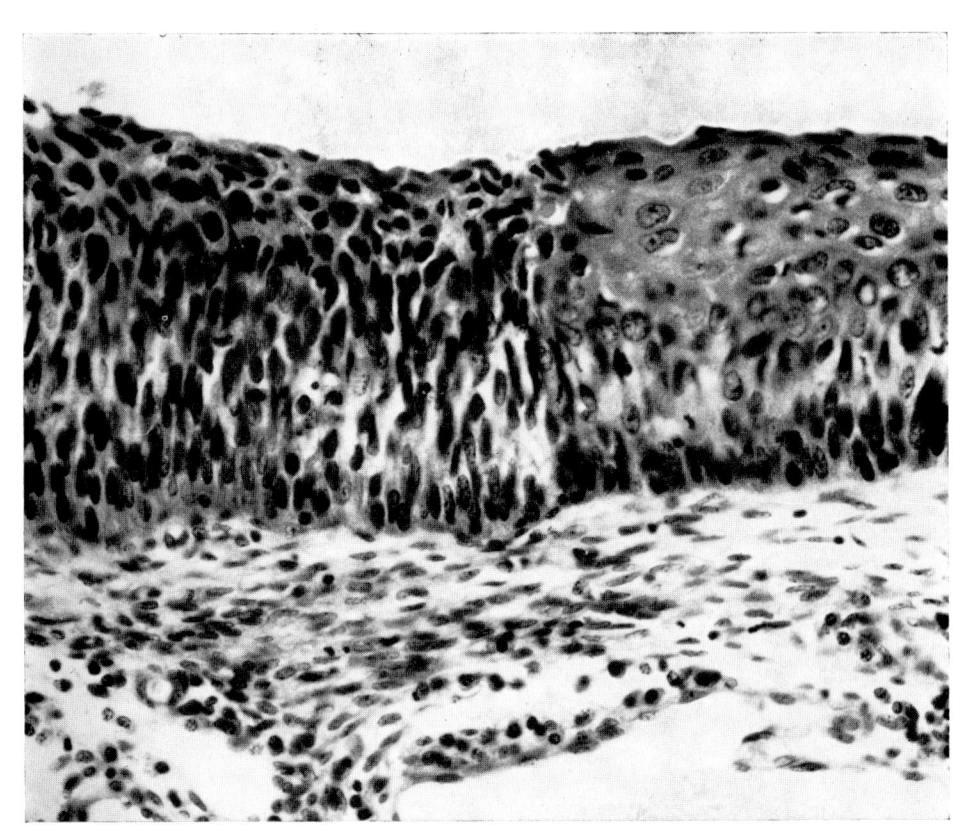

Figure 113. Photomicrograph of biopsy of atypical transformation zone (Grade II lesion). The epithelium shows loss of differentiation, variation in nuclear size, and hyperchromatism. The appearances are those of carcinoma in situ on the left and dysplasia on the right. Such a picture can be frequently expected with Grade II atypical colposcopic findings.

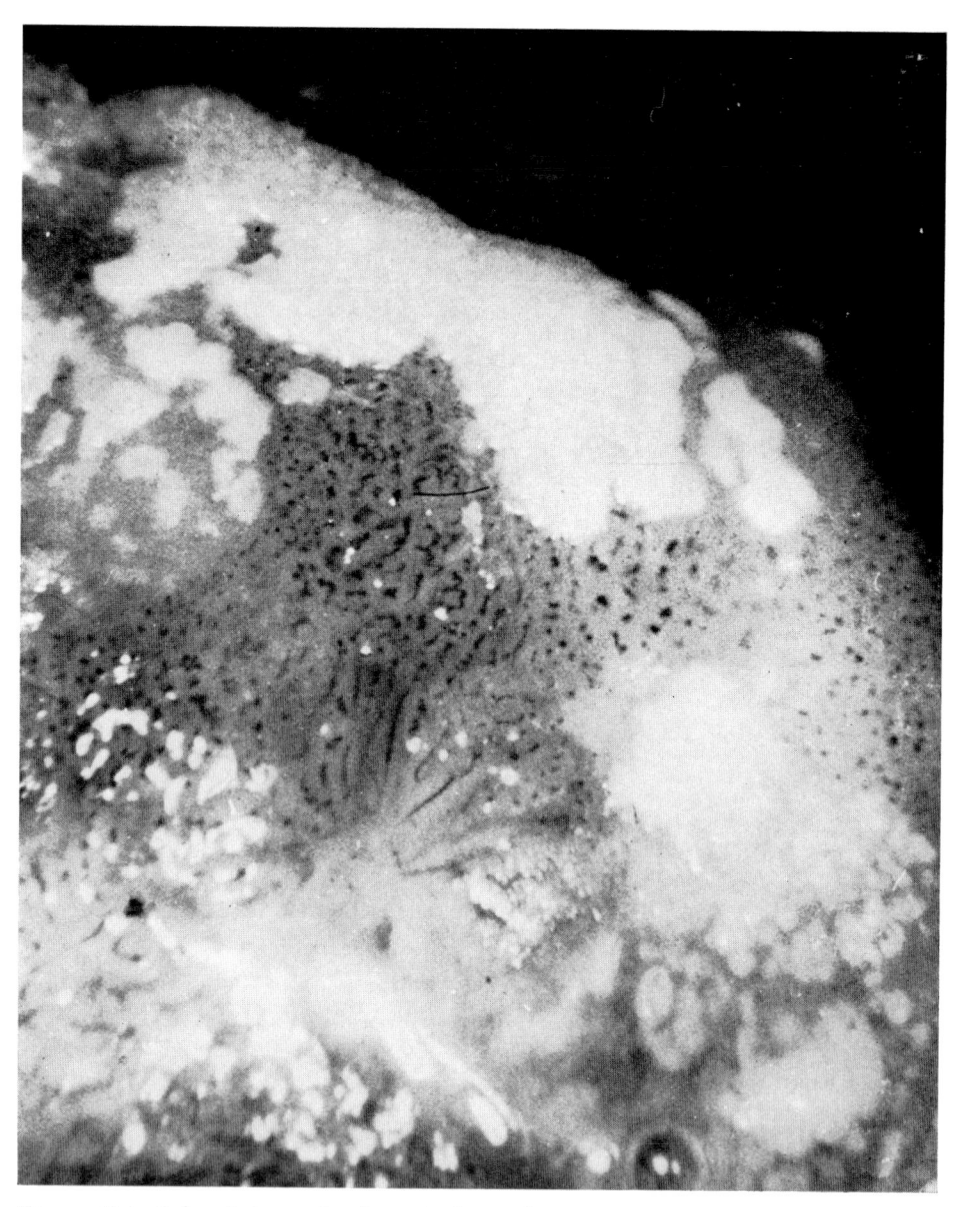

Figure 114. Colpophotograph of atypical transformation zone (Grade III lesion). An atypical transformation zone exhibits coarse irregular punctation with widely spaced, coarse and coiled vessels, thick keratosis, and minute variations in surface level. This Grade III atypical colposcopic lesion showed carcinoma in situ, an expected diagnosis on histological examination.

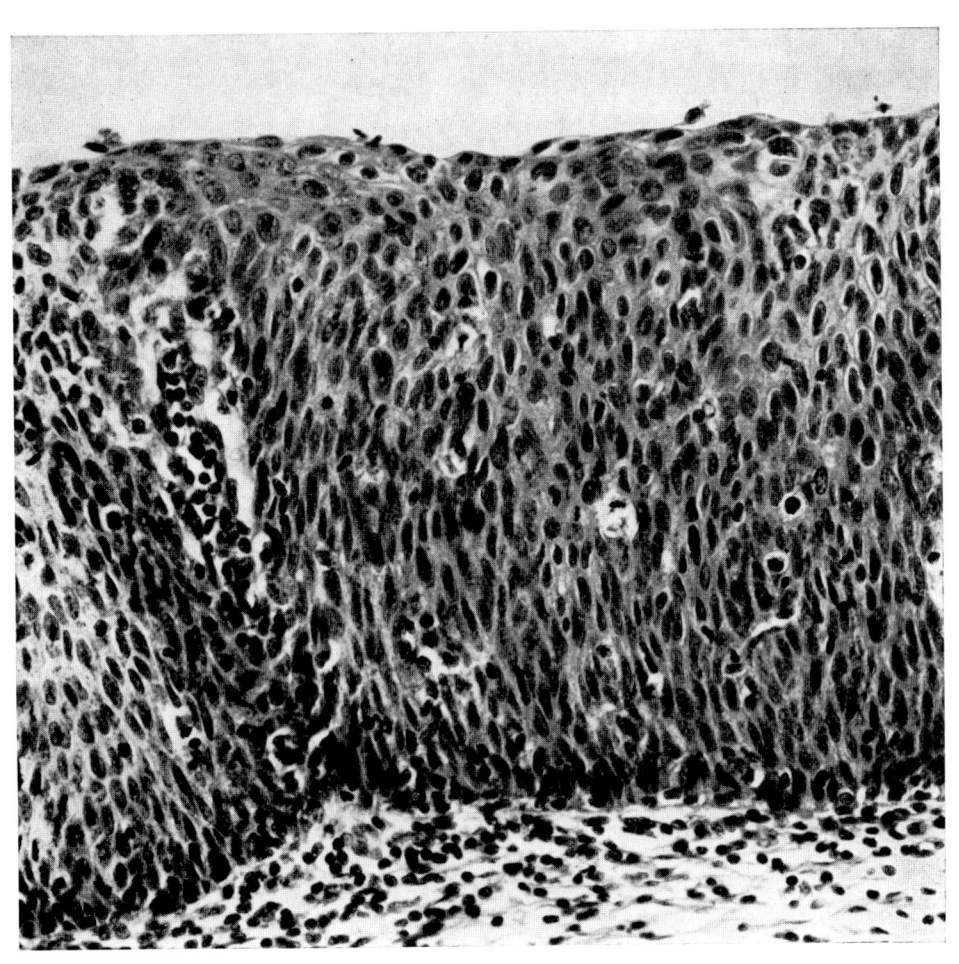

Figure 115. Photomicrograph of atypical transformation zone (Grade II or Grade III lesion). Full-thickness loss of differentiation of epithelium is seen. This finding frequently occurs with Grade II and Grade III atypical transformation zones, especially when the cervical smear is positive.

At the present level of knowledge, it would be bold to speculate on the reasons for discrepancies. Depending on his training and experience, the observer questions either the histological or colposcopic opinion. Conversely, there may be real biological significance underlying such discrepancies, the nature of which is presently obscure. For example, it could be that an epithelium showing full-thickness loss of differentiation has hyperaemia of superficial capillaries no greater than that to be expected of tissue which is histologically normal. That the same condition occurs in association with great hyperaemia is undisputed. A reasonable conclusion from this seeming impasse is that the histological entity of a full-thickness loss of differentiation represents two conditions; one with and one without an associated blood vessel response. Thus, these two conditions may have different prognostic significance (p. 403). Considerations of this kind bring to mind conclusions of other authors, very speculative at the present time though they may be, that the real biological significance of many of these histological appearances is unknown and that, like so many other indivisible elements in the course of the history of medical science, such as anaemia or virilism, many different conditions may lie beneath a single, conventionally sound label, in this instance, carcinoma in situ.

PART III

Technique

Chapter 6

THE TECHNIQUE OF COLPOSCOPY

THE INSTRUMENTS

THE CLINICAL MATERIAL and illustrations upon which this text is based have been examined and recorded with two types of colposcope, the Leisegang, series 111b, and the Zeiss (Figs. 116 and 117). Each provides the essential: magnification, high-intensity illumination, stereoscopic viewing, and photographic recording. As the colposcope has gained popularity, new instruments with important innovations have become available.

Illustrations have been chosen from a wide range to show the variety of instruments, attachments, and mounting systems available to the gynaecologist (Figs. 118-121). Surgical laser units are being used more frequently for therapy in gynaecology, and two models are illustrated (Figs. 122 and 123).

The requirements of some gynaecologists are met by the more basic instruments, whereas others who wish to keep more accurate clinical records, teach, consult, or undertake research require more elaborate instruments with photographic, teaching, and consultation attachments. Another consideration in selection is the type of mounting required, which is determined by the specific features of the examination room in the consulting suite.

Magnification available on the various models is in keeping with arbitrary figures recommended by experienced colposcopists. Systems provide a magnification range from ×5 to ×40, but ×5 to ×16 is adequate for viewing the fine morphological detail on which the colposcopic method is based. Higher magnifications yield small fields of vision, loss of resolution, and are unnecessary.

Provision of the green filter on the colposcope is mandatory. Many physicians currently using and teaching the method rarely undertake colposcopic examination without having the green filter in place. Despite a small loss of intensity of illumination, several aspects of morphology are enhanced. In particular, the terminal angioarchitecture becomes etched in black, allowing a degree of discrimination not otherwise achieved. The contrast also extends to the features of surface configuration, and there is a useful diminution in the reflections of the light source. We recommend the routine use of the green filter. Colour blindness is no bar to good colposcopy.

Stereoscopic vision is essential, and each instrument allows adjustments

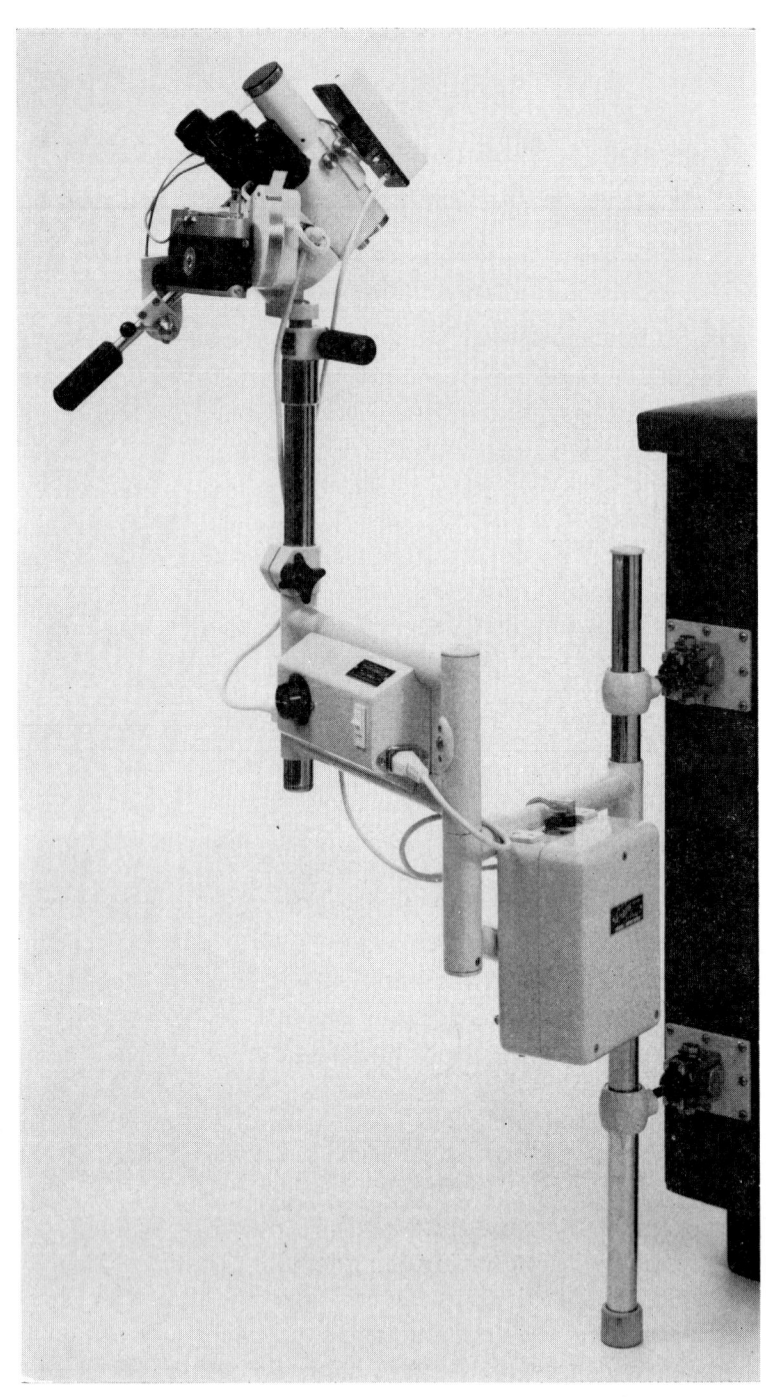

Figure 116. The 111B Leisegang model is illustrated. The magnification is 13.5×. This model offers attachments for stereoscopic photography with film identification system. A Polaroid camera is incorporated, and surgical laser is intended for attachment. Teaching ocular is also available (Photograph courtesy of Gynemed Inc., Palo Alto, California).

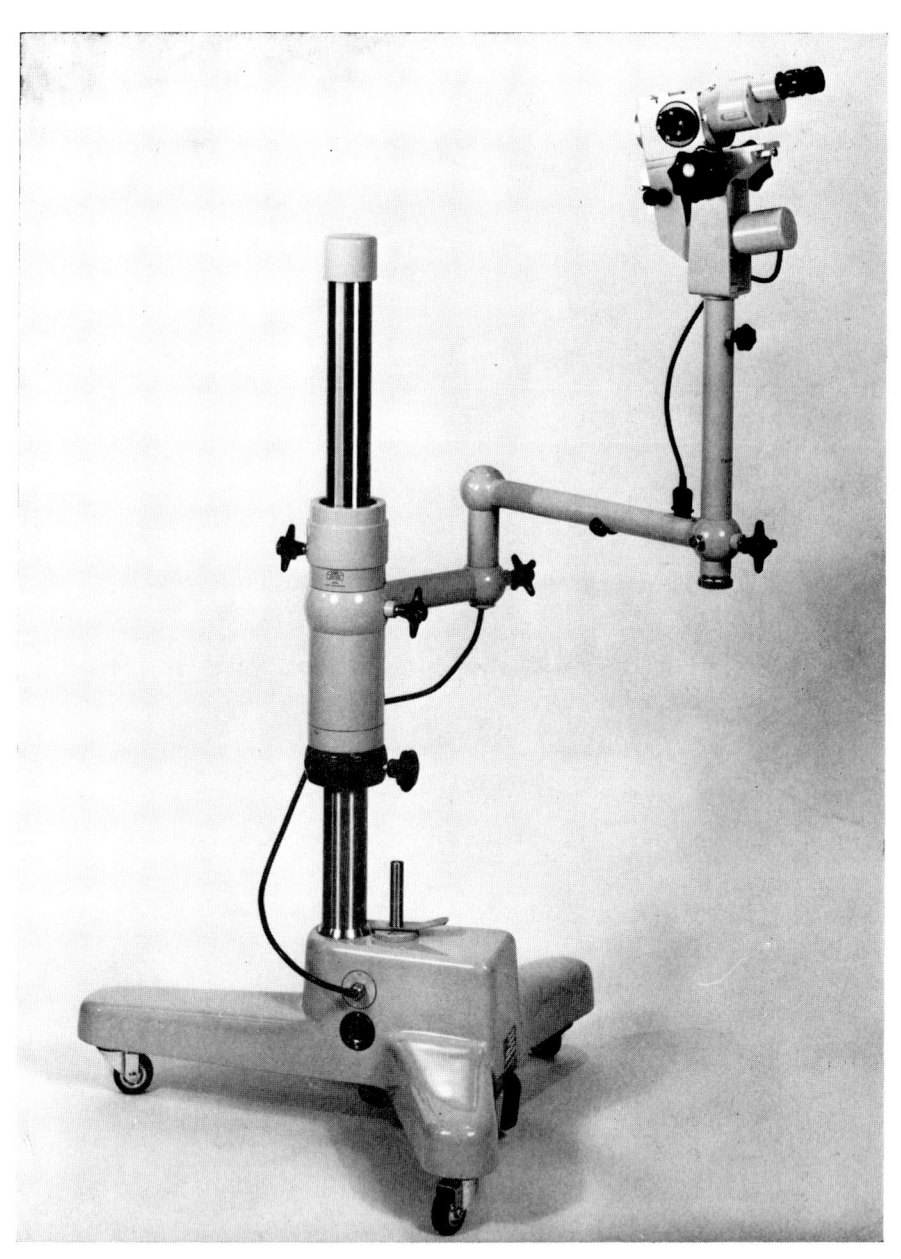

Figure 117. A recent Zeiss colposcope is illustrated. The magnification available is 6× to 40×. Attachments include devices for still photography, cinematography, television, teaching consultation eyepiece, and surgical laser. A zoom lens is available for one model (Carl Zeiss).

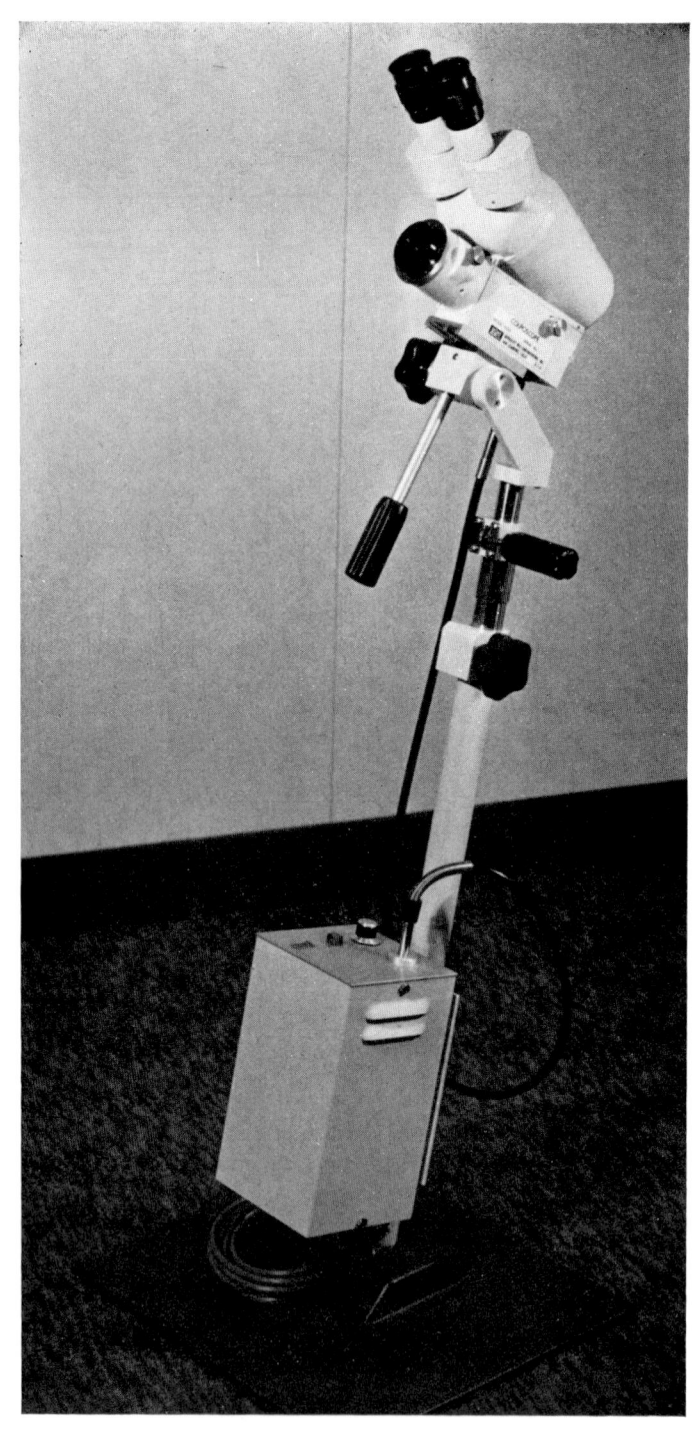

Figure 118. This model demonstrates the system of mounting of the colposcope on a tilting arm hinged to a heavy base. Photographic attachments are available on a larger model. Magnifications available are 12.5× and 16×. (Berkeley Bioengineering Inc., San Leandro, California)

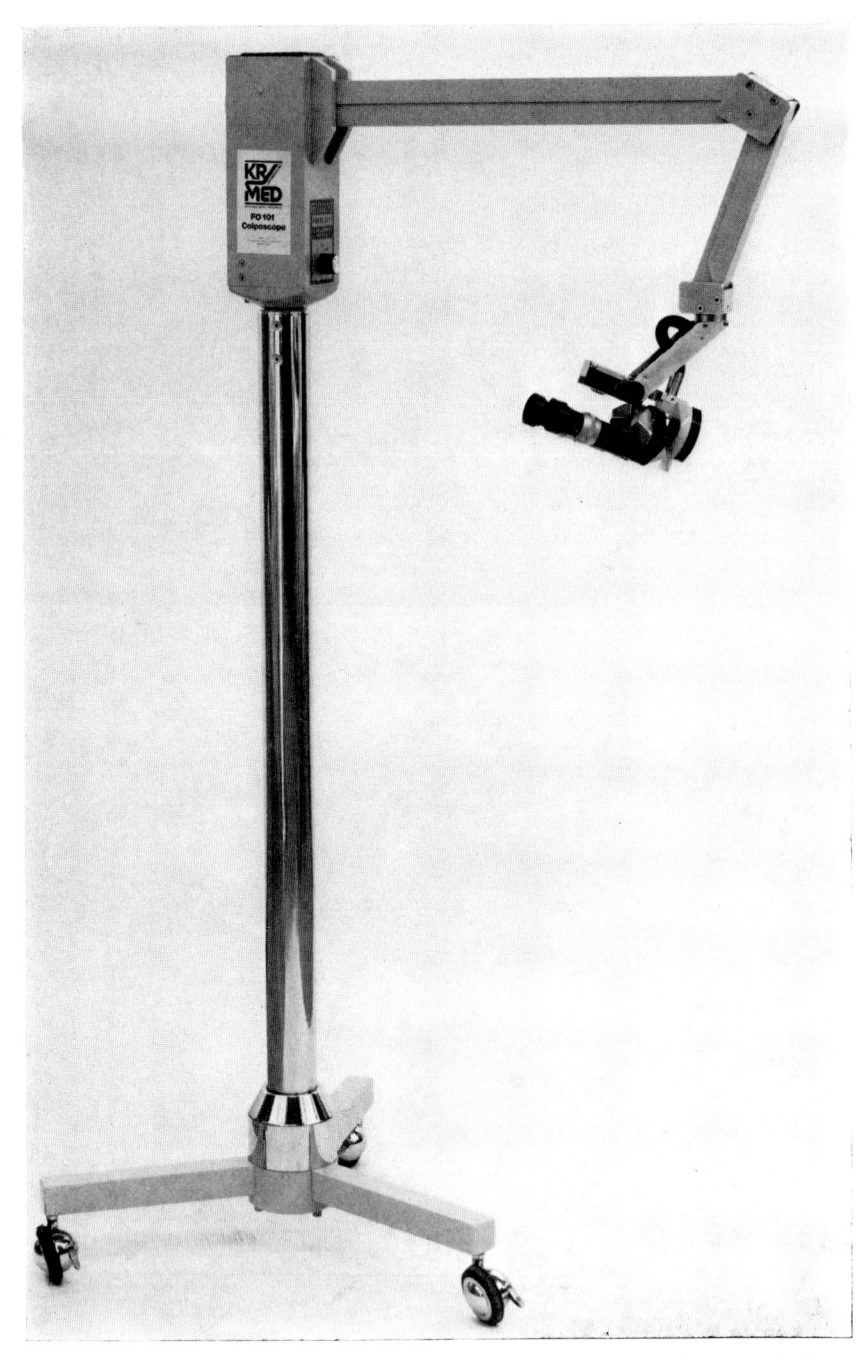

Figure 119. This model allows two mounting systems, wall and floor, and allows suspension of the colposcope above the observer. Magnifications are 10×, 13× and 16×. (Cryomedics Inc., Bridgeport, Connecticut)

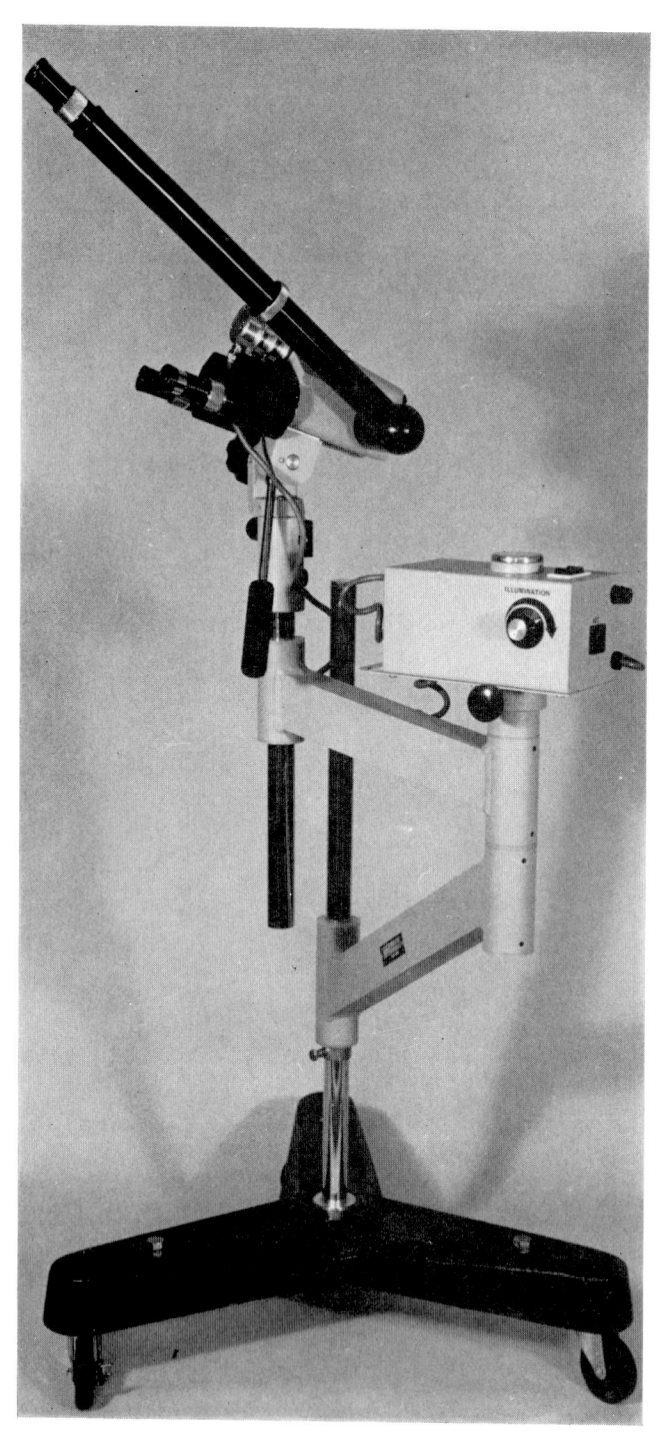

Figure 120. This colposcope illustrates a teaching attachment allowing simultaneous viewing by physician, consultant, or student. Photographic attachments are available. Magnification is 16×. Alternative oculars are available and allow magnification from 10× to 40×. (Frigi-scopes Inc., Shelton, Connecticut)

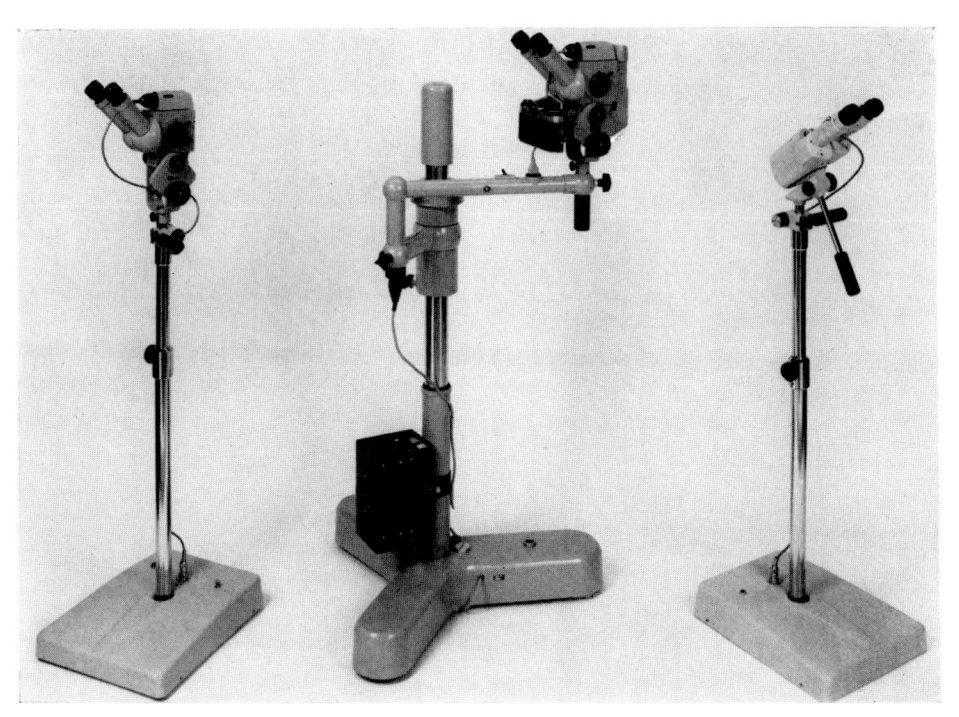

Figure 121. This illustration shows the Dynatech-Jena range of colposcopes. The two larger colposcopes have a built-in five-step magnification changer (5×, 8×, 12.5×, 20×, 32×). Most suppliers provide such a range, which allows the physician or hospital to choose a model to suit the individual requirements. (Dynatech Cryomedical Co., Burlington, Massachusetts)

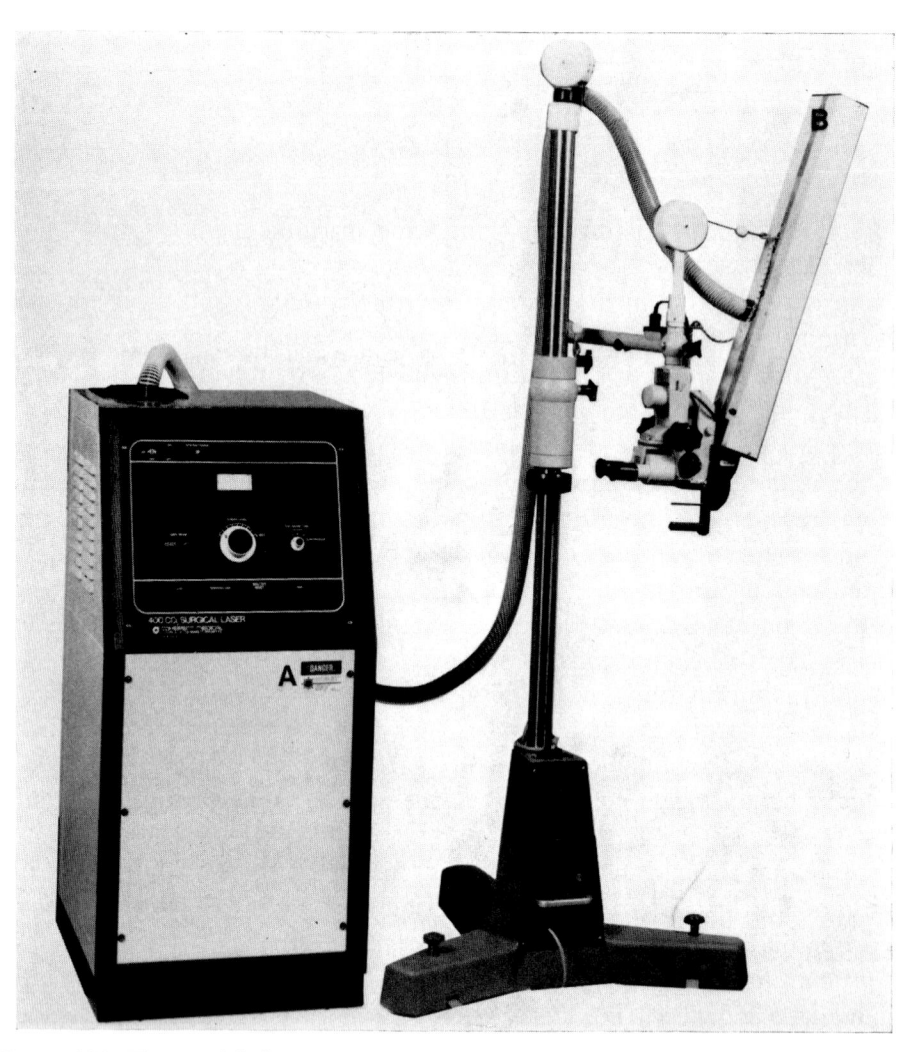

Figure 122. This model demonstrates a surgical laser unit attached to the Zeiss model 1 colposcope. (Coherent, Medical Division, Palo Alto, California, and Gynemed Inc., Palo Alto, California)

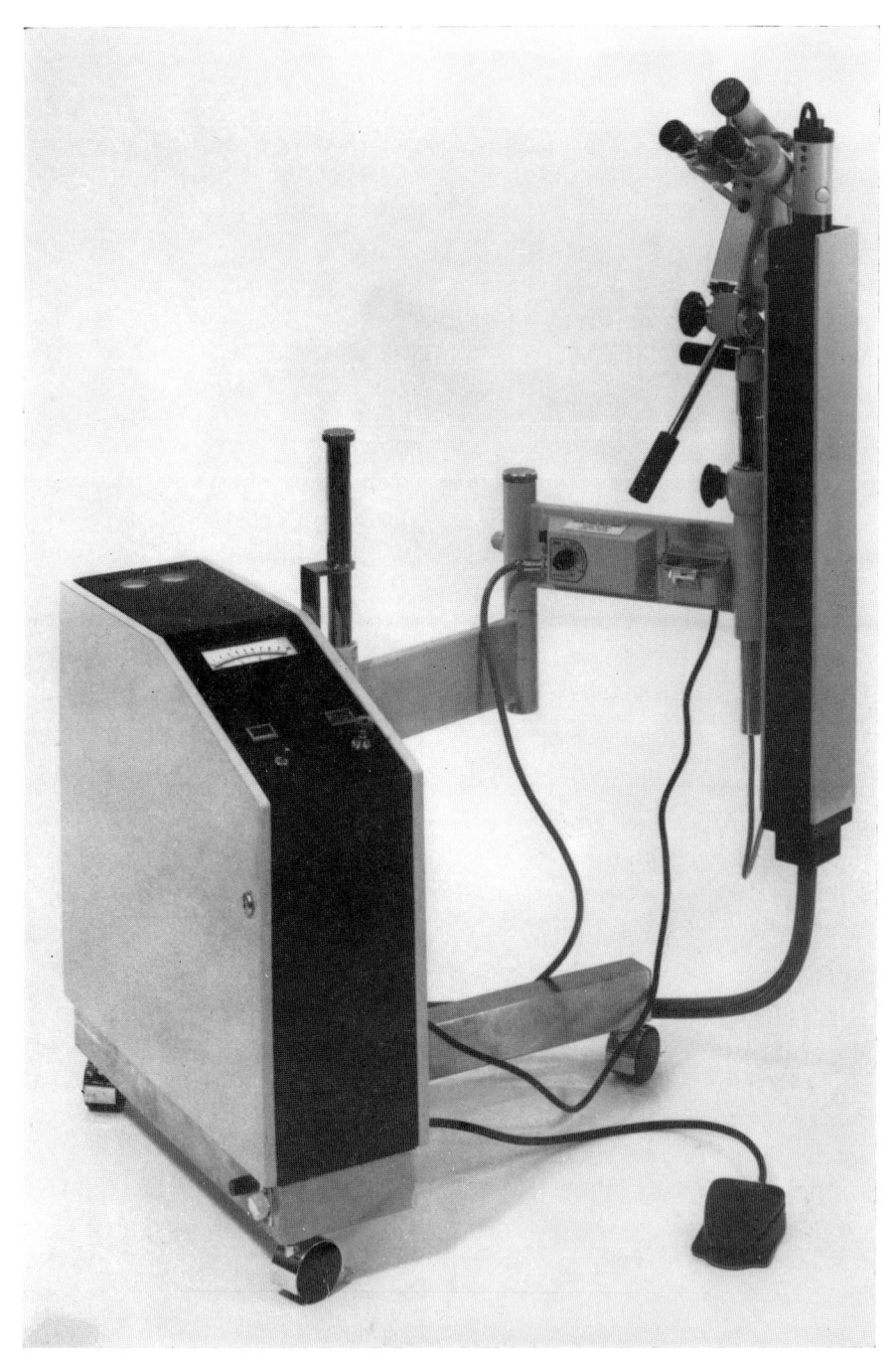

Figure 123. This colposcope (Gynetech-Toitu) is one of the range of instruments available. Various eyepieces allow magnifications of 6× to 20×. The laser device is attached, and a swing mount is illustrated. Photographic attachments are available. (Gyne-Tech Instrument Corporation, Burbank, California)

of the interpupillary distance of the eyepieces to suit the individual observer. At the start of each series of examinations, it is necessary to make this adjustment and to render the focus of the eyepiece lenses coincident so that optimal viewing is obtained.

The physician using an instrument for the first time should quickly develop an easy familiarity with the operation of the instrument. Before using a recently acquired instrument on patients, he should practice manipulating the controls upon a suitable object placed at the end of his examination couch.

OFFICE REQUIREMENTS

Great stress is given to the position of the patient and examiner for the colposcopic examination. The standard examination couch with stirrups used in most physicians' offices allows positioning of the patient in the dorsal position with exposure of the vulva and vaginal introitus. A means of tilting the patient to align the axis of the introduced vaginal speculum with the optical axis of the instrument is an advantage. A tray containing the speculae and other equipment required for the colposcopic examination should be within reach of the examiner (Fig. 124A and B).

EXPOSURE OF THE CERVIX

The choice of a range of self-retaining vaginal speculae is important. The metal varieties are superior to the disposable plastic types; those designed by Graves and Cusco are the most suitable. When colpophotography is contemplated, the disposable plastic design is best, since it offers fewer surfaces for reflection of the light source. These can cause light streaks on the exposure.

TECHNIQUE OF EXAMINATION

Following positioning of the patient, the appropriate vaginal speculum is slowly introduced. A lubricant is desirable and not contraindicated. The blades are separated soon after introduction, allowing exposure of the cervix. Eventually, they should be adjusted to expose as much of the cervix and upper vagina as possible. The taking of smears for cytological examination before colposcopy should be avoided. This point is further discussed (p. 396).

The colposcope is then placed in position to illuminate the cervix, advancing the objective lens to its approximate focal distance from the cervix so that the optical axis of the system coincides with the vaginal speculum. The optical system is then adjusted for the individual and the hand control used finally to position the instrument and bring the cervix into fine focus.

The nature of any discharge is noted. The cervix is lightly cleansed with

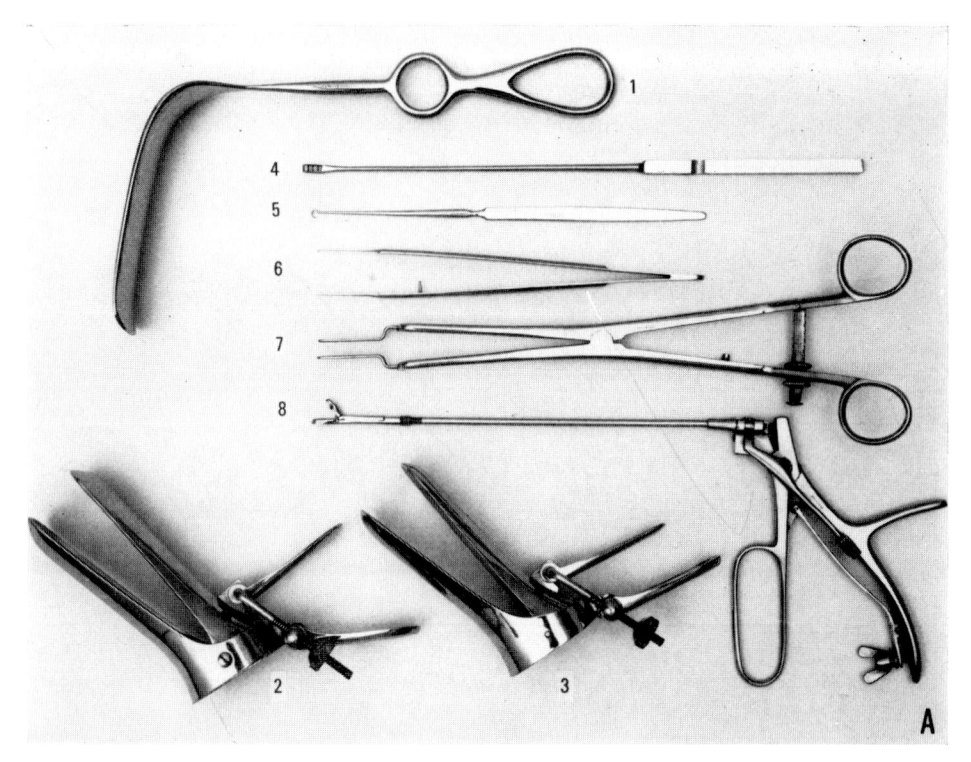

Figure 124A. Instruments for colposcopic examination: (1) Jackson's retractor, which assists exposure of the vagina and fornix in difficult cases. (2) Cusco's vaginal speculum, to be used mainly in the multiparous subject. The square end, though slightly more difficult to introduce exposes the cervix and vaginal vault to best advantage. (3) Cusco's vaginal speculum (medium) to be used in the nulliparous subject. (4) The Kevorkian endocervical curette for evaluation of the endocervix. It may also be used to sample the endometrium. (5) The iris hook, which is useful to steady an area for application of the punch biopsy forceps. (6) The fine rat-tooth forceps, used as in (5) above. (7) The endocervical speculum. Several designs, attributed to Kevorkian, Sims, and Chanen of Melbourne, enable the epithelium of the canal to be visualized. (8) The Eppendorfer biopsy forceps is preferred for critical sampling of the cervical epithelia.

a dry swab and its appearance evaluated with the unaided eye. Acetic acid application is then undertaken. During all of these stages, great care should be taken to avoid trauma, which can cause troublesome bleeding from both normal and abnormal areas.

PREPARATION OF THE CERVIX

Careful atraumatic cleansing of the cervix is an essential prelude to the colposcopic evaluation. Hinselmann (1955), in his empirical search for mucolytic preparations, found a dilute solution of acetic acid in water (2%-4%) to be satisfactory. In addition, this solution evokes a change in colour

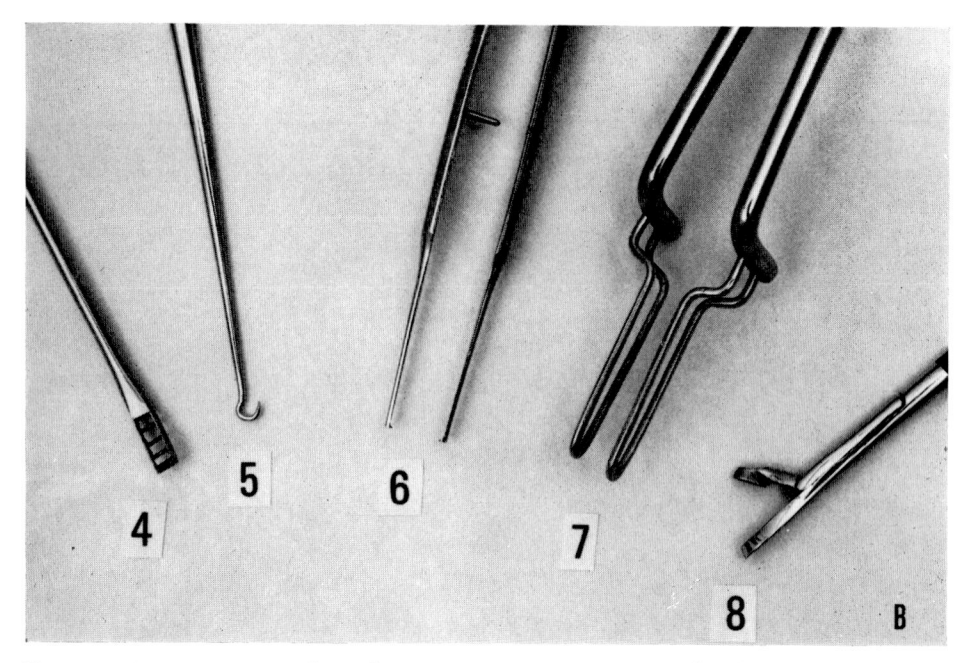

Figure 124B. Instruments for colposcopic examination. Finer detail of some of the instruments presented in Figure 124A.

tone of epithelium, which is extremely useful in categorising the types of epithelium present. Koller (1963) and Kolstad (1964) rely on preparation with a solution of normal saline. Ideally, the cervix should be prepared first with saline, examined, and then re-examined following application with dilute acetic acid. Our preference is for the acetic acid technique, as we think it superior in allowing appreciation of detailed surface morphology and in its evocation of the colour changes in atypical epithelia.

Acetic Acid Application

The acetic acid solution is initially applied with a standard cotton-wool ball or swab. It should be liberal in amount and carefully applied by soaking rather than rubbing, to avoid any degree of trauma. Usually all but the most tenacious cervical mucus undergoes changes which allow its removal from the surface structures. In pregnant subjects and those using combined oestrogen-progestogen contraceptive preparations, the mucus is most resistant to change, and repeated application and cleansing is often necessary. Mucus within the endocervical canal is best removed with a cotton-wool-tipped applicator. Occasionally, it is necessary to draw out the mucus plug and sever it with a biopsy forceps.

The minutiae of surface morphology become immediately evident, but the evanescent colour changes take a variable amount of time to develop. Columnar epithelium becomes pale and its villous and papillary character strikingly evident. More importantly, squamous epithelia which are nonglycogenated, less than well differentiated, or keratotic are rendered opaque, pale, or white; this appearance emerges in areas not previously distinguishable. The change boldly etches the site of atypical transformation zone within which the precursors of cancer are found. The physician may have to wait up to two minutes for the change to occur, and tissues resume their normal colour after several minutes. Frequently, it is necessary to apply further acetic acid to sustain the changes. A freshly prepared solution appears to be important in eliciting this series of changes in surface and colour morphology. During extended examinations in live teaching sessions, which involve frequent acetic acid application, there is a gradual emergence of traumatic and inflammatory appearances in response to chemical injury.

The Saline Technique

In most circumstances, mucus can be adequately cleansed from the surface epithelia with normal saline solution. This allows close evaluation of the vascular structures and original colour variations. The method is essential to the technique of colpophotography detailed in the monographs by Koller (1963) and Kolstad (1964). Such studies involve the use of an object lens of 12.5-cm focal length and specially adapted vaginal speculae, in order to produce a high degree of resolution and contrast on special photographic emulsion. These requirements cannot be applied to standard clinical practice, in which standard lens and speculae are used.

COLPOSCOPY OF THE ECTOCERVIX AND ENDOCERVIX

Systematic evaluation can now start. Essentially, the purpose of colposcopic examination of the cervix is to determine the presence and extent of the transformation zone. This can be fulfilled in most subjects by scanning the surface circumferentially to define the original squamocolumnar junction, which is usually visible. Within its boundary, the character of the transformation zone can be determined. In most subjects, the new squamocolumnar junction or upper limit of the transformation zone can be seen, whether ecto- or endocervical (Fig. 125). In discussion on topography, we have already emphasized the effect of the bivalve speculum, which effectively reveals a useful portion of the endocervical canal epithelia (*see* Figs. 3, 43, and 44).

The colposcopic examination which fails to identify the upper limit of the transformation zone, the new squamocolumnar junction, is termed *unsatisfactory*, for it may contain the area of most significance. For those subjects in whom this junction remains obscured, techniques have evolved which can at times display the junction and allow further evaluation of the canal epithelia.

It is helpful to use a cotton-tipped applicator to evert the canal further. The posterior portion of the canal can often be exposed by pushing the applicator into the posterior vaginal fornix (Fig. 126A and B).

In those instances where the transformation zone extends far into the canal, the endocervical speculum is of value (Fig. 127). Examples of this instrument include the Kogan and Chanen models. At times most, if not all the cervical canal may be seen. Traumatic bleeding sometimes results, especially as one attempts to remove tenacious mucus from the canal.

Some authorities recommend endocervical curettage with either Kevorkian's, Sims', or Chanen's endocervical curettes to provide material for histological examination, especially when colposcopic examination has been indecisive. This is fully discussed later (p. 414).

Examination of the cervix is completed by allowing the blades of the speculum to collapse so that the real (p. 17) view of the cervix can be seen and recorded. Much of what has been exposed, the apparent view, is seen to revert to its endocervical situation (*see* Figs. 3, 43, and 44).

COLPOSCOPY OF THE VAGINA

Systematic examination of the lower genital tract is completed during withdrawal of the speculum. Adequate evaluation may tax the dexterity of the examining physician and the subject's patience. This has become a special problem in young girls who have become exposed *in utero* to nonsteroidal oestrogens. Generally, by exposing the upper vagina widely and retracting with applicators and additional instruments, a full view can be obtained.

SCHILLER'S IODINE SOLUTION

The application of iodine solution to depict areas likely to contain cervical intraepithelial neoplasia is well established and is used by many gynaecologists (Fig. 128). Its basis is largely determined by the response of fully differentiated squamous epithelium which, due to its glycogen content, stains deeply with the iodine and is designated generally as iodine-positive. Most other forms of epithelia, including columnar, immature metaplastic epithelium, cervical intraepithelial neoplasia, and colposcopically overt and clinically overt cancer usually fail to stain and are recognised as iodine-negative. Regenerating epithelium occurring after electrocautery, electrodiathermy, and cryosurgery gives a variable stain response.

Iodine should not be applied immediately prior to colposcopic examination, for it almost totally obscures morphological detail. It may be used to confirm the site and extent of atypical transformation zone prior to undertaking biopsy. In particular, the technique should be employed in the

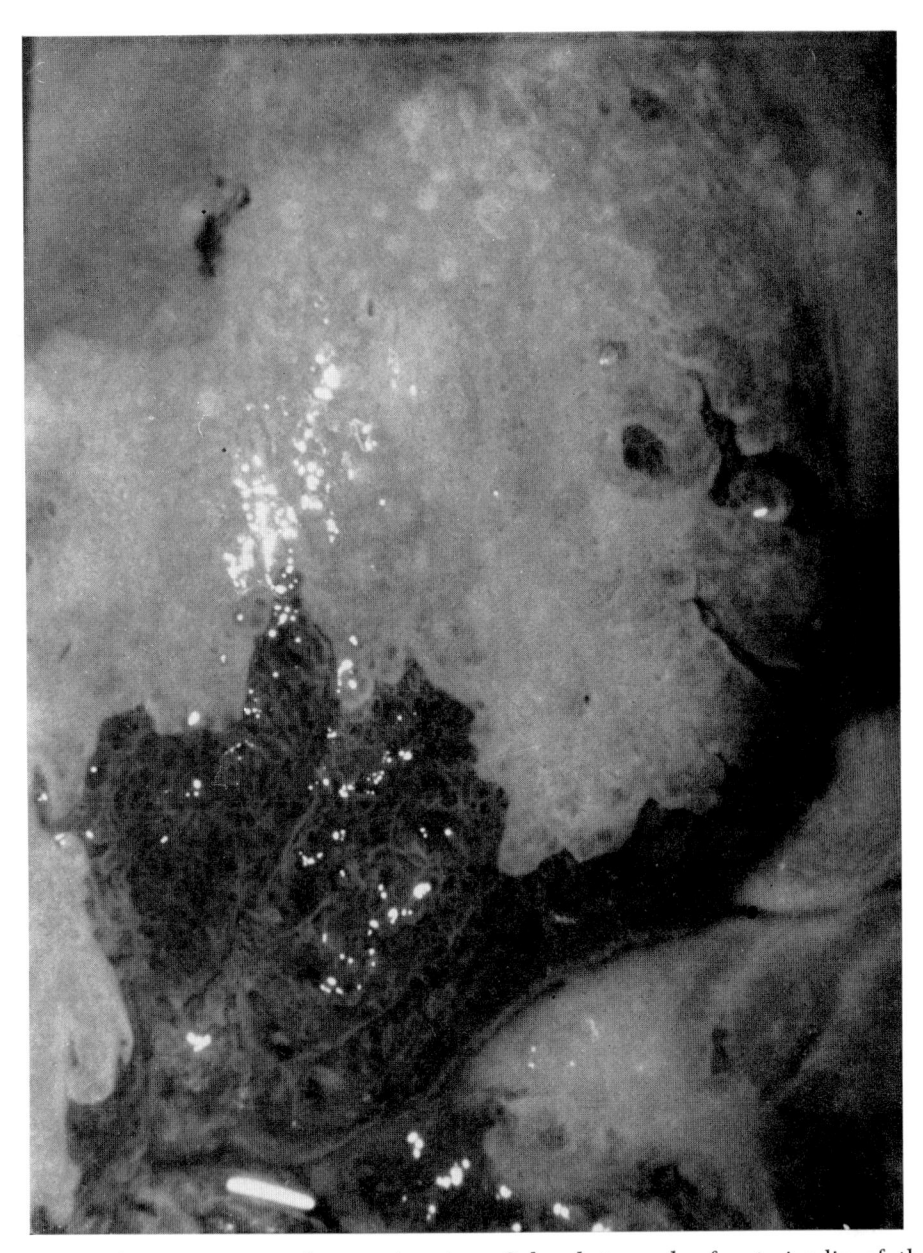

Figure 125. New squamocolumnar junction: Colpophotograph of anterior lip of the cervix with cervical canal running diagonally across the lower right quadrant of the photograph. Both limits of an atypical transformation zone are seen; the cephalad limit in the middle of the photograph adjoins columnar epithelium at the new squamocolumnar junction. This latter junction was equally well displayed on the posterior lip by minimal eversion with the speculum. In such cases, the colposcopic examination is termed *satisfactory*.

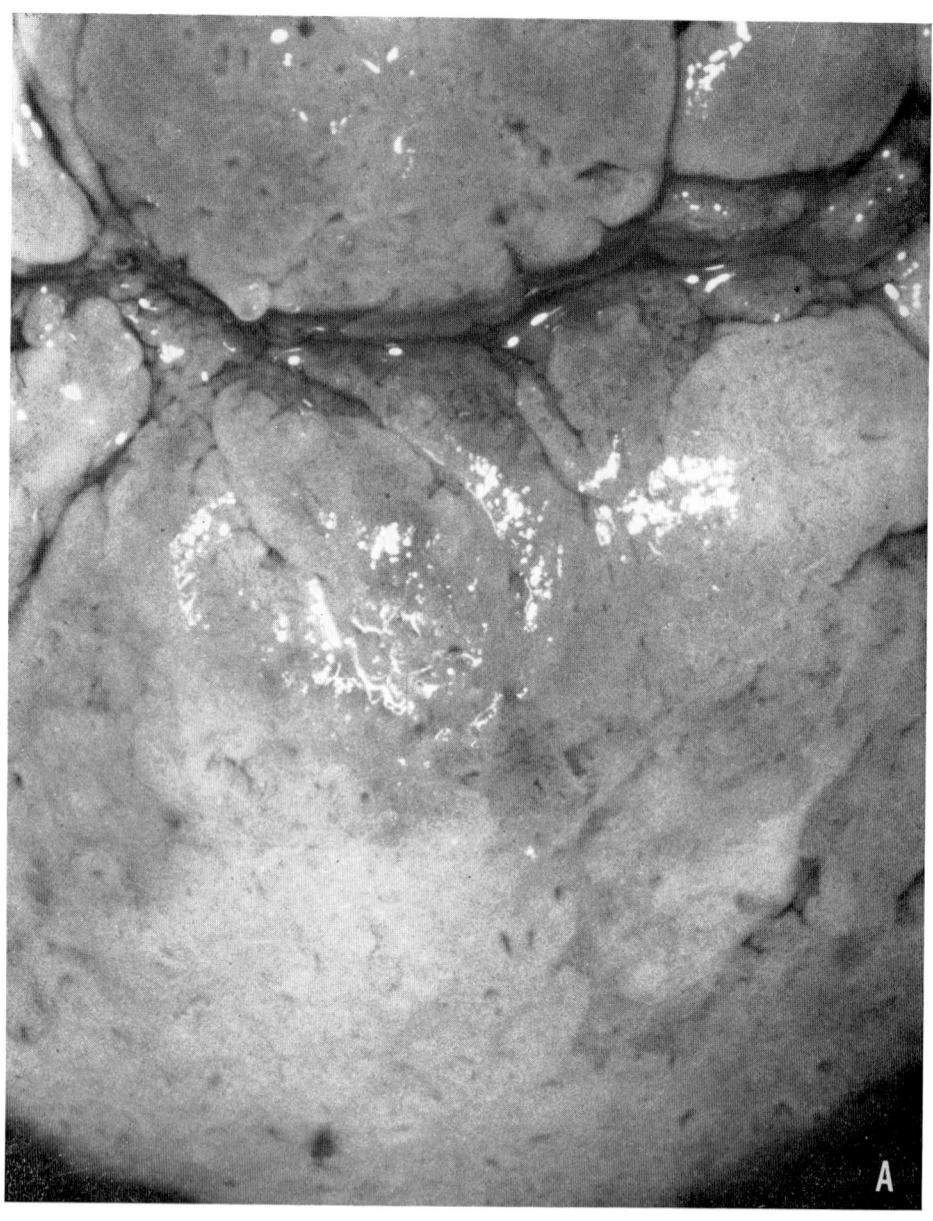

Figure 126A. In apparently *unsatisfactory* colposcopic examinations, eversion with the vaginal speculum may fail to expose the new squamocolumnar junction.

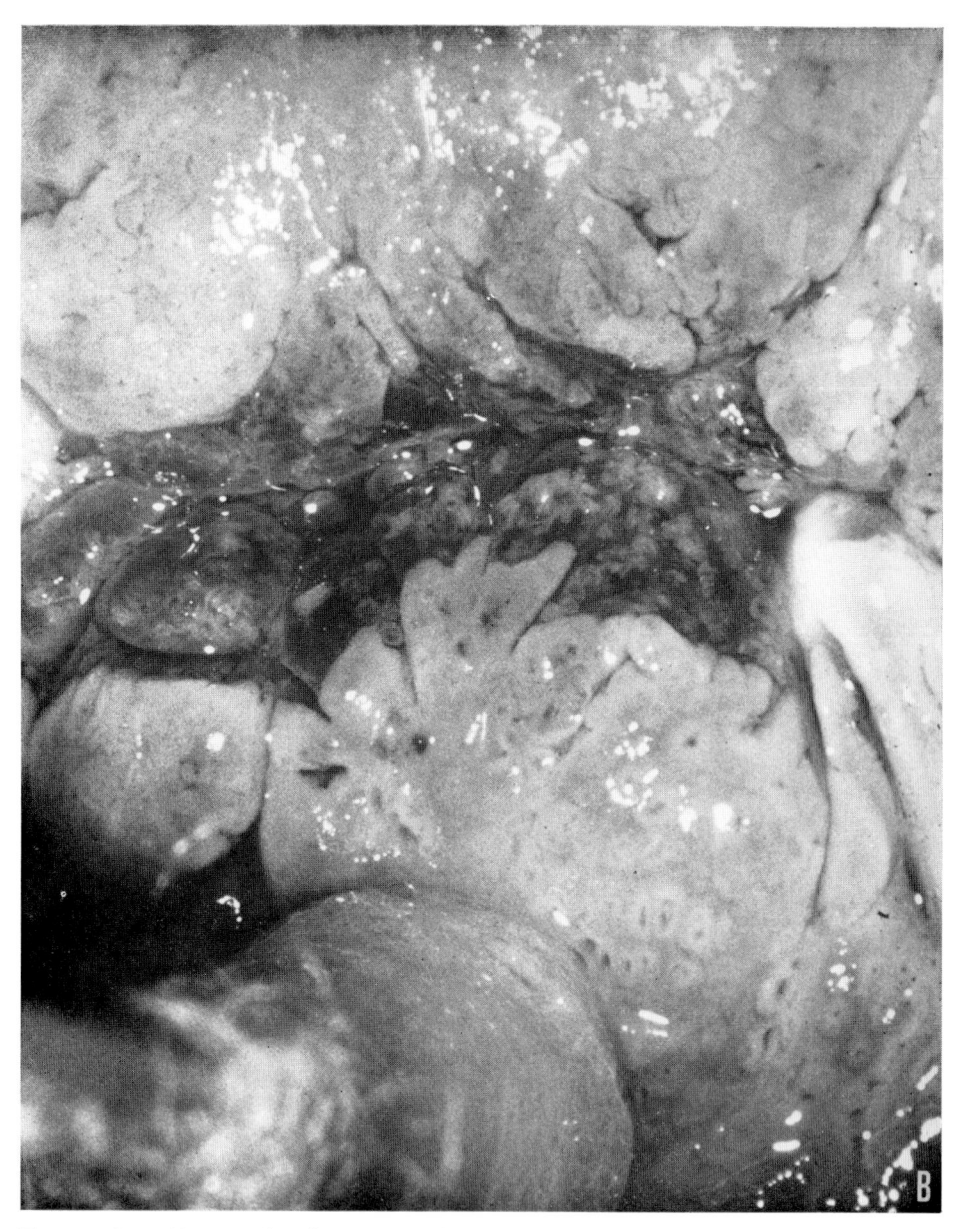

Figure 126B. Frequently, distraction of either cervical lip with a cotton-tipped applicator (seen in the bottom of the photograph) reveals the new squamocolumnar junction.

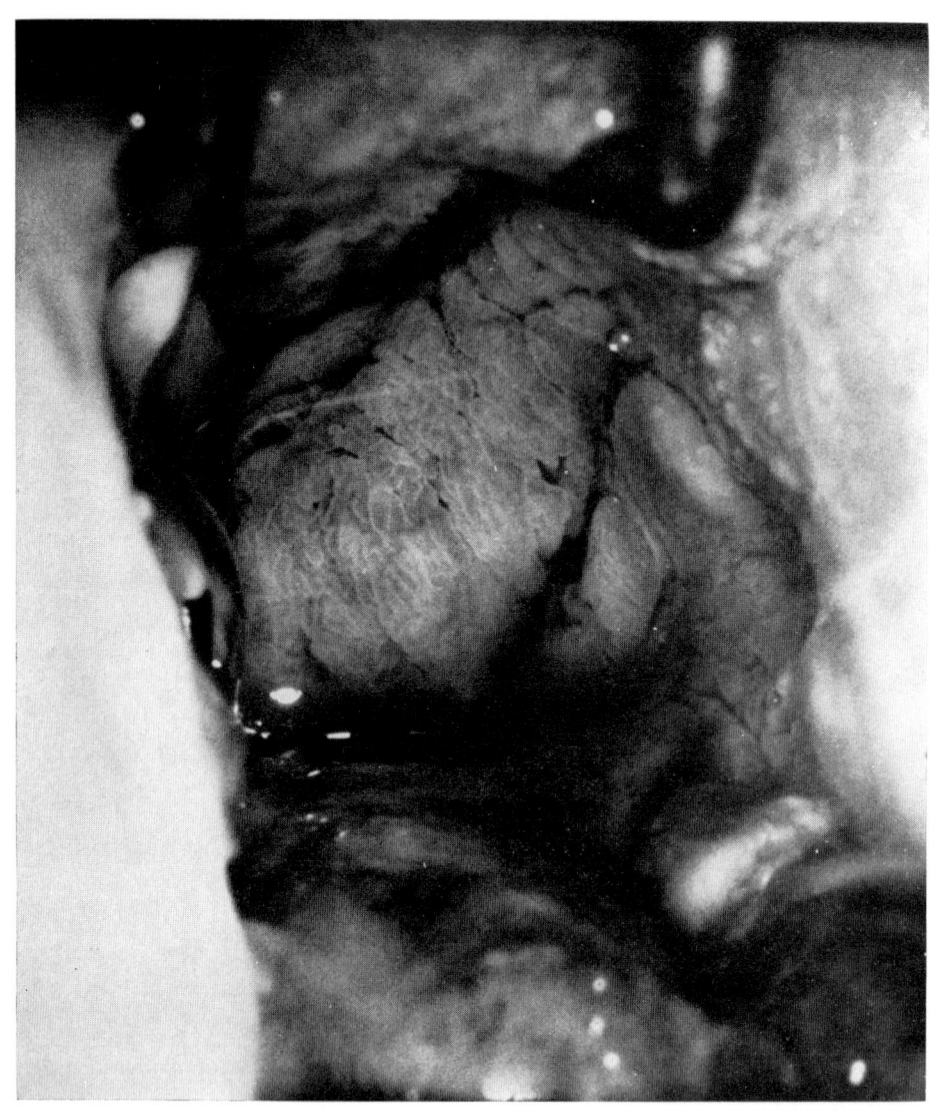

Figure 127. The endocervical speculum. Epithelia of the endocervical canal and the new squamocolumnar junction are revealed in many cases by the use of this instrument. In this picture, the blades expose columnar epithelium deep in the cervical canal.

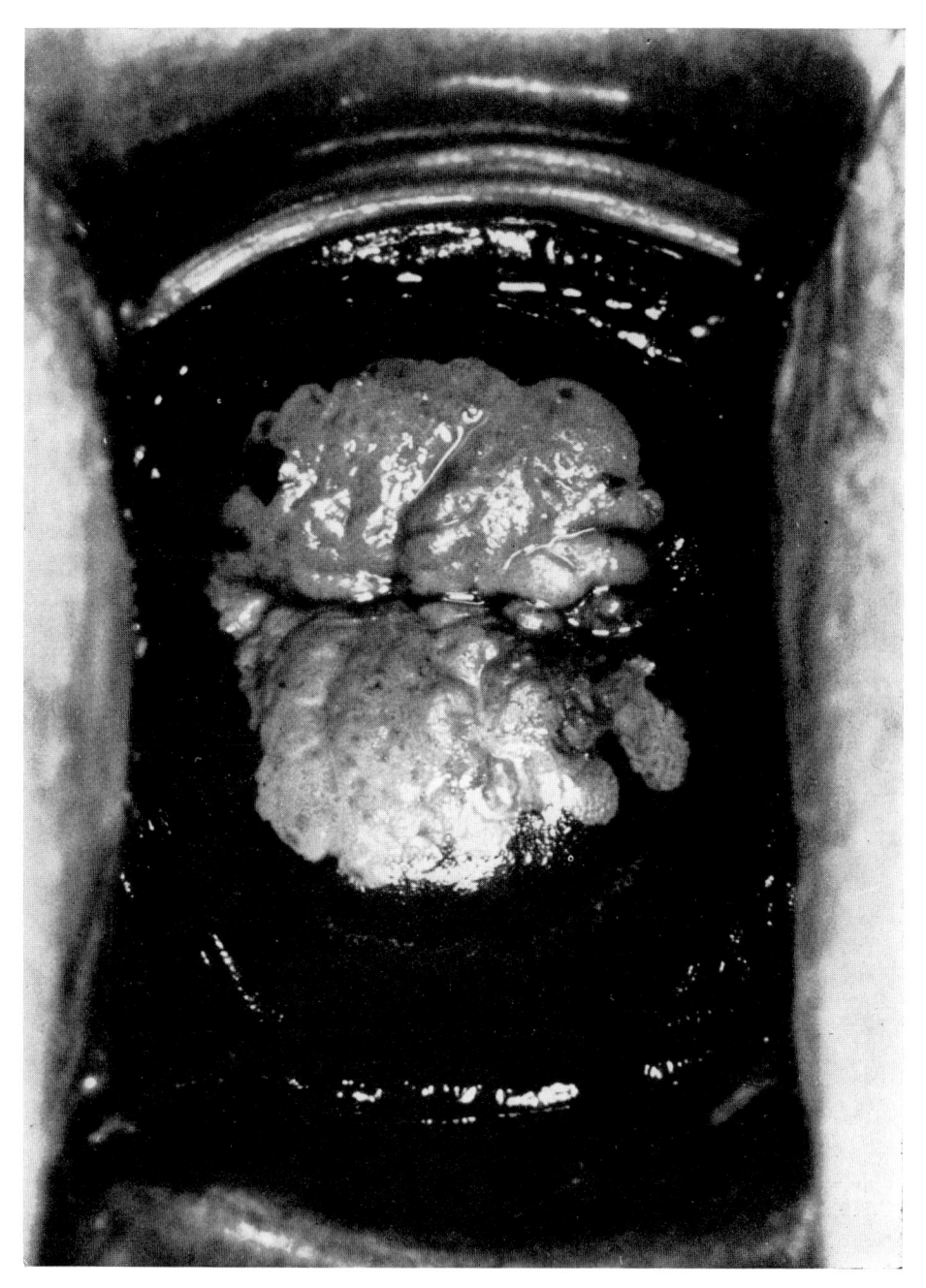

Figure 128. Schiller's iodine solution. This technique is of most value in delineating the limits of excision for conisation or eradication of lesions by physical destruction.

operating room prior to making the annular incision on the cervix to start a conisation procedure. Occasionally, it is useful to distinguish between certain inflammatory disorders and punctation (p. 278). Schiller's solution should be applied at the end of colposcopic examination in order to correlate both methods of examination.

A reliable iodine solution contains 300 g iodine, 6 g potassium iodide, and up to 1,000 ml distilled water.

BIOPSY INSTRUMENTS

The technique and indications for cone, wedge, and colposcopically directed biopsy and for endocervical curettage are discussed later (*see* Chap. 16). Several instruments have become standard for the latter procedures (*see* Fig. 124A and B). The Eppendorfer, the Kevorkian, and the Yeoman varieties are most commonly used for punch biopsy and the Kevorkian and Sims for endocervical curettage.

The iris hook and the slightly longer Emmett tenaculum are valuable aids to accurate punch biopsy. The cervix may be painlessly transfixed and selected areas steadied as the biopsy forceps are employed. Use of the hook generally enables a good bite to be obtained, for occasionally the biopsy instrument, especially if not sharp, slips off the desired site. Bleeding is usually minimal but may be controlled by the application of Monsel's Solution® (ferric subsulphate) or, if necessary, by insertion of a vaginal tampon for a few hours.

RECORDING OF COLPOSCOPIC FINDINGS

The recording of colposcopic appearances is an essential part of the procedure. The variety of individual requirements dictated by the nature of a gynecologist's practice or the demands of an institute or department does not allow a standardised approach. There are differences between a written report on diagnosis, prognosis, and projected therapy and a data-collecting device suitable for research which seem irreconcilable. We have used a complicated system (Fig. 129A and B) but now have reverted to a simple verbal and diagram report, which is intended later to be based on photography. An example may read, "atypical transformation zone, Grade II with white epithelium and punctation consistent with a diagnosis of carcinoma in situ or major dysplasia. Columnar epithelium is visible in the canal, and the lesion is suitable for colposcopically directed punch biopsy and eradication by electrodiathermy under anaesthesia or cryosurgery." The appropriate area is hatched on the diagram of the cervix. Such reports are purely for communication between clinicians and for inclusion in clinical notes.

HISTOLOGY RECORD No.	WARD or DEPT.
BACTERIOLOGY RECORD No.	
PHOTOGRAPHIC RECORD No.	RECORD No.
DISPOSAL:	SURNAME
a. Follow Up e. Diathermy	CHRISTIAN NAMES
b. Conization	STREET
c. Hysterectomy	TOWN
d. Radical	PUBLIC ☐
	PRIVATE ☐

COLPOSCOPIC REPORT

Signature..

Figure 129A

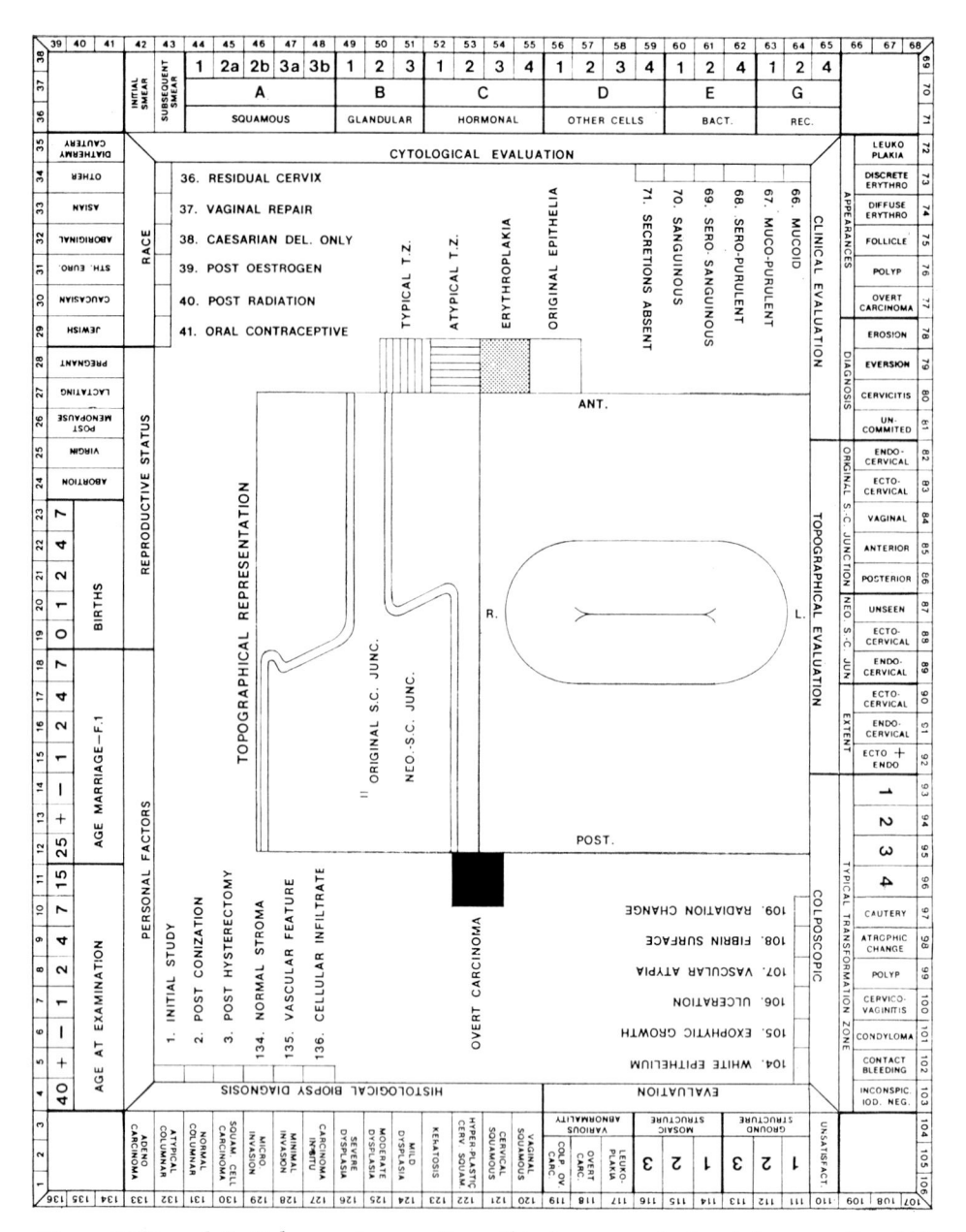

Figure 129A and B. Colposcopic recording. This form was designed for reporting (A) and recording (B). In practise, this form has proved unsatisfactory and has been replaced by a simple description and diagram as described in the text.

Colpophotography

Still Photography

Recording of colposcopic appearances has contributed substantially to the development of the concept of the cervical epithelia now available. Transmission of these concepts has largely been achieved through demonstration of colour transparencies exposed during routine clinical practice. At present, the large library of appearances recorded in many centres offers the best exposure to the colposcopic morphology the learner can have. Excellent sets of teaching slides for both monocular and stereoscopic viewing are available. Recent advances in photographic chemistry allow direct colour prints to be made from transparencies, which then become available for inclusion in record systems. It has been our experience that Kodachrome® transparencies are superior to all other available products. Black-and-white prints do not convey colour characteristics but are most suitable for recording fine detail of angioarchitecture, using the special lenses in the techniques of Koller and Kolstad. Polaroid® systems have recently been introduced. Recording of appearances with colour print systems have proved disappointing in the poor resolution obtained.

Careful selection of subjects and detailed preparation of the cervix are important in obtaining good photographic record. Undoubtedly, certain subjects display cervical morphology that is bold and photographs well. Women using sequential contraceptive preparations invariably provide the best photographic results. Our library is composed of a selection made from many thousands of exposures, many disappointing, and the physician entering the field cannot expect invariably to achieve a good result.

Cinematography

At many conferences, outstanding colour films demonstrating the essentials of colposcopic technique and morphology have been shown. These have served as excellent introductory teaching enterprises for physicians attending courses.

Television

In some North American centres, the advantages of television display systems are being exploited with great success. The image transmitted can be stored on video tape and displayed to small groups on standard television screens or to large groups when projected. Television is becoming an important resource for teaching.

PART IV

Colposcopic Morphology

Chapter 7

COLPOSCOPIC APPEARANCES OF THE ORIGINAL EPITHELIA

THE ORIGINAL EPITHELIA represent a residual embryological contribution to the covering of the ectocervix and lining of the endocervical canal of the adult. Their morphological features are important in the understanding of the more significant neosquamous epithelia of metaplastic origin.

ORIGINAL SQUAMOUS EPITHELIUM

Continuous with and nearly identical to the stratified squamous epithelium of the vagina is the original squamous epithelium. From a purely colposcopic viewpoint, this is the least important and variable of the epithelia to be described. It is not subject to the process we have postulated to be the precursor of squamous cancer. It is, however, most evidently affected by vaginal infections and variations in hormonal levels. For these reasons its disorders become significant, especially to the exfoliative cytologist.

Origin

Colposcopic entities are established during the middle months of intrauterine existence. In all specimens, recognisable original squamous epithelium is seen lining the vagina and various portions of the cervical surface.

Prime Morphological Features

Topography

The extent of the original squamous epithelium on the cervical surface is inversely proportional to the contribution of the columnar and metaplastic epithelia. When the original squamocolumnar junction is observed near the vaginal fornix, only a small portion of this epithelium is evident, whereas in other cervices, the whole of the ectocervix is original squamous in origin and is coextensive with similar epithelium within the lowermost portion of the canal (Fig. 130). The most common type of cervix, however, exhibits amounts of this and the other types of epithelium on the ectocervix (Fig. 131).

Colour

Original squamous epithelium presents a characteristic pinkish hue that is paler than that of the metaplastic epithelium and contrasts markedly with the darker red of columnar epithelium. Variations in colour are seen principally in inflammatory states, and paler shades are characteristic of the oestrogen-deprived postmenopausal era and of thick epithelium. Occasionally, a pale stippling is seen (Fig. 132).

Surface Configuration

Original squamous epithelium is smooth and featureless and, at or near the reflection onto the vaginal surface, gradually assumes the rugose character of the vagina. This is most characteristic of the reproductive and postmenopausal years.

Angioarchitecture

Examination of original squamous epithelium for vascular patterns reveals little variation and is often unrewarding, as the epithelium may be opaque and obscure all but major vessels (Fig. 130).

When the capillary pattern is evident, two fairly characteristic arrangements are seen, and both may coexist. Fine-calibre capillary loops reach towards the surface. Situated in fingerlike papillae, these are single loops sometimes twisted, disposed both obliquely and perpendicularly to the surface (Fig. 133). A fine, punctate appearance is evident when such vessels are seen end-on (Fig. 131). When papillae are absent, no intraepithelial vessels are apparent, and the second common pattern is then evident. This consists of a fine network of capillaries beneath the epithelium (Fig. 134), and deeper vessels serving this capillary bed may be seen branching terminally (Fig. 135).

THE COLUMNAR EPITHELIUM

The columnar epithelium zone of the uterine cervix exhibits perhaps the greatest variation in its colposcopic features, yet within its range of variation is invariably characteristic. Some portions of it, including its cephalic limits and those lying deep in the cervical stroma, are not seen by colposcopic examination. The general structure of the cervical columnar epithelium is the architectural framework upon which the metaplastic covering develops. An understanding of this tissue is, therefore, a prerequisite for a proper appreciation of the metaplastic epithelium and in turn for the behaviour of squamous dysplasia and preclinical carcinoma. This folded sheet of mucus-secreting epithelium is found in its manifold variations in areas clinically determined to be erosion, pseudoerosion, cervicitis, and ectopy. It is puzzling that such normal and highly functional tissue continues to be described by so many as abnormal, the eradication of which becomes a therapeutic objective. Our appreciation of the distribution of this epithelium holds that it is partly ectocervical in a majority of instances and that this observation renders the adjective *ectopic* invalid. We recognise it in its variations as the cervical columnar epithelium.

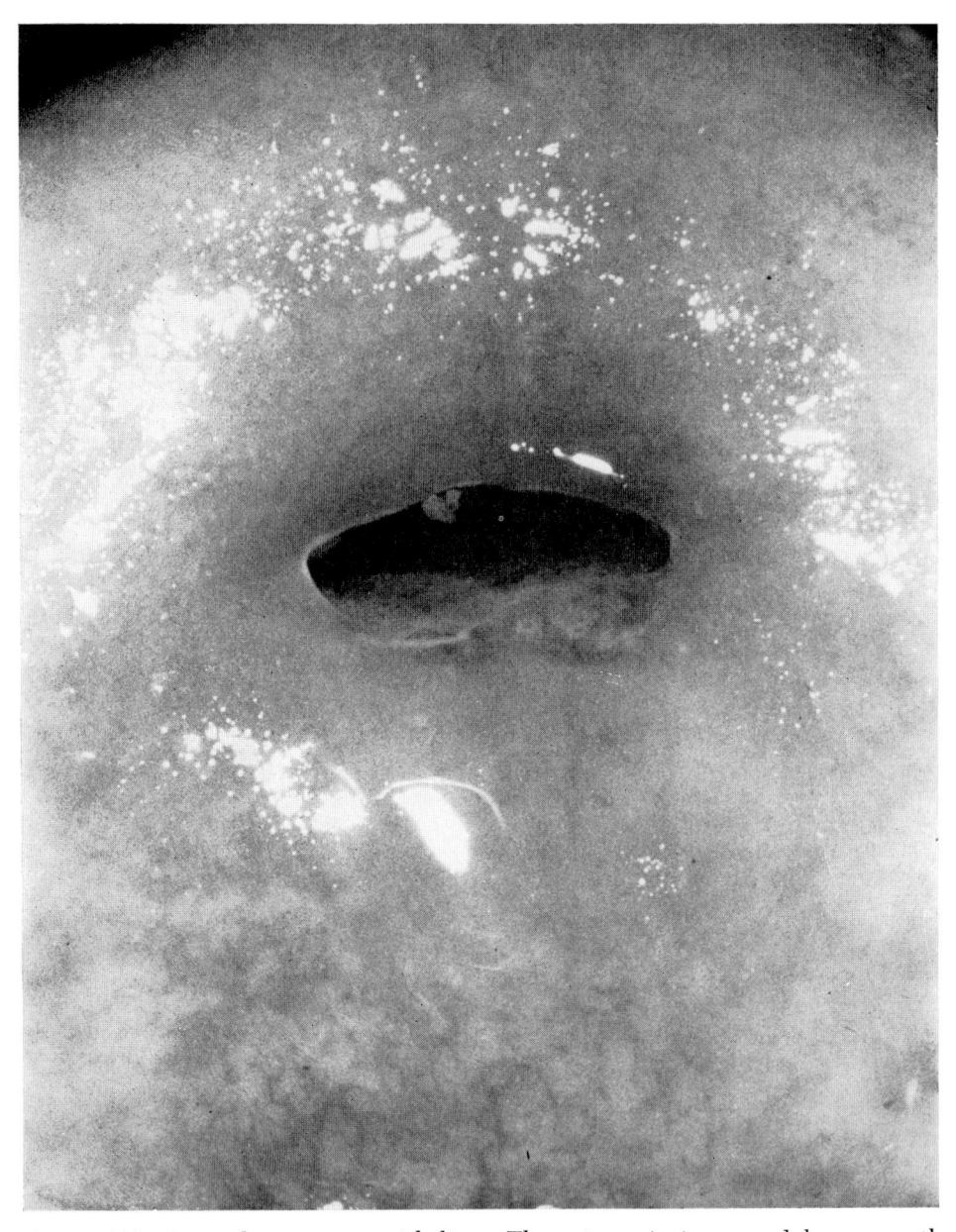

Figure 130. Original squamous epithelium. The ectocervix is covered by a smooth featureless epithelium that reaches to the central external os. Few distinct vascular markings are seen, but there are many light reflexes, presumably from high points. Within the endocervical canal, the small typical transformation zone is seen on the posterior wall.

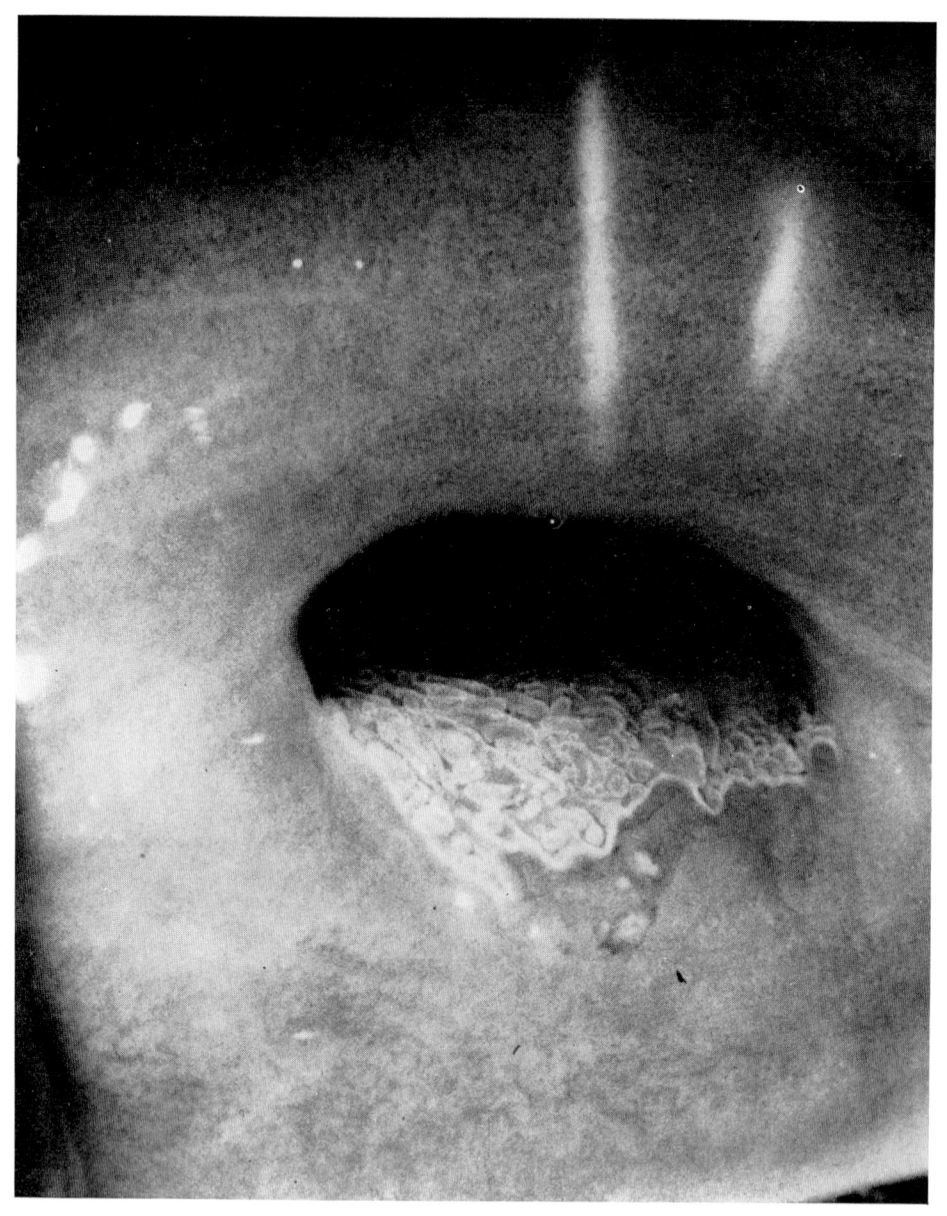

Figure 131. Original squamous epithelium. Most of the ectocervix shown in the photograph exhibits the characteristic smooth surface. Minute looped capillaries are clearly seen on the anterior lip. Posteriorly, a small typical transformation zone, with some columnar epithelium, forms part of the ectocervical covering.

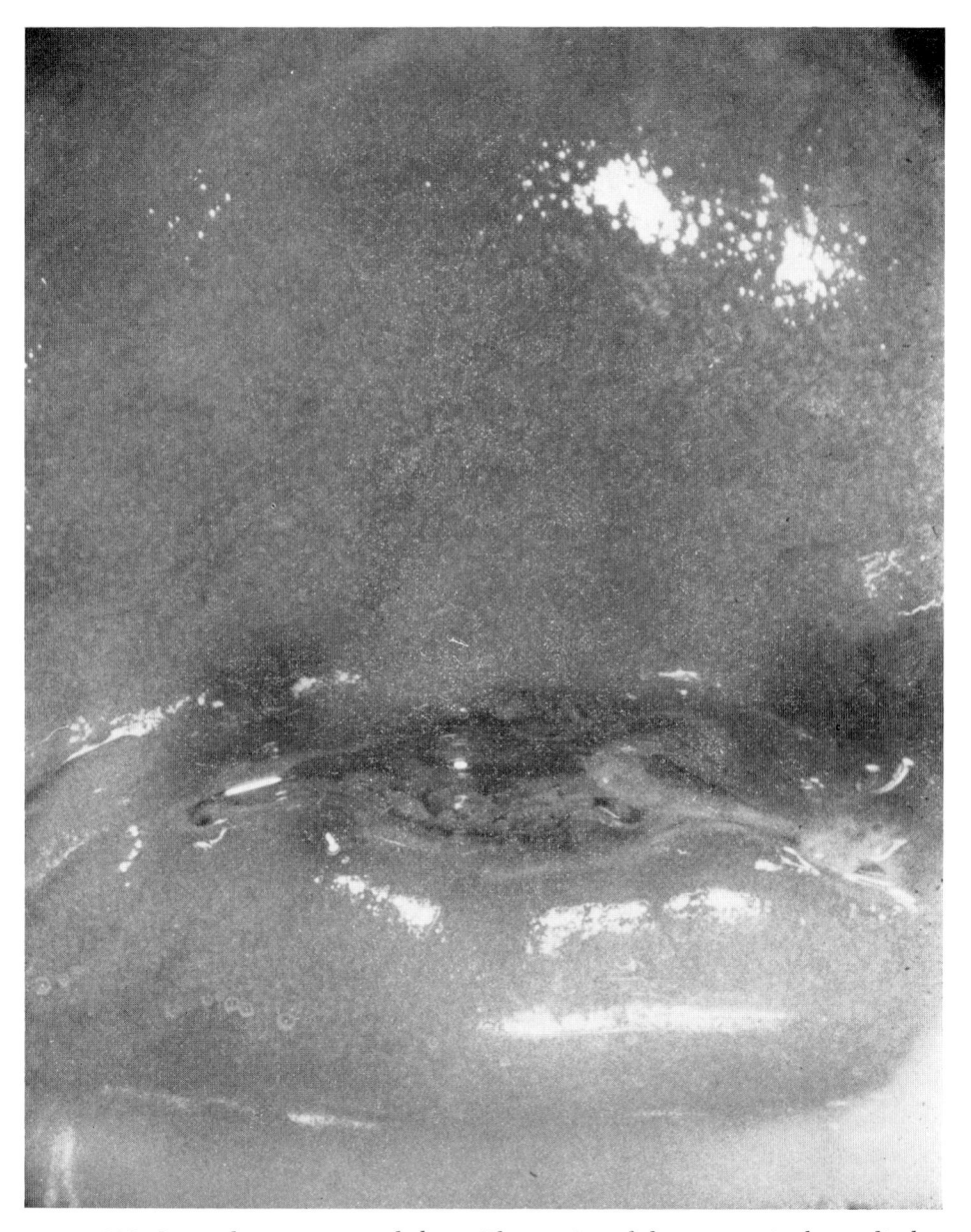

Figure 132. Original squamous epithelium. The portion of the ectocervix shown displays original squamous epithelium which appears stippled. Such stippling probably represents stromal papillae containing inconspicuous vessels.

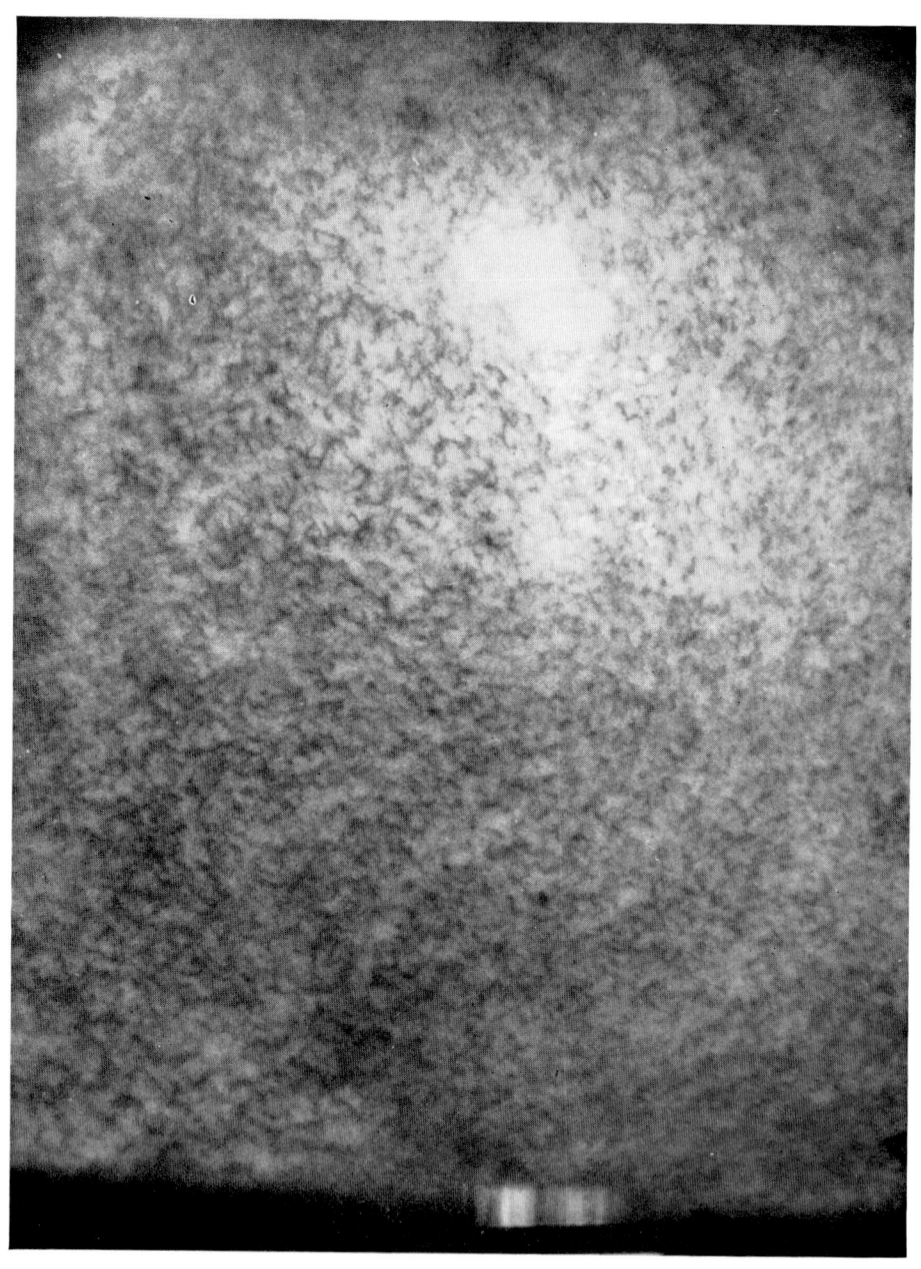

Figure 133. Original squamous epithelium. Angioarchitecture. The vascular structures depicted on this small portion of the anterior lip constitute a dense arrangement of terminal capillary loops, each of which courses upwards through the stratified epithelium within the core of a stromal papilla.

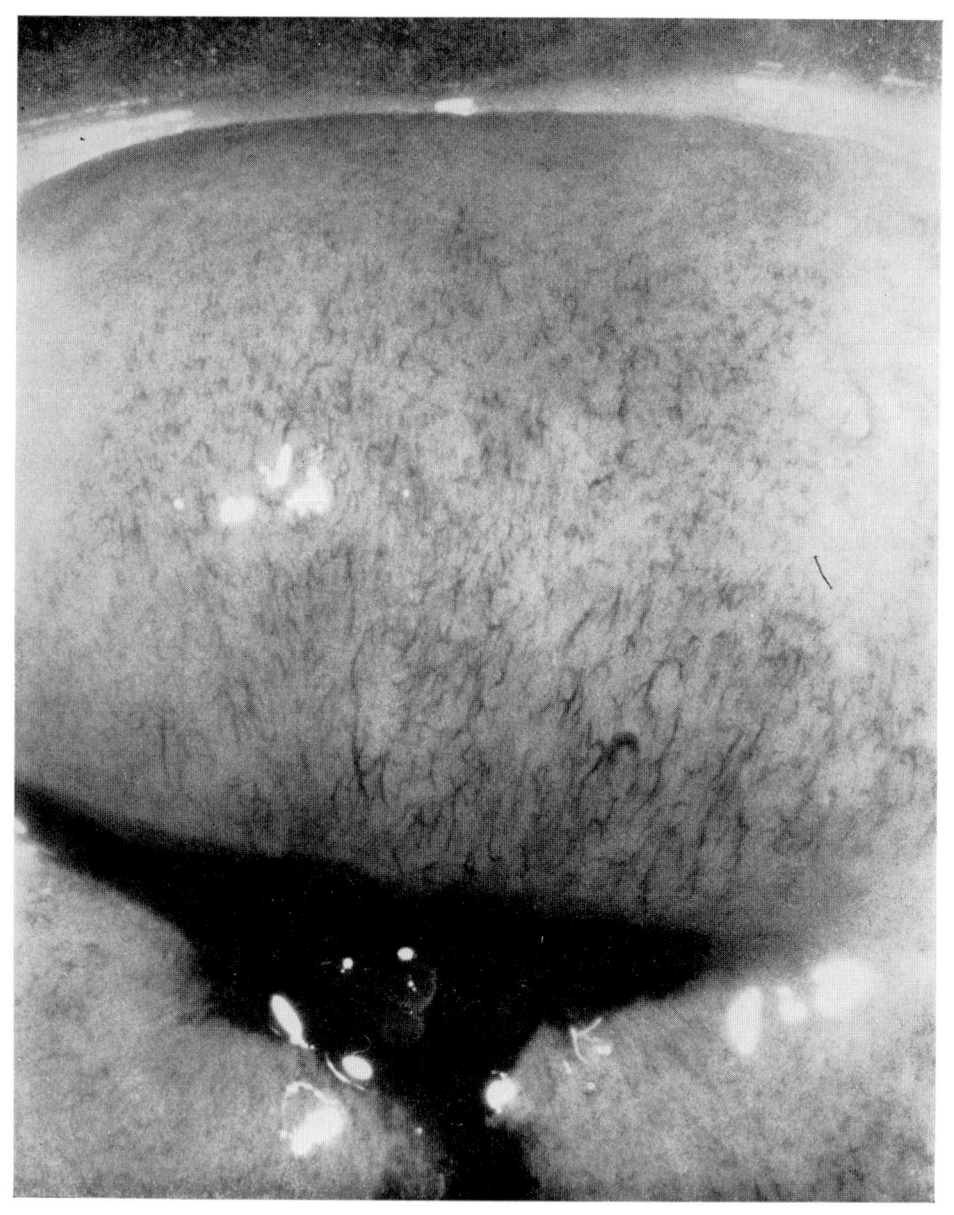

Figure 134. Original squamous epithelium. Angioarchitecture. Intradermal looped capillaries can be seen in the upper portion of the anterior lip of the cervix. In the lower portion, the predominant pattern is a network of fine vessels branching tangenitally beneath the epithelium.

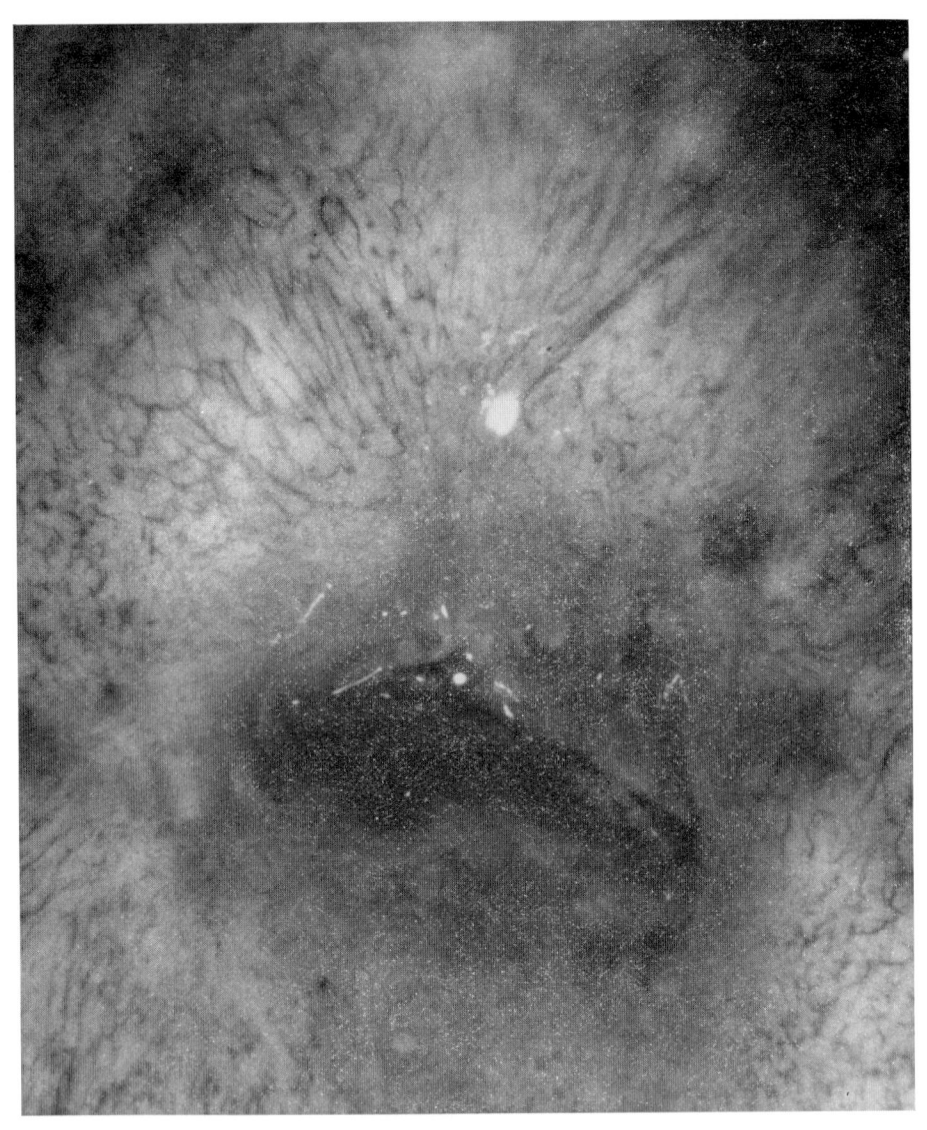

Figure 135. Original squamous epithelium. Angioarchitecture. The deeper vessels of the cervical stroma form a prominent network. Such a display of the subepithelial network is unusual with standard methods of colposcopy and suggests that either the vessels are hyperaemic or the epithelium thin.

Origin

The extensive topographical variations and folding of the columnar epithelium are not evident in the foetus of less than thirty weeks gestation. Specimens display increasingly complicated arrangements after this age, and it is apparent that between thirty-two and thirty-six weeks gestation there is great development in this area. In the last month, the embryological process appears complete, and the foetal arrangements are those which are seen to persist into adult life (Fig. 136).

Prime Morphological Features

Topography

The introduction to topographical aspects provided in Chapter 3 suggests that no particular epithelial form (original squamous, columnar, or metaplastic) is proper to any region of the cervix. It is rare for an area of the ectocervix to be composed entirely of columnar epithelium. In fact, in most subjects such areas of original columnar epithelium have undergone metaplasia over much of their exposed extent.

The original squamocolumnar junction defines the embryologically determined caudal extent of the columnar epithelium. This junction or line, if traced, varies in both situation and course. The most cephalic situation occurs some distance within the endocervical canal, whereas in exceptional instances, the most caudal limit encountered has been in the lower half of the vagina, even to the introitus. These limits are the uncommon boundaries, the most common being those circumscribing an area of columnar epithelium upon the ectocervix (Figs. 137 and 138). The new squamocolumnar junction defines the new caudal extent of columnar epithelium where it adjoins squamous epithelium resulting from the metaplastic process (Fig. 139). Although most areas of this type of tissue are elliptical, some demonstrate irregular and asymmetrical arrangements (*see* Fig. 136). It is apparent that from subject to subject the extent of the columnar epithelium varies widely, and the capacity for mucous secretion has equally wide physiological limits.

Colour

The intervention of only one cell thickness between the observer and the vasculature of the stroma insures that stromal hues are clearly transmitted. Columnar epithelium is dark red and contrasts sharply with other forms. The application of acetic acid solution reduces this contrast. In almost all instances, aspects other than colour are the useful diagnostic features of this form. There is no reason to ascribe to such redness an inflammatory origin.

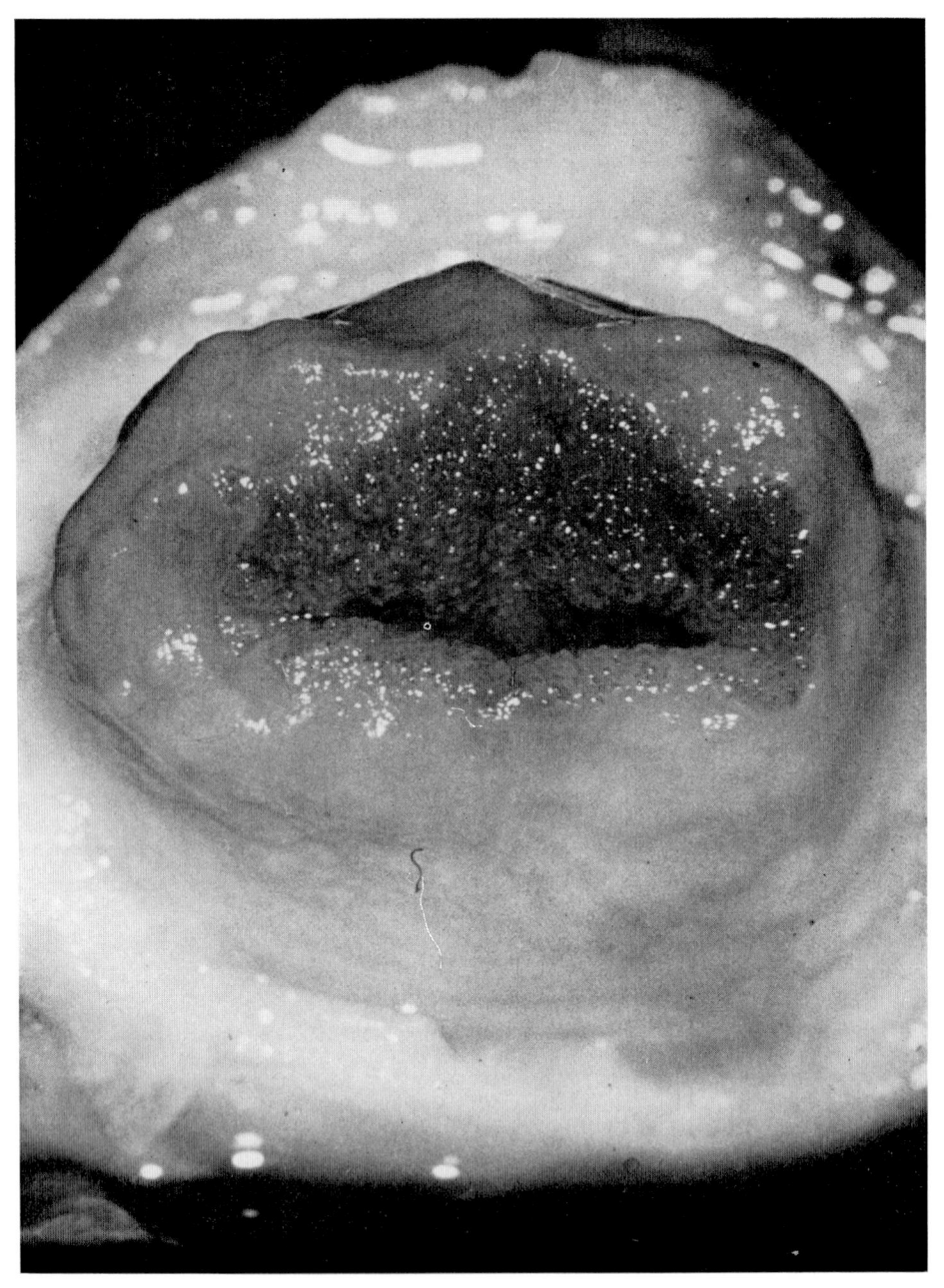

Figure 136. Colpophotograph of a preserved specimen of cervix from a week-old neonate. The surface of the cervical columnar epithelium is characteristically villous. Blood vessels can be seen in some villi. Note how the morphology in the newborn constitutes the basis of the structure of the adult cervix.

Surface Configuration

The most variable characteristic and yet distinctive quality of the cervical columnar epithelium is the folding of surface form. In most subjects, the presence of the characteristic villous and papillary outgrowths make recognition of this tissue immediate (Figs. 137-139). The columnar epithelium resembles grapes, and this resemblance is enhanced markedly when acetic acid solution is applied, especially in pregnancy. On the other hand, columnar epithelium in its most simple arrangement is seen in the form of an almost flat sheet (Fig. 140). Almost invariably, clefts extend deeply into the cervical substance. These clefts usually extend obliquely, diverging on each side from the midline (Figs. 140 and 141).

There is an ill-defined subdivision of the columnar epithelium into two morphological zones. The more distal or caudal zone contains mainly villiform or grapelike processes, whereas the cranial zone, the area of the arbor vitae uteri,* is deeply cleaved in many directions but is covered by the almost smooth or flattened villous epithelium. Between the zones, transition from one to the other is seen. In each subject, most of the arrangements described are found. Differences are usually in degree. Sometimes the features of this epithelium may be obscured by bleeding, as the thin covering is easily damaged by the introduction of the speculum or even by gentle application of solutions.

Angioarchitecture

For colposcopic recognition of columnar epithelium, the vascular arrangement is not of fundamental importance and is difficult to reproduce with our equipment. However, the importance of this arrangement is its contribution to the eventual patterns observed in metaplastic epithelia. It seems that the basic vascular forms present in the columnar epithelium from foetal life onwards become incorporated with some remodelling into the new epithelial form. The characteristic angioarchitecture which usually allows easy distinction between the metaplastic and the original squamous epithelia is thereby acquired.

When the stromal core of a villus is narrow, a single, central, looped vessel is present (see Fig. 88), whereas the broader villous structures may exhibit several vessels in a peripheral subepithelial network pattern forming as it were a basket network. When the columnar epithelium is not villous, but almost flat, a simple, fine network is seen. Deeper than these vessels the large terminal veins may be seen in some subjects (see Fig. 87).

---

* Arbor vitae uteri = A series of folds of the cervical columnar epithelium. They consist of anterior and posterior longitudinal folds from which secondary folds branch off obliquely upwards and laterally.

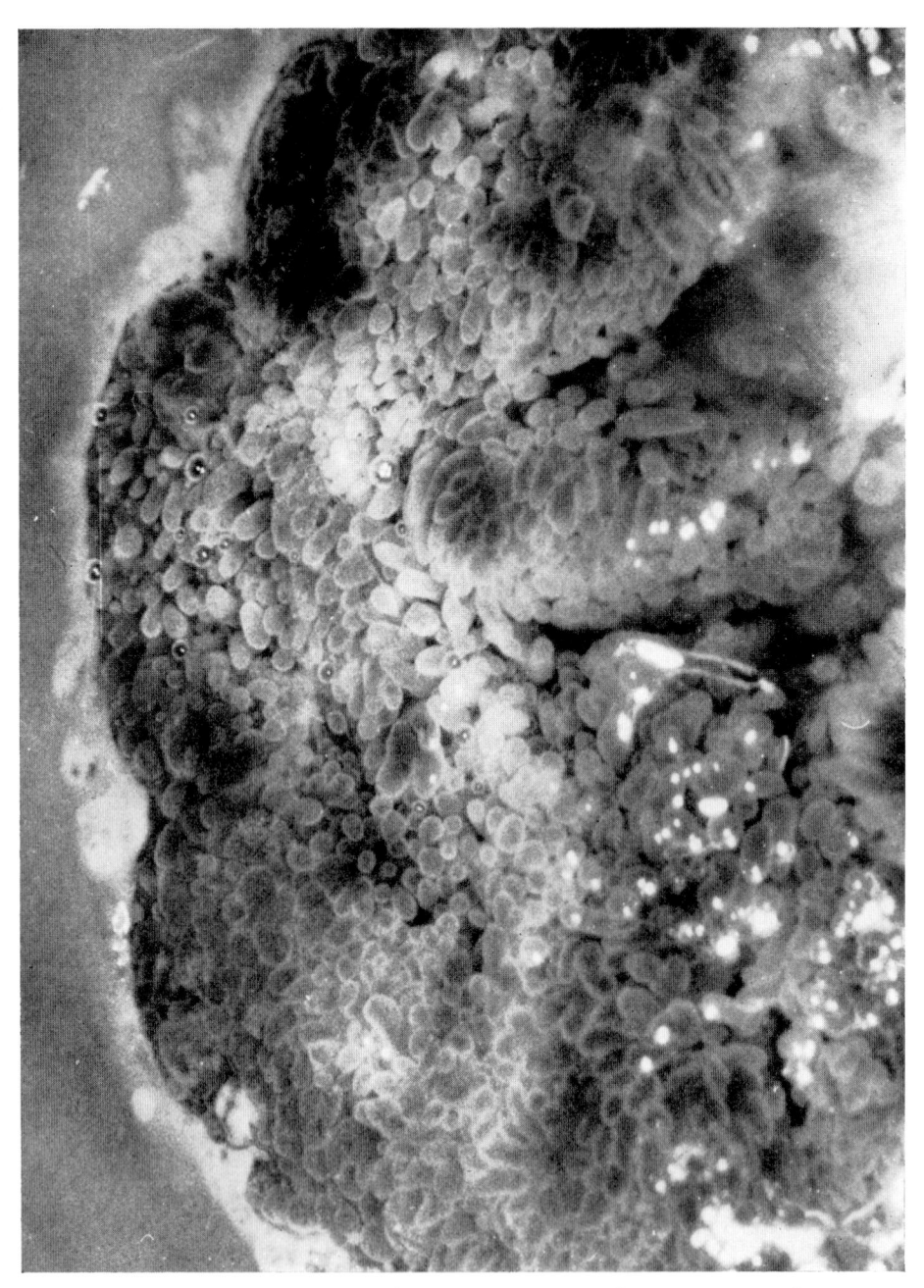

Figure 137. Columnar epithelium. The original squamocolumnar junction has circumscribed a nearly circular area on the cervix, most of one lateral half of which appears in the photograph. Within it is a small margin of transformation zone. The remainder is columnar epithelium displaying numerous villi and grapelike structures.

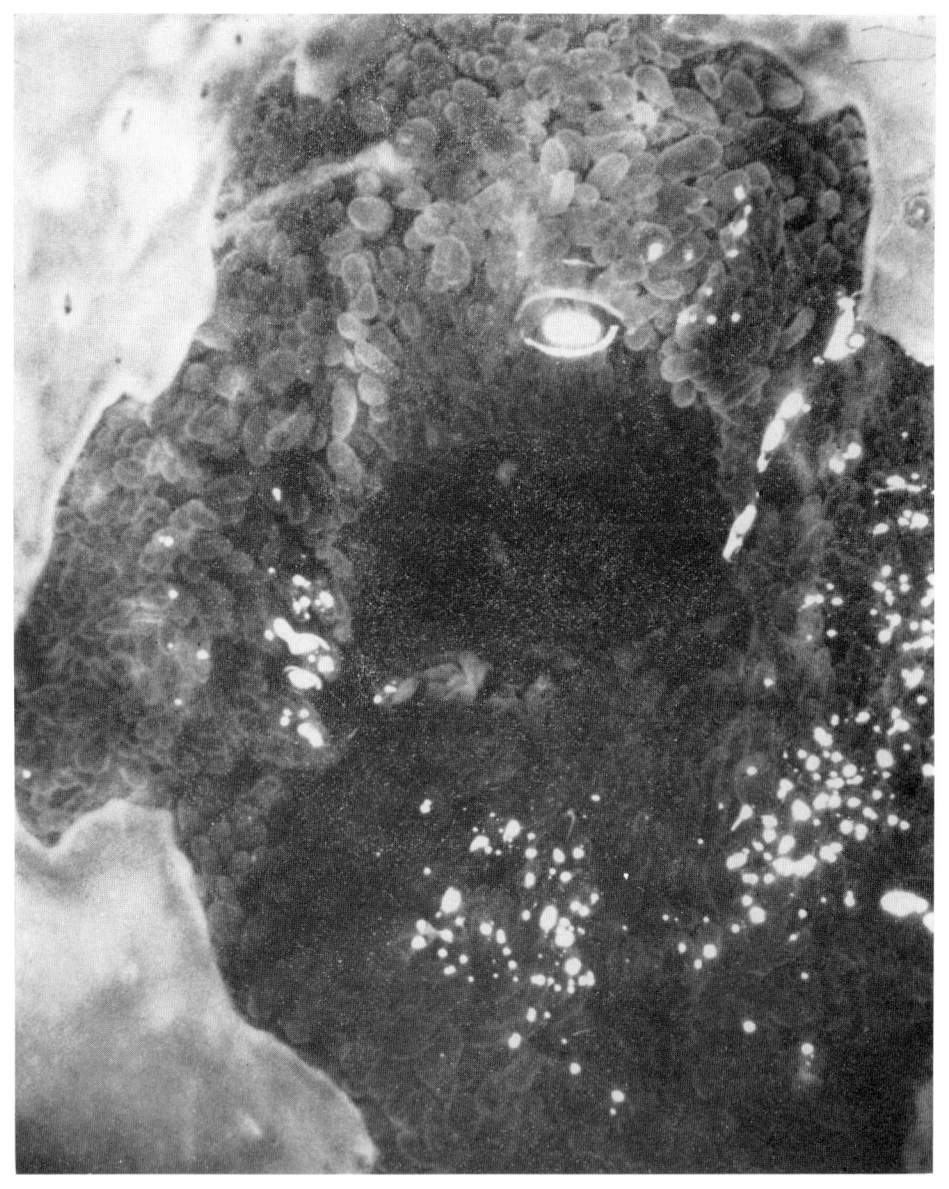

Figure 138. Columnar epithelium. The original squamocolumnar junction is less regular, and a non-symmetrical area of columnar epithelium is outlined surrounding the canal in the centre of the photograph.

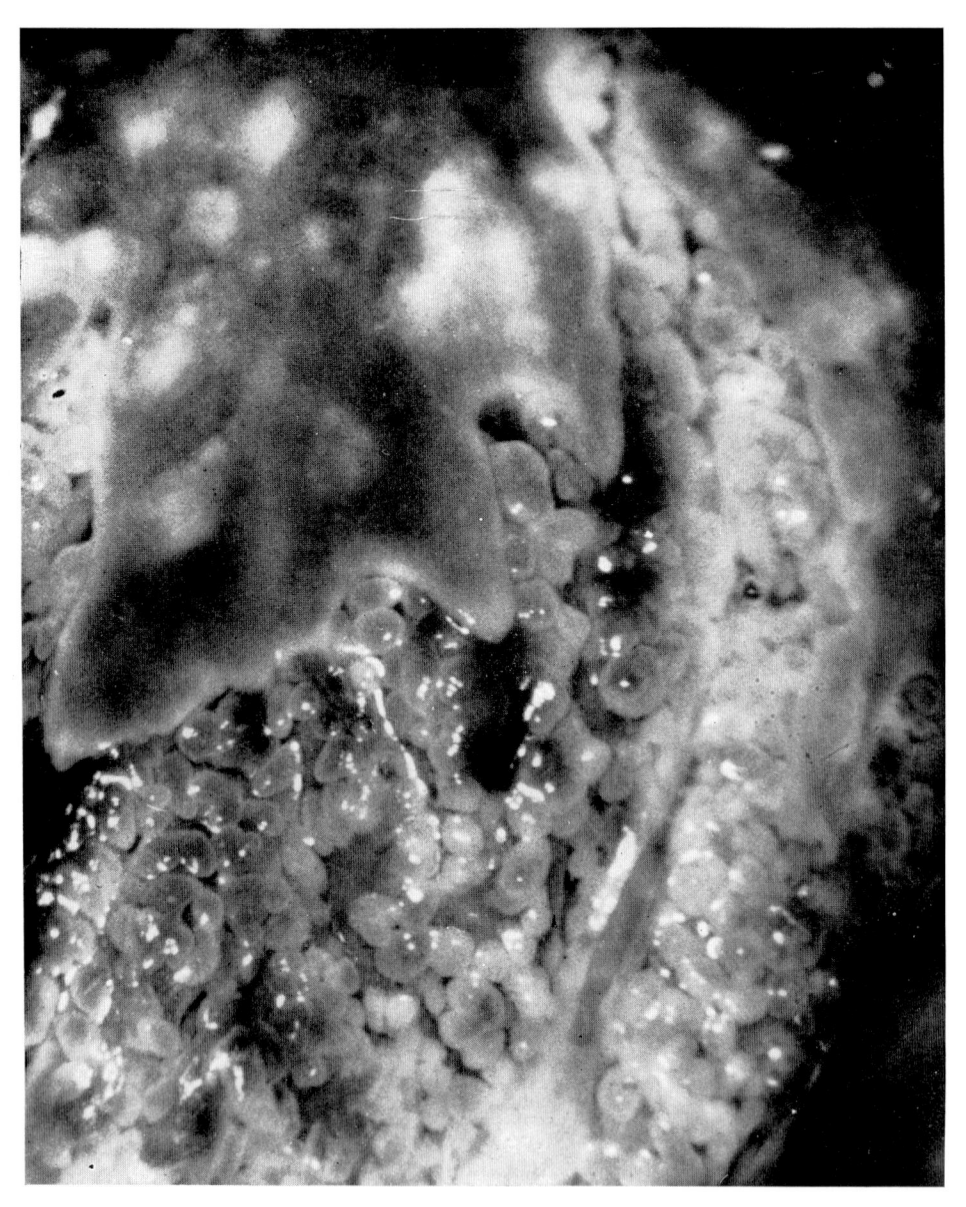

Figure 139. New squamocolumnar junction. The mature metaplastic squamous epithelium of the upper left quadrant joins the columnar epithelium at a sharply demarcated line, the new squamocolumnar junction.

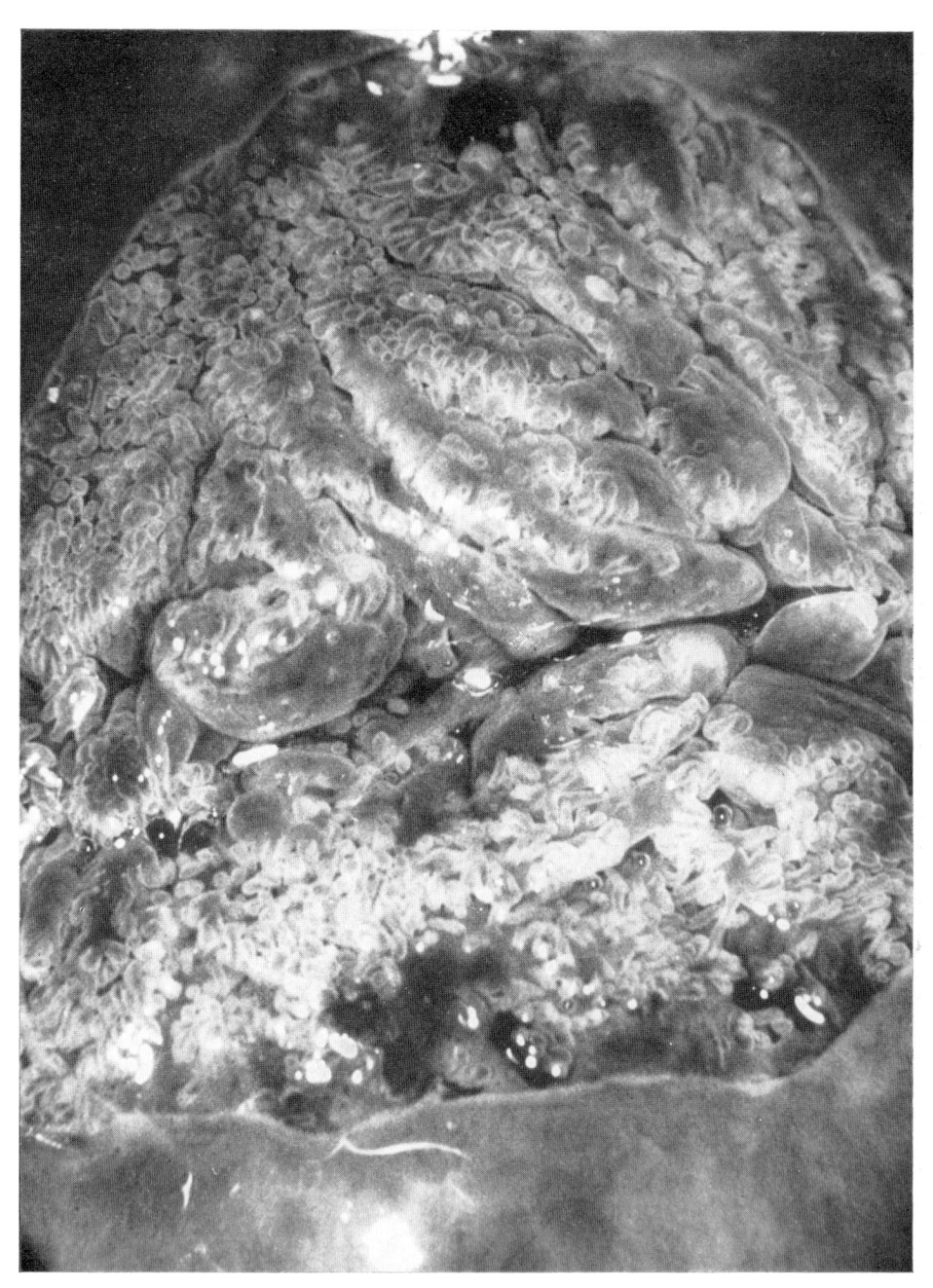

Figure 140. Columnar epithelium. Several characteristics of the columnar epithelium are present. Villi are present in most areas, and clefts cross the surface transversely and obliquely, circumscribing ridges in which the villi have fused. In a few areas, this has progressed to a flat covering, especially near the entrance to the canal, seen as a transverse slit across the centre of the photograph. The fused villous and flat surface appearances indicate early metaplasia.

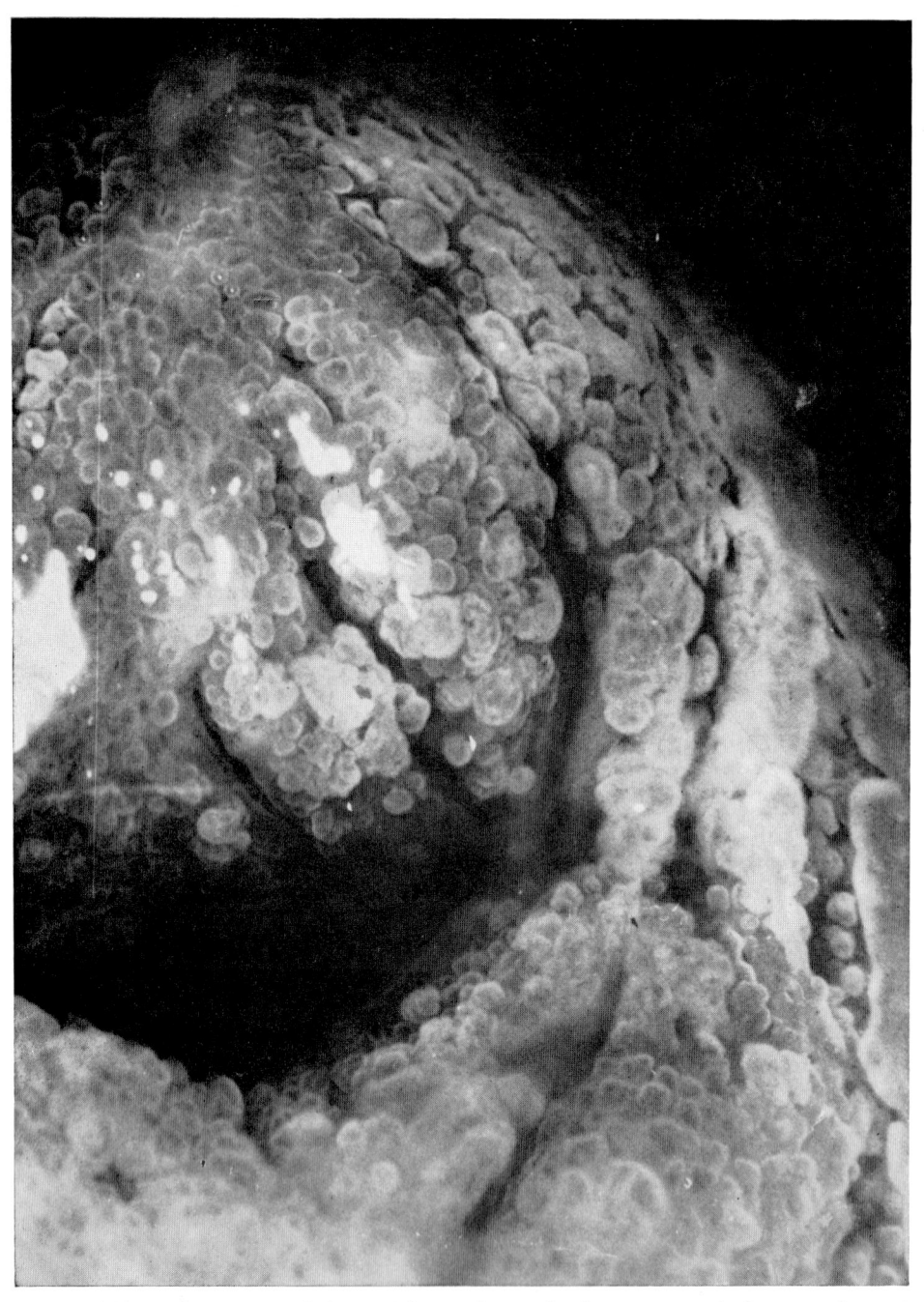

Figure 141. Columnar epithelium. This subject displays some of the complicated arrangements of villi, clefts, and rugae which makes each area of columnar epithelium individual in its appearance.

Chapter 8

COLPOSCOPIC APPEARANCE OF THE TYPICAL TRANSFORMATION ZONE

THE TYPICAL TRANSFORMATION zone represents the contribution of physiological metaplasia to the cervical coverings. In this section, the wide range of variations in the colposcopic features of this tissue is described. The existence in this zone of variable vascular patterns, as well as the fate of residual columnar glands and clefts, whether entrapped and cystic or opening to the surface, determines the great variety of patterns.

Origin and Development

The early stages of the dynamic phase of the transformation zone have been dealt with earlier (p. 81). Three stages of the physiological metaplastic process indicative of increasing maturity are recognised colposcopically, as follows (Figs. 142 and 143).

STAGE I: The original papillary surface of the columnar epithelium is still evident, but there is a loss of translucency so that the villi assume a ground glass appearance (Fig. 142a).

STAGE II: The original papillary or grapelike conformation is still vaguely evident, as successive villi are fused and the intervening spaces filled in (Figs. 142b and 143).

STAGE III: The villous appearance is lost, and the new surface takes on the appearance of a decreasingly translucent, vascular, pearly tongue of tissue, apparently growing over the tissue folds (Figs. 142c and 143).

These *early stages of the typical transformation zone* are usually most evident at the summit of the villi, while in the less exposed adjacent clefts, unchanged columnar epithelium is present. This arrangement offers the basis for a common variety of transformation zone in which fingerlike ridges of metaplasia are present separated by longitudinal clefts of columnar epithelium (Fig. 144). Other arrangements are seen. The earliest phases of metaplasia are represented as discrete patches which eventually become confluent in random fashion (Fig. 145). In this way, so-called islands of columnar epithelium remain untransformed in the transformation zone.

In the cervix that displays *well-developed transformation zone* with more mature forms of metaplastic epithelium, the epithelial surface is usually smooth and its colour now reddish rather than pale. Raised above the level of other elements, the metaplastic epithelium has become thick

(Fig. 146). Other arrangements are seen, obviously representing maturation in the original tongues of metaplasia laid down during the dynamic phases (Figs. 147 and 148).

At various stages in the life history of the cervix, cystic inclusions and gland openings are seen. Usually in the peripheral, more mature zone, gland or cleft openings remain to allow mucus discharge onto the surface (Figs. 149-151), whereas the less mature stages exhibit more extensive persistence of columnar epithelium. Occlusion of the glands results in the formation of potential cysts. Continued secretion results in cystic inclusions of various size, which have long been termed *nabothian follicles* (Figs. 152 and 153).

It is difficult to forecast an end point for any particular area of metaplastic epithelium, but it seems that increasing maturation of the metaplastic zone tends towards a *fully developed (or healed) transformation zone* with a relatively smooth epithelium. As a result of the interposition of the various elements described, glandular and squamous, the appearances of the definitive mature transformation zone is highly variable, displaying a range of gland openings, nabothian cysts, and characteristic vessels. Sometimes there is complete replacement of the columnar elements, so that only branching vascular structures may remain as evidence of metaplasia (Figs. 154 and 155).

Prime Morphological Features

Topography

Topography of the transformation zone has been exhaustively treated in Chapter 3. The importance of topography in relation to the area of transformation zone available for detailed inspection by colposcopy is further stressed. The caudal limit of the zone is the original squamocolumnar junction, and the cephalic limit is the new squamocolumnar junction (*see* Figs. 23 and 139).

Colour

Generally, the colour of the typical transformation zone is paler than that seen in the original squamous epithelium and contrasts too with the dark red columnar zone and the white colour of the atypical transformation zone. Within the typical transformation zone, variations that depend upon the presence of other factors are encountered. When inclusion cysts are present, the area overlying it may be translucent or yellowish. About the openings of glands, a pale or white opaque ring is present (Figs. 150 and 151) (p. 361).

Surface Configuration

In the early phases of existence, the surface contour of metaplastic epithelium reflects the characteristics and disposition of the original columnar epithelium. These are evident in minute papillary projections, in remnants of clefts or glands, and in the presence of cystic inclusions, large and small (Figs. 152 and 153). Gradually, surface contours become less apparent, and in time, the metaplastic epithelium is smooth.

Angioarchitecture

The range of vascular structures evident in the typical transformation zone remains throughout the life of the individual as a most distinctive feature. It has been previously stated that the vascular structures of the original columnar epithelium are incorporated in the transformation zone as metaplasia occurs. Modification of the original structures can arise, and a widely variable set of appearances may be encountered.

Most typical of the structures are the branching terminal vessels probably inherited from the original columnar tissue (Figs. 154 and 155). These are always most strikingly displayed in the zone where cystic inclusions provide a translucent background for contrast (Figs. 152 and 153). As inclusion cysts enlarge through distension, vascular structures from deeper layers are displaced towards the surface. Thus, branching vessels are seen, diminishing uniformly in calibre as branching proceeds and terminating in a fine capillary network beneath the epithelium. The narrow capillaries and closeness of the network contrast with patterns encountered in abnormal epithelia.

When columnar tissue persists as glands opening onto a metaplastic surface, terminal circular vessels are seen about the openings. Several such vessels in proximity may resemble a mosaic structure.

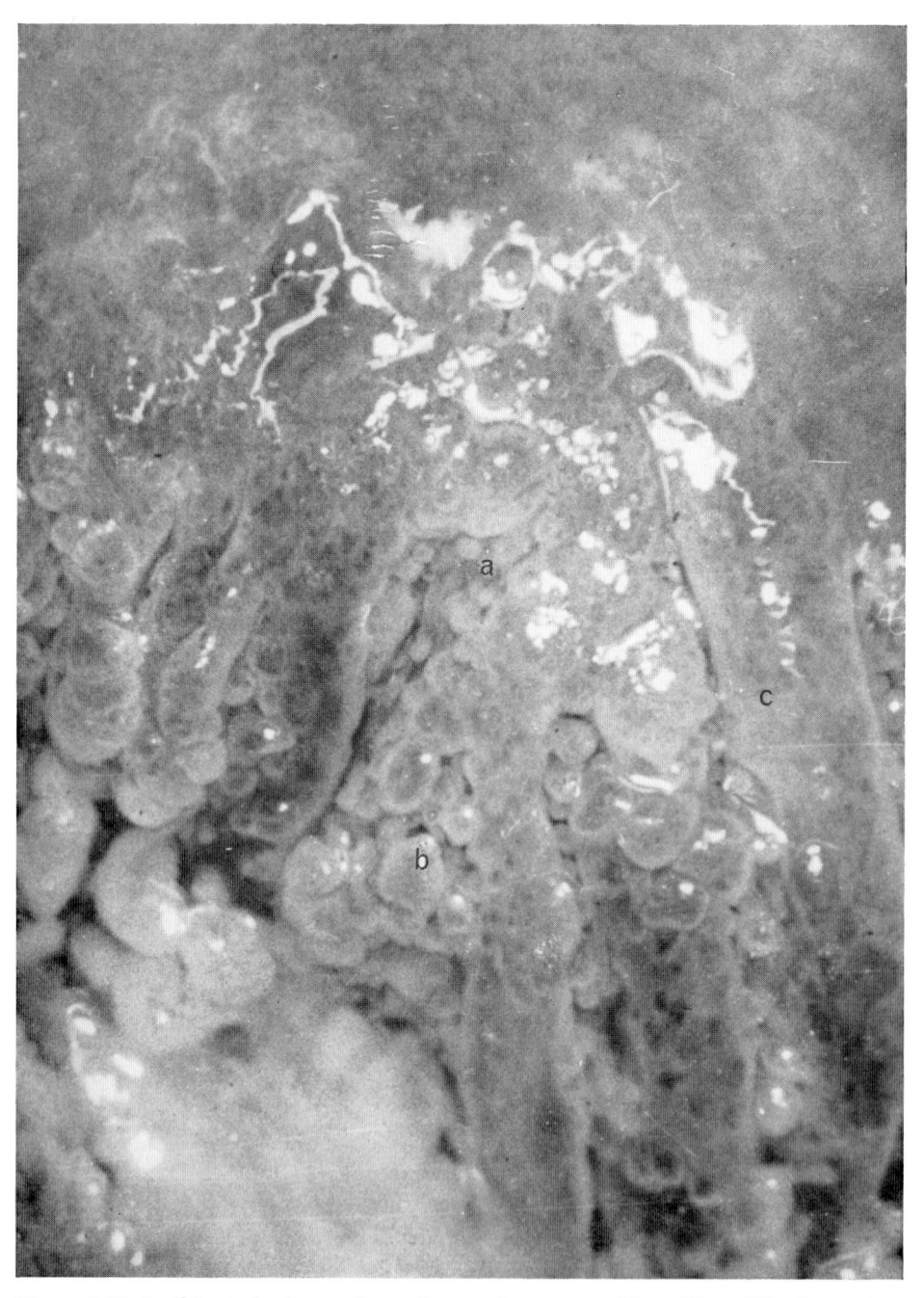

Figure 142. In this study drawn from the previous series (Figs. 73 to 76), the various colposcopic features of early metaplasia are displayed. Glazed (a) and fused (b) villi are seen gradually to form fingerlike ridges of new physiological metaplastic squamous epithelium (c).

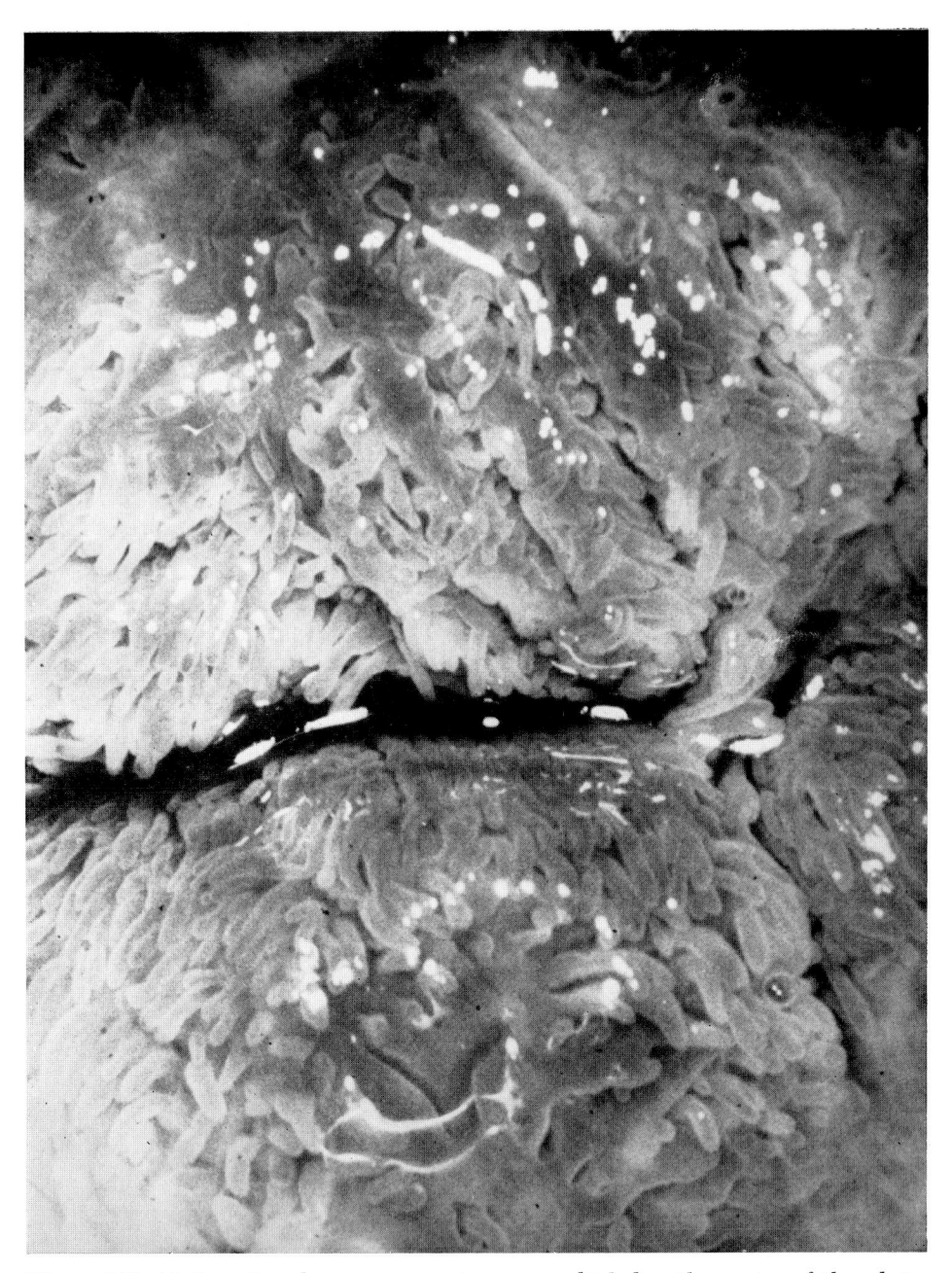

Figure 143. At the external os, seen as a transverse slit below the centre of the photograph, unaltered columnar epithelium is arranged in typical villi. Peripherally the surface is restructured by early metaplasia so that villi, especially in the more prominent ridges, have fused.

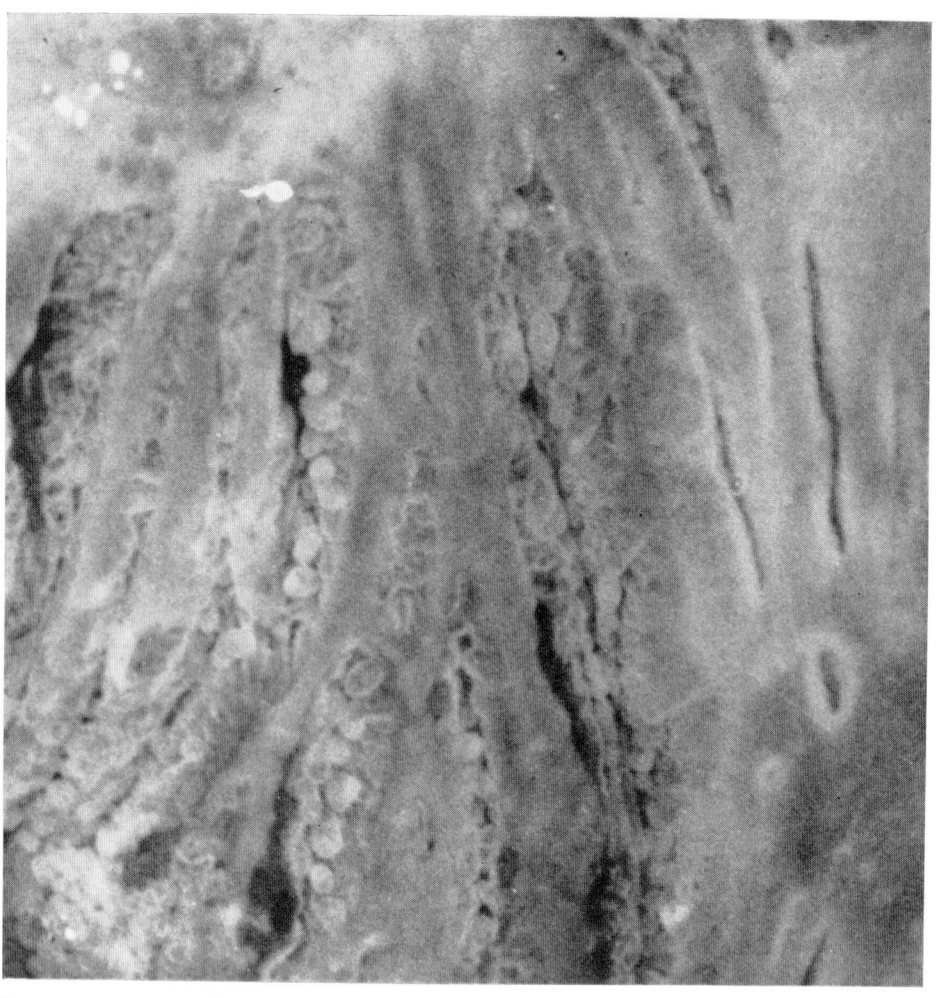

Figure 144. Fingerlike ridges of early metaplasia are seen separated by longitudinal clefts of columnar epithelium.

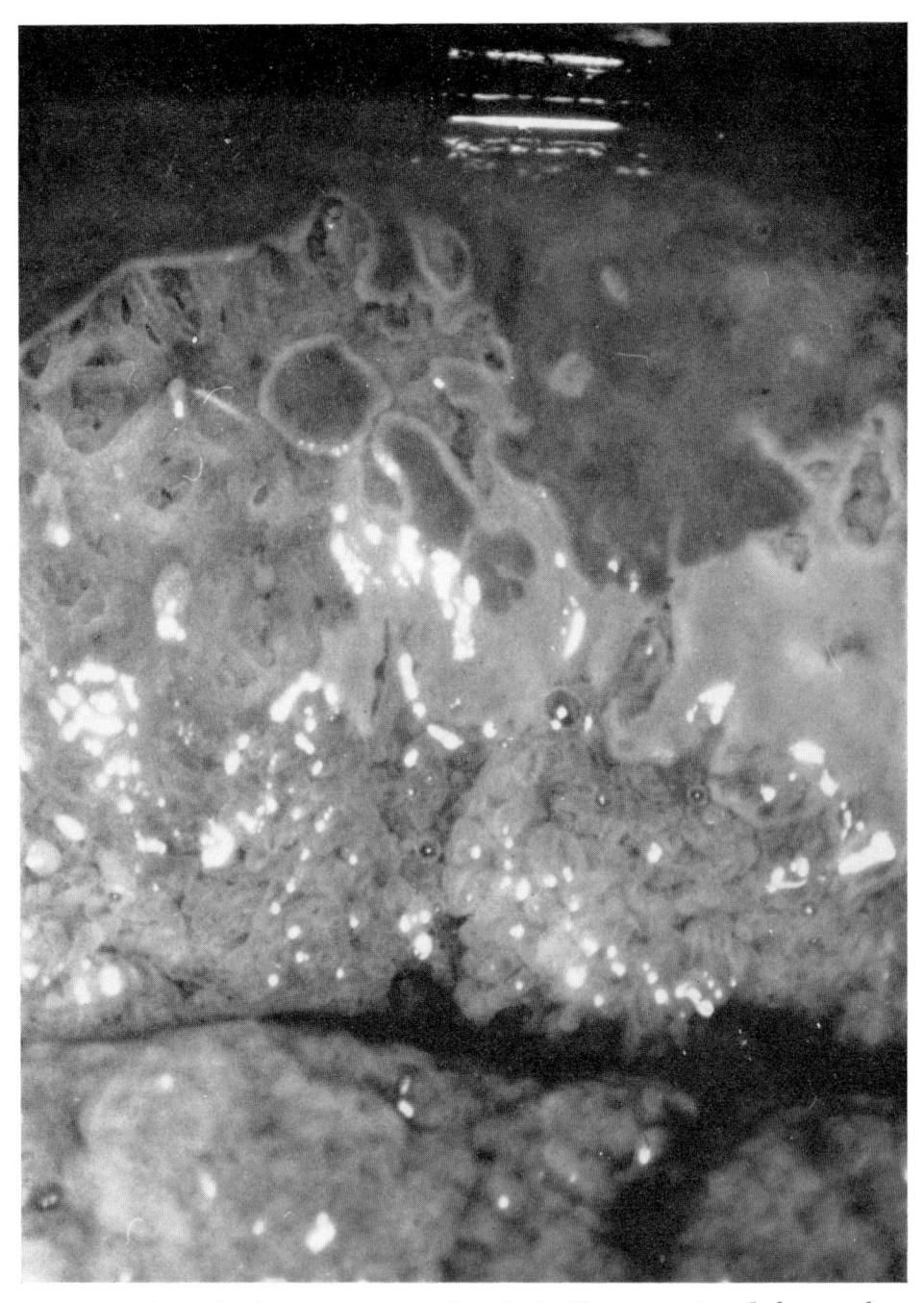

Figure 145. Areas of pale, immature metaplasia lie beside more mature dark areas above the centre of the photograph on the anterior lip of the cervix. Note the undoubted insularity of a small patch above and to the left of the centre of the photograph. The distribution of the metaplastic epithelium emphasises the discrete origin of areas of metaplasia.

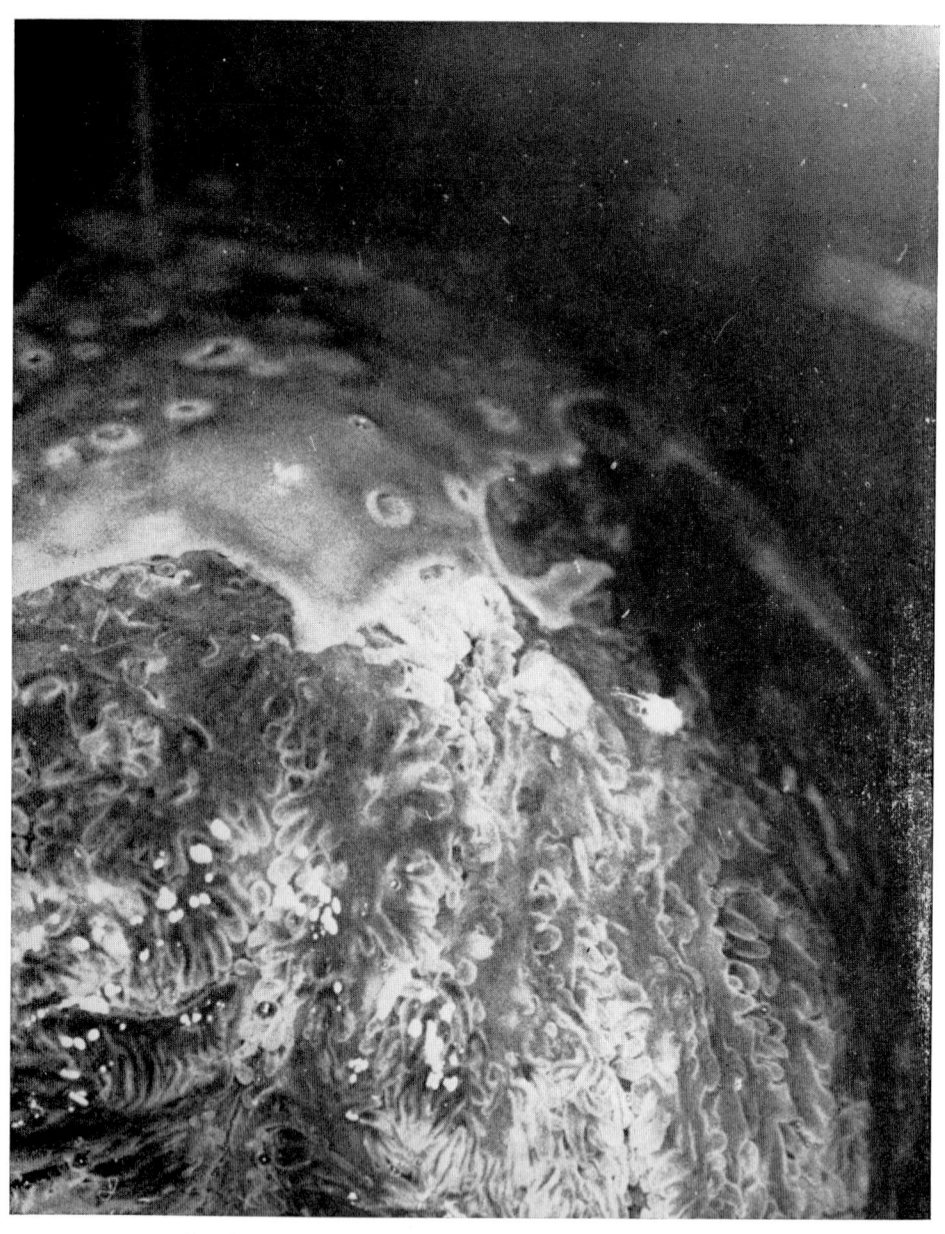

Figure 146. Study showing two contrasting areas. Below, columnar epithelium and fused villi representing immature stages of metaplasia adjoin the upper mature metaplastic plate containing gland openings.

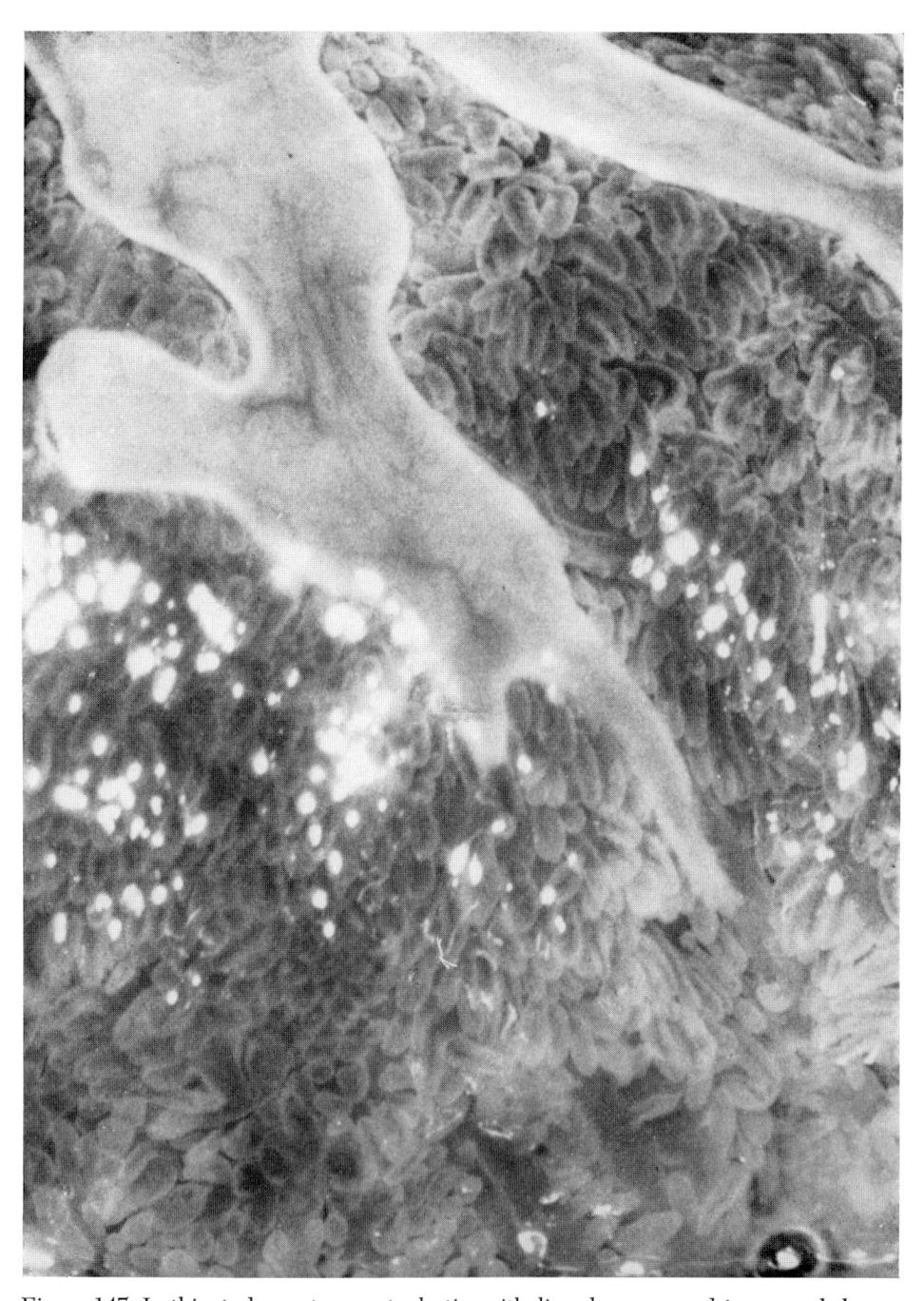

Figure 147. In this study, mature metaplastic epithelium has emerged in unusual shapes.

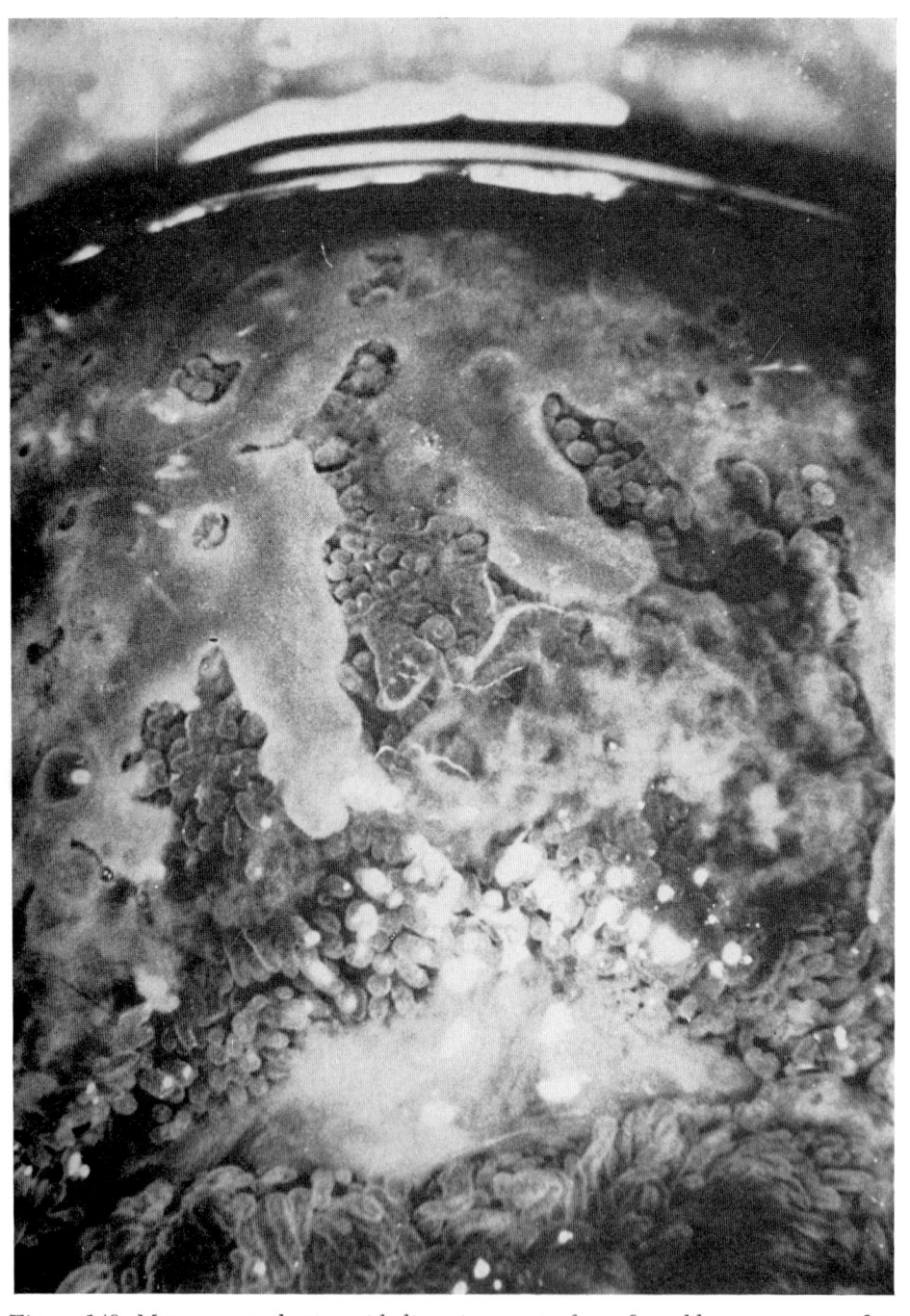

Figure 148. Mature metaplastic epithelium is seen to form fingerlike processes and to enclose islands of columnar epithelium and smaller gland openings.

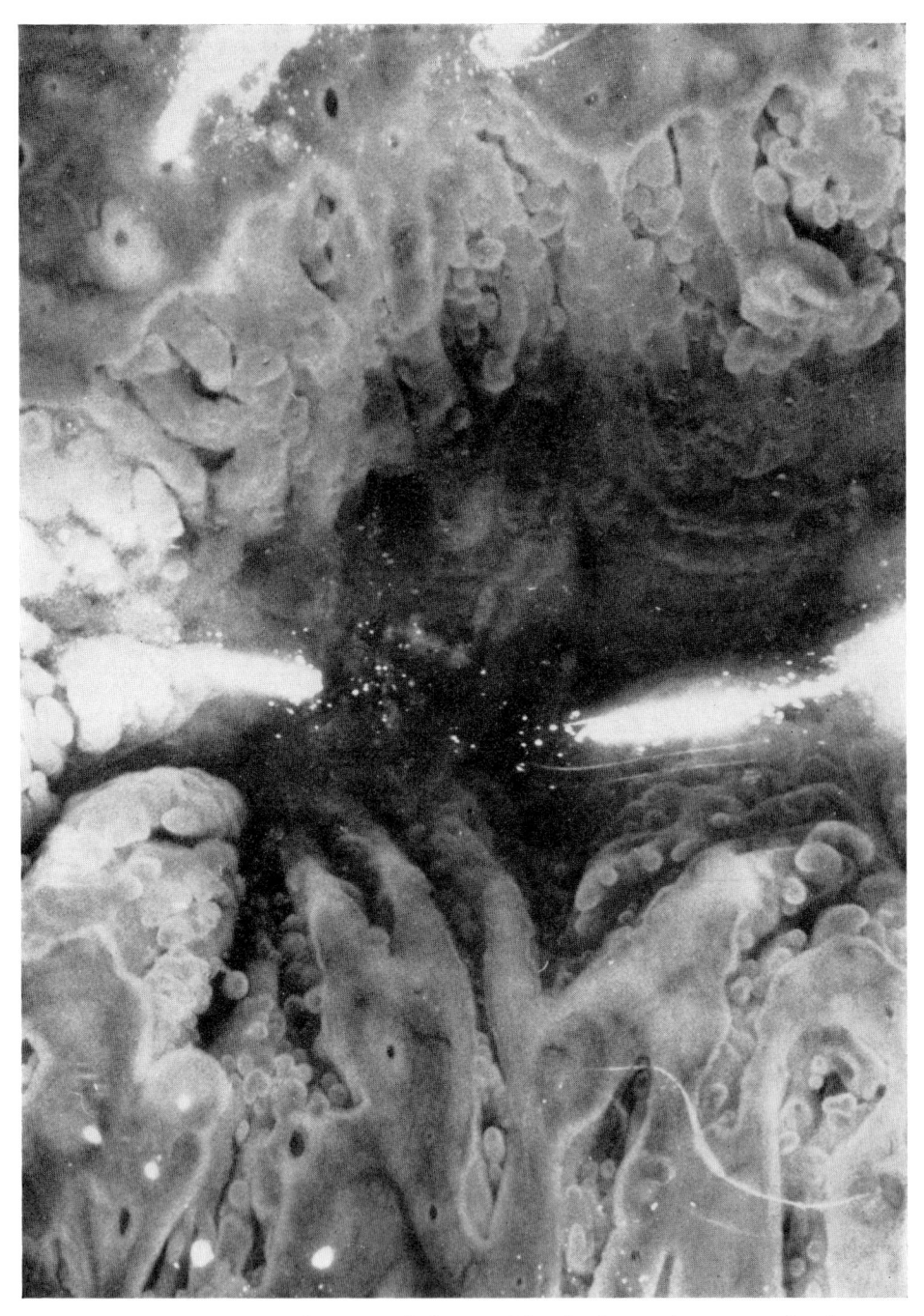

Figure 149. Mature metaplastic epithelium with gland openings extends almost to the cervical canal.

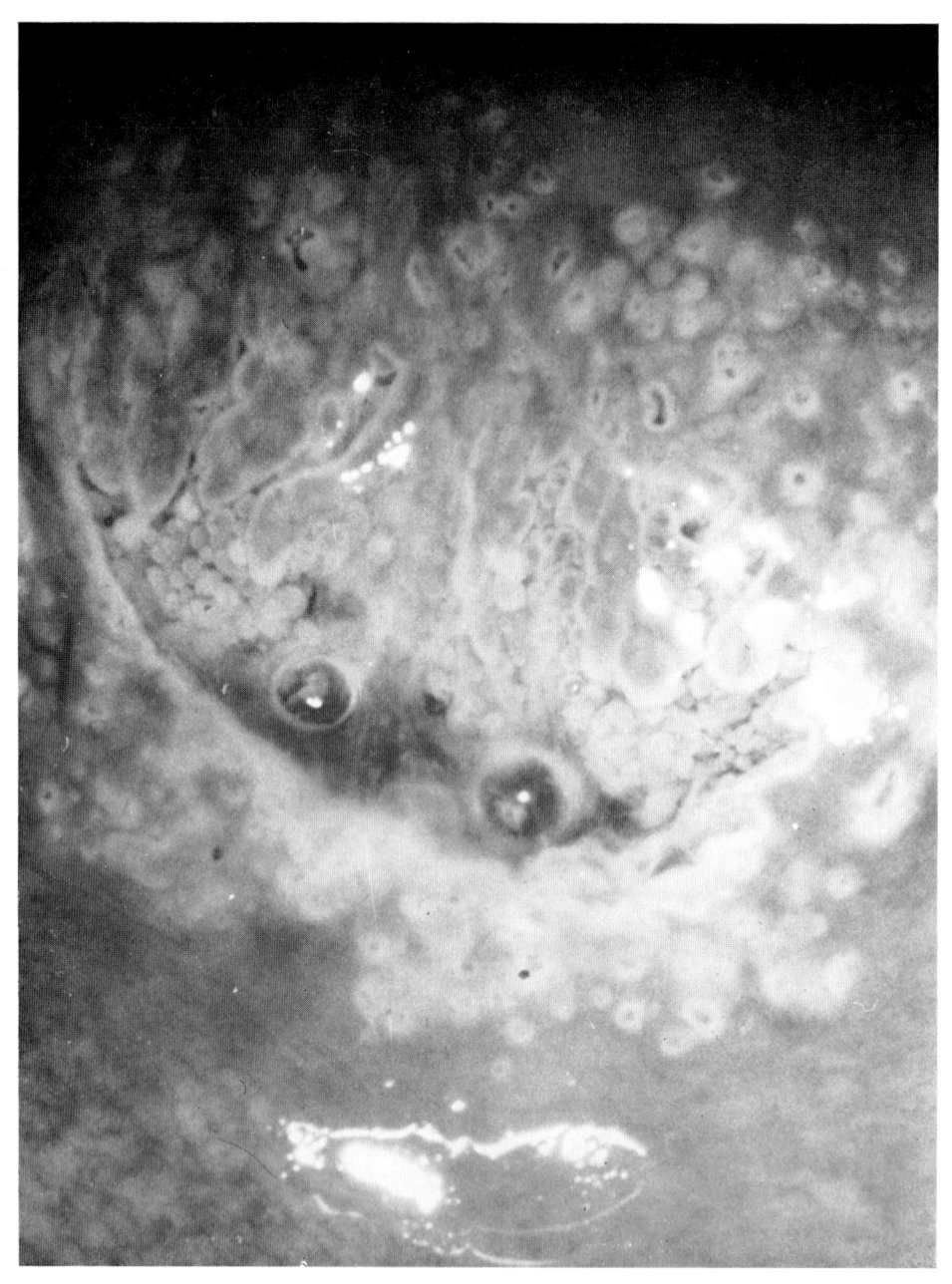

Figure 150. An almost fully developed transformation zone exhibits gland openings with ridges of metaplasia on the anterior lip near the cervical canal. The white ring around the gland opening is a common appearance and does not indicate atypical epithelium.

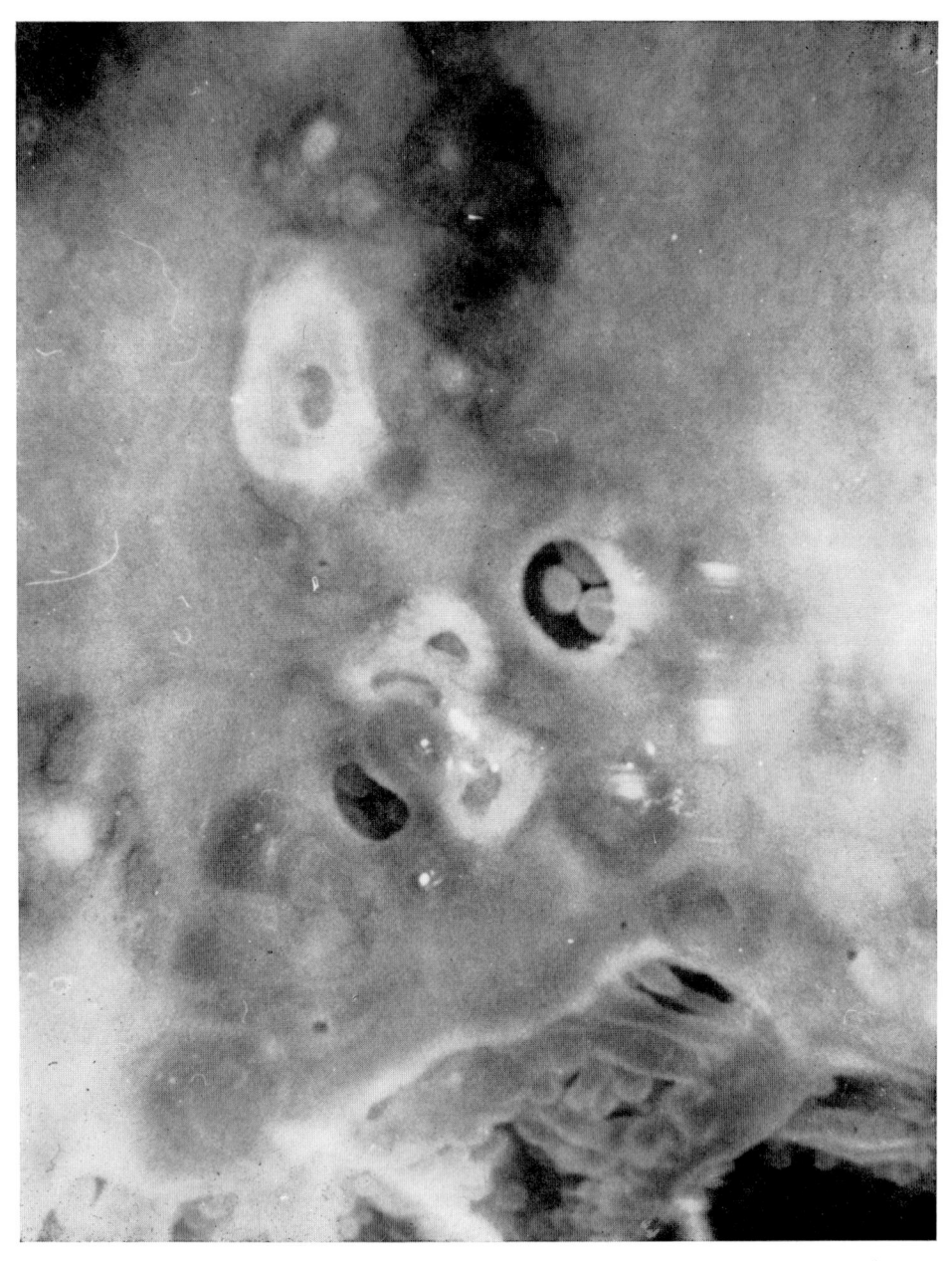

Figure 151. Through gland openings in a well-developed transformation zone, columnar epithelium-covered villi can be seen.

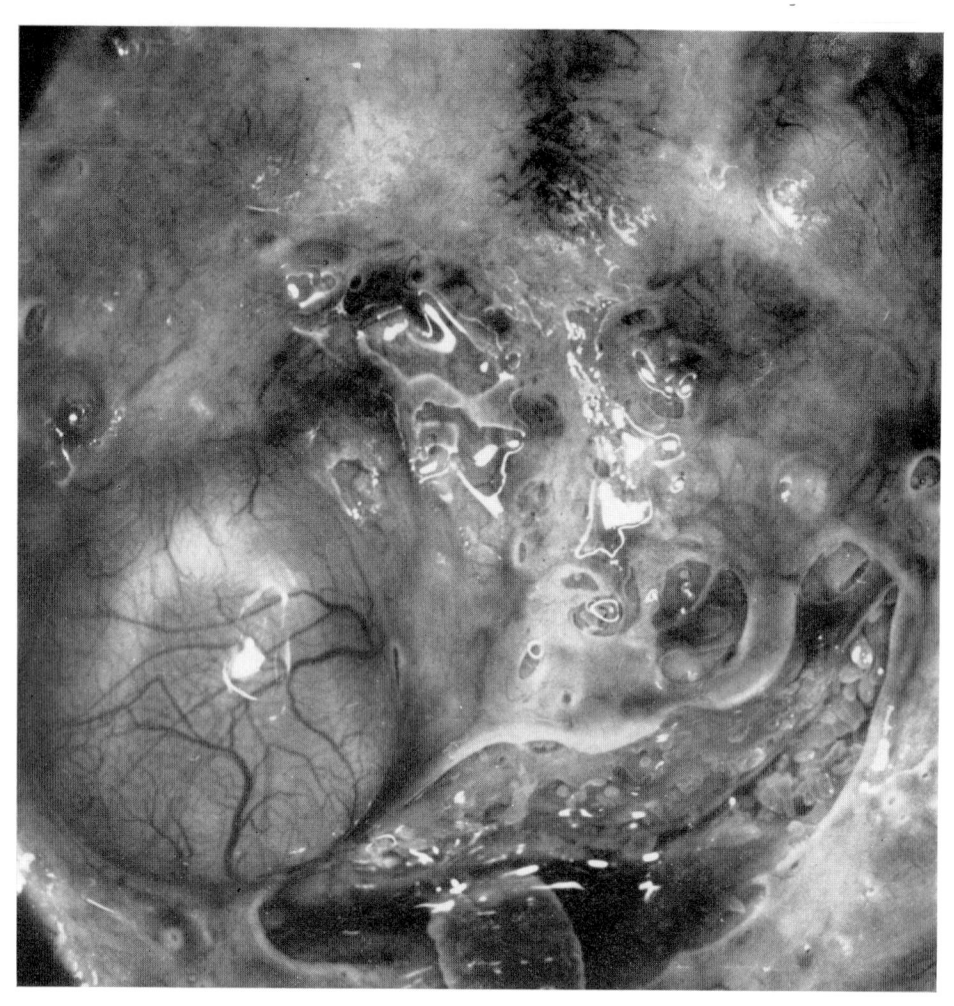

Figure 152. Several of the features of an almost fully developed typical transformation zone are seen. A large inclusion cyst above and to the left of the cervical os, gland openings, and typical variations of vasculature are present. The contribution of these three features to the appearances of the typical transformation zone varies in different cervices.

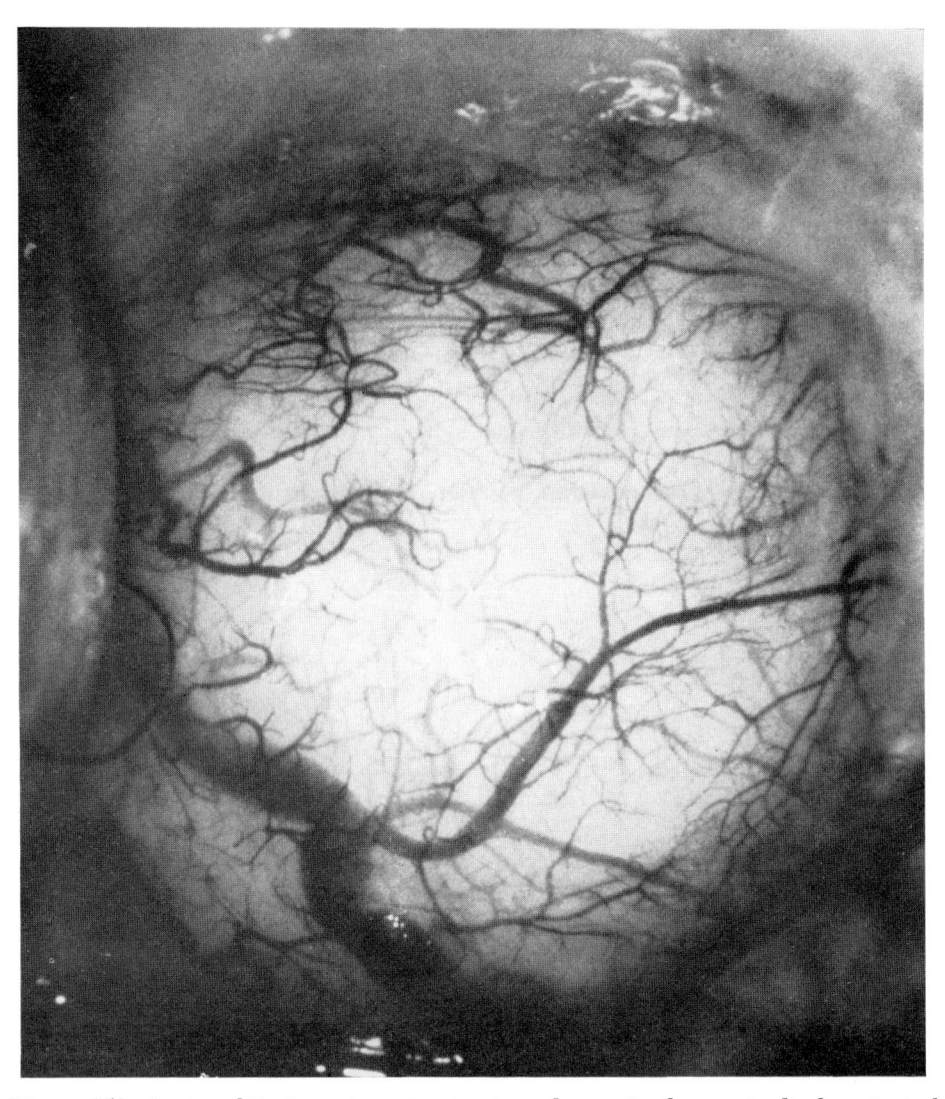

Figure 153. Angioarchitecture. A cystic structure deeper in the cervix displays typical vessels coursing over its surface. They are regular, branching, diminishing in calibre to terminate in a capillary network.

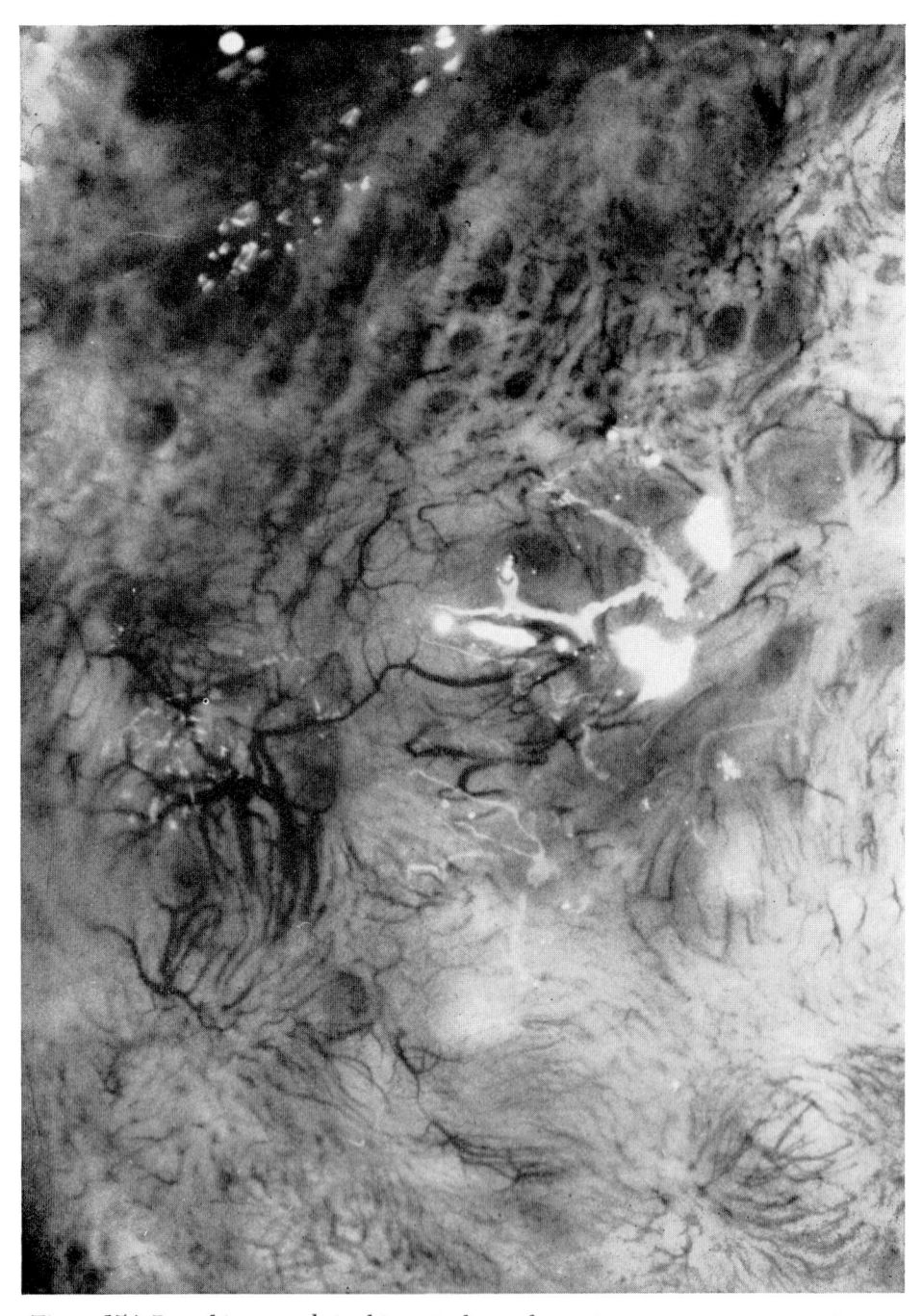

Figure 154. Branching vessels in this typical transformation zone are most conspicuous.

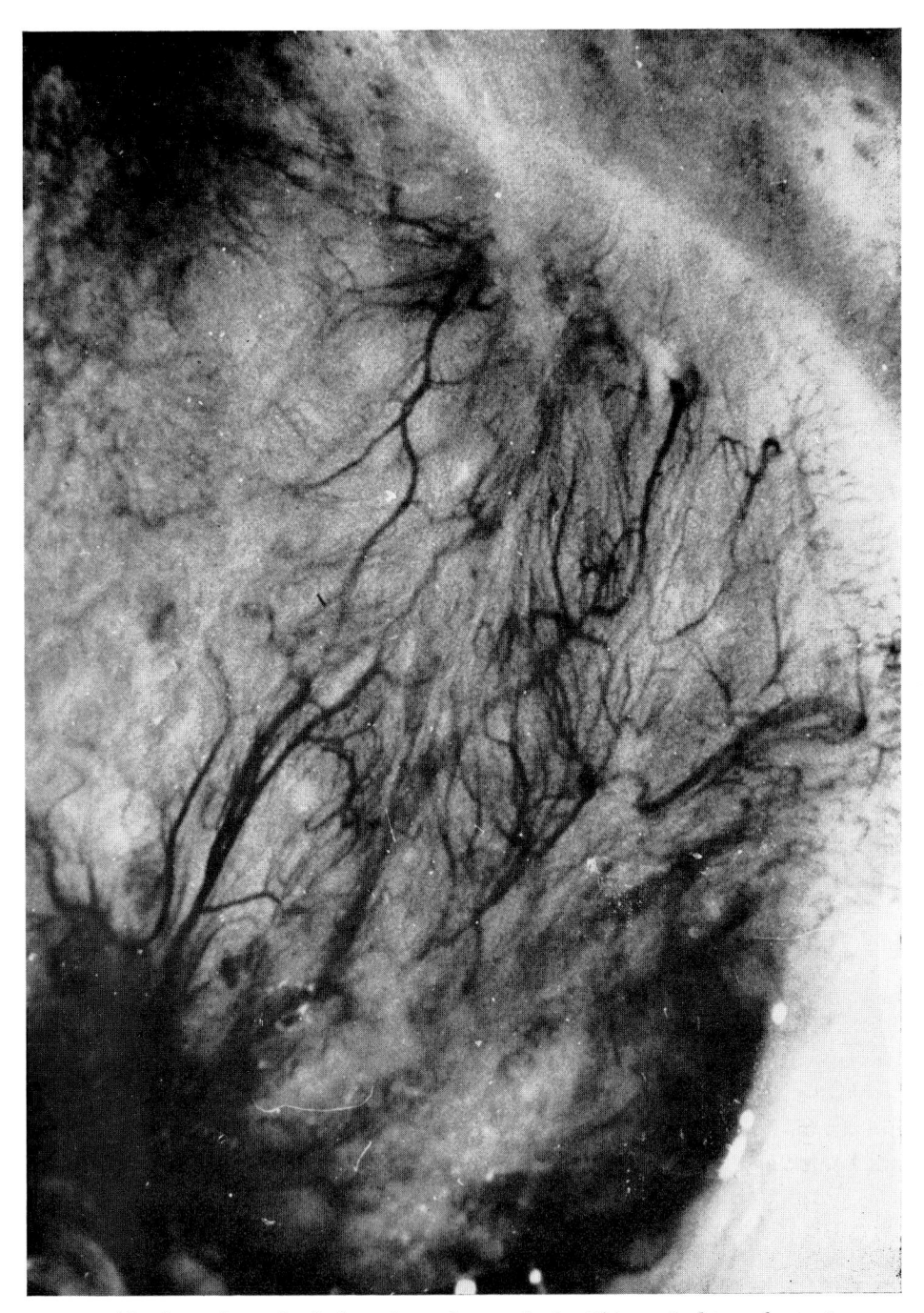

Figure 155. The end-result of physiological metaplasia. This typical transformation zone has proceeded to full development with replacement of all columnar tissue. The branching vessels remain as the only evidence of the origin of this squamous area.

Chapter 9

COLPOSCOPIC APPEARANCES OF THE ATYPICAL TRANSFORMATION ZONE

THE ATYPICAL TRANSFORMATION zone is the distinctive area of the cervix that includes and, indeed, delimits the site of dysplasia and preclinical cancer. The essential value of the colposcopic method is determined by its ability to distinguish these changes from the physiological. An appreciation of the finer structure of the area revealed by the colposcope aids the clinician in understanding some otherwise unavailable aspects of preneoplasia and neoplasia of the cervix. Such an understanding must of necessity be reflected in the planning of the therapeutic approach and in an overall increase in the knowledge of these contentious conditions.

No single colposcopic appearance of dysplasia or preclinical carcinoma is summary and incontrovertible evidence for the presence of either lesion. The real value of the colposcope lies in its ability to detect a variety of quite different appearances, all of which are consistent with the same histological diagnosis.

The transformation zone can exhibit, in whole or in part, singly or in combination, the features of white epithelium, with or without the specific vascular arrangements of punctation, mosaic, and atypical vessels, or keratosis. These appearances are collectively termed the *atypical transformation zone* (Table III).

Although the atypical transformation zone identifies the site and extent of major dysplastic and cancerous epithelia, there are numerous exceptions. It is a matter of disappointment even disillusion to many clinicians that so many atypical transformation zones show on histological examination only the most minor disturbances, even normal appearances in the cervical epithelium, and have no apparent clinical significance (*see* p. 157 and Chap. 15).

A means of assessing the more serious lesions, no matter how unrefined

TABLE III
ATYPICAL TRANSFORMATION ZONE

White epithelium	Increased cellular density
	± Subepithelial vessels
+ or – Punctation	Alterations in epithelial capillaries
Mosaic	
Atypical vessels	
+ or – Keratosis	A keratin covering thickened beyond the normal

at this stage, is therefore of paramount importance. In this respect, a concept of *grading* stemming simply from degrees of difference observable in the prime morphological features is proposed (p. 156). Major grades suggest (1) a correlation with the more severe histological grading of dysplasia or preclinical cancer (p. 157) and (2) a declared potential for progression to invasion (p. 403). Our approach in promoting such a scheme is quite tentative, because of its probable oversimplification of a complex situation but draws attention to an urgent need for a better scheme in the near future.

Origin and Development

The appearance of the well-developed atypical transformation zone can be best understood by observing the zone during its initiation or dynamic phases. Originating in columnar epithelium, the undifferentiated, opaque, and white epithelium is seen capping the original villous structure (Fig. 156). The new squamous epithelium may exhibit white epithelium with emerging punctation (Fig. 157), which at a later stage becomes more pronounced (Fig. 158). Mosaic (Figs. 159 and 160) may also be seen evolving from the original columnar epithelium.

During colposcopic examination, the tissue colour of the earliest phases of the metaplastic change is often white. Correlative studies with histology show this to be immature metaplastic epithelium. The subsequent fate of this white epithelium is, at present, under investigation as to the frequency with which this epithelium becomes atypical or persists as physiological. This series (Figs. 156-160) is not assembled as an authoritative forecast of a course that metaplasia would take. This is in view of our subsequent experience with serial colposcopic observations that similar patterns can have, as an end-result, the appearance of mature typical transformation zone (*see* Fig. 263). These early phases, in which the epithelial cells are mainly undifferentiated, may proceed no further towards maturity and differentiation during the lifetime of the individual and continue to display low-grade colposcopic atypical features.

Early phases are usually followed by a maturation process as in the typical transformation zone. The maturation phases constitute the classical appearances of the atypical transformation zone. As such, they represent an intermediate phase in the ultimate development of cancer, and as with a typical transformation zone, they can become arrested at any phase for shorter or longer periods up to a lifetime.

Prime Morphological Features

Topography

It must be emphasized that the site and extent of the atypical transformation zone determines the area in which lesions are initially sought and

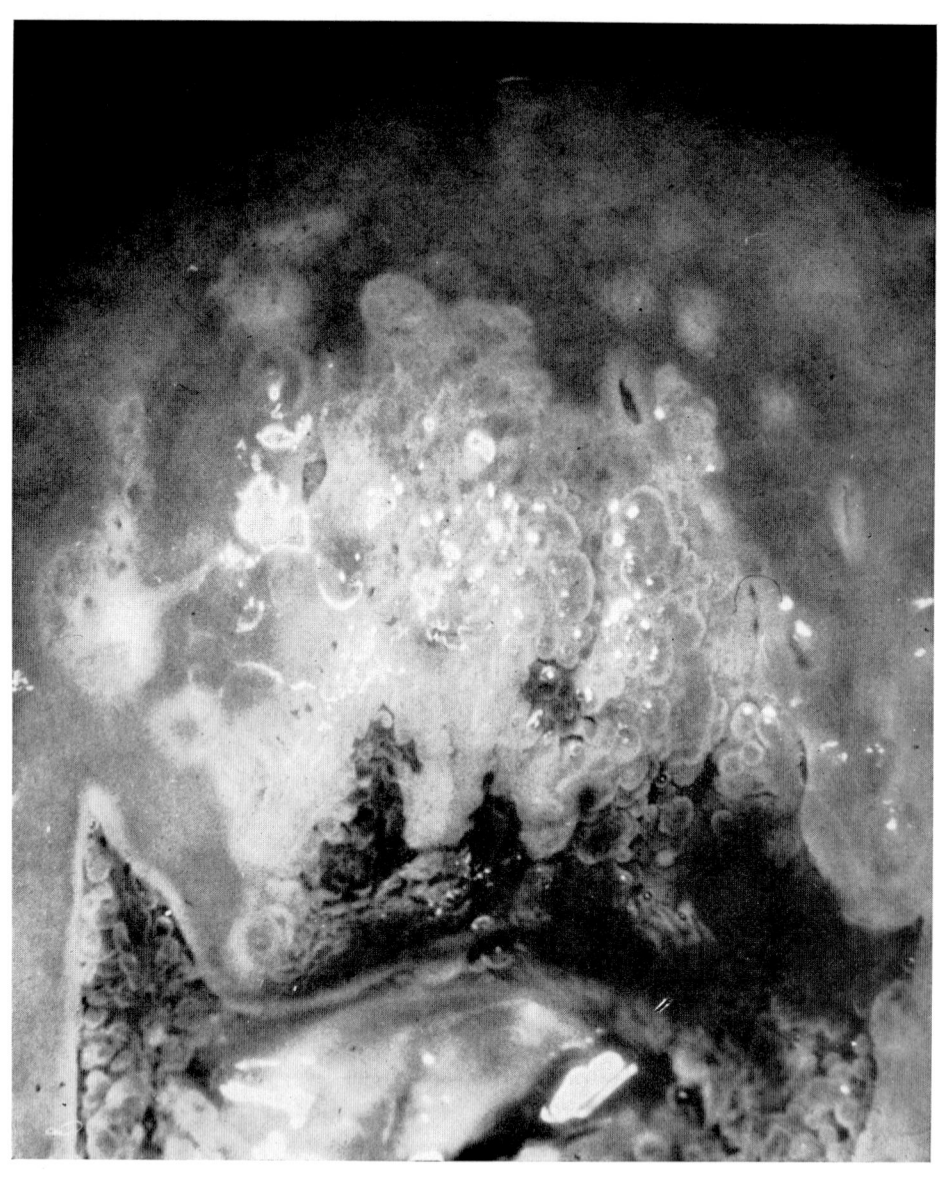

Figure 156. White epithelium. At an early stage after fusion of the columnar villi, the new squamous epithelium has an irregular surface which reflects its origin. Histologically an undifferentiated epithelium would be expected.

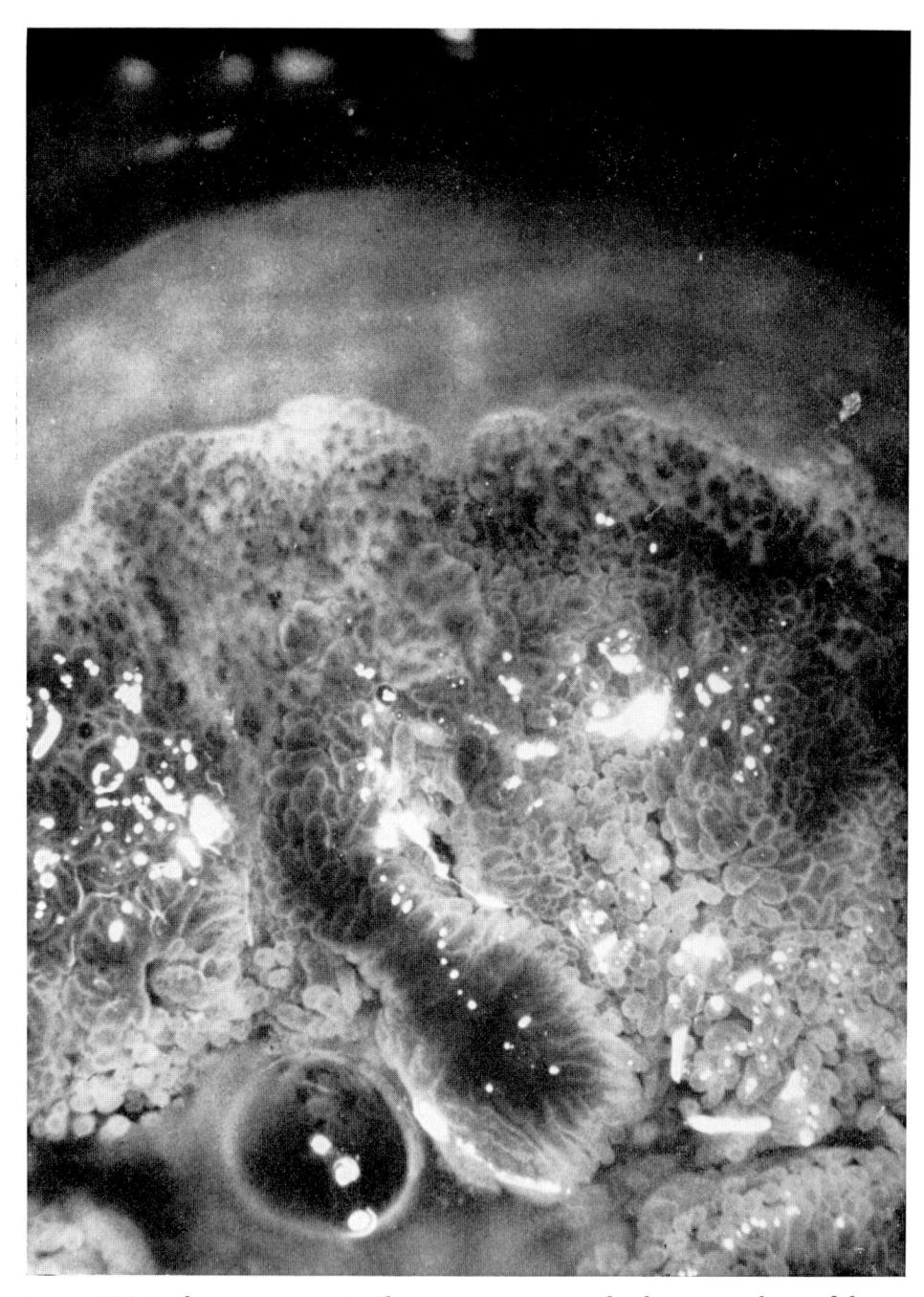

Figure 157. Early punctation. Developing punctation is clearly seen in the caudal zone of the columnar epithelium abutting original squamous epithelium in the upper third of the photograph. The original capillary loops of the columnar epithelium show through a pale epithelium of metaplastic origin.

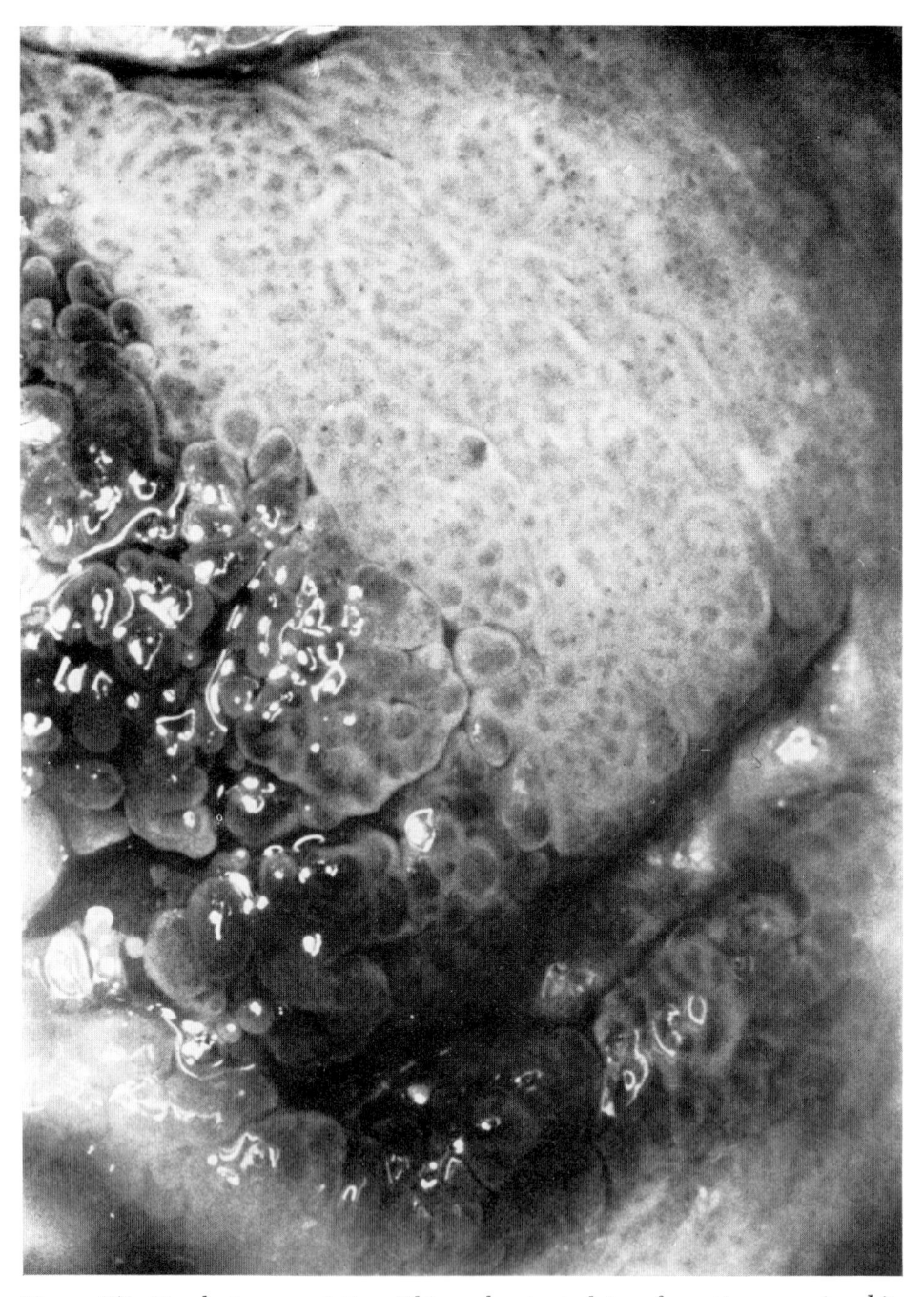

Figure 158. Developing punctation. This early atypical transformation zone is white and contains punctate arrangements of its capillary loops, which are somewhat more marked than in Figure 157.

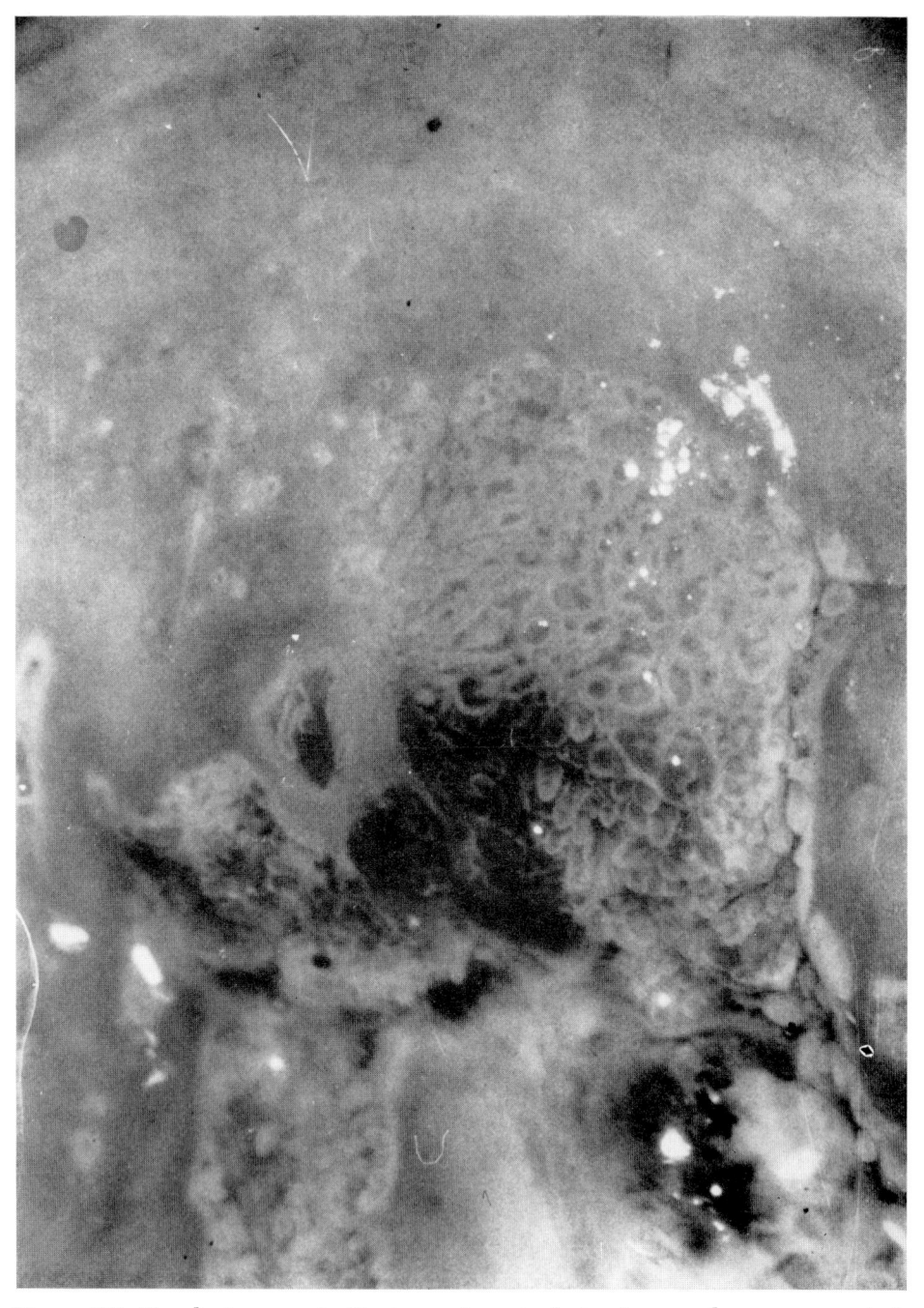

Figure 159. Developing mosaic. During early metaplasia, the vascular arrangements in some instances are suggestive of evolution towards a mosaic structure.

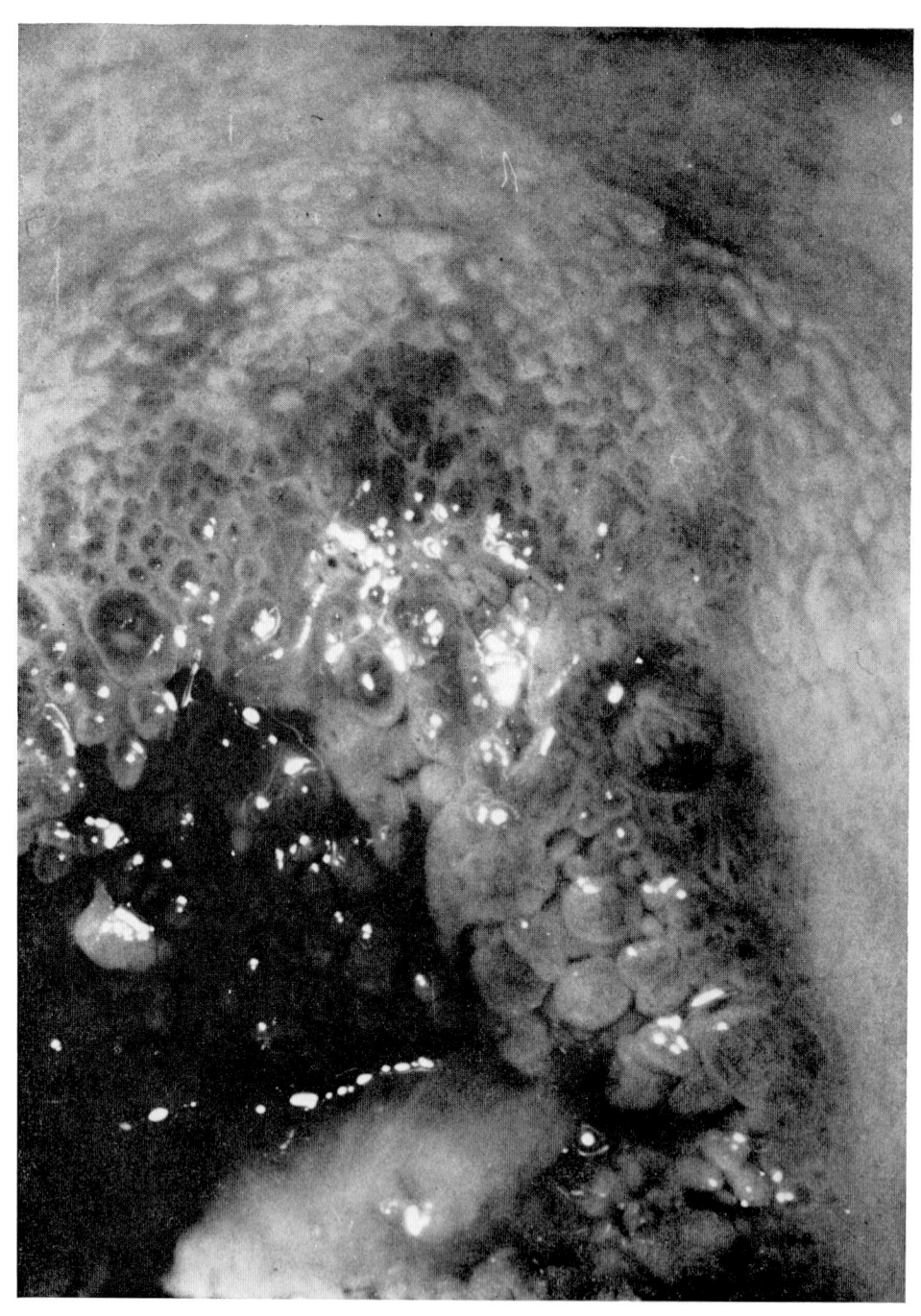

Figure 160. Developing mosaic. In this better developed atypical transformation zone, metaplasia has generated a definite mosaic structure. Note the abrupt junction with original squamous epithelium in the upper right corner.

the limits of any proposed excision. The atypical transformation zone may be wholly visible or partly visible due to its presence in the cervical canal out of sight of the colposcope. The clinical significance of these variations is discussed later (Chap. 16).

As in the typical transformation zone, the original squamocolumnar junction serves as the caudal limit enclosing the atypical transformation zone. Its sharp delineation (Fig. 161) contrasts somewhat with the more vague line of demarcation in typical forms. In some accounts of dysplasia and preclinical carcinoma, there seems to be an understanding that this limit is subject to change, as the atypical epithelium gradually extends outwards, replacing the adjacent original squamous epithelium. We have never observed such outward extension and believe that it does not occur unless as part of an invasive carcinoma. The atypical changes encountered on the vaginal wall, in about 4 per cent of cases, represent the embryologically determined extent of the original squamocolumnar junction and not an outward extension of a proliferating lesion (Fig. 161). The proximal limits of the atypical transformation zone are variable.

Topographically, in different areas of the same zone, there is frequently a combination of both atypical and physiological colposcopic appearances (Fig. 162). Within the atypical areas, a combination of different appearances may also occur. Likewise, histological appearances varying from dysplasias to carcinoma may occur in the same zone.

Colour and Opacity

WHITE EPITHELIUM: With the routine application of acetic acid solution, the principal characteristic is the tendency for the atypical transformation zone to display an area of sharply delineated white or grey colour which is substantially opaque or shows faint vascular markings (Figs. 163-165). In our experience, the changes following the acetic acid application allow the most useful diagnostic interpretation, and the whiter the change, the more extreme is the histological abnormality. The reason for this temporary change, which fades within several minutes of the application of acetic acid, is unknown.

Colours prior to the application of acetic acid are not distinctive and are of little diagnostic value. Colour in these discussions refers to those developed upon the addition of acetic acid.

KERATOSIS: Within areas of atypical transformation zone, white keratotic elevations may occur and do not need the application of acetic acid to render them apparent (Figs. 166 and 167). Areas of keratosis may be extensive or patchy and, when relatively thick, are evident with the unaided eye. They express some disorder of keratin synthesis, a process which may or may not be related to preneoplastic events. The presence of abnormal

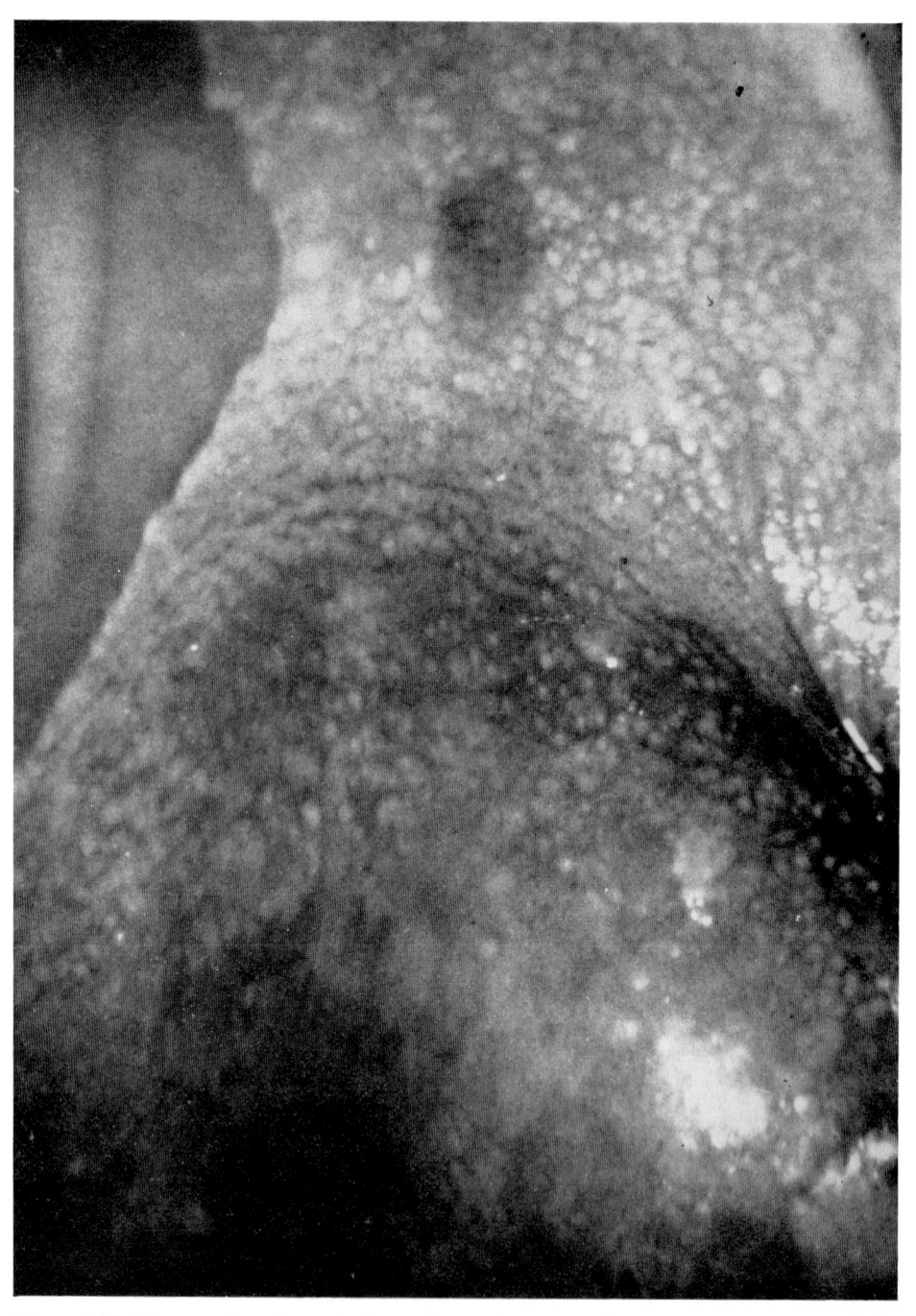

Figure 161. Topography of atypical transformation zone. An important variation of the distribution of the atypical transformation zone is shown. The atypical epithelium with mosaic structure extends from cervical canal to the lower portion of the photograph across the fornix onto the anterior vaginal wall.

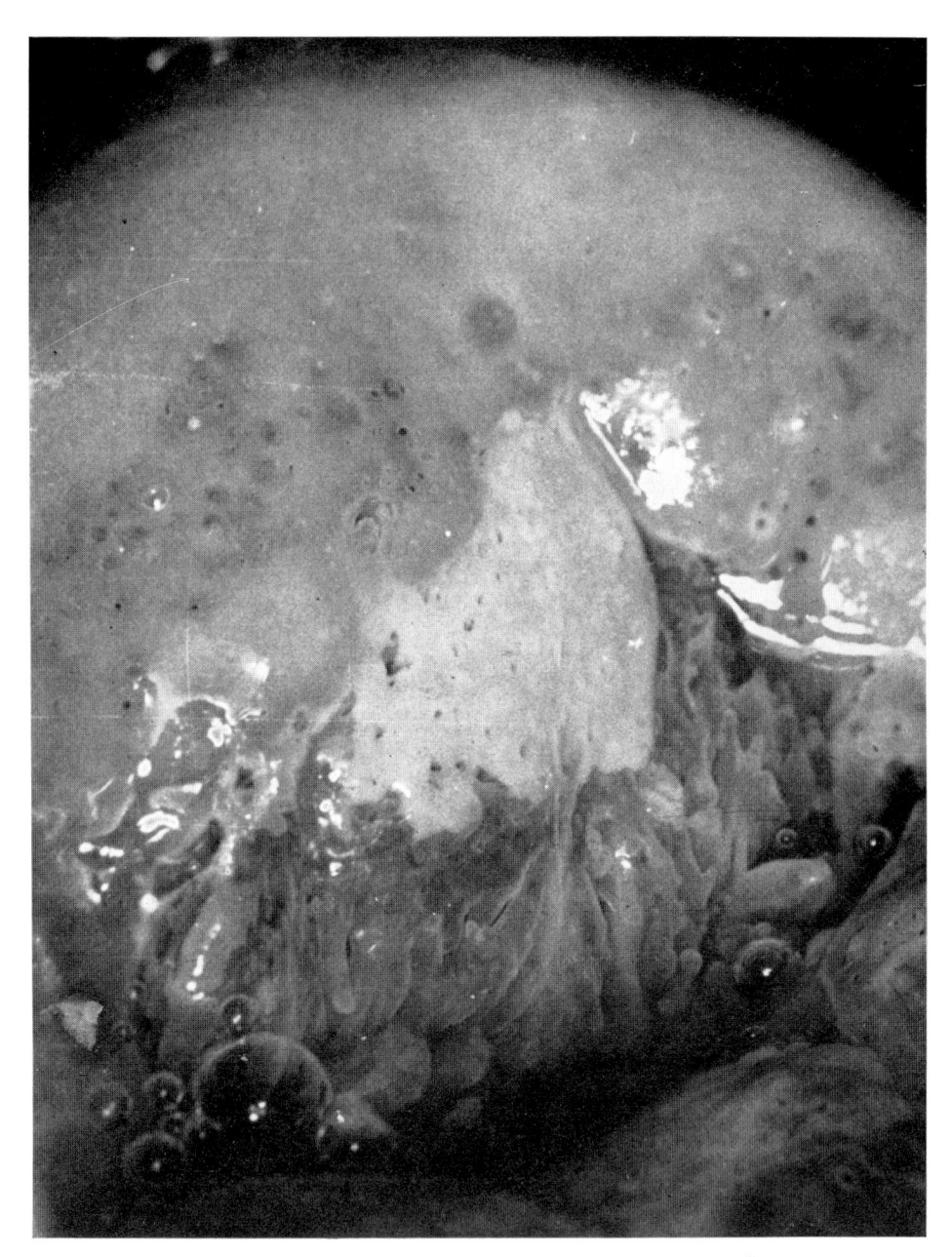

Figure 162. Topography of atypical transformation zone. An atypical area may constitute the whole or portion of the transformation zone. In this example, white epithelium forms part of the cephalic extent of a transformation zone and represents an episode of metaplasia occurring at a different time.

amounts of keratin obscures other underlying morphological features, such as mosaic and punctation. Also, an appreciation of the more important aspects of grading is prejudiced.

Keratosis is also seen in the original squamous epithelium, in the original transformation zone (p. 374), where it has no clinical significance, and in some forms of condyloma (*see* Fig. 212).

Surface Configuration

Some surface configurations imply underlying abnormal epithelial states and are important in the system of grading in use, but other surface features of physiological origin need to be recalled. These latter features are the possible legacy of the original columnar epithelium which the atypical metaplastic form has succeeded and may represent the persistence of cleft remnants, cystic inclusions (*see* Fig. 152), and even the persistence of villiform structures (*see* Fig. 156). With these basic variations in surface configuration in mind, appreciation of the more important appearance suggestive of neoplasia is possible.

The essence of gross atypical change is the presence of minute papillary elevations. Each elevation is associated with a stromal papilla enclosing the intraepithelial capillary (*see* Fig. 171). In a gradation of changes, small protuberances or excrescences become evident in more advanced lesions. The size and irregularity of the excrescences becomes increasingly evident until these changes are clinically manifest and form the basis for a clinical suspicion of invasive cancer.

Angioarchitecture

The range of appearances of vascular variations occurring within the atypical transformation zone are discussed in angioarchitecture. Intraepithelial capillaries of varying pattern and calibre constitute some of the most striking colposcopic appearances. However, atypical transformation zone is not necessarily associated with the presence of intraepithelial capillaries; in fact, large areas of white epithelium are often devoid of blood vessels (*see* Figs. 163-165).

PUNCTATION: The basic unit of this structure is the single, looped capillary lying within the stromal papilla, seen end-on as a dot and coursing obliquely or perpendicularly towards the surface of the epithelium. This arrangement confers the pattern so characteristic of punctation, which in its minimal degree is extremely fine, with closely spaced, looped capillaries of narrow calibre forming a mainly regular pattern. The distance between each capillary is minimal (Fig. 168A). More marked degrees affect the course and calibre of the looped capillaries and intercapillary relationships. The vessels then display increasing calibre, showing increased and

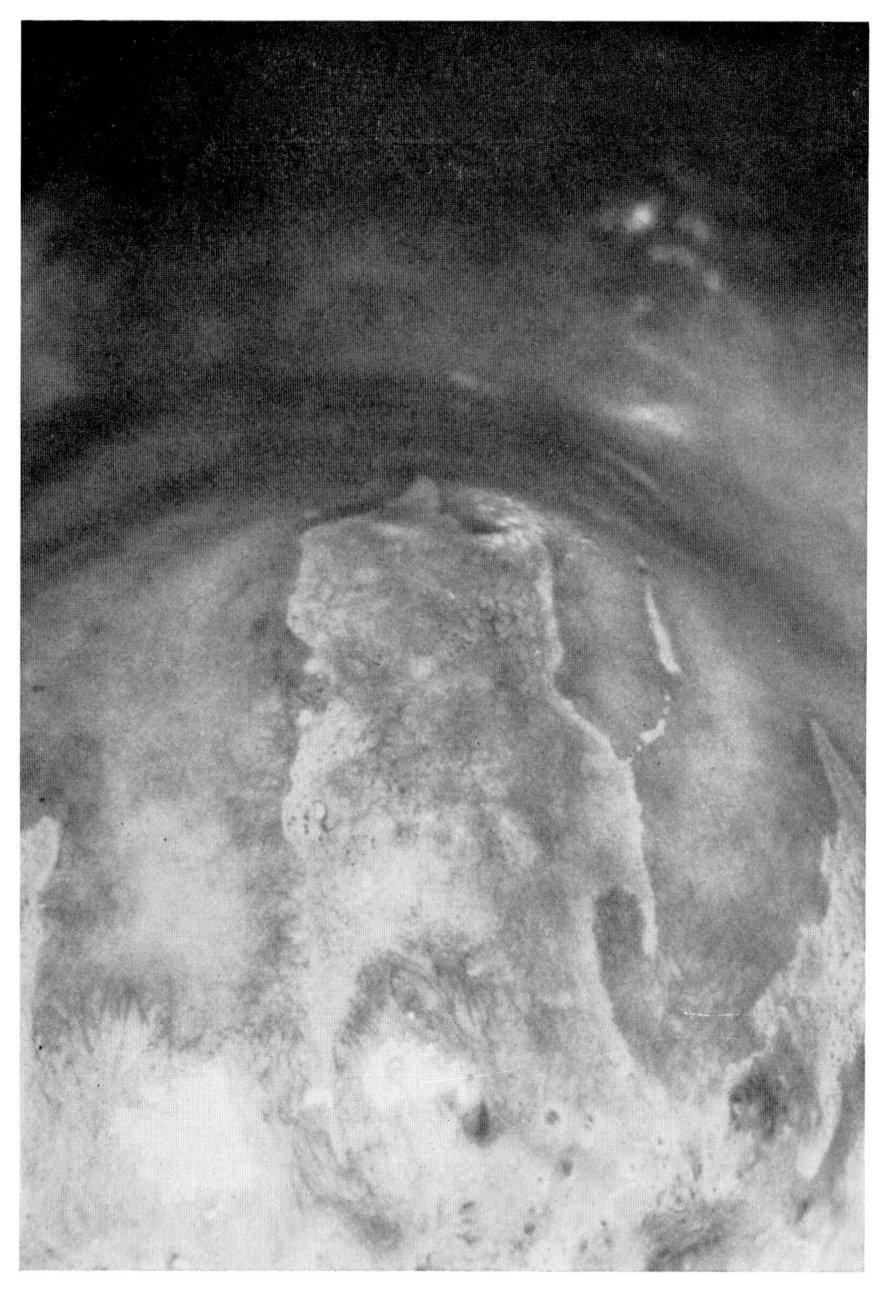

Figure 163. White epithelium. The atypical transformation zone on the anterior lip displays few vascular structures. The field displays the least degree of whiteness in atypical lesions and no histological abnormality is expected. The area extends almost to the vaginal fornix.

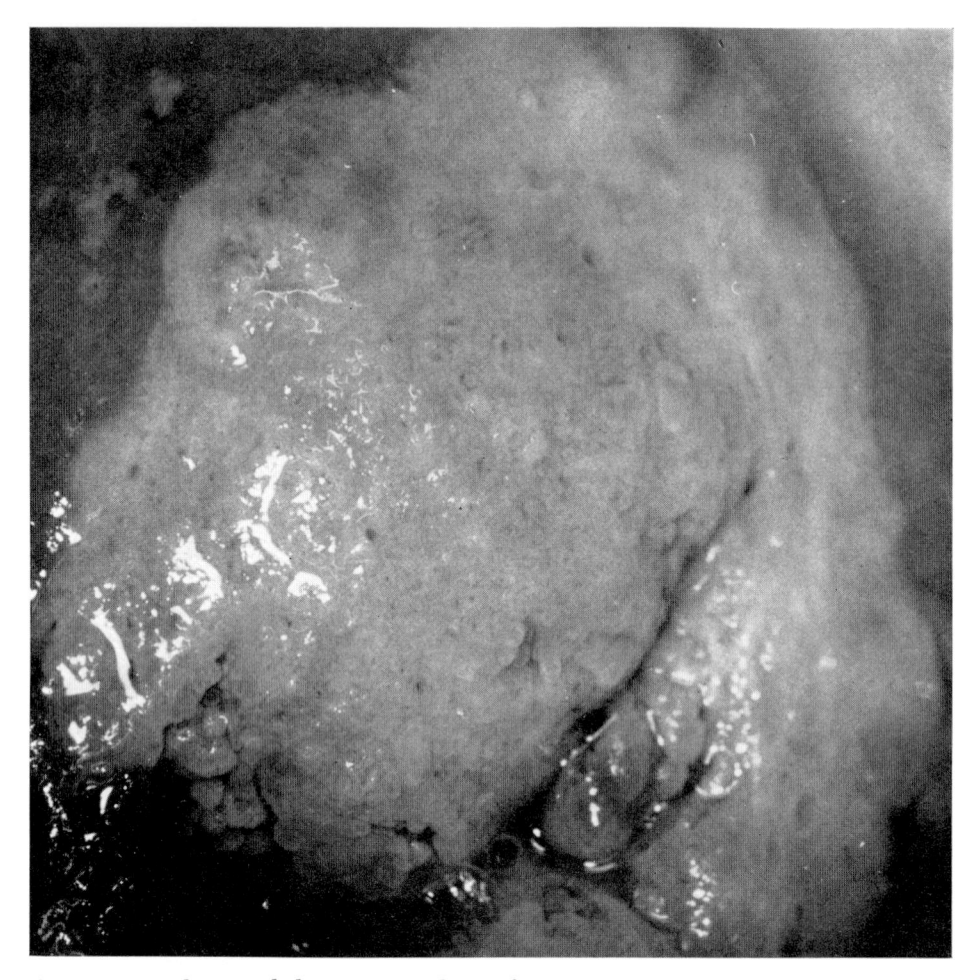

Figure 164. White epithelium. Atypical transformation zone has evolved as white epithelium with gland openings but no vascular markings. The degree of whiteness is more pronounced than in Figure 163, and histological disorders of moderate degree would be expected.

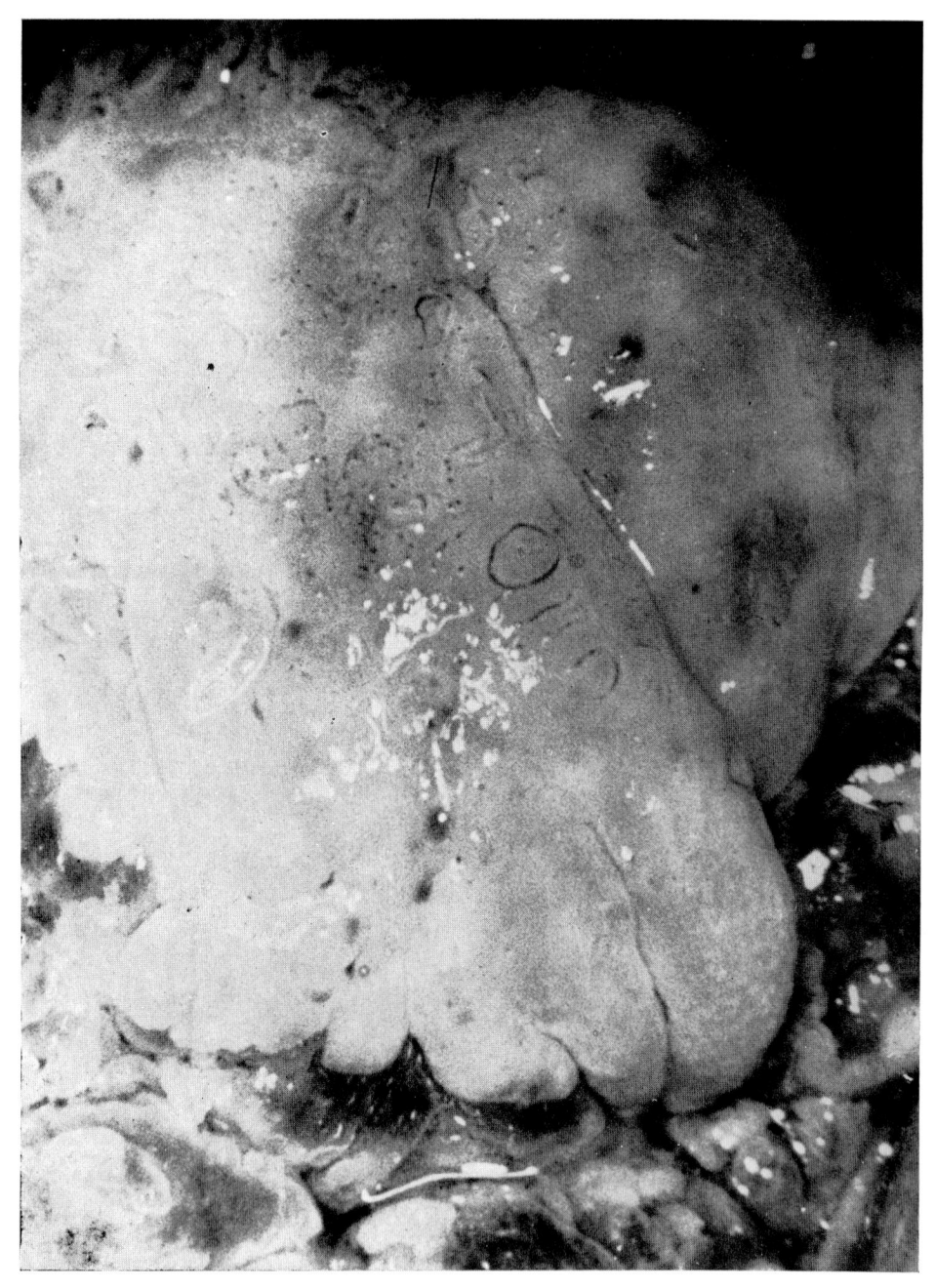

Figure 165. White epithelium. The cervix displays an extensive area of very white epithelium on the anterior lip of the cervix in some parts of which a vascular pattern is evident. The appearances are consistent with a histological diagnosis of carcinoma in situ.

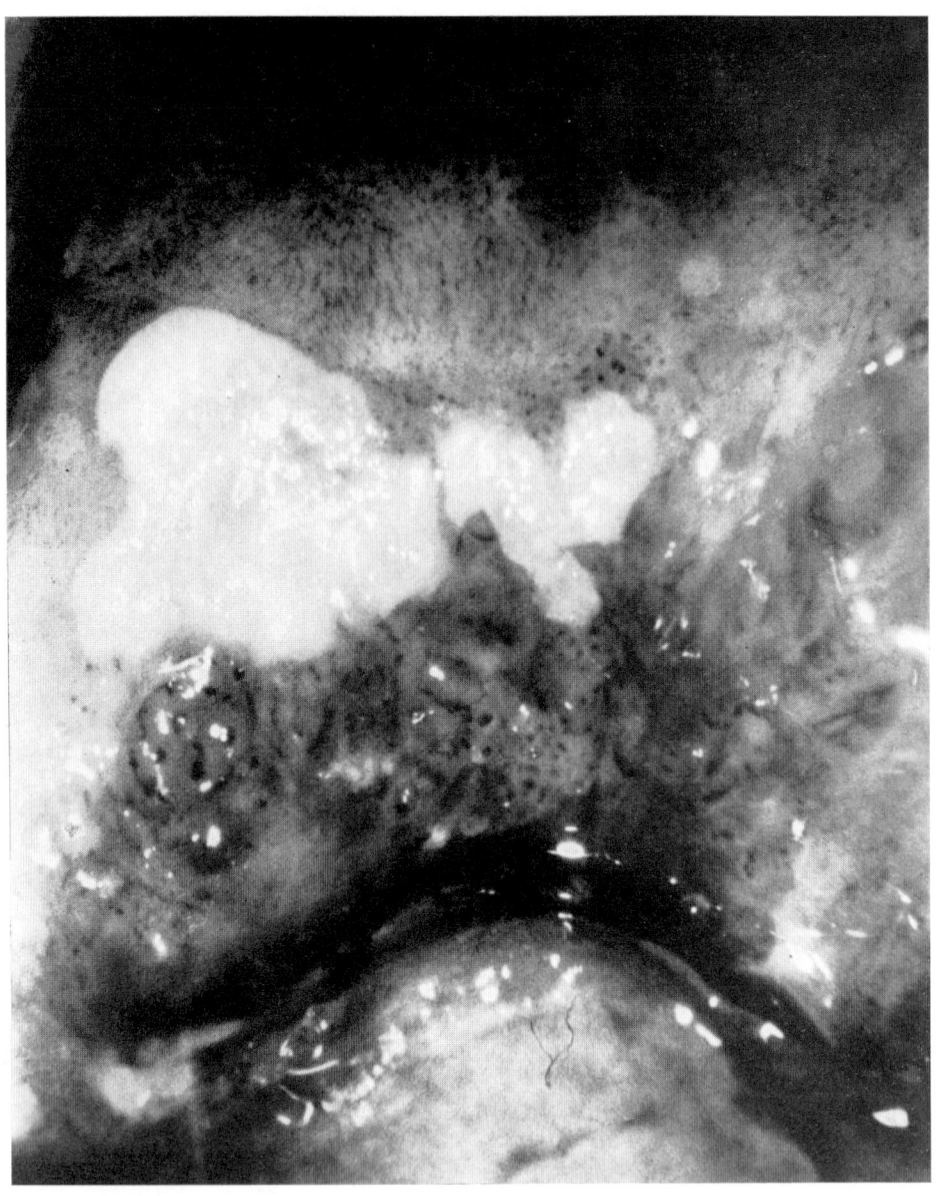

Figure 166. Keratosis. Metaplastic epithelium may produce excessive keratin, seen as keratosis. This colpophotograph shows portion of the anterior lip with the cervical canal in the lower portion of the photograph. The atypical transformation zone displays coarse-calibre punctation above and below a circumscribed patch of keratosis.

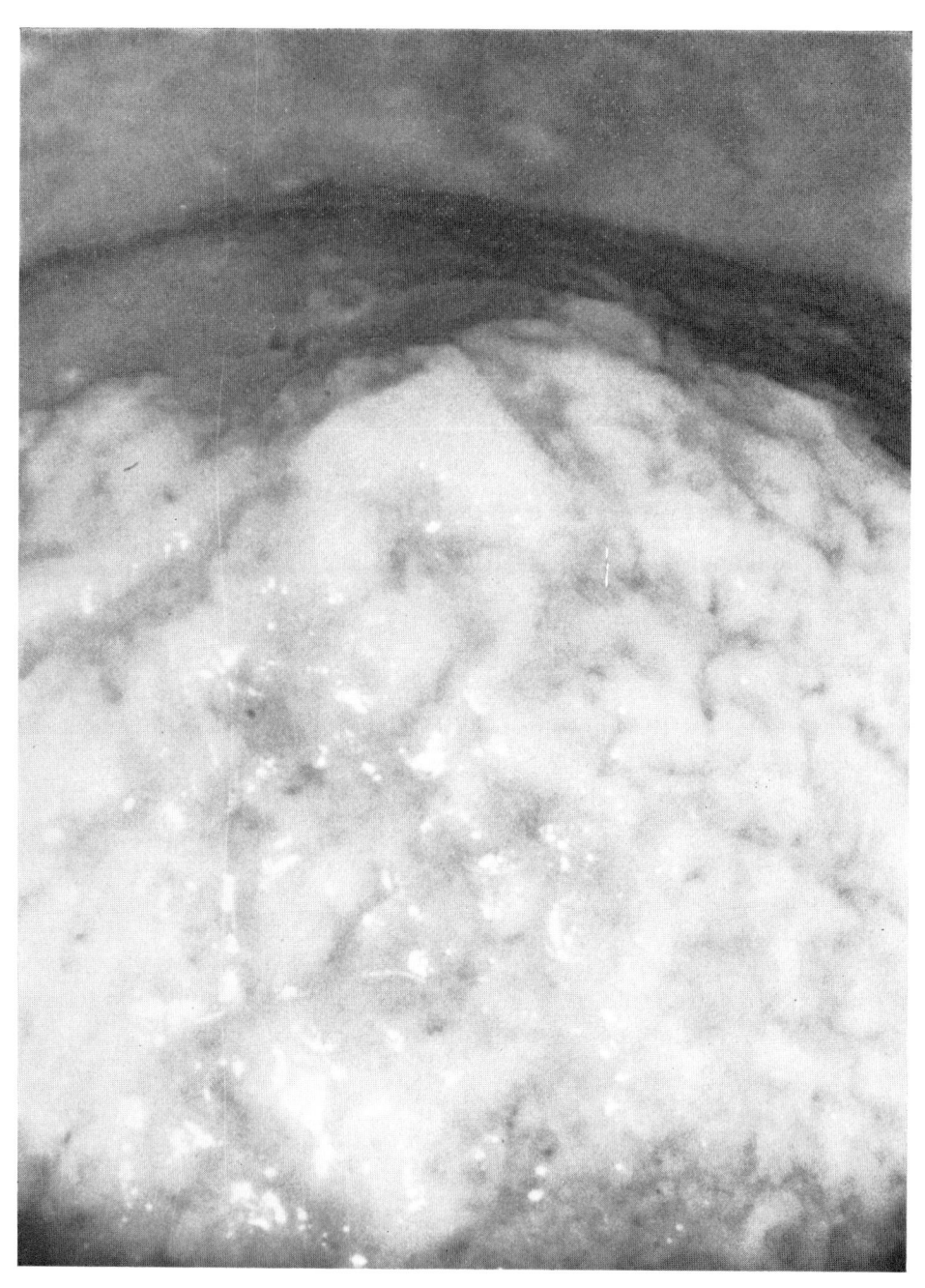

Figure 167. Keratosis. Colpophotograph of the upper portion of the anterior lip adjoining the vaginal fornix. The whole transformation zone is covered and obscured by keratosis. No cytological or histological abnormality was found.

irregular spacing (Fig. 169). The most marked degrees show terminal vessels which are coarse calibre and coiled, often resembling corkscrews, widely spaced with irregular intervals, randomly directed and sometimes raised (Figs. 170-174).

Mosaic: The regular mosaic arrangements of terminal vessels have always been recognised as an important attribute of atypical forms of epithelia. Several variations contribute to this appearance. In its minimal development, mosaic pattern shows fine-calibre vessels surrounding small areas of regular size and shape (Figs. 168B and 175). Increasing through intermediate stages (Figs. 176 and 177) to its maximal development (Figs. 178-180), the pattern shows coarser, more superficial vessels surrounding fields which may be grossly irregular in size and shape, so that overall intercapillary distances are increased.

Often, combinations of both punctation and mosaic structure intermingle (Figs. 181-183).

Occasionally, in typical transformation zone, a pattern often mistaken for mosaic structure is evident. This is merely an arrangement of the circular vessels often seen surrounding gland openings.

Atypical Vessels: In some lesions, especially those in which invasive changes have occurred, new vessel formation results in branching vessels demonstrating gross variation in calibre and course with bizarre, irregular branching. These appearances are most characteristic of overt carcinoma but may occur in the major grade of atypical transformation zone (Figs. 184 and 185).

The transition of this new formation from pre-existing punctation or mosaic may be seen at times, so that differentiation between these major vascular abnormalities is difficult. More often, the degree of aberration is sufficiently clear cut to make the categorization straightforward. Atypical vessels as a rule are strikingly different from the vascular patterns seen in typical transformation zones, except for the occasional presence of large vessels in the typical zone which may have complicated branching. However, even in these cases, close inspection reveals a finer terminal arborization, which does not occur with atypical vessels. A wide intercapillary distance is not a sufficiently constant finding to be diagnostic in these cases.

Grading

As experience is gained in the technique of colposcopy, the observer becomes aware of a range of variation of the prime morphological features. This is termed *grading*. The criteria upon which atypical transformation zones are classified by degree, and their histological correlations have already been discussed (p. 156). The importance of grades in assessment of

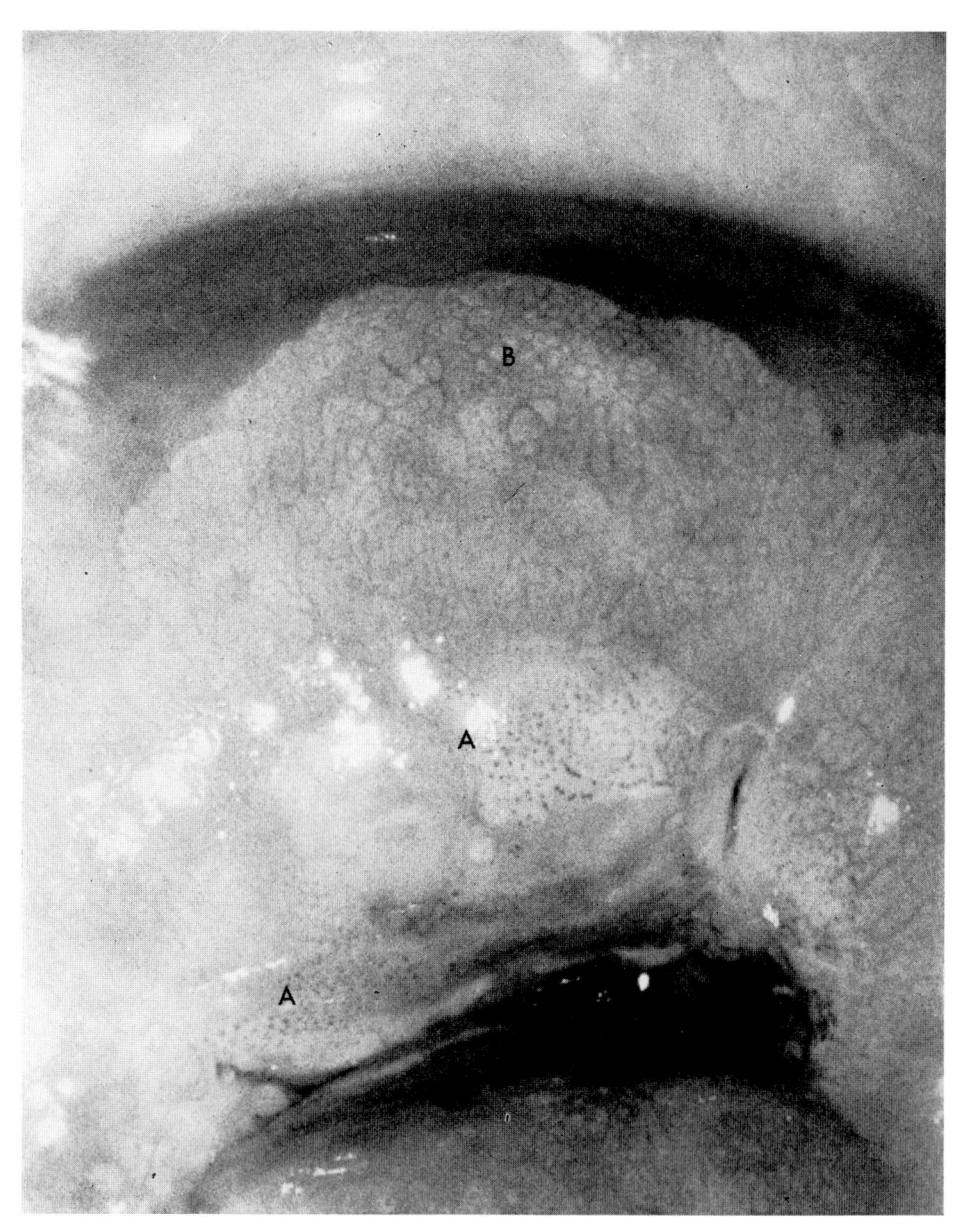

Figure 168. Punctation. Colpophotograph of anterior lip of cervix displaying extensive atypical transformation zone. At the sites A, closely spaced intraepithelial capillaries of small calibre can be seen. At site B is fine regular mosaic structure.

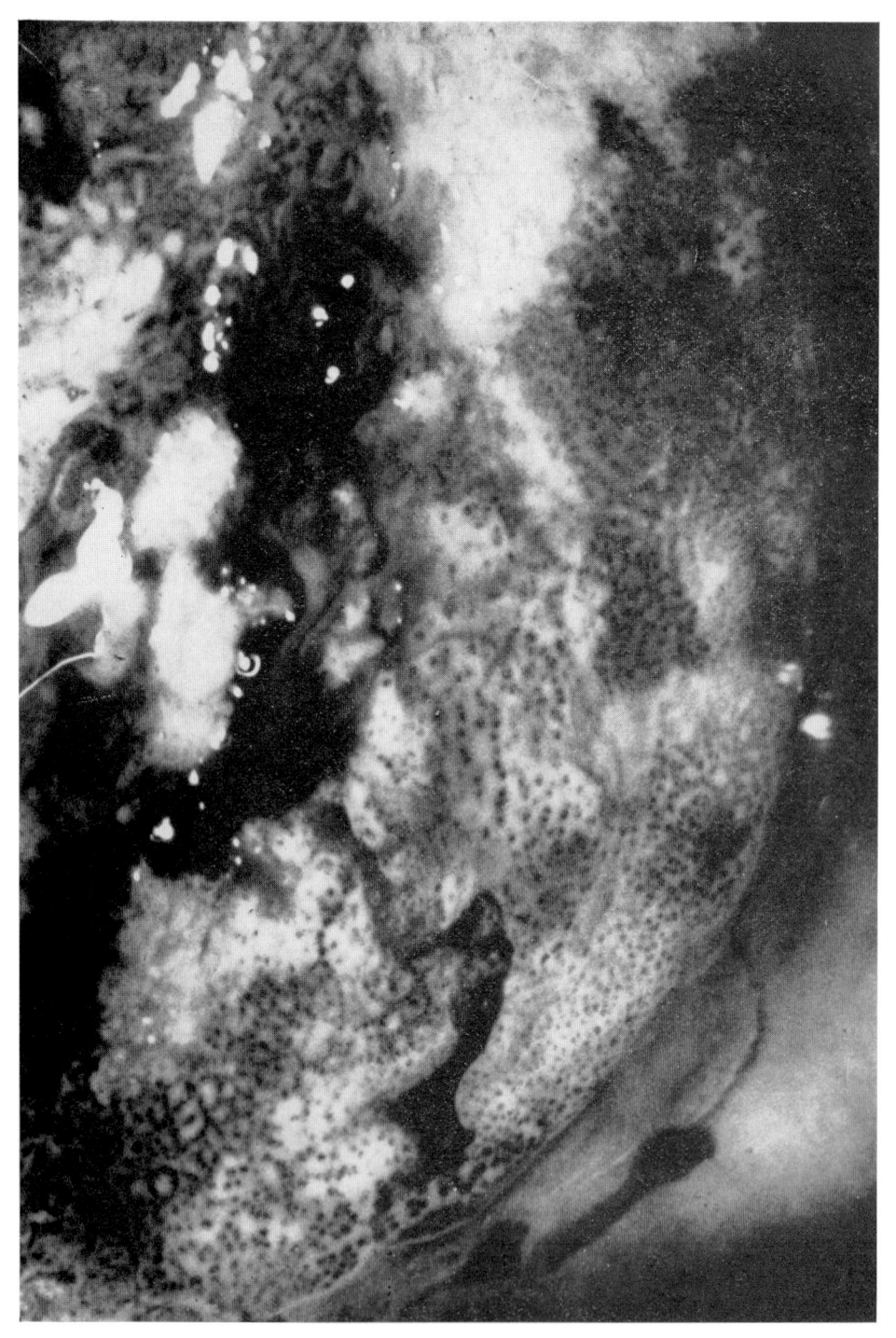

Figure 169. Punctation. Colpophotograph of portion of anterior lip showing an extensive atypical transformation zone. The capillary loops display increased calibre and spacing compared to that seen in Figure 168. A significant histological disorder is expected.

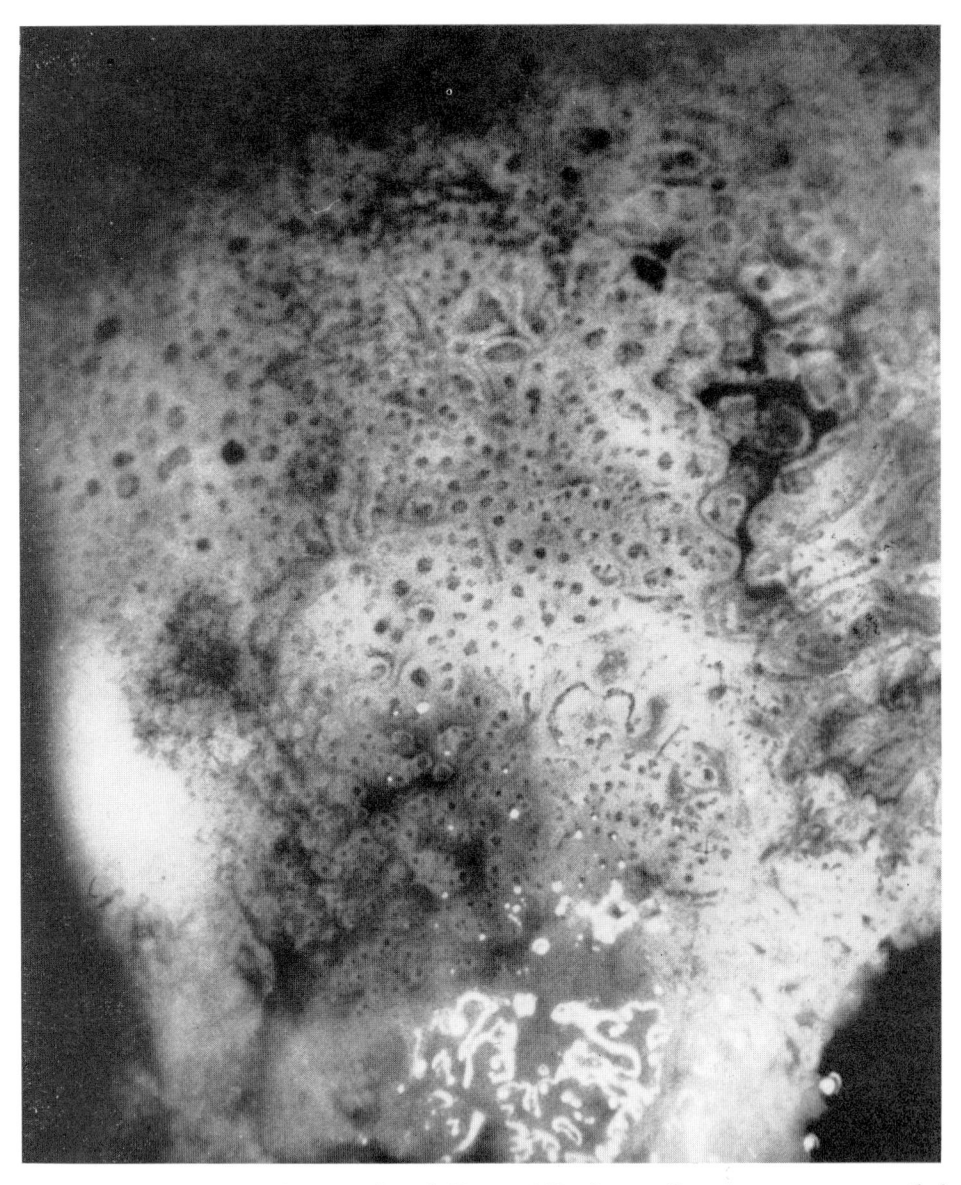

Figure 170. Punctation. Compared with Figure 169, the capillary loops are now coiled and dilated as they approach the surface. Some are seen coursing horizontally and obliquely through the epithelium. Carcinoma in situ or early invasion can be predicted. The area adjoined frank invasive cancer.

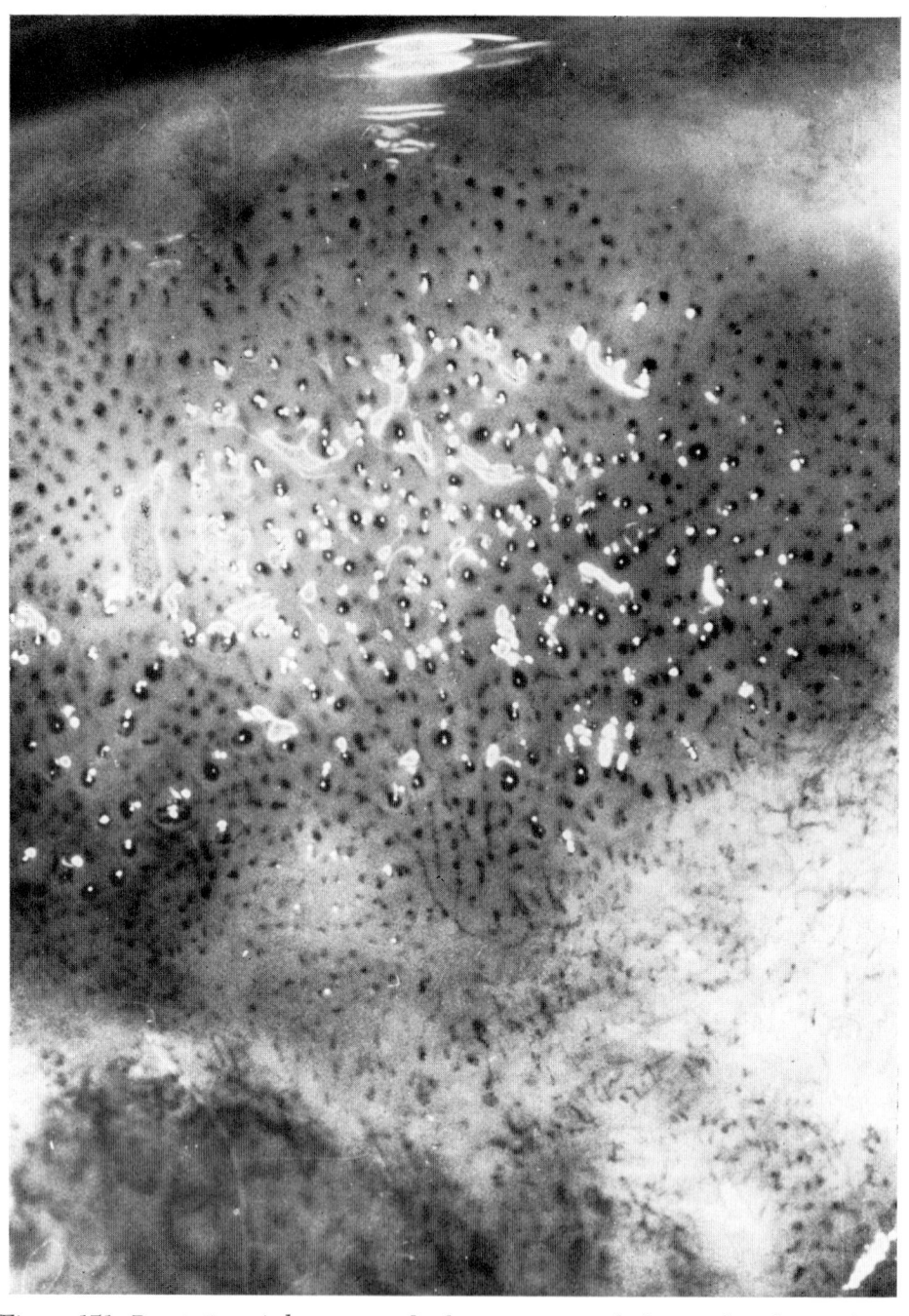

Figure 171. Punctation. A large area displaying very marked vascular abnormalities. The capillaries are dilated, raised, and widely spaced. The characteristic sharp edge of the atypical transformation zone is evident at the top of the photograph.

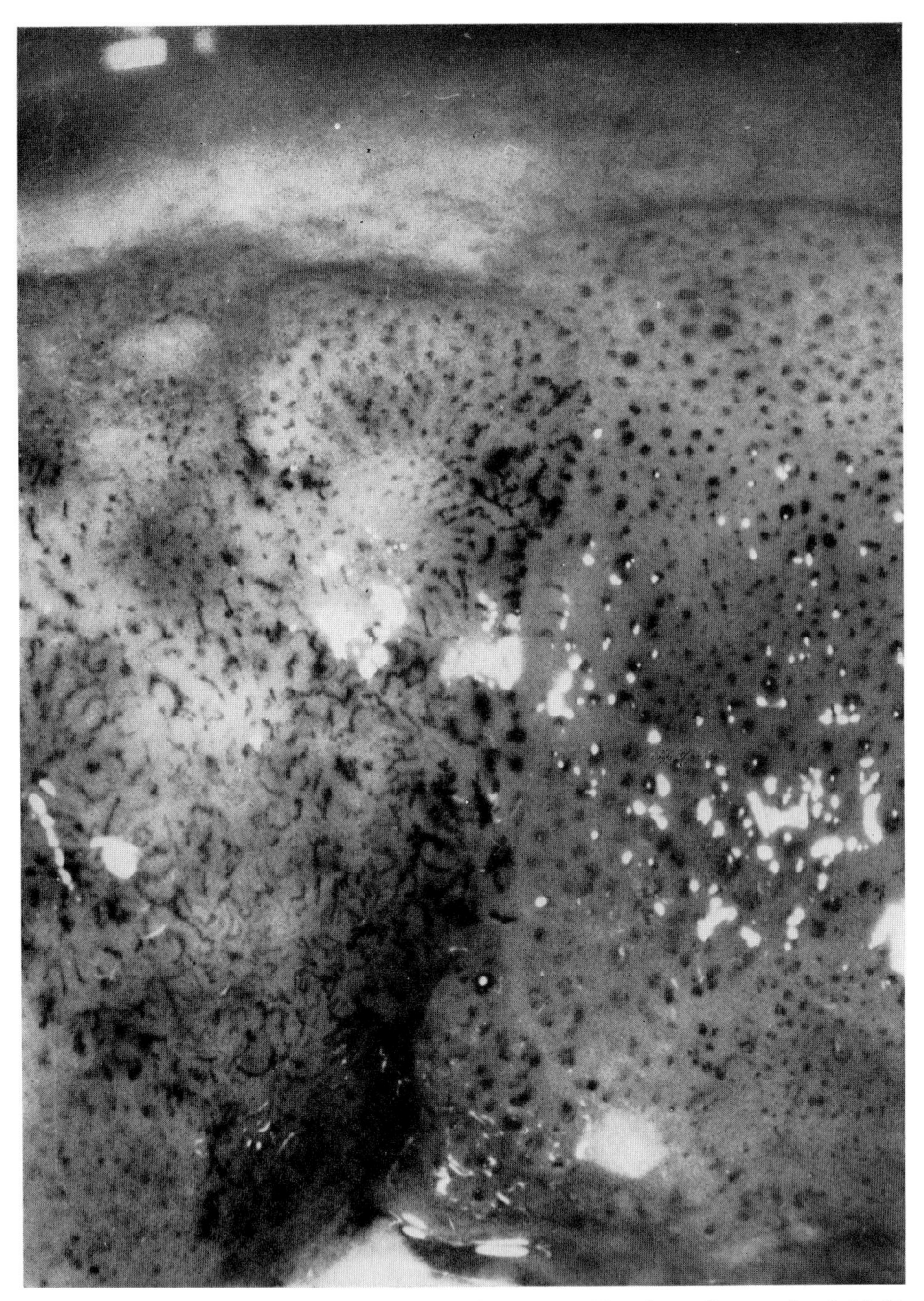

Figure 172. Punctation. In addition to widely spaced dilated capillaries, the field displays atypical vessels occurring amidst punctation. The vascular structures course in many directions and are dilated and irregular. The appearance was associated with carcinoma in situ.

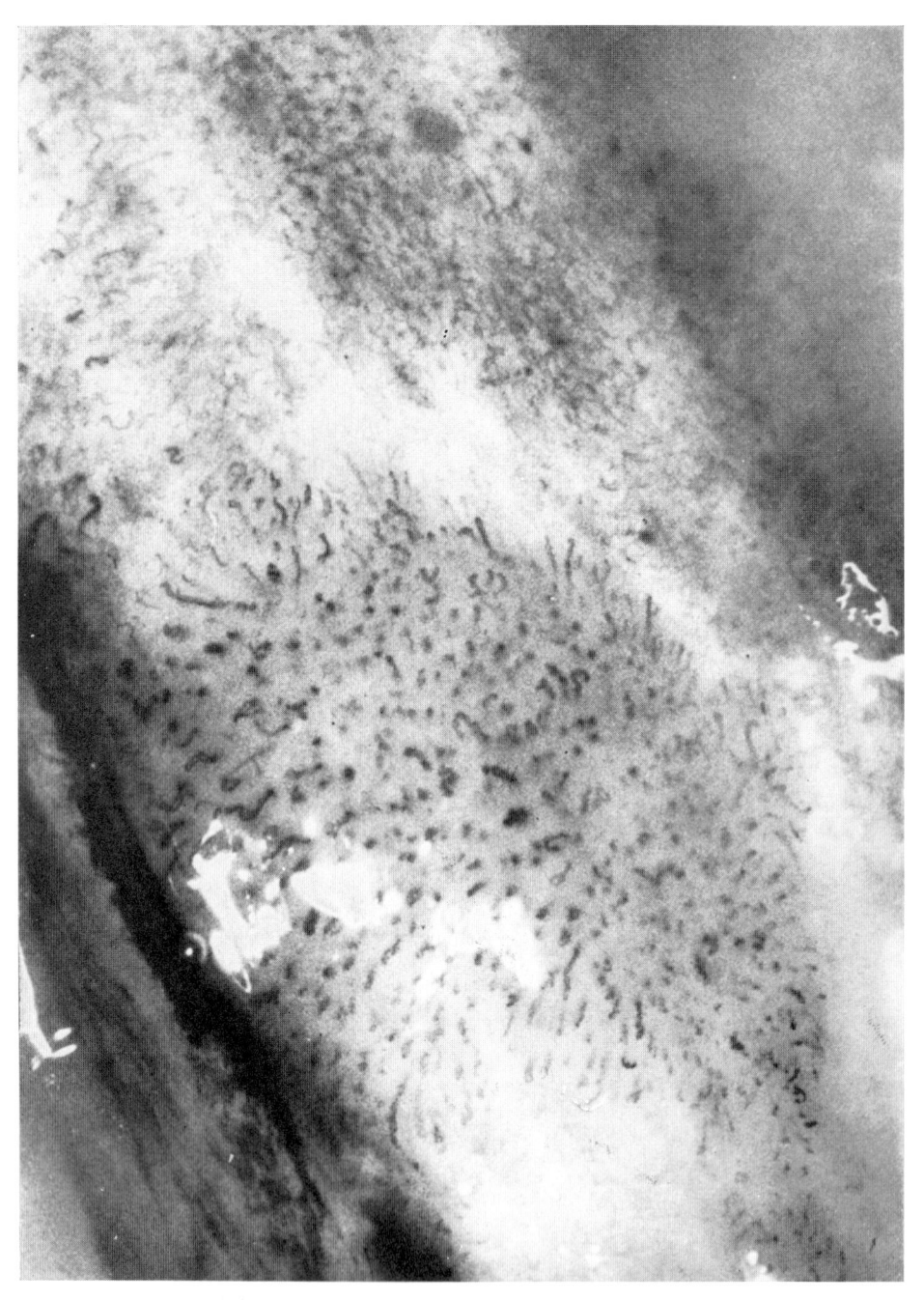

Figure 173. Punctation. In the vessels of the lower half of the photograph dilatation, coiling, and wide spacing of capillaries is evident. Vessels course obliquely and horizontally in many directions within the epithelium.

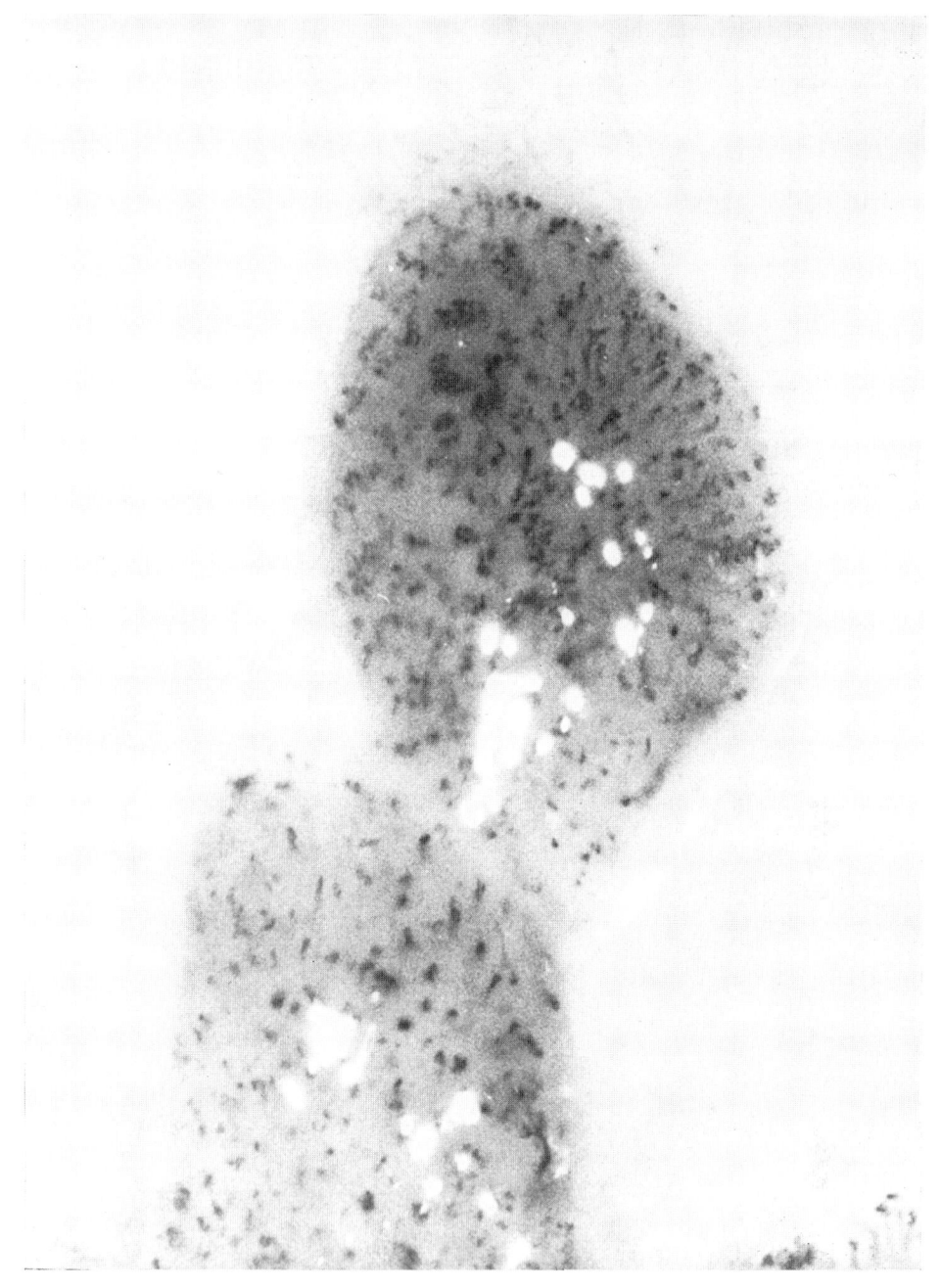

Figure 174. Punctation. In this study, Grade III punctation was found in association with invasive cancer elsewhere on the cervix. The large intercapillary distance is striking in the lower portion of the area.

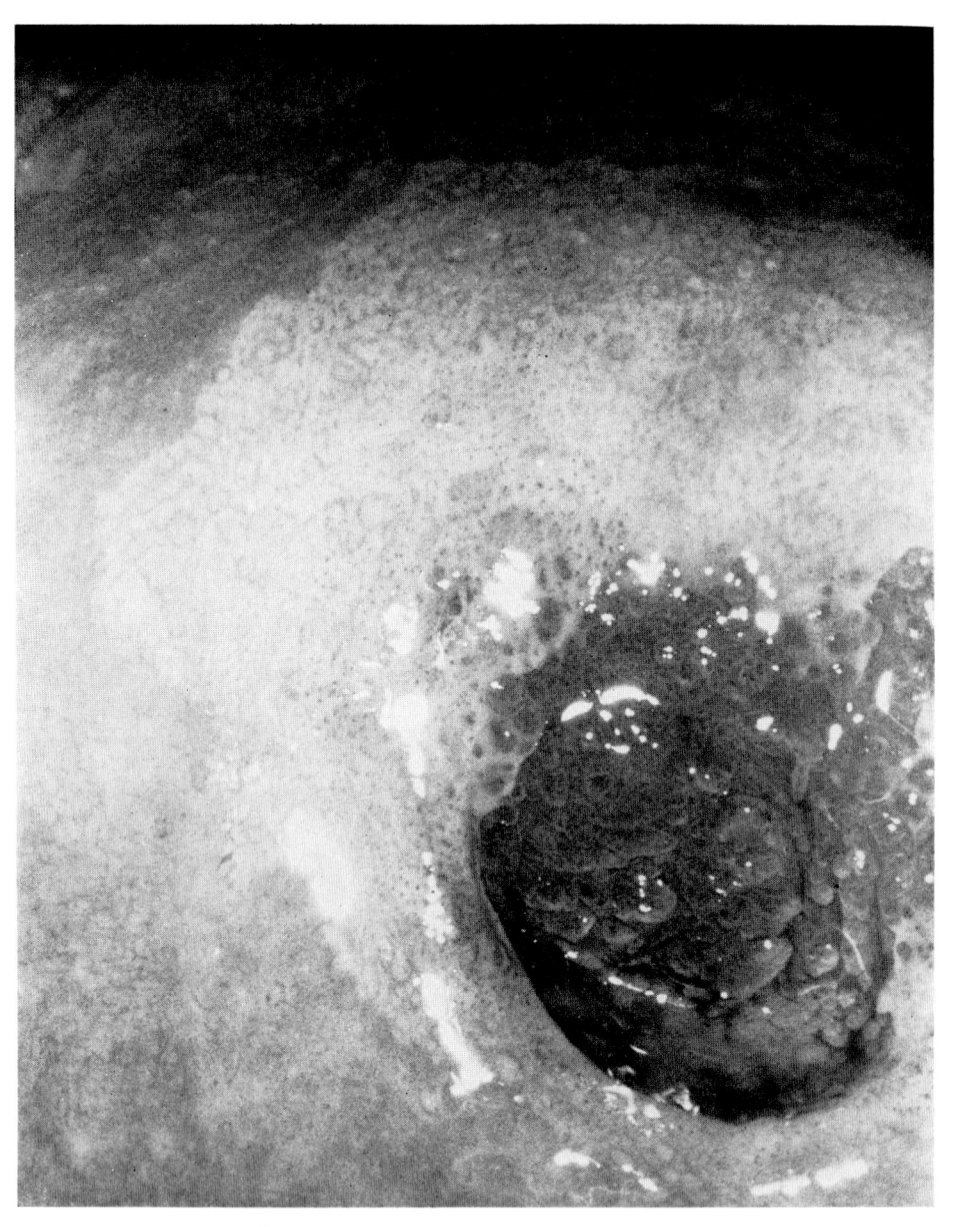

Figure 175. Mosaic. This study shows atypical transformation zone which is principally mosaic, but contains some punctation. The vessels forming the mosaic pattern are of small calibre and circumscribe blocks of regular size. Columnar epithelium of the lower canal can be seen in the rounded area of the lower right quarter of the photograph. No histological abnormality was present on biopsy.

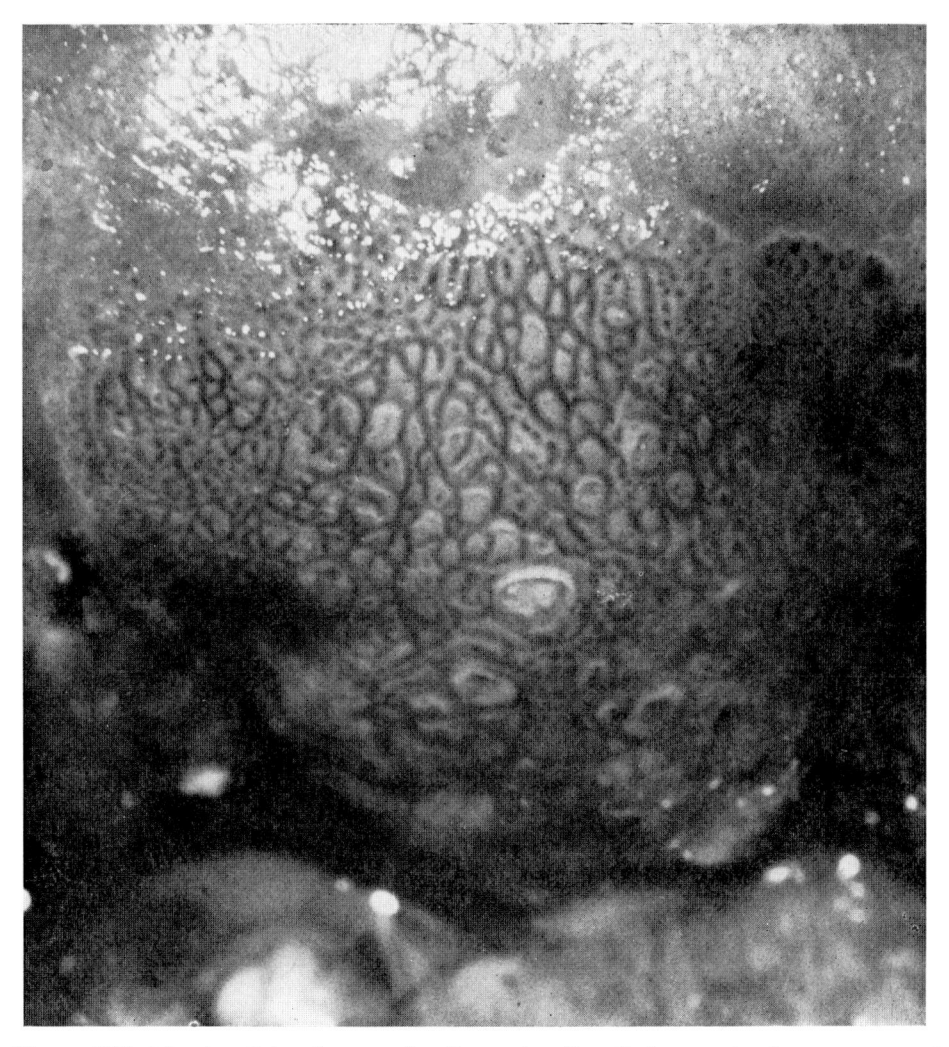

Figure 176. Mosaic. Colpophotograph of anterior lip of the cervix showing atypical transformation zone. The mosaic pattern is more striking than that of Figure 175. The vessels are of larger calibre and are more evident, being closer to the surface. Generally, the pattern is regular. Biopsy showed major dysplasia.

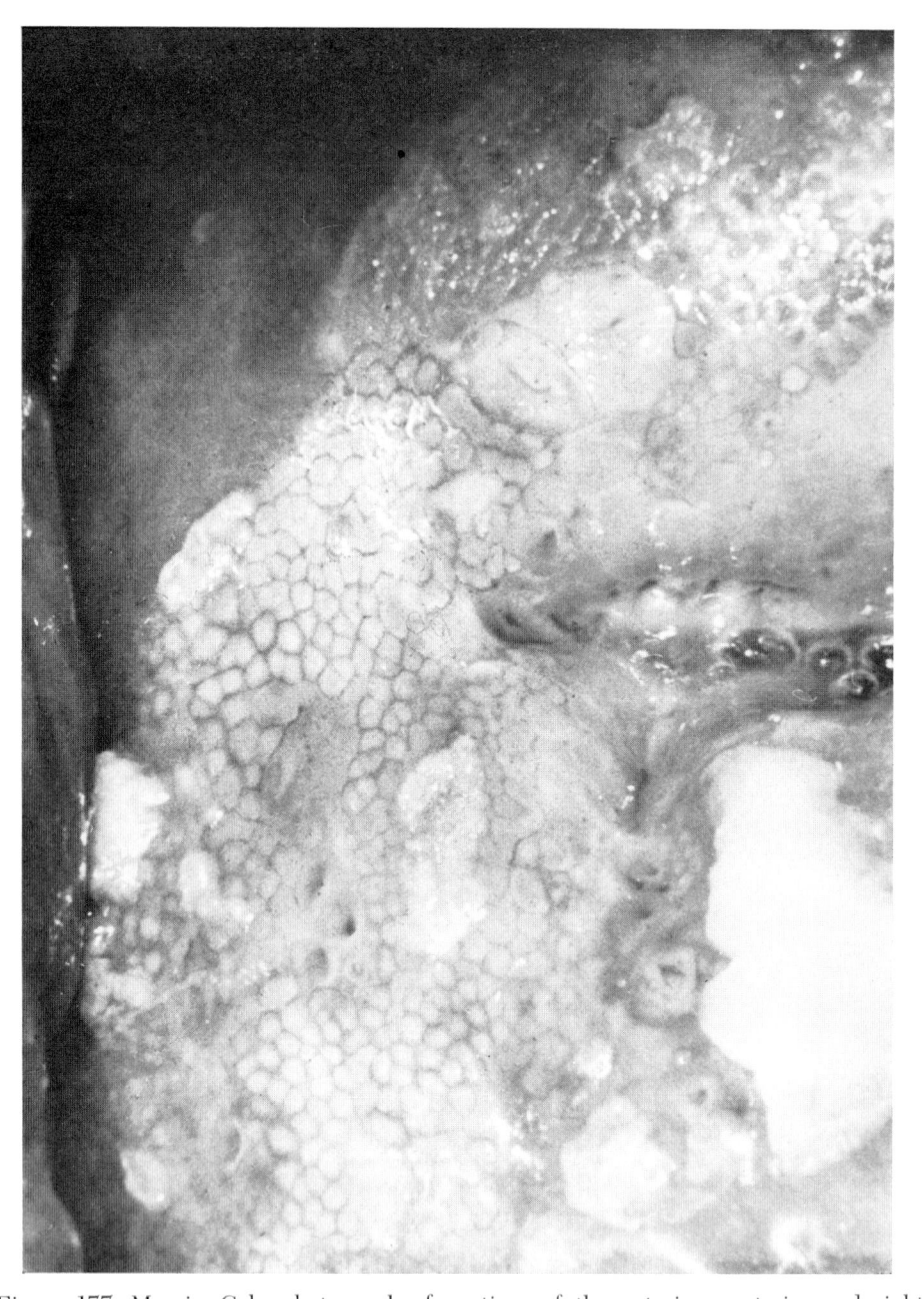

Figure 177. Mosaic. Colpophotograph of portions of the anterior, posterior and right lateral lips of the cervix. A striking mosaic has evolved in epithelium shown to contain carcinoma in situ. Patchy keratosis is present. The epithelium is very white, and the vessels surround regular mosaic blocks. An extensive area including the endocervix is involved.

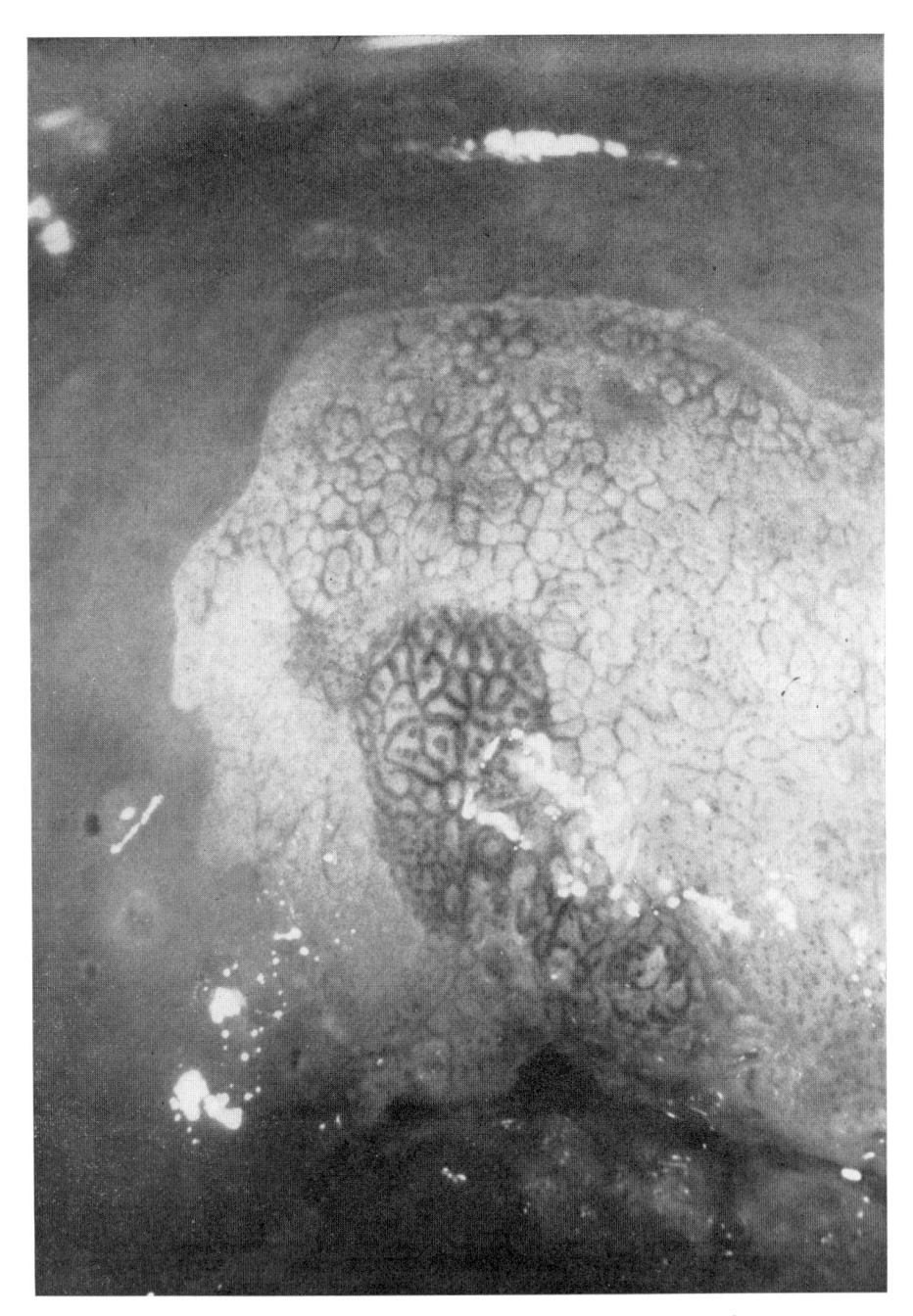

Figure 178. Mosaic. Colpophotograph of an extensive atypical transformation zone on the anterior lip of the cervix. A variable pattern is seen. Much of the atypical transformation zone is composed of a fine mosaic with vessels which are not very prominent. In one patch close to the middle of the picture, the mosaic is rendered more evident by more dilated vessels, which are closer to the surface. Predictably, the histological appearances of the central area will be more significant than those of the peripheral mosaic.

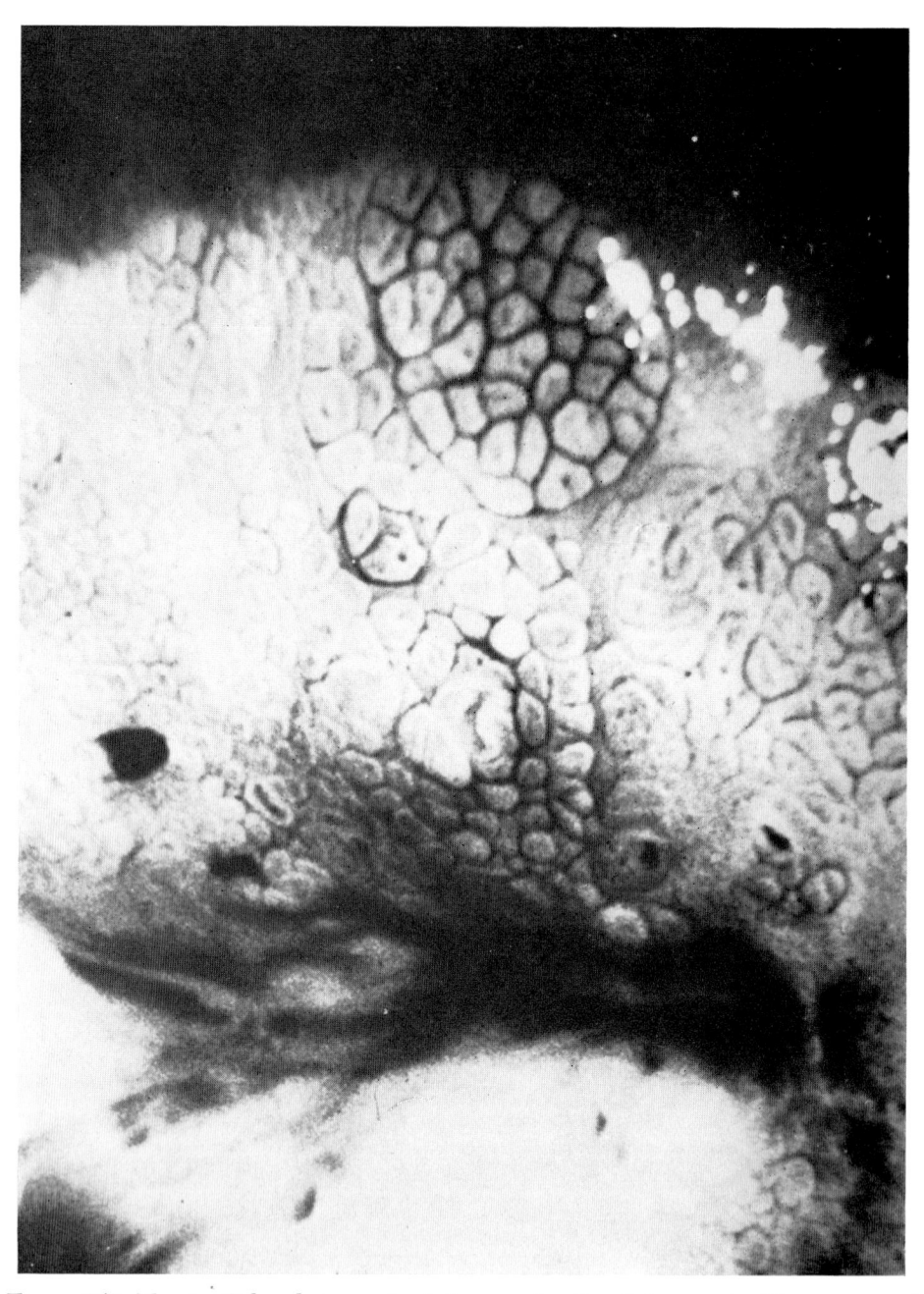

Figure 179. Mosaic. Colpophotograph of the anterior lip of the cervix. The pattern of mosaic blocks is irregular and is produced by prominent, dilated vessels. Under the stereoscopic view provided by the colposcope, the surface contour was irregular. Significant histological disorder is expected.

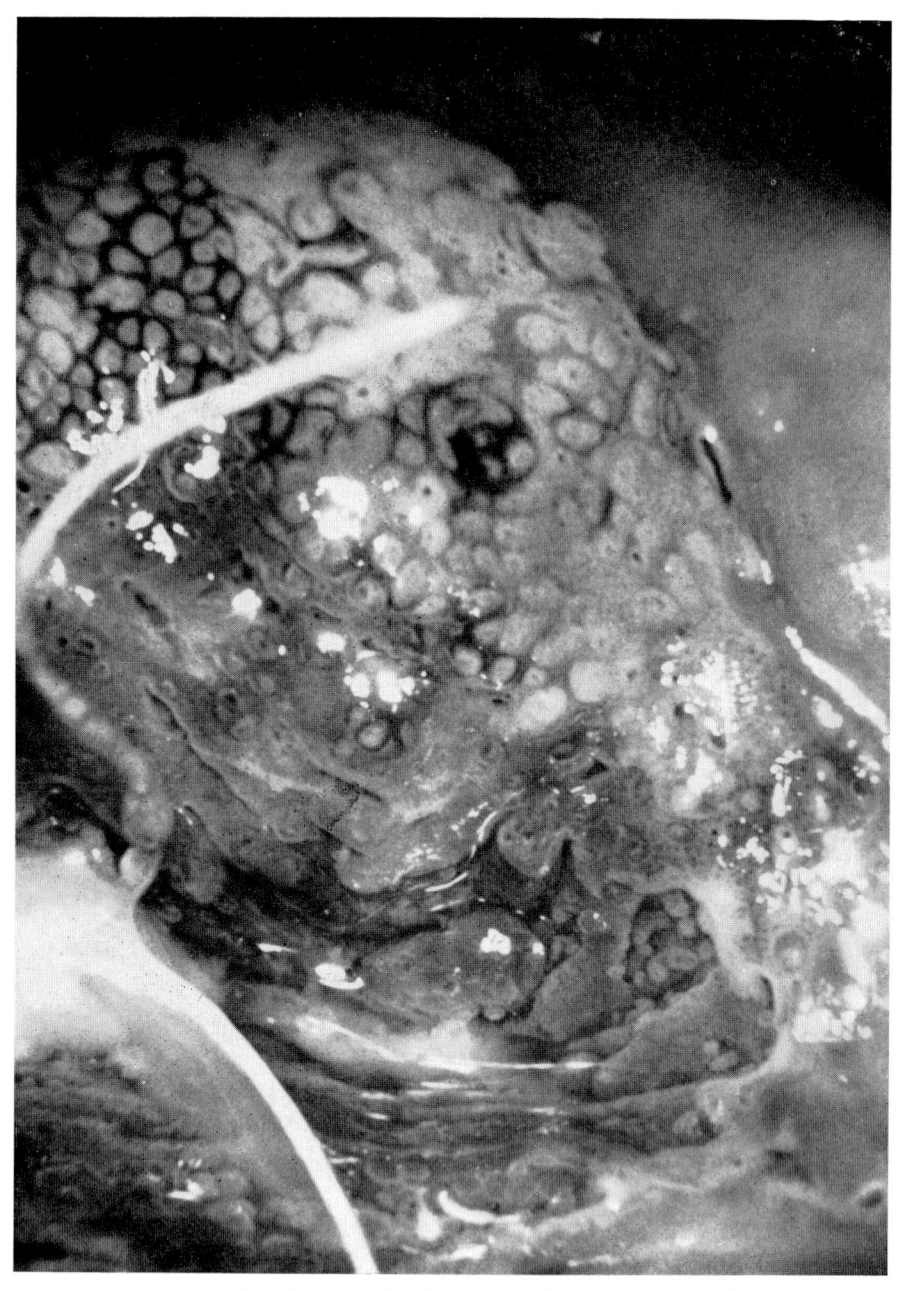

Figure 180. Mosaic. Colpophotograph of most of the anterior lip of the cervix. This transformation zone displays an area toward the left with an irregular surface contour containing prominent dilated vessels approaching the surface. The white streaks originating from the os are cervical mucus.

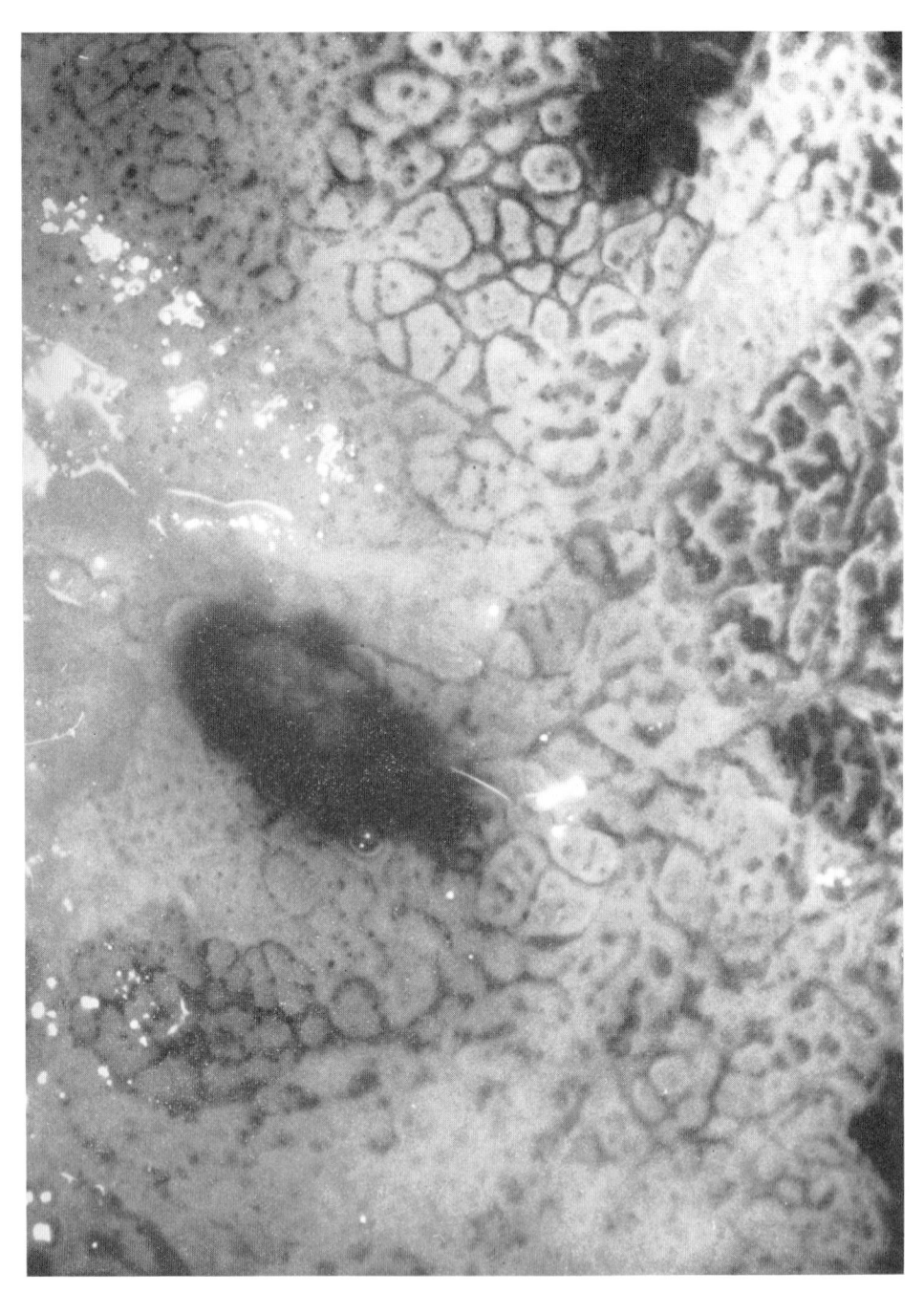

Figure 181. Mosaic and punctation. Colpophotograph of an area of atypical transformation zone surrounding the cervical os to the left of centre in the picture and exhibiting a combined pattern of mosaic and punctation. The vessels are very prominent in most areas, being greatly dilated and close to the surface. The whole picture strongly suggests a major histological disturbance.

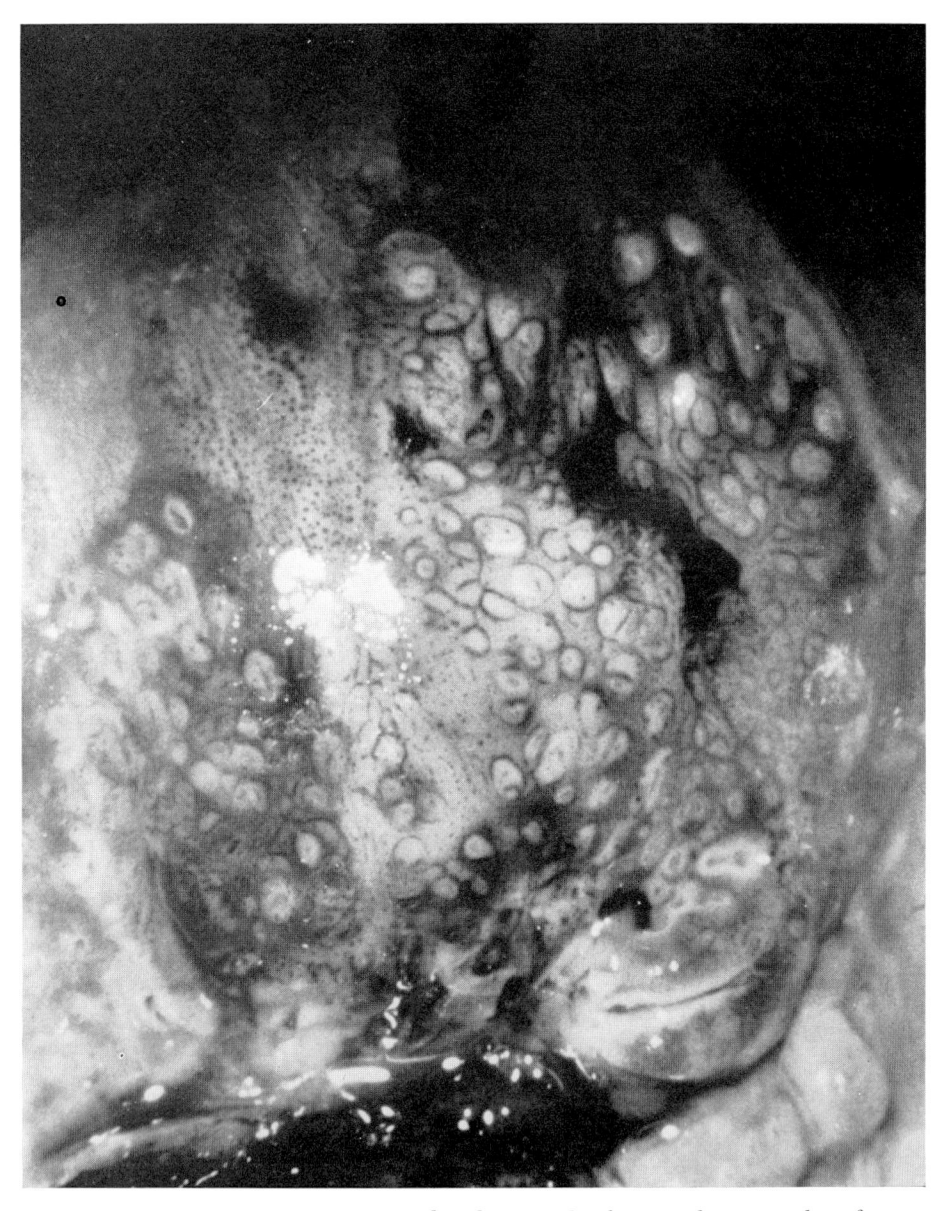

Figure 182. Mosaic and punctation. Colpophotograph of most of anterior lip of cervix. In this study, punctation with dilated capillary loops is interspersed with mosaic which is irregular with prominent vessels. Contact bleeding seen in the upper right is common with such fragile epithelium.

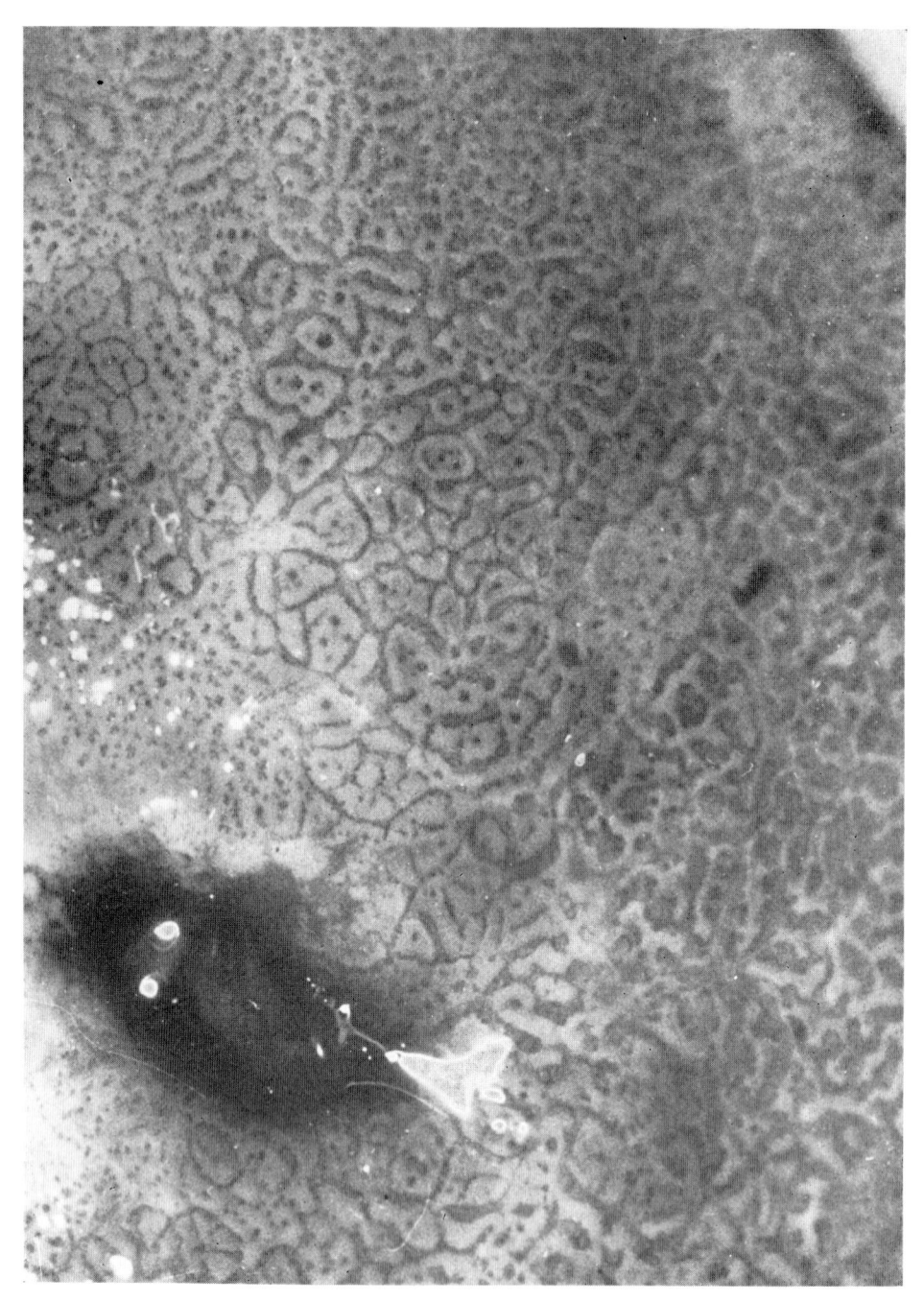

Figure 183. Mosaic and punctation. Colpophotograph of atypical transformation zone surrounding the cervical os shown in the lower left corner. The mosaic and punctation patterns are characterised by a striking dilatation of the intraepithelial capillaries.

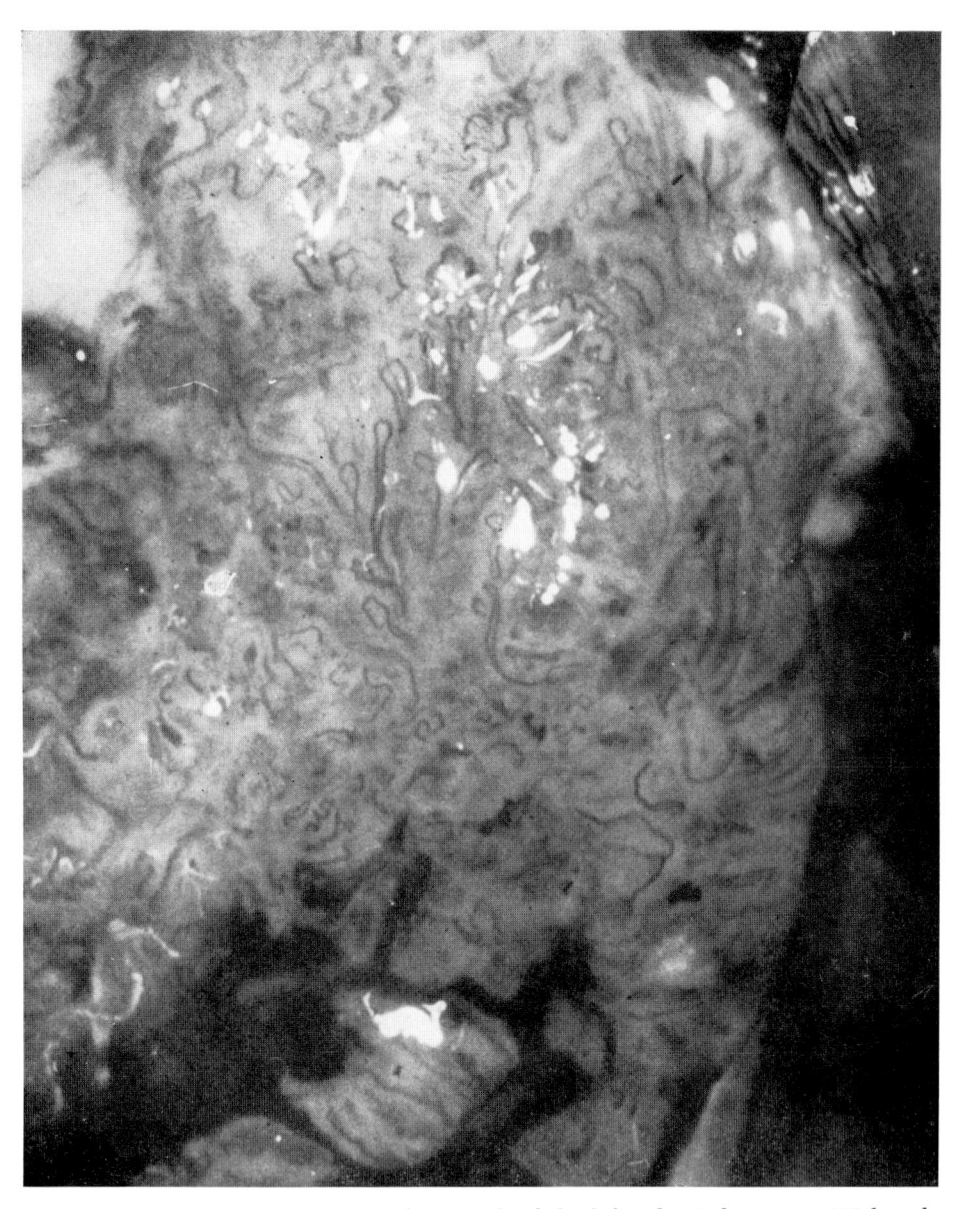

Figure 184. Atypical vessels. Colpophotograph of the left side of the cervix. Within this field, the irregular development of capillary loops has become extreme, with no semblance of mosaic or punctation. There is gross variation in calibre, and characteristically, most vessels are now coursing tangential to the surface. These features give a strong indication that this lesion is invasive.

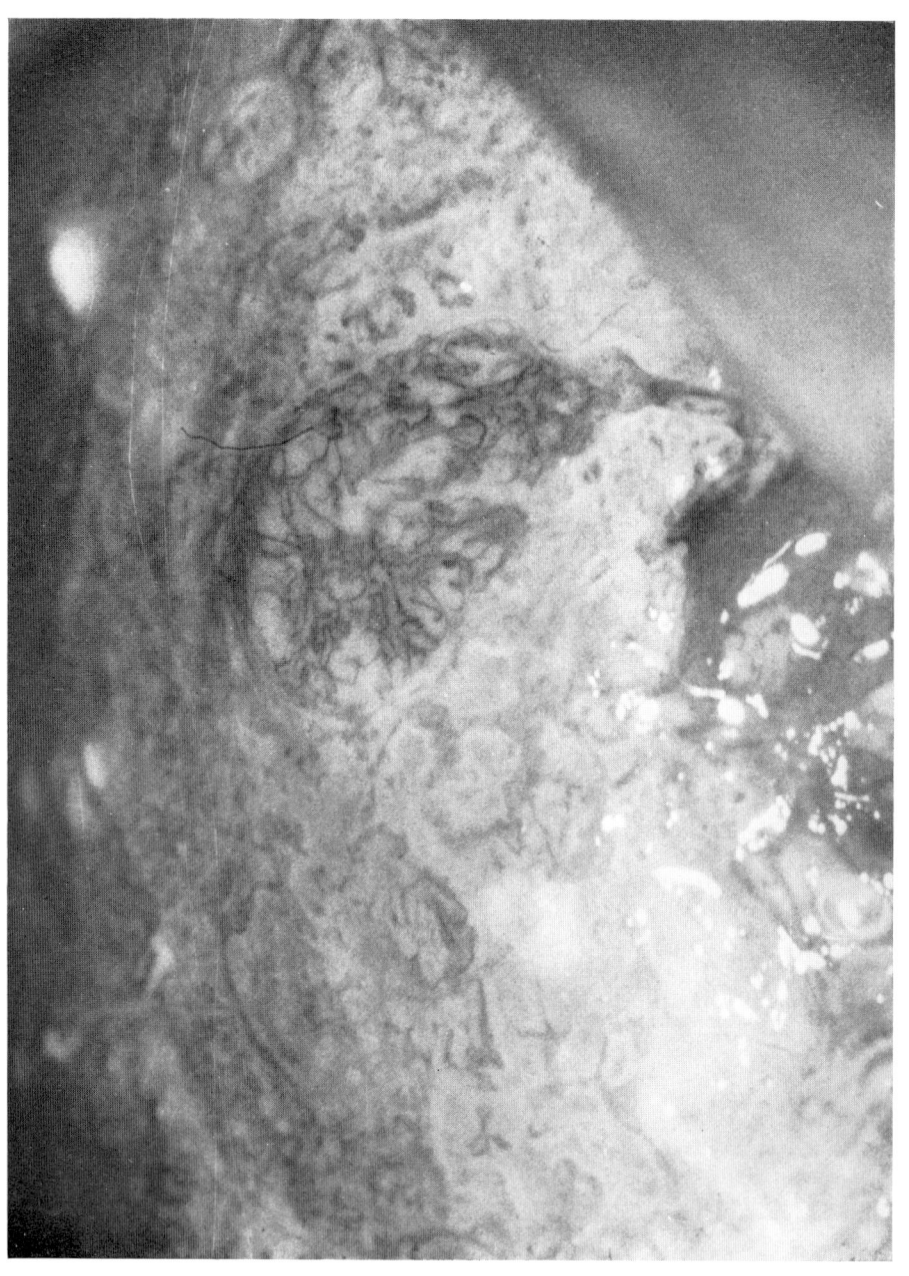

Figure 185. Atypical vessels. Colpophotograph of portion of the right side of the cervix showing atypical transformation zone. In the prominent patch seen above the centre of the photograph, the vessels have assumed a tangential distribution with bizarre shapes, patterns, and directions. In such cases, the prediction of invasive cancer is warranted.

problems of management is discussed in Chapter 16. The grades are defined as follows.

GRADE I: Flat, white epithelium, fine calibre, regularly shaped vessels, absence of atypical vessels, small intercapillary distance (Figs. 163, 168, and 175).

GRADE II: Flat, whiter epithelium, dilated calibre, regularly shaped vessels, absence of atypical vessels, usually increased intercapillary distance (Figs. 164, 169, 176, and 177).

GRADE III: Very white epithelium, dilated calibre, irregularly shaped often coiled, often atypical vessels, increased but variable intercapillary distance and usually irregular surface contour—*papillary epithelium* or *microexophytic epithelium* (Figs. 165, 170-174, and 179-185).

In most cases, the variations of surface and vascular features are coincident. However, gross vascular atypia may exist without obvious changes in surface contour. The appearance of atypical vessels in association with an irregular surface contour is of the greatest significance and usually indicates invasive carcinoma.

Irregularities of surface due to persistence of villous pattern of the pre-existing columnar epithelium (p. 209) imposes some irregularity on its contour, but differentiation from irregularity of more serious significance is usually a simple matter to the experienced colposcopist. The irregular surface of the epithelium as seen by stereoscopic examination with the colposcope cannot be adequately demonstrated by colpophotographs.

The development of the parameter, increasing intercapillary distance, is variable and not necessarily consistent in the major grades with increasing significance to lesions. Although minor grades have a narrow intercapillary distance, major grades can also be associated with a narrow intercapillary distance either throughout or in areas of the lesion.

Chapter 10

COLPOSCOPIC APPEARANCES OF OVERT CANCER

W̶HEN LARGE SECTIONS of the female population are screened using exfoliative cervical cytology, a range of possible histological abnormalities is uncovered. In addition to dysplasia, carcinoma in situ, and preclinical invasive carcinoma, overt carcinoma is occasionally apparent on clinical examination. If all cases with abnormal findings in the cervical smear are submitted to colposcopic examination, another highly significant entity emerges, the *colposcopically suspect overt carcinoma.*

OVERT CARCINOMA

Carcinoma obvious on the basis of inspection, palpation, and probing has little clinical significance for the colposcopist other than in the following instance. The grossly abnormal appearance of the carcinoma to both naked eye and colposcope is but an exaggeration of the appearances to be seen in that form inapparent to the naked eye but obvious through the colposcope.

Squamous Carcinoma

Gross irregularities in surface contour occur, including nodulation, smaller papillary elevations, and ulceration in squamous carcinoma (Figs. 186-188). The surface usually bleeds readily on contact (Fig. 189). The blood vessel pattern shows great individual variation from one tumour to another. Great variations occur in disposition and calibre of the vessels, which may course for long distances without branching (Figs. 190 and 191). Occasionally, the dilatation of these vessels is gross (Fig. 192).

Adenocarcinoma

The colposcopic appearances of squamous cell carcinoma and adenocarcinoma are superficially similar (Fig. 193), although subtle differences have been described. Villous outgrowths, resembling normal columnar epithelium and normal intercapillary distance in vessels, which are nevertheless atypical, are features of the colpophotographs of Kolstad and Stafl (1977). Although these villous outgrowths may occur in invasive lesions, they are always present in adenocarcinoma in situ, where they may closely mimic the surface configuration of normal columnar epithelium (Fig. 194). The distinguishing feature of the villi after application of acetic acid is their striking white colour. White villous epithelium is also characteristic of the rarer histological type, adenosquamous carcinoma in situ.

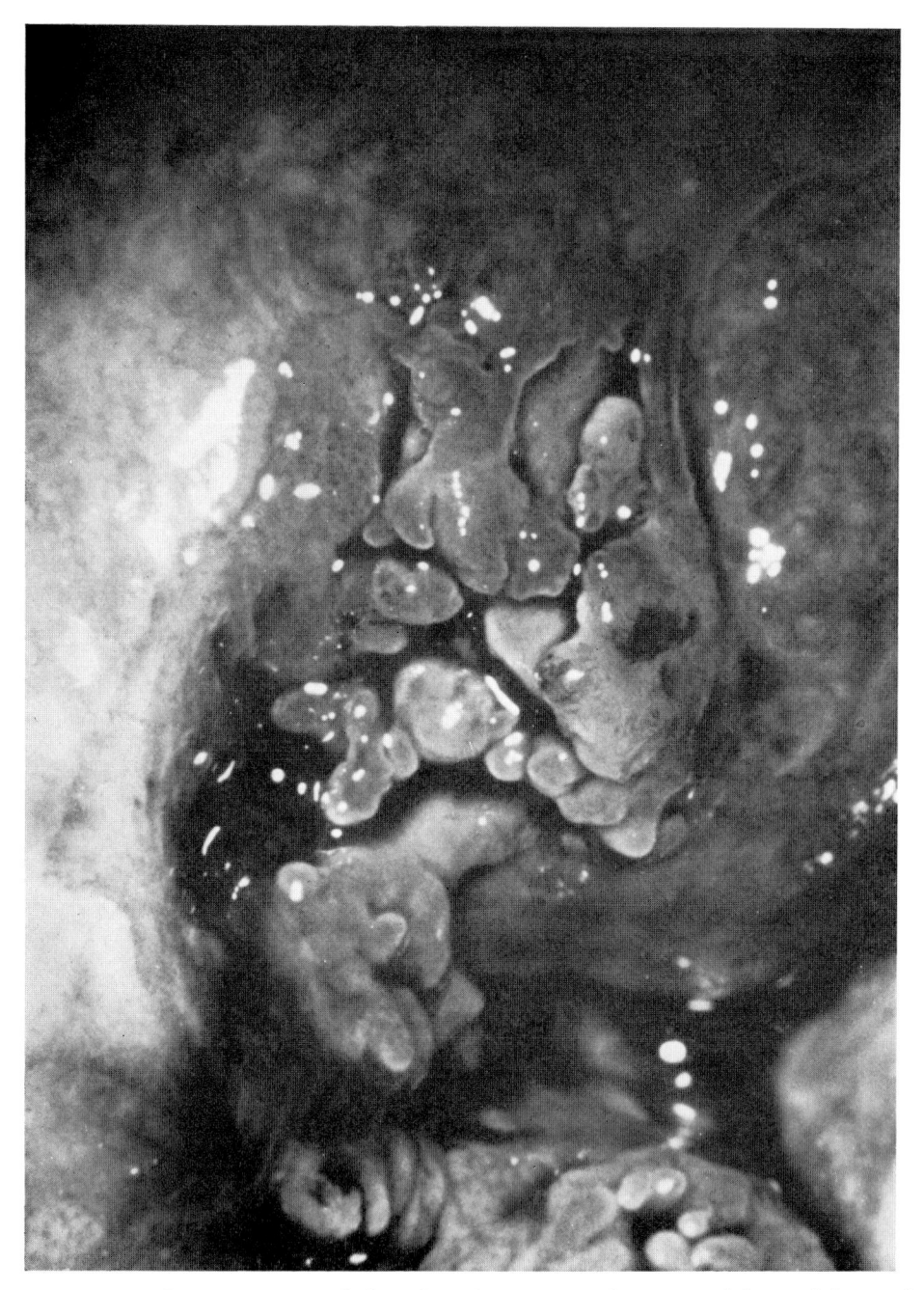

Figure 186. The appearance of this clinical cancer is characterised by nodular and papillary elevations that are unlike any physiological structures.

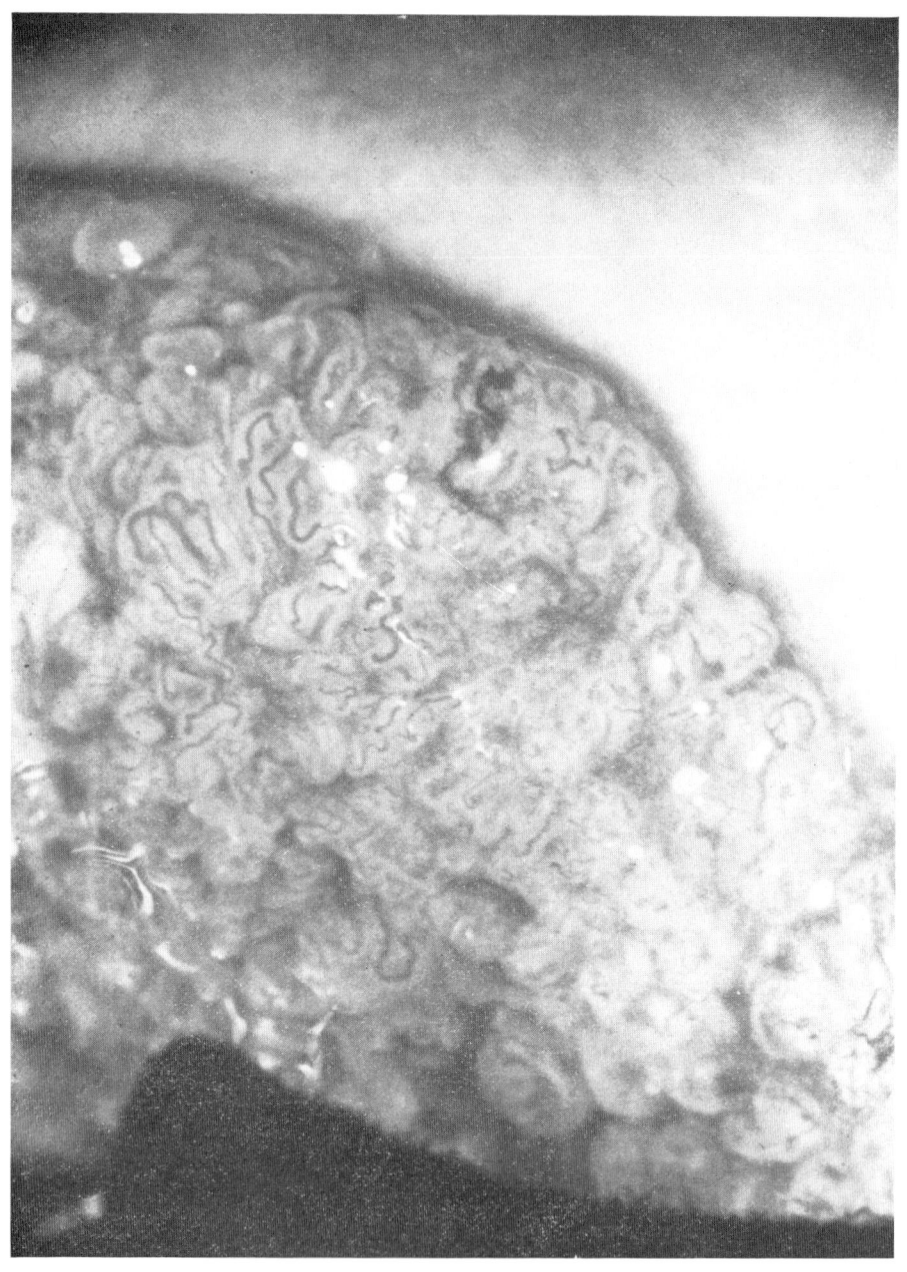

Figure 187. Overt squamous cancer presenting mainly as a diffuse excrescence with papillary surface. Atypical vessels are present.

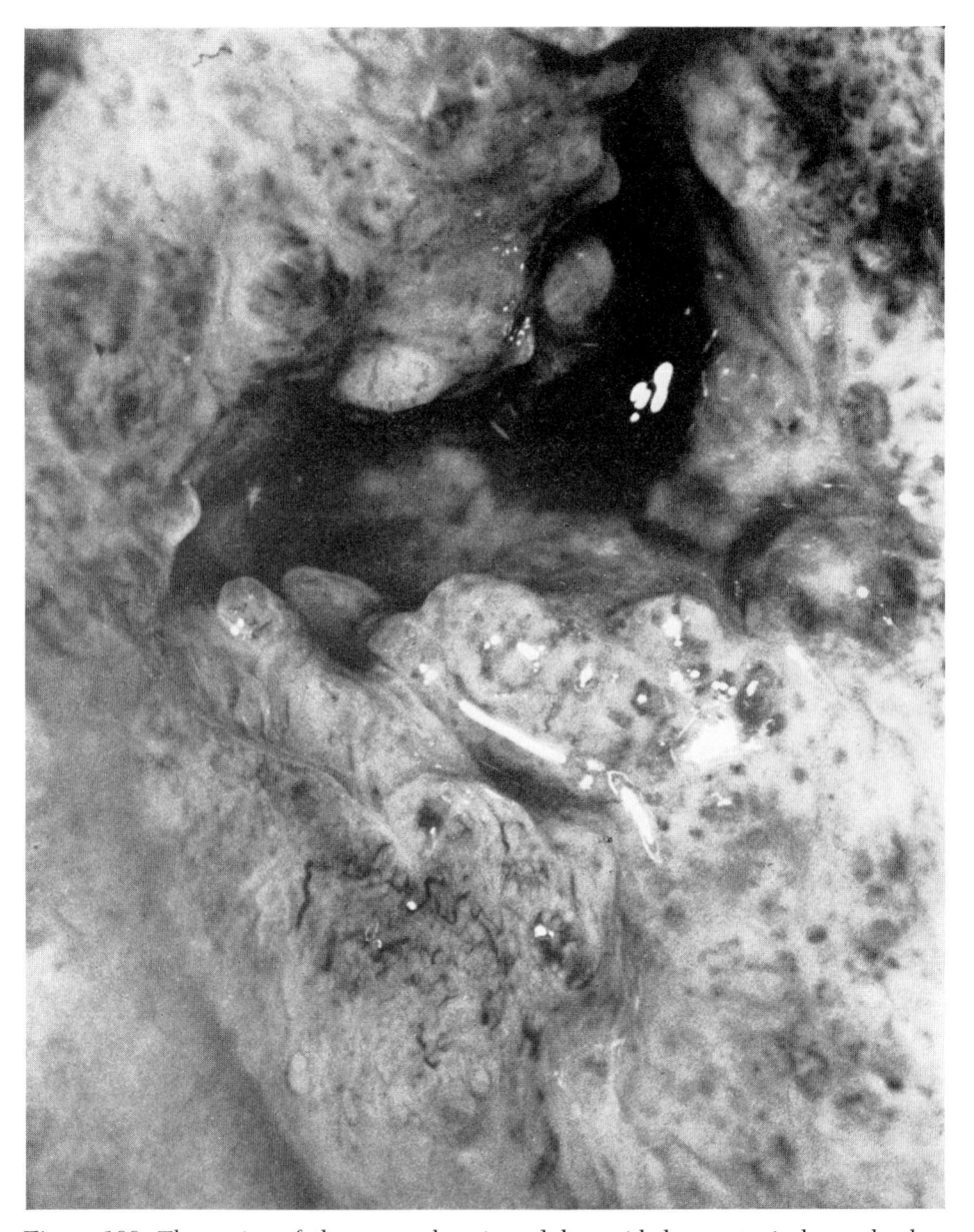

Figure 188. The region of the external os is nodular, with large atypical vessels characteristic of overt cancer.

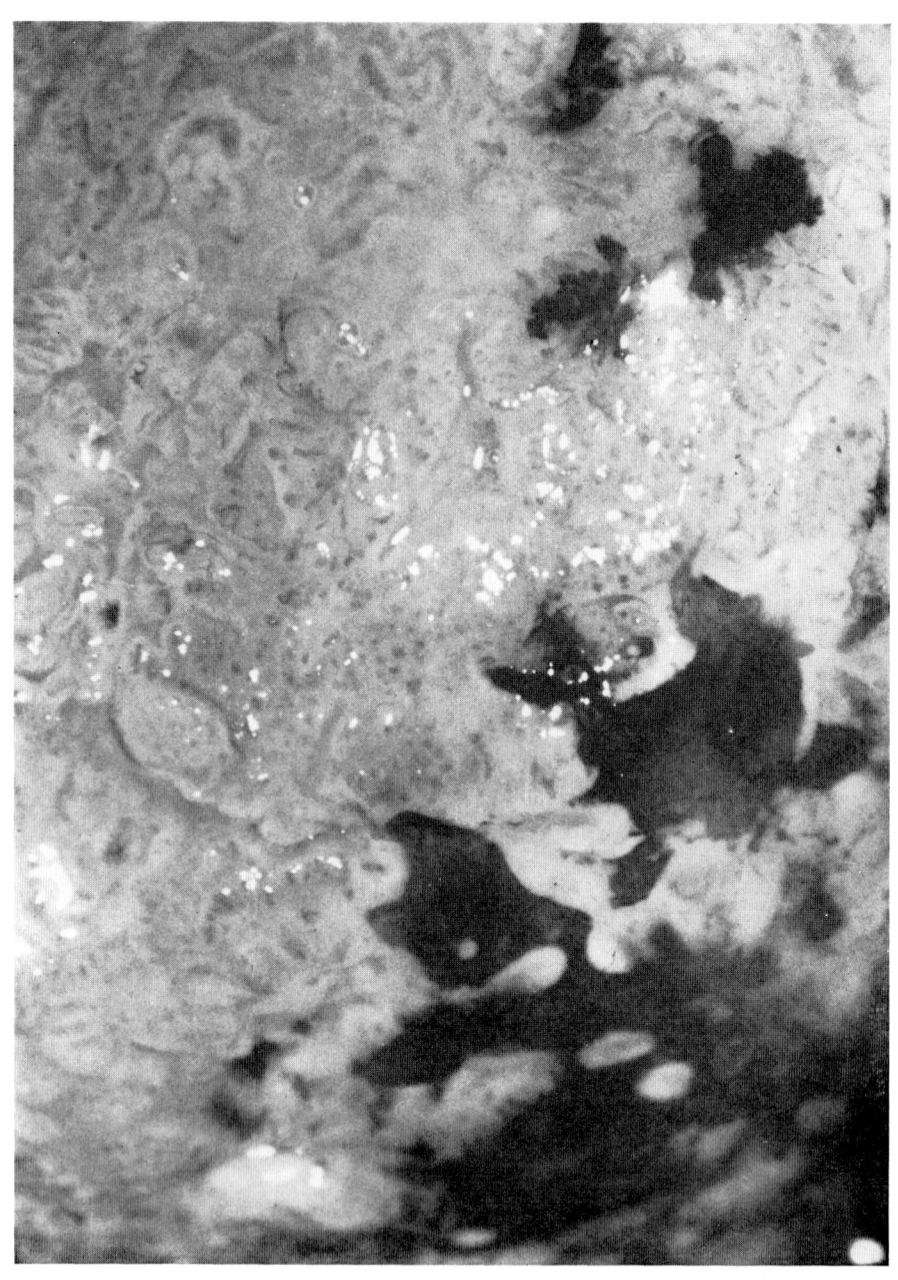

Figure 189. Colpophotograph of the surface of part of a large invasive cancer displaying atypical vessels in its white surface. Bleeding points are evident, and surface ulceration is starting.

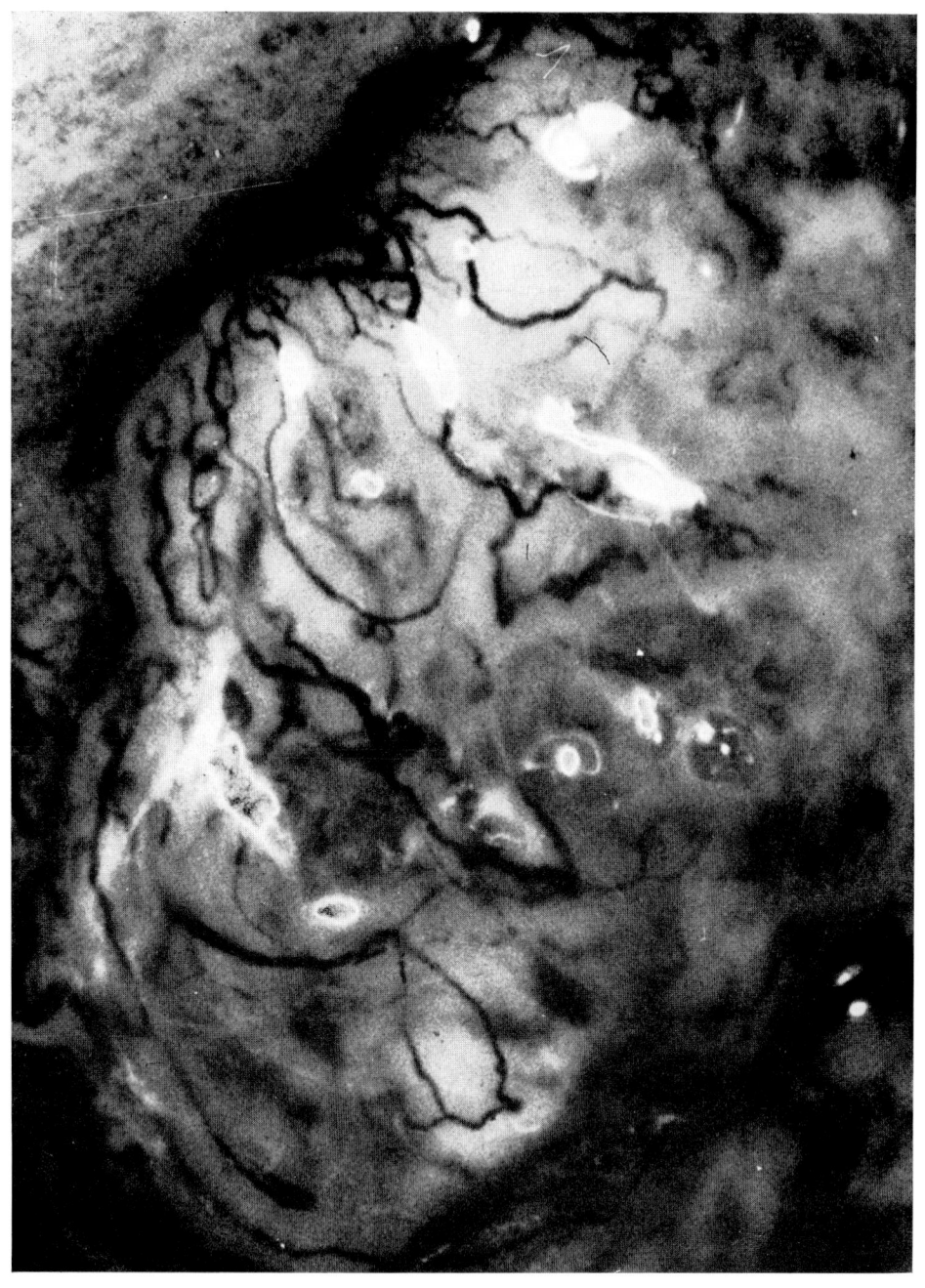

Figure 190. An exophytic squamous carcinoma of the cervix obvious on clinical examination. The gross irregularity of the terminal vasculature is evident on colposcopic examination.

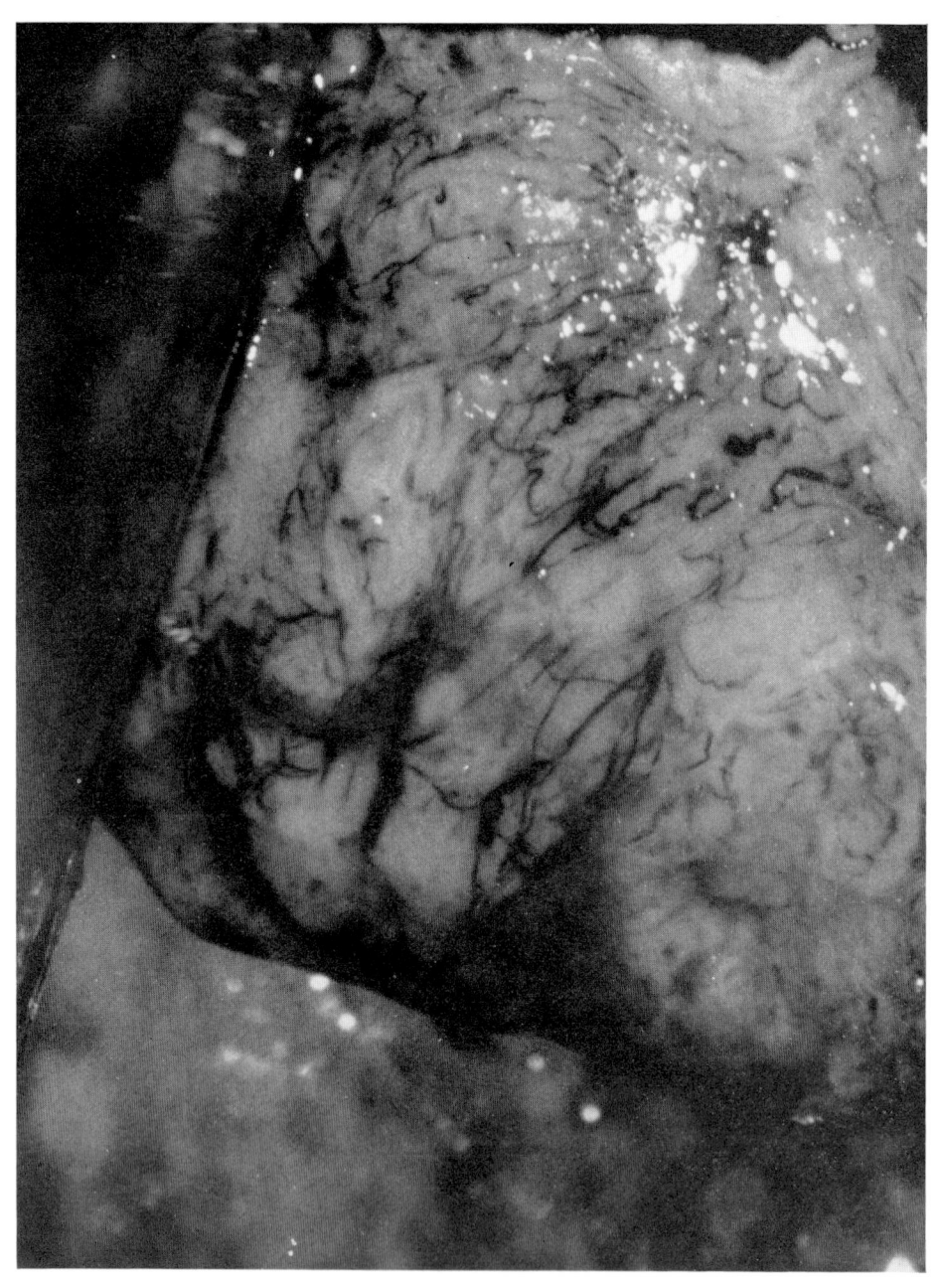

Figure 191. An obvious exophytic carcinoma of the cervix. Grossly atypical vessel formations characteristic of invasive carcinoma are seen.

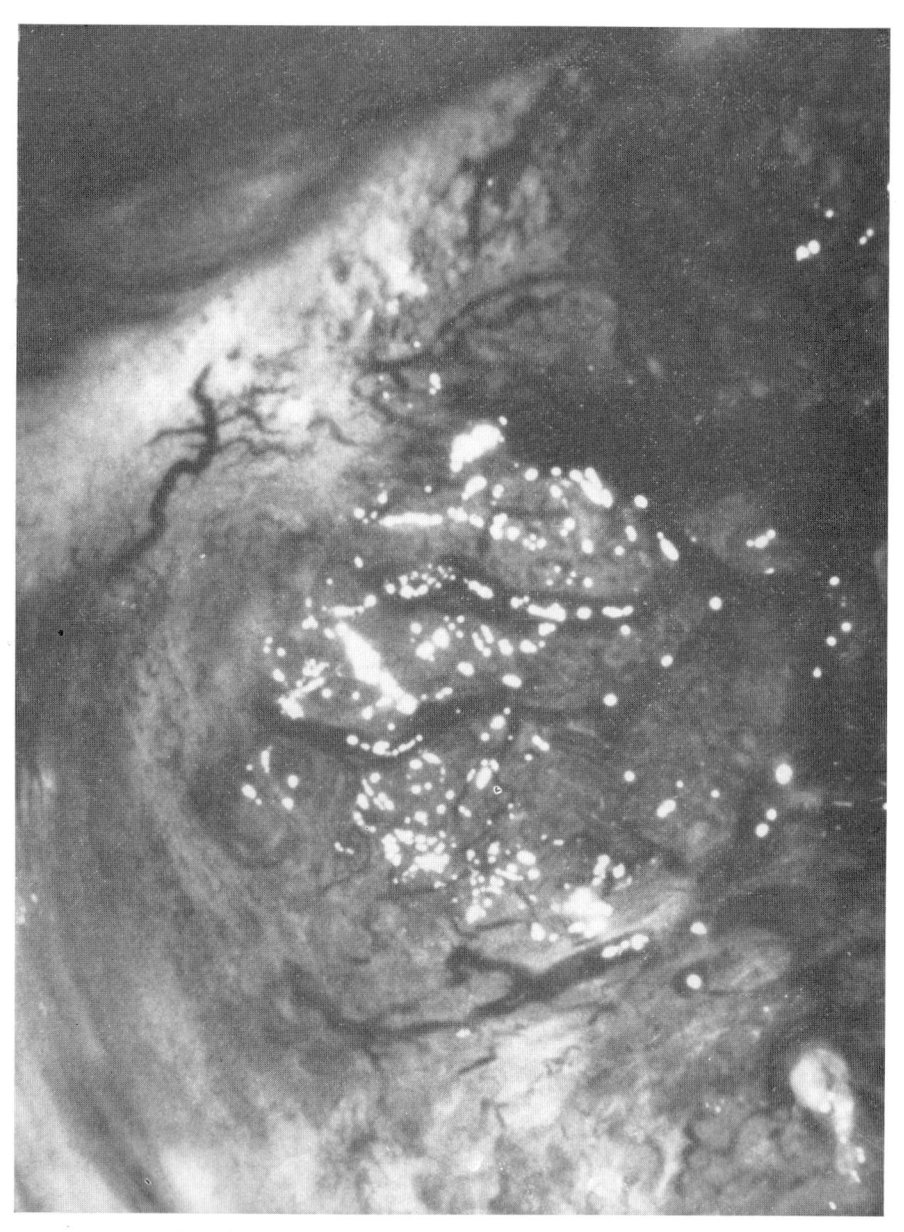

Figure 192. Grossly dilated vessels are often seen on and near the surface of invasive cancer.

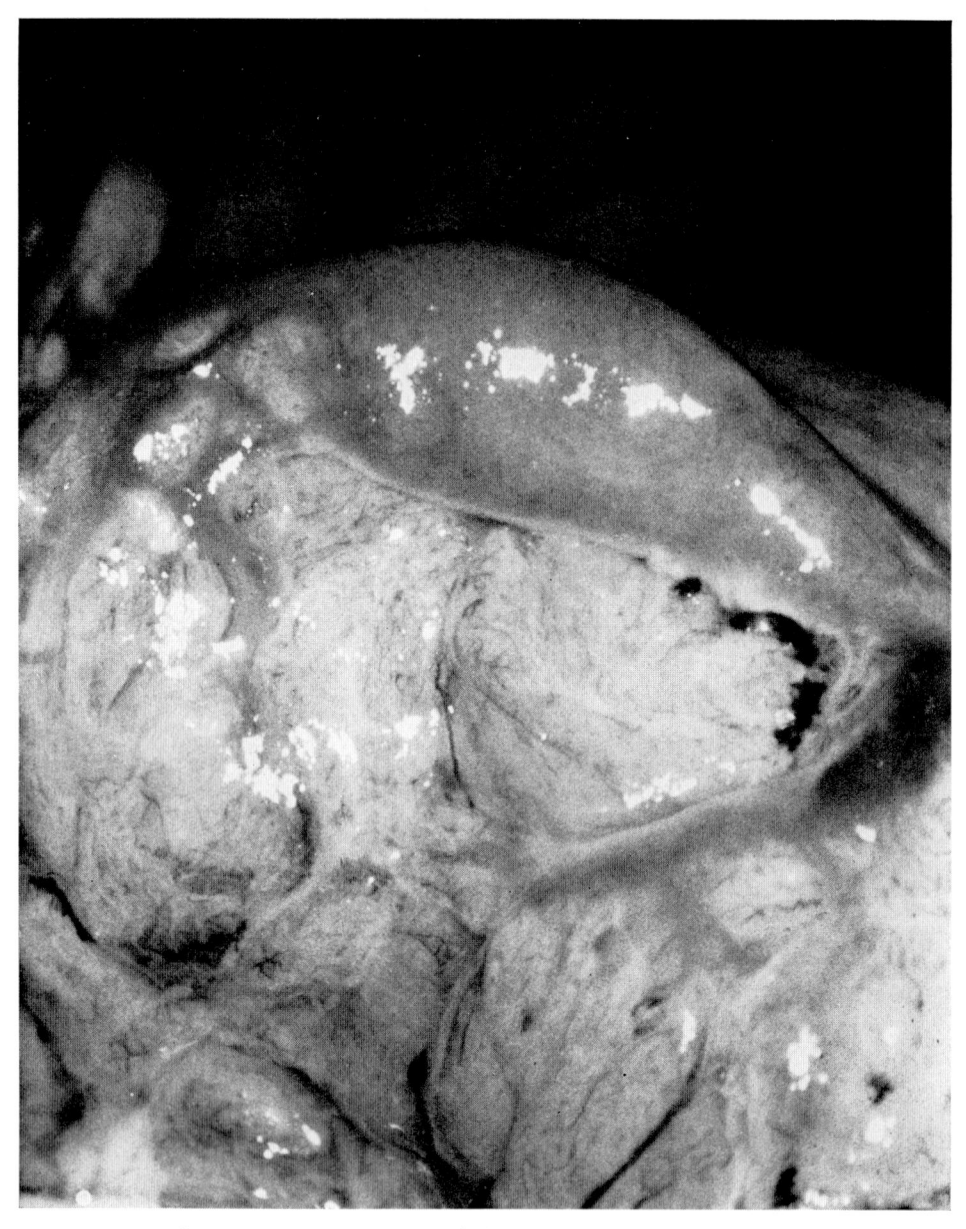

Figure 193. Adenocarcinoma. No special features distinguish this example from the more common squamous type. Gross surface variations and atypical vessels are present.

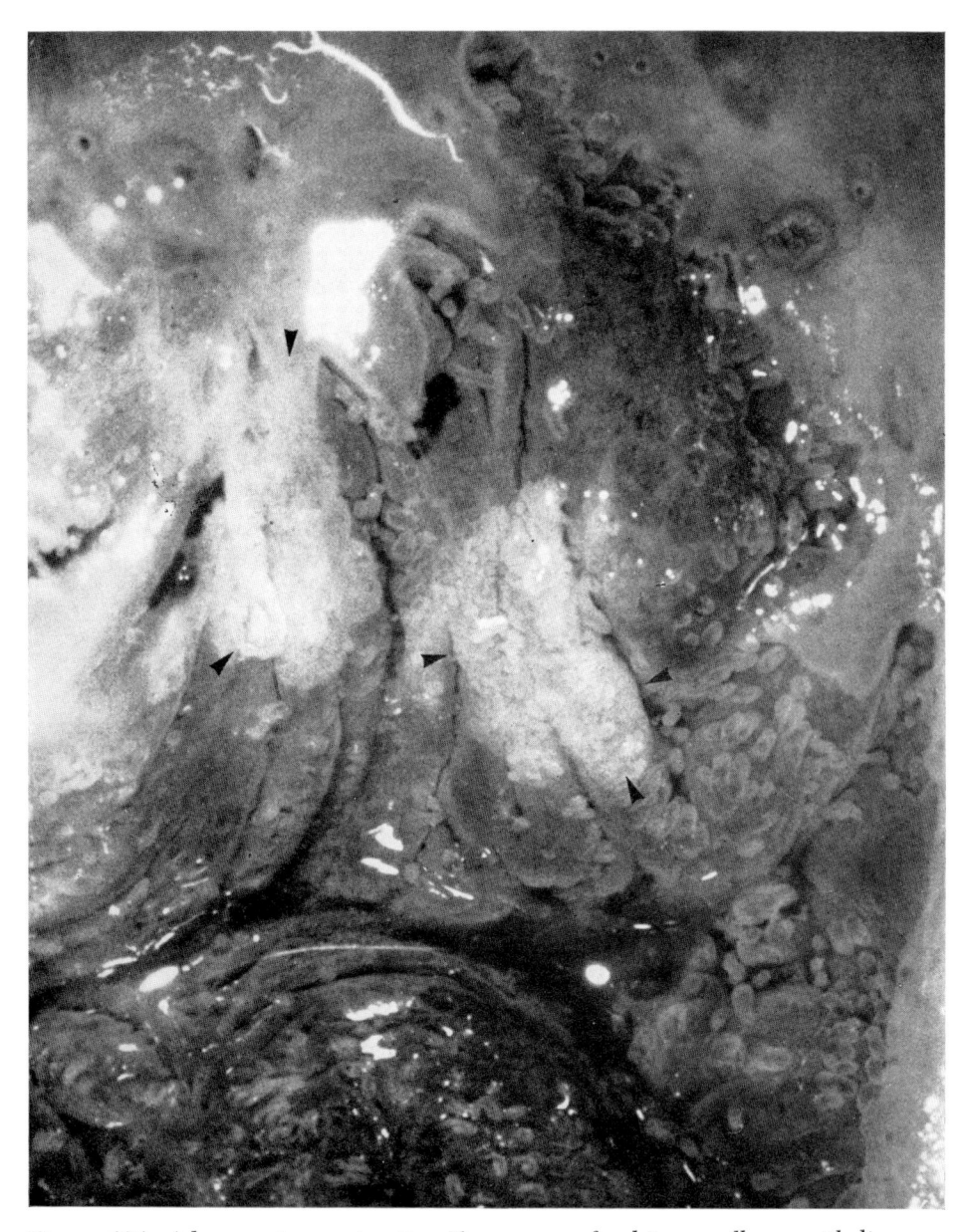

Figure 194. Adenocarcinoma in situ. Two areas of white papillary epithelium are present in the columnar epithelium (arrows). Abnormal glandular cells were present in the smear and histological examination showed adenocarcinoma in situ.

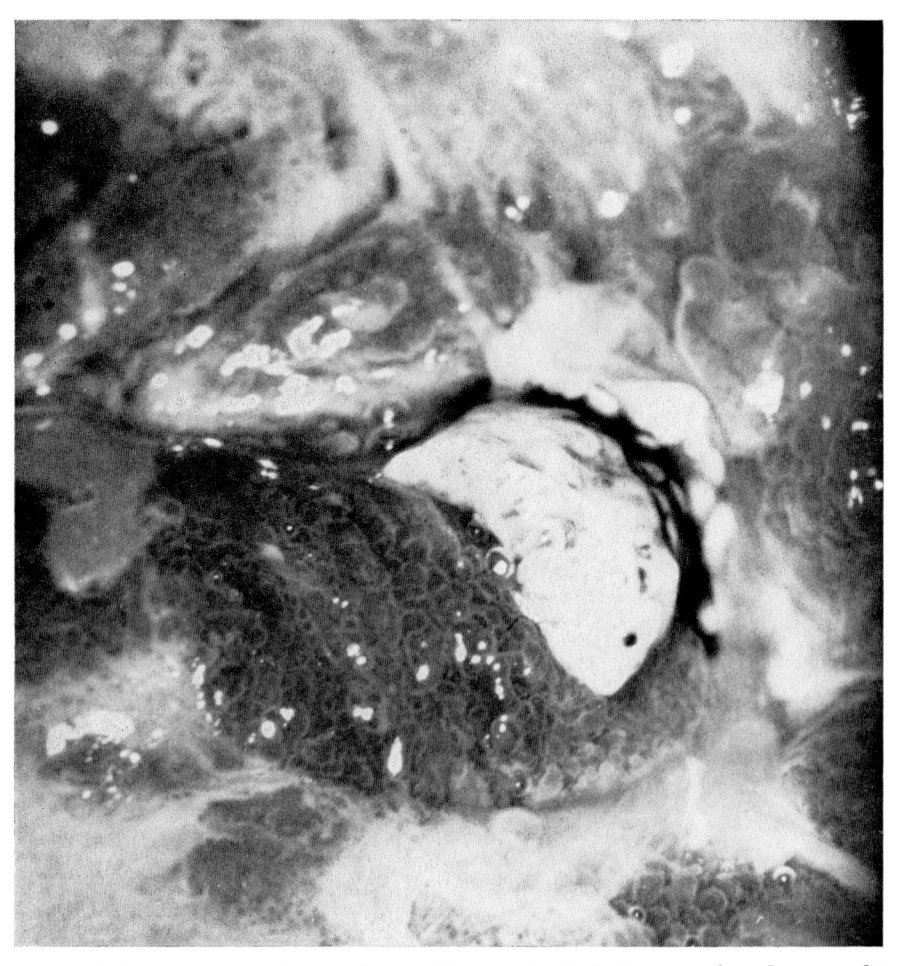

Figure 195. Verrucous carcinoma. This white exophytic lesion was found in a subject with an abnormal smear.

Clear Cell Adenocarcinoma

Clear cell adenocarcinoma is discussed in Chapter 14.

Verrucous Carcinoma

Verrucous carcinomas, rare, well-differentiated squamous cancers with a low incidence of lymph node metastases and no reports of distant metastases, have a well-developed papillary surface contour. An example of a microinvasive verrucous cancer is shown in Figure 195.

COLPOSCOPICALLY SUSPECT OVERT CARCINOMA

Overt carcinoma may be unsuspected when clinical examination fails to reveal the classic macroscopic characteristics of cancer. At colposcopic examination, the diagnosis of invasive cancer may be immediately obvious (*see* Figs. 30, 196, 197, and 285). Invasive carcinoma so diagnosed is the colposcopically suspect overt variety.

Colposcopically suspect overt carcinoma is rare but merits the most special consideration. It represents a clinical situation in which the colposcope immediately warns of unsuspected invasion, and it identifies a type of lesion, the recognition of which is regarded as essential in problems of management (Chap. 16).

In some cases, preclinical carcinomatous areas in which invasion started are still present. Grade III atypical transformation changes are almost invariably seen in such areas and thereby demonstrate the serious prognosis attaching to appearances within this grade (Fig. 196).

Topography

Whereas preclinical carcinoma invariably terminates distally at the original squamocolumnar junction, the frankly invasive form may bypass this junction. Although remnants of the pre-existent atypical transformation zone may be in evidence, the edge of the overt lesion often invades the original squamous epithelium.

Colour and Opacity

The *exophytic* tissue after the application of acetic acid is white or yellow. Contact bleeding is occasionally present.

Surface Configuration

Stereoscopic appearances after the application of acetic acid solution show a characteristic irregular surface contour or "mountain range" appearance typical of an invasive exophytic growth. The whole area of the invasive lesion is uniformly of this appearance, so that gross differences in surface level are widespread (Figs. 196 and 197). After the application of

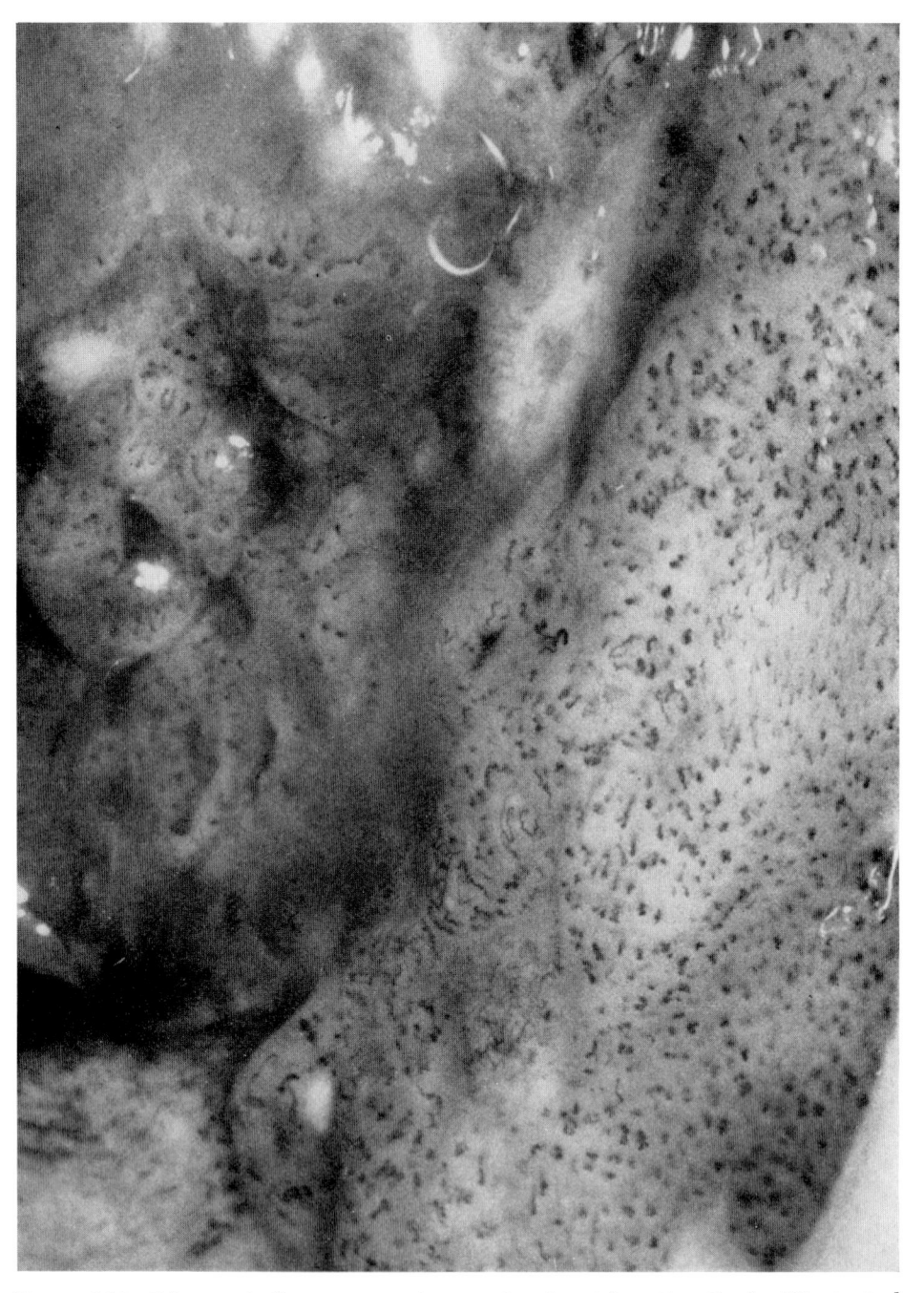

Figure 196. Colposcopically overt carcinoma. On the right side, Grade III atypical transformation zone is present. On the left, the now colposcopically overt cancer displays characteristic variations of surface contour but still retains recognisable punctation.

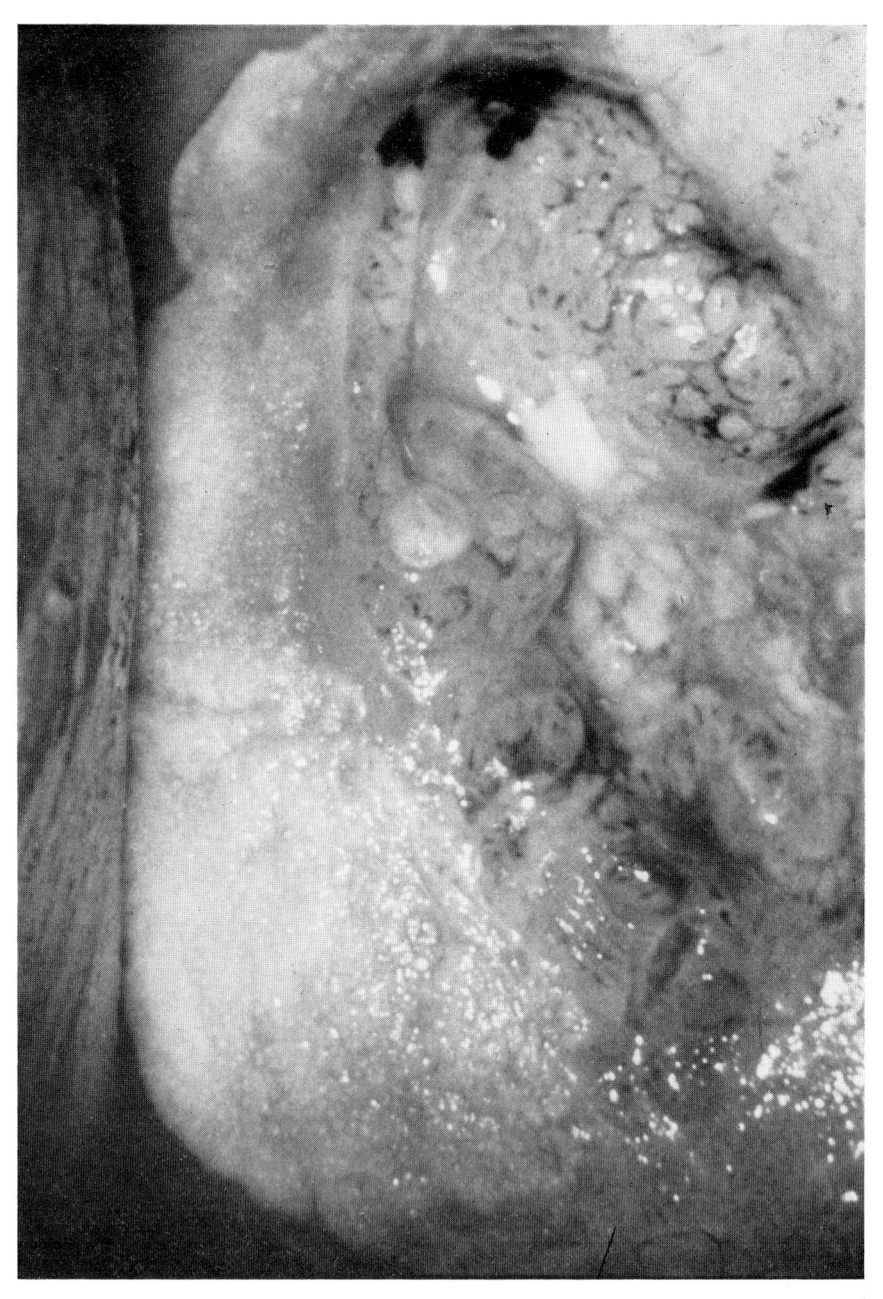

Figure 197. Colposcopically overt carcinoma. Within atypical transformation zone, slight contact bleeding, early exophytic growth, and atypical vessels with persistent mosaic-like pattern strongly suggest invasive cancer.

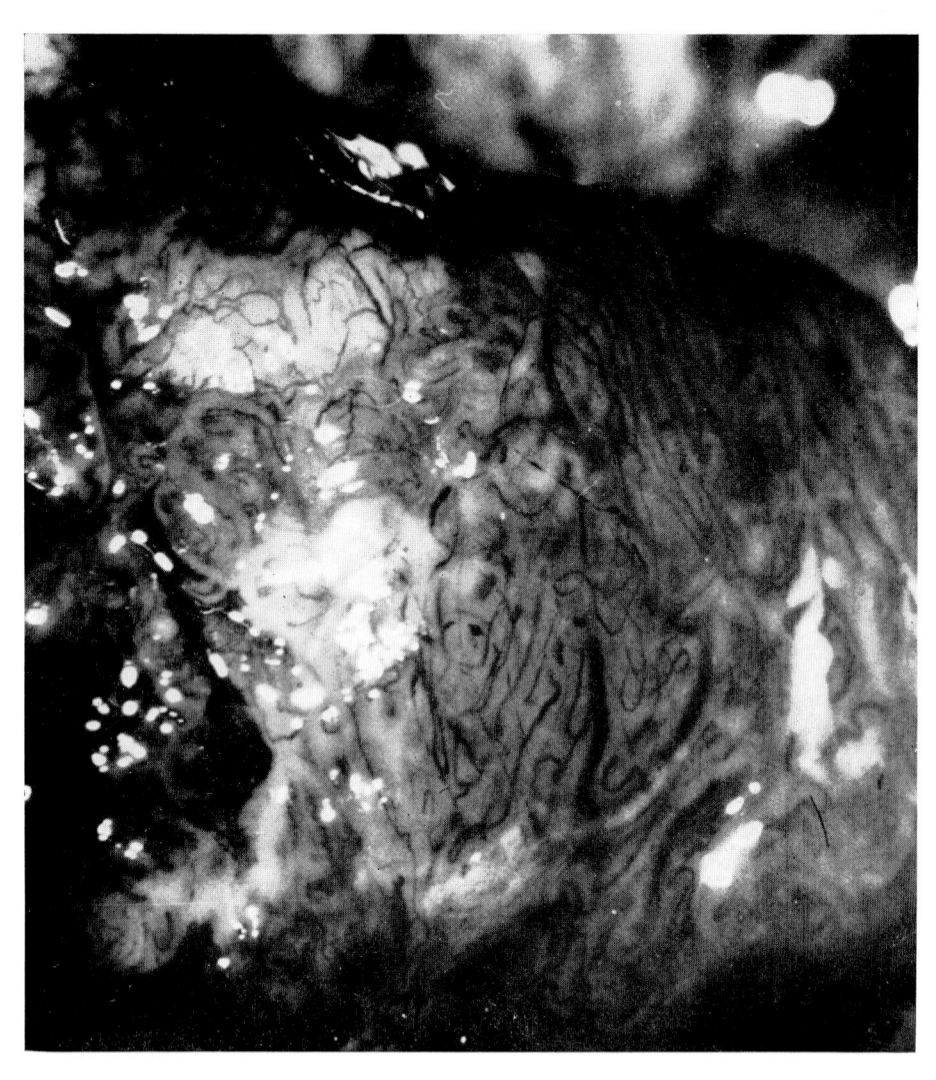

Figure 198. Unsuspected clinically, colposcopy reveals an obvious cancer with gross disturbance of vascular pattern and irregularity of surface contour.

acetic acid, the junction of the lesion with the uninvolved epithelium shows a striking raised edge (*see* Fig. 30).

Angioarchitecture

Equally striking and characteristic are the changes in the terminal vasculature. Branching vessels displaying the most marked variations in size, shape, calibre, direction, and arrangement occupy much of the field of view (Fig. 198). In some cases, this atypical branching of vessels is not a feature or may be absent. The vessels then display maximum grades of punctation and mosaic (Figs. 196 and 197).

Chapter 11

COLPOSCOPIC APPEARANCES OF MISCELLANEOUS CONDITIONS

VARIOUS DISORDERS unrelated to metaplasia, typical or atypical, are encountered during colposcopic examination. Some of these may produce abnormalities in vaginal cytology. Most are host responses to injury due to micro-organismal infestations or trauma. The basis of the colposcopic appearances is seen most commonly as some form of vascular response. The epithelium itself may exhibit appearances resulting from increased proliferation, oedema, fragility, ulceration, and exophytia.

VAGINOCERVICITIS

Responses are produced to many micro-organisms, including fungi, protozoa, bacteria, viruses, and viruslike organisms, and no particular form of response is specific for any particular form of infection. In our population, *Candida albicans* is the most common organism. *Trichomonas vaginalis* and *Neisseria gonorrhoeae* evoke the most outstanding response when they are clinically evident.

Colposcopic examination reveals the reaction to be principally within the vascular capillary bed. Terminal capillaries undergo hypertrophy by dilatation, coiling, and duplication. This change occurs in the original vascular structures of the original epithelia as well as in the transformation zone. Vertical intraepithelial capillary loops present in the original squamous epithelium become hyperaemic and produce a pronounced punctate-like appearance, diffuse or patchy, which frequently confuses the learner (Figs. 199-201). Table IV lists the characteristics that help distinguish true atypical transformation zone from the inflammatory disorder. Similar responses developing within the transformation zone can generate mosaic-like appearances closely resembling the atypical variety (Fig. 202).

TABLE IV
DIFFERENTIAL DIAGNOSIS
ACUTE VAGINOCERVICITIS AND PUNCTATION

	Acute Cervicitis	*Punctation*
Colour	Normal to red	Pale to white
Spacing of capillaries	Dense	Sparse
Vascular hypertrophy	Minor to moderate	Minor or moderate or major
Border	Diffuse	Sharp
Extension to vagina	Common	Uncommon
Iodine staining	Partly stains	Non-staining
Microbiology study	Usually positive	Usually negative

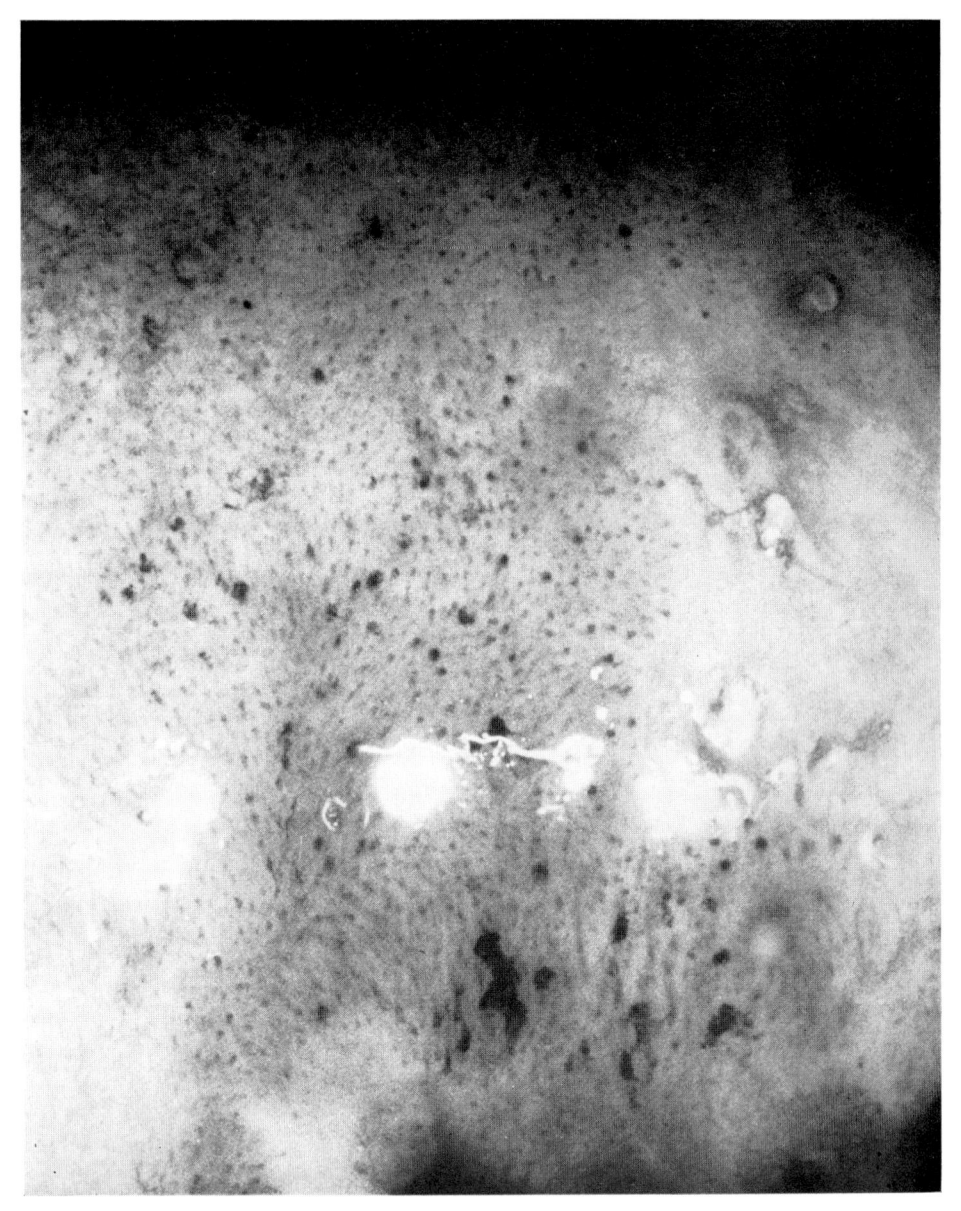

Figure 199. Vaginocervicitis. A diffuse response is present in the terminal capillary bed. Varying dilatation and some multiplication of capillary loops is evident, producing overall a punctate-like appearance. Such appearances can indicate the presence of Candida species, *Neisseria gonorrhae, Trichomonas vaginalis,* and *Chlamydia.*

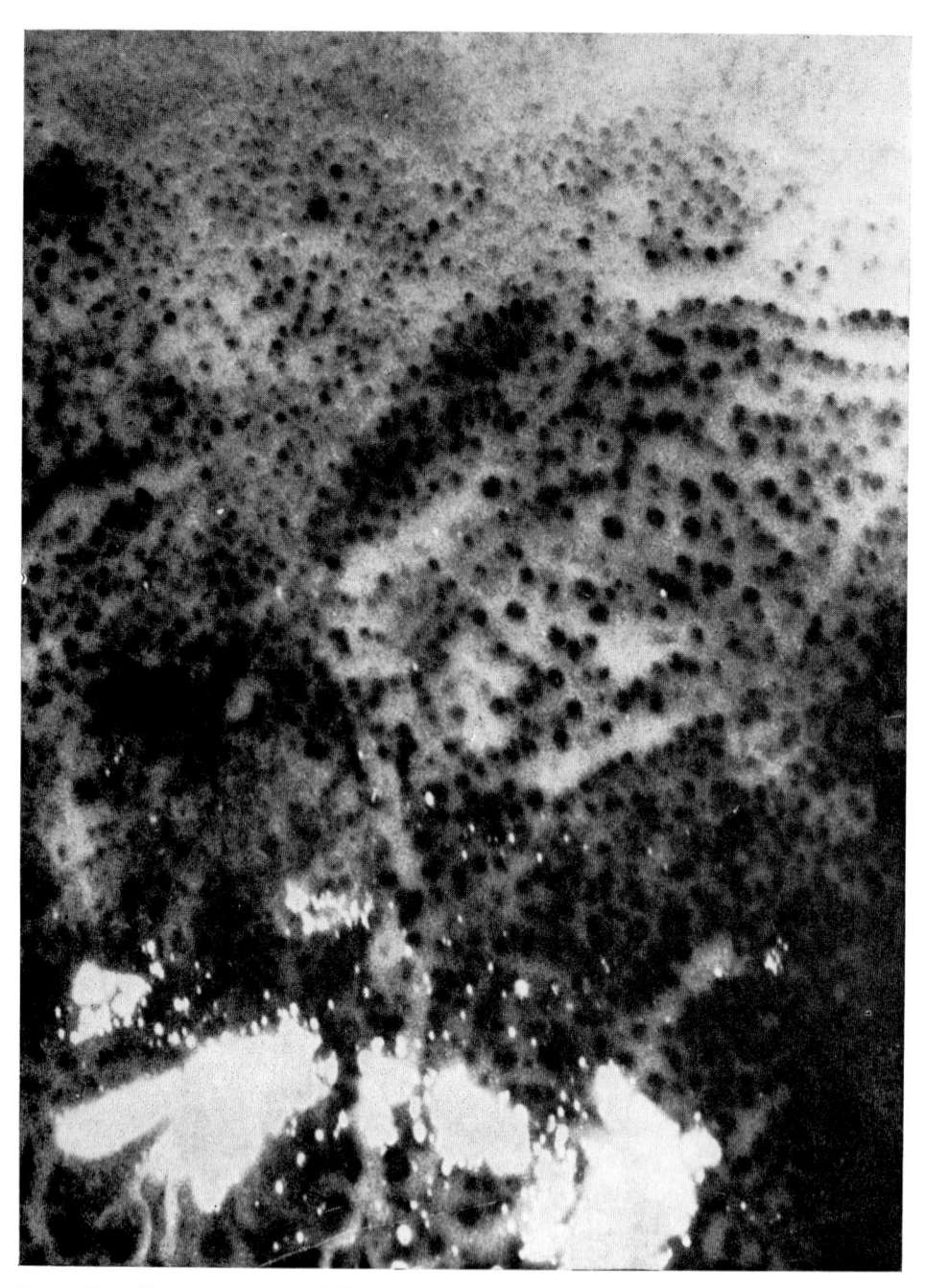

Figure 200. Vaginocervicitis—diffuse. *Trichomonas vaginalis* infestation was responsible for this appearance. Terminal vessels are dilated diffusely over the epithelial surface.

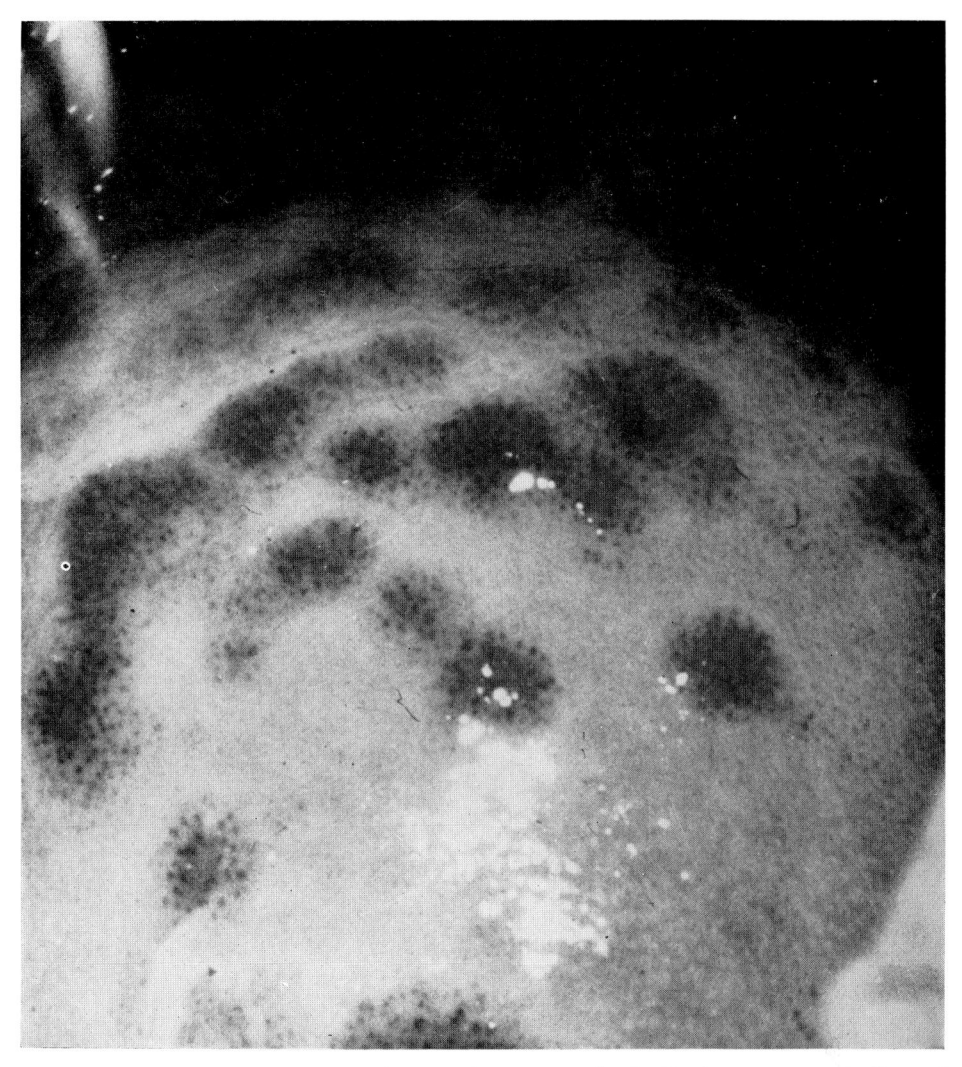

Figure 201. Vaginocervicitis—patchy. In this patient both *Trichomonas vaginalis* and *Neisseria gonorrhoeae* were detected. The vascular response is punctate and patchy, compared with Figure 200.

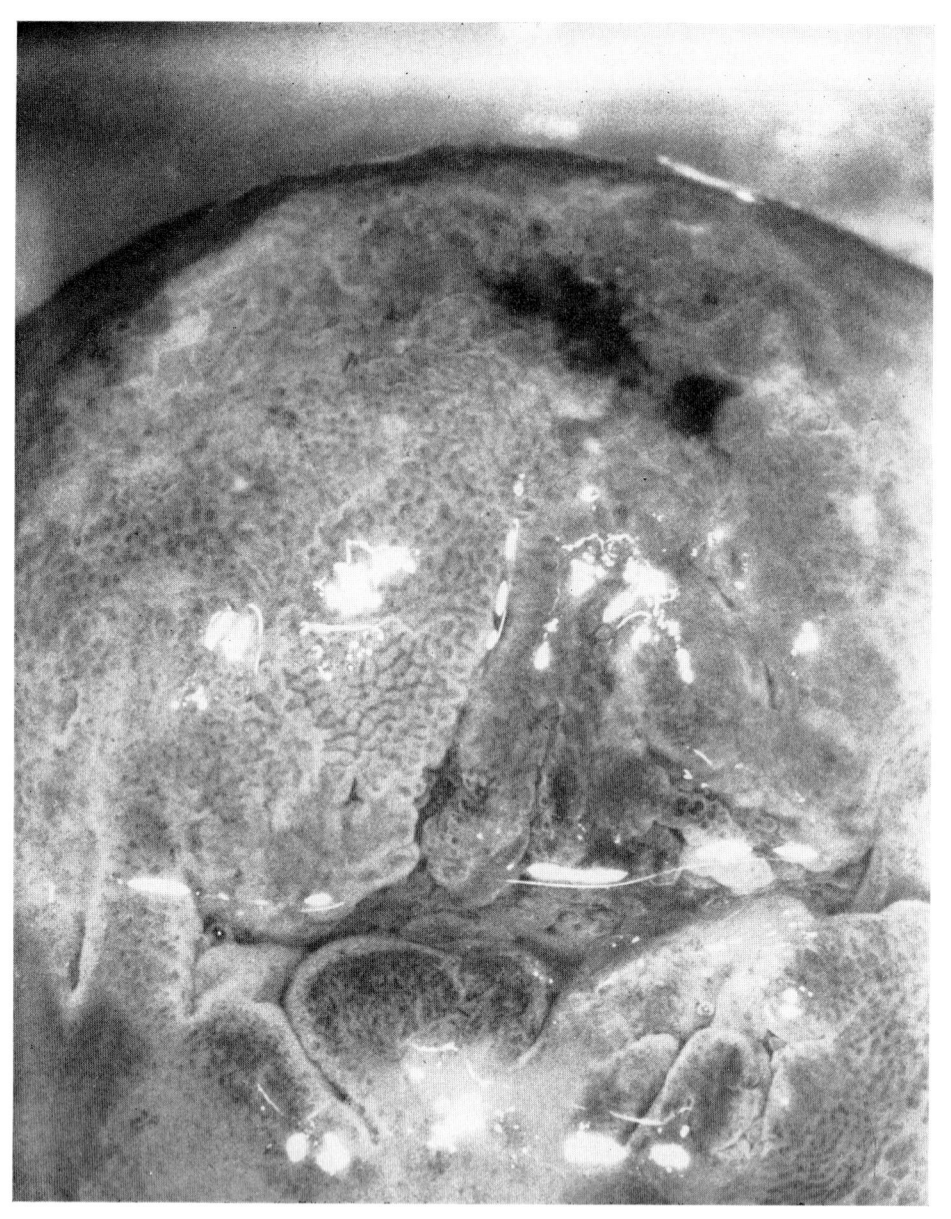

Figure 202. Vaginocervicitis. A mosaic-like arrangement of vessels associated with proven neisserian infection is seen on the anterior lip to the left of the photograph. The appearances faded as the infection subsided.

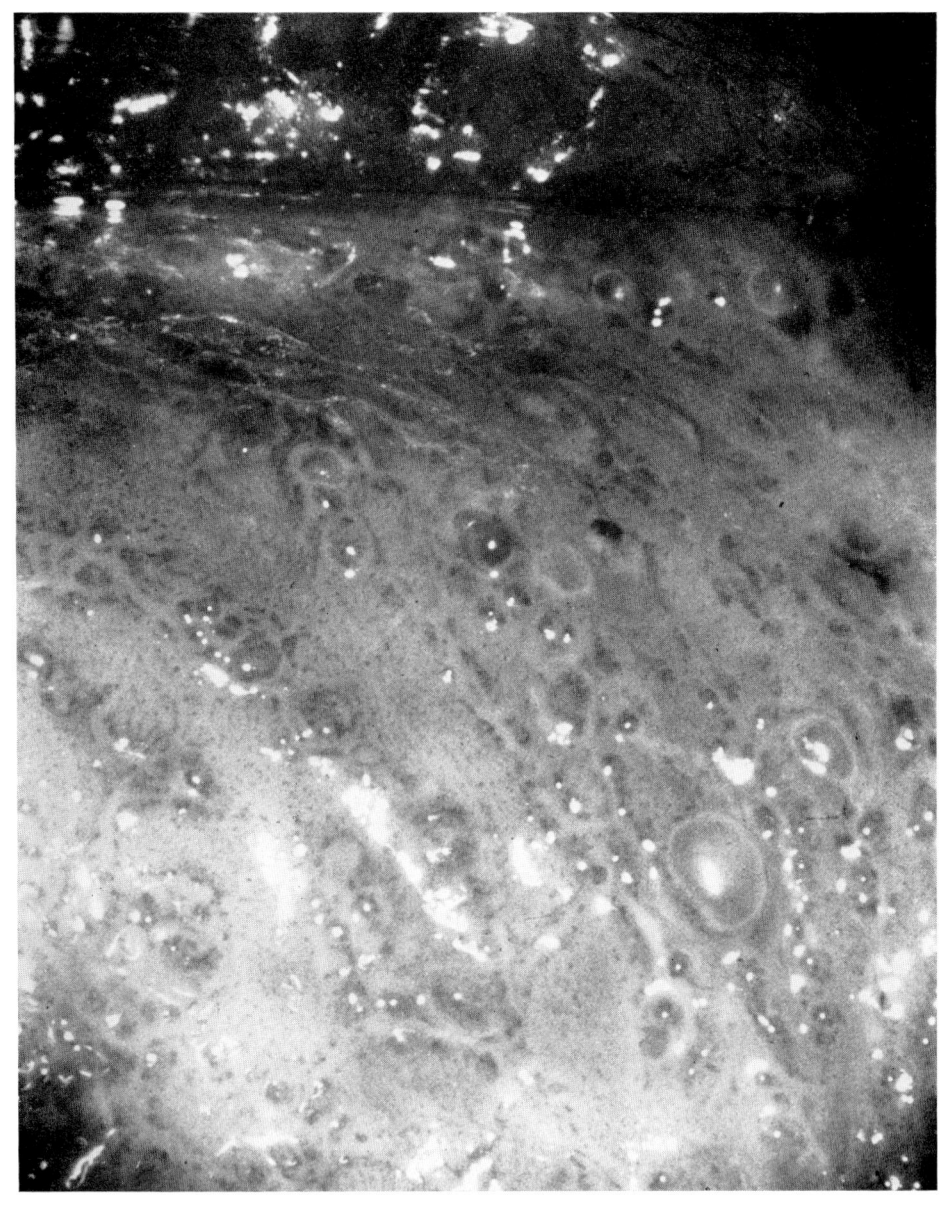

Figure 203. Vaginocervicitis. A marked response to trichomonas infestation is present. Vascular dilation and bubbling of the discharge are commonly seen.

284 Colposcopy

The more marked responses to bacterial inflammation cause diffuse red appearances; yellow spots, possibly lymphocyte collections; and ulceration, which can obscure the features usually seen with the colposcope (Fig. 203). No colposcopic diagnosis should be attempted until the response has subsided.

Chronic cervicitis has been commonly attributed to the state in which a *mucopurulent* discharge exudes from the glandular structures of the cervix. Commonly, no inflammatory response is observed through the colposcope, and only unaffected typical transformation zone is identified.

ATROPHIC CERVICITIS
(Oestrogen-deficient Vaginocervicitis)

Invariably, the vaginal and cervical epithelia show certain changes after

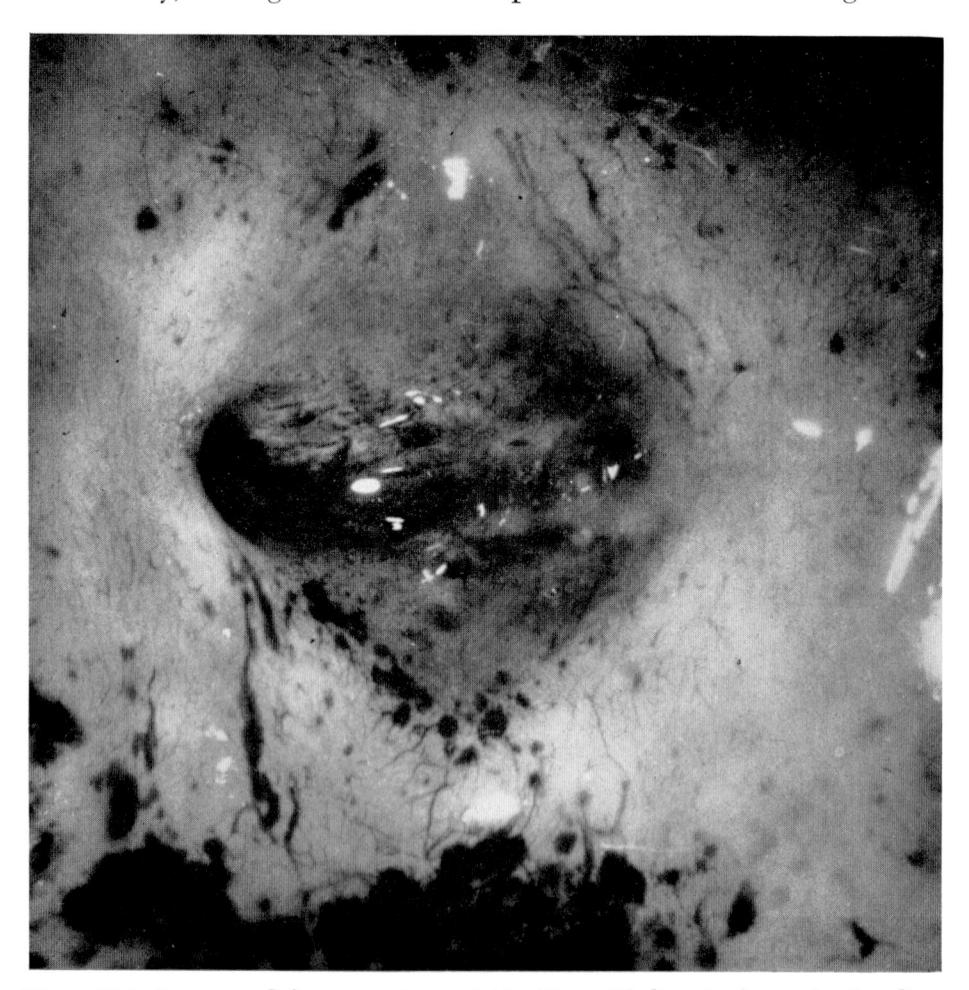

Figure 204. Oestrogen-deficient vaginocervicitis. The epithelium is thin and pale, allowing the subepithelial vessels to be seen. Petechial haemorrhages are often caused by trauma of the examination.

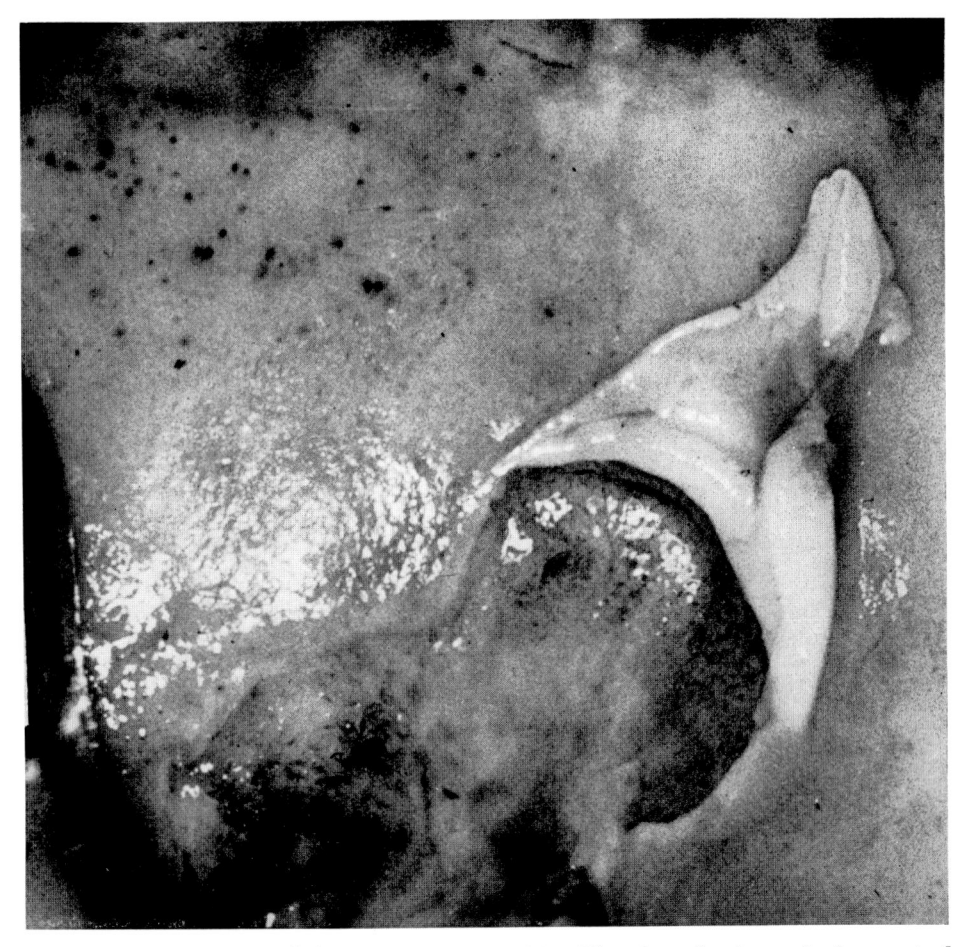

Figure 205. Oestrogen-deficient vaginocervicitis. The introduction of the vaginal speculum has resulted in lifting up a portion of the fragile epithelium. A so-called true erosion results.

the menopause. The epithelium becomes paler and even white, and at times, there may be difficulty in distinguishing the colour from that of the atypical transformation zone. Surface contours are reduced, and the epithelium becomes thin. Intraepithelial vascular structures become narrower in calibre, and the subepithelial terminal network is visible through the translucent epithelium (Figs. 204, 205, and 261). Some subepithelial petechiae are usually seen, apparently of spontaneous origin. The trauma of examination often causes multiple petechiae to become immediately evident. These changes, which can be a source of an abnormal cervical smear, are usually reversed by the use of local or systemic oestrogen therapy.

TRUE EROSION

Provided care is taken during introduction of the vaginal speculum and no examination has recently been undertaken, true erosion of the surface of the cervix is rare. In early literature on colposcopic technique, this entity was regarded as possibly indicating the presence of fragile, cancerous epithelium and the need for biopsy. We now believe that most true erosions usually have a straightforward traumatic explanation.

Fragile squamous epithelium, especially in postmenopausal women and in atypical transformation zone, is easily lifted by trauma. The resultant effect is seen as an exposed red area in which the stroma with its characteristic terminal vessels is highly visible. The edge is sharp and may be surrounded by the rolled, lifted epithelium originally covering the area (Fig. 205). These appearances are found in all varieties of typical and atypical transformation zone at all ages but are most characteristic of postmenopausal women. Of importance in the interpretation of a true erosion is the nature of the epithelium at its edge. Normal squamous epithelium or normal columnar epithelium may adjoin a true erosion, or true erosion may lie within an area of colposcopically atypical epithelium such as white epithelium, punctation, or mosaic, where it is of more significance (Fig. 206).

CONDYLOMA AND PAPILLOMA

Opinion on the terminology applied to lesions having a papillary surface configuration is divided. One group uses the term *papilloma* for a solitary outgrowth and reserves the term *condyloma* for multiple outgrowths; the other makes no clinical, histological, or aetiological distinction between the two. We support the second group and prefer the generic term *condyloma*.

More by clinical impression than laboratory characterisation, the conditions are thought to be due to wart viruses transmitted by sexual contact. Possibly for this or other reasons, these conditions recently seem to have become prevalent, warranting a more detailed discussion of their colposcopic appearances.

The clinical and colposcopic characteristics of a few examples of condyloma may be virtually impossible to differentiate from overt cancer, even for the experienced colposcopist. The resemblance to neoplastic vascular patterns may be striking, but there is usually a regularity in vessel spacing which is absent in true malignancy. Some condylomata exhibit cytological and histological disorders and may coexist with cervical intraepithelial neoplasia and minimal forms of invasive cancer. In such circumstances, it may be necessary to await the result of careful biopsy before undertaking treatment of these usually benign disorders. Condylomata arising in the transformation zone are of particular interest, suggesting another possible stimulus to cellular activity with potential neoplastic consequence. In this connection, it is possible that some atypical transformation zones without papillary surface changes may be of wart viral origin. Electron

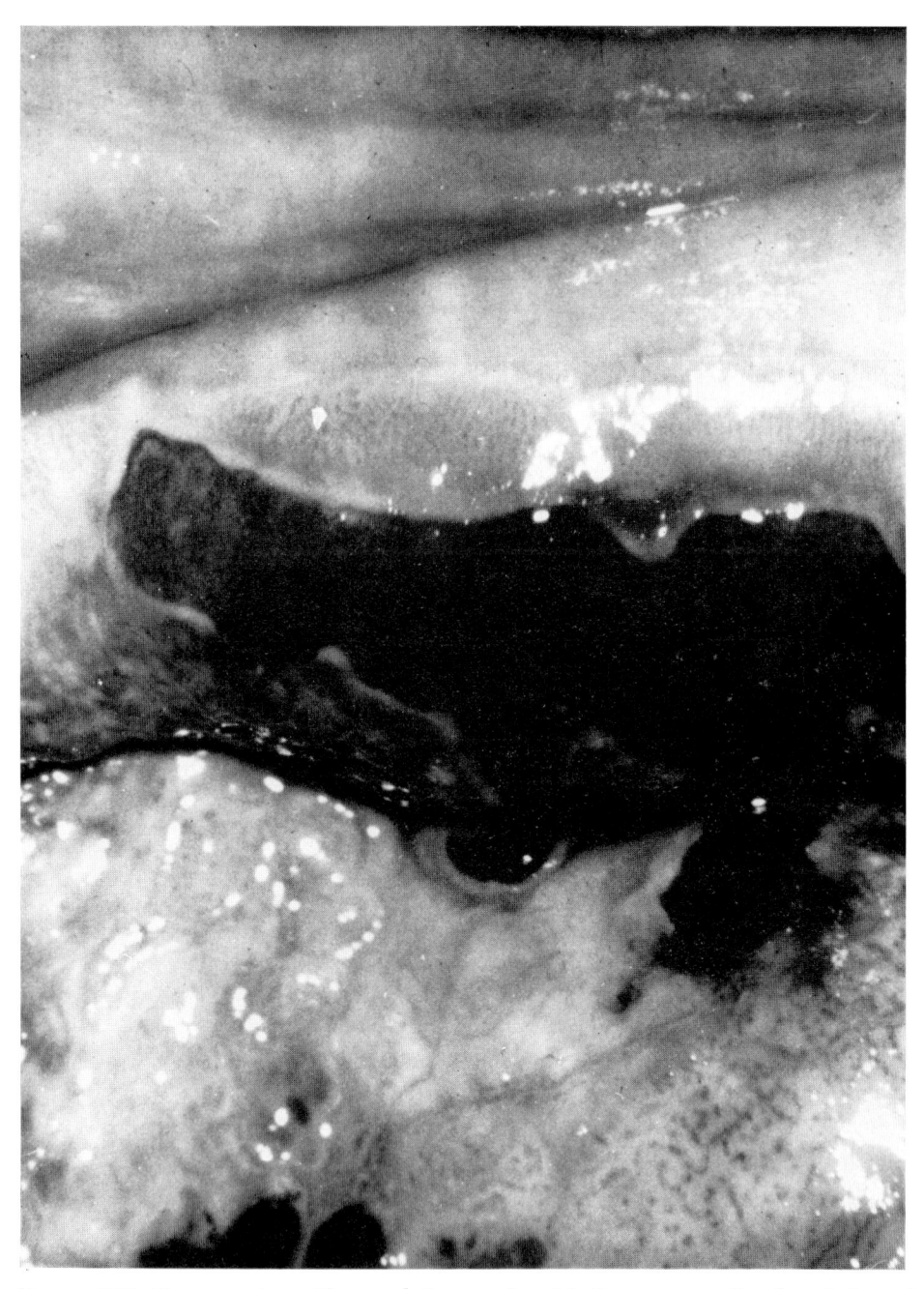

Figure 206. True erosion. Abnormal forms of epithelium are easily denuded, and atypical transformation zone with white epithelium and punctation is seen above and below the denuded area.

micrographs of biopsy material may sometimes reveal virus particles as an aid to diagnosis.

Several types of condylomata occur, some of which are uncharacteristic and raise a suspicion of more serious disorder:

1. Most commonly, the disorder is seen in the form of multiple, discrete papillary outgrowths present in the vulval epithelium and in the original squamous epithelia of the vagina and cervix. There is an accompanying characteristic type of angiogenesis with multiple coiled capillary loops (Fig. 207).

2. In some instances, the appearances are restricted to epithelia of the transformation zone (Figs. 208 and 209).

3. Some varieties exhibit long, fingerlike outgrowths with long capillary loops that, clinically and colposcopically, are not unlike overt cancer (Figs. 210 and 211).

4. Occasionally, the vaginal and/or the cervical epithelia are involved diffusely to produce a sheet of epithelium that clinically resembles keratosis. No vessels can be seen (Fig. 212).

CERVICAL ULCER—NON-MALIGNANT

Ulceration of the cervix is occasionally encountered from mechanical pressure, chemical trauma, or self-infliction, or the cause may not be apparent (Fig. 213). Currently, the more common lesions are of microbial origin, and because they may at first sight evoke some confusion with ulcers of a possible malignant origin, some detail is warranted in their description. Of current interest are the lesions of herpes simplex virus type 2 (HSV2). When characteristic lesions are present on the vulva, they may also be found on the vagina and cervix. Occasionally, cervical involvement can occur without vulval involvement. Ulcers may be single or multiple, shallow or deep, and the edge is often necrotic. Confluent types are seen (Figs. 214 and 215). After healing, no evidence of the pre-existing infection may be seen. Even when clinically evident, laboratory confirmation is difficult, whether by serological, cytological, or ultrastructural studies.

Syphilitic ulcers may occur on the cervix in the form of a primary chancre three weeks after infection. Single or multiple small ulcers can resemble those of herpes. Typically, the syphilitic ulcer has regular edges and a flat regular base that does not bleed on contact. Diagnosis is made by a search for the organism by darkfield microscopy. Serology is less helpful in the early stages of the disease. Tuberculous ulcers are described on the cervix.

CERVICAL POLYPS

Benign new growths of the columnar epithelium, seen as orderly exophytic structures reproducing the character of the parent tissue, are common. They persist, primarily unchanging for long periods, and have

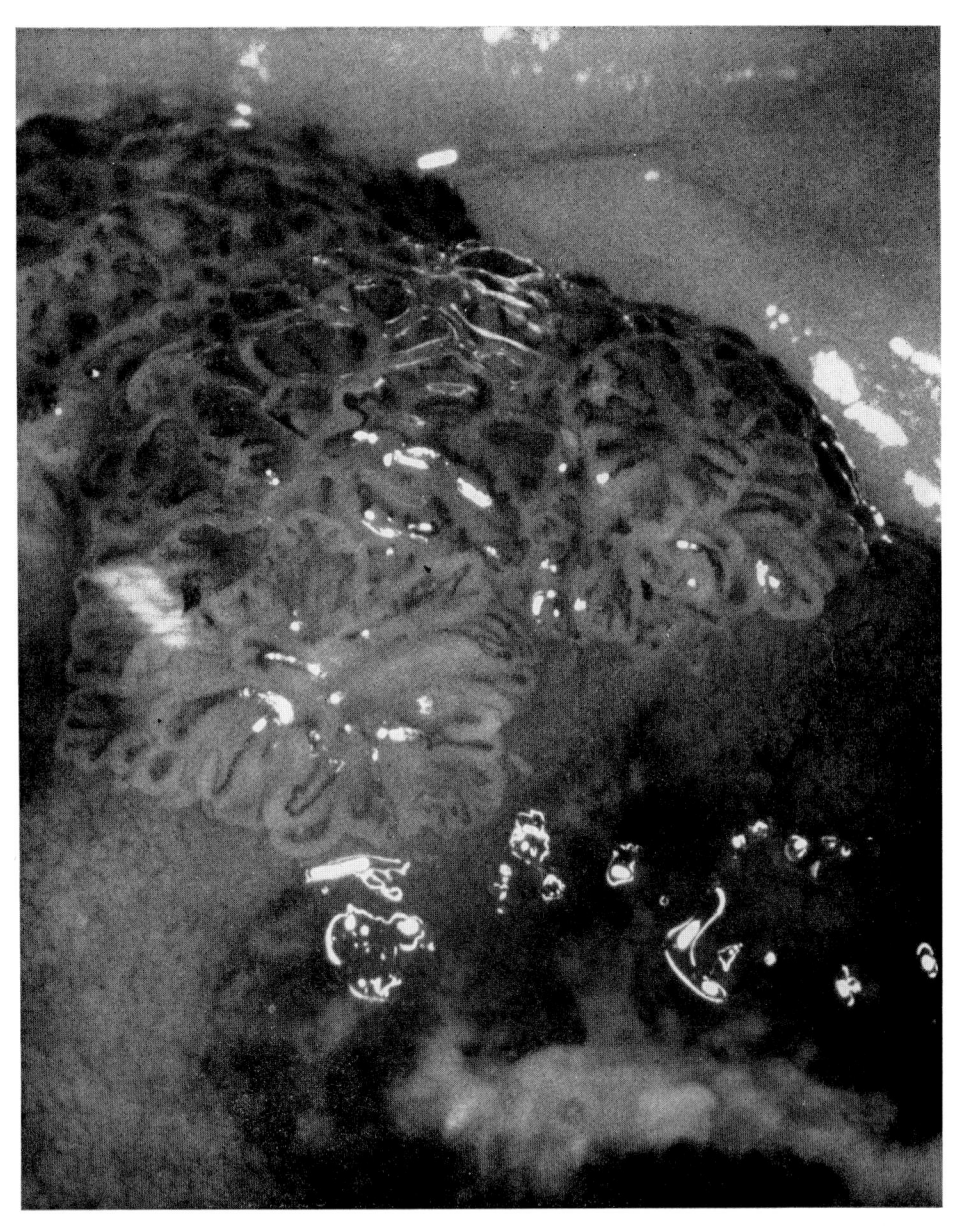

Figure 207. Condyloma. A characteristic type of condyloma is seen extending from the ectocervix onto the vagina. The surface is grossly papillary, and the complicated vascular structures are not unlike those present with malignancy.

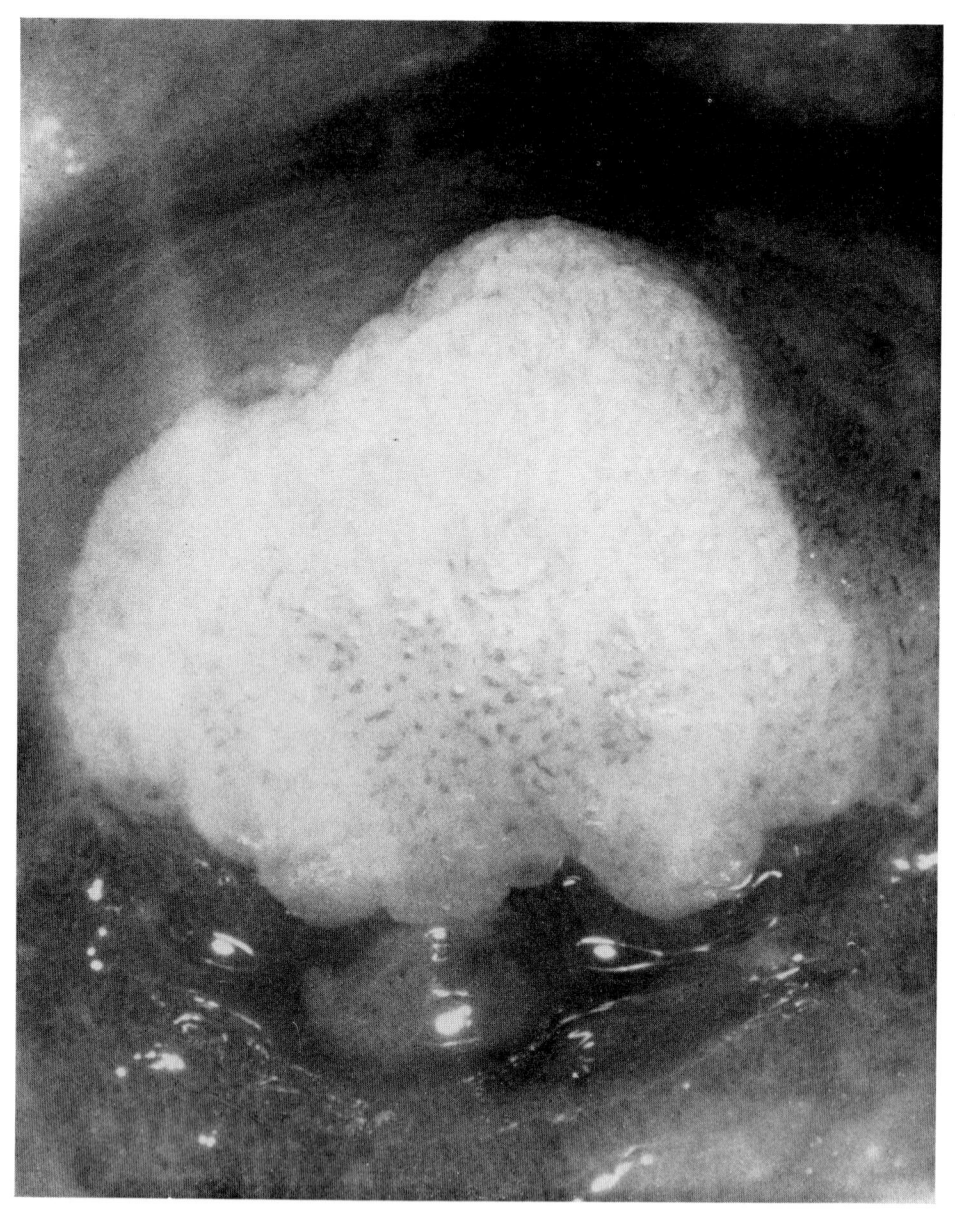

Figure 208. Condyloma. Involvement of a large portion of the transformation zone by confluent condylomata is sometimes seen. This example was white before the application of acetic acid, and the terminal vessels are almost obscured.

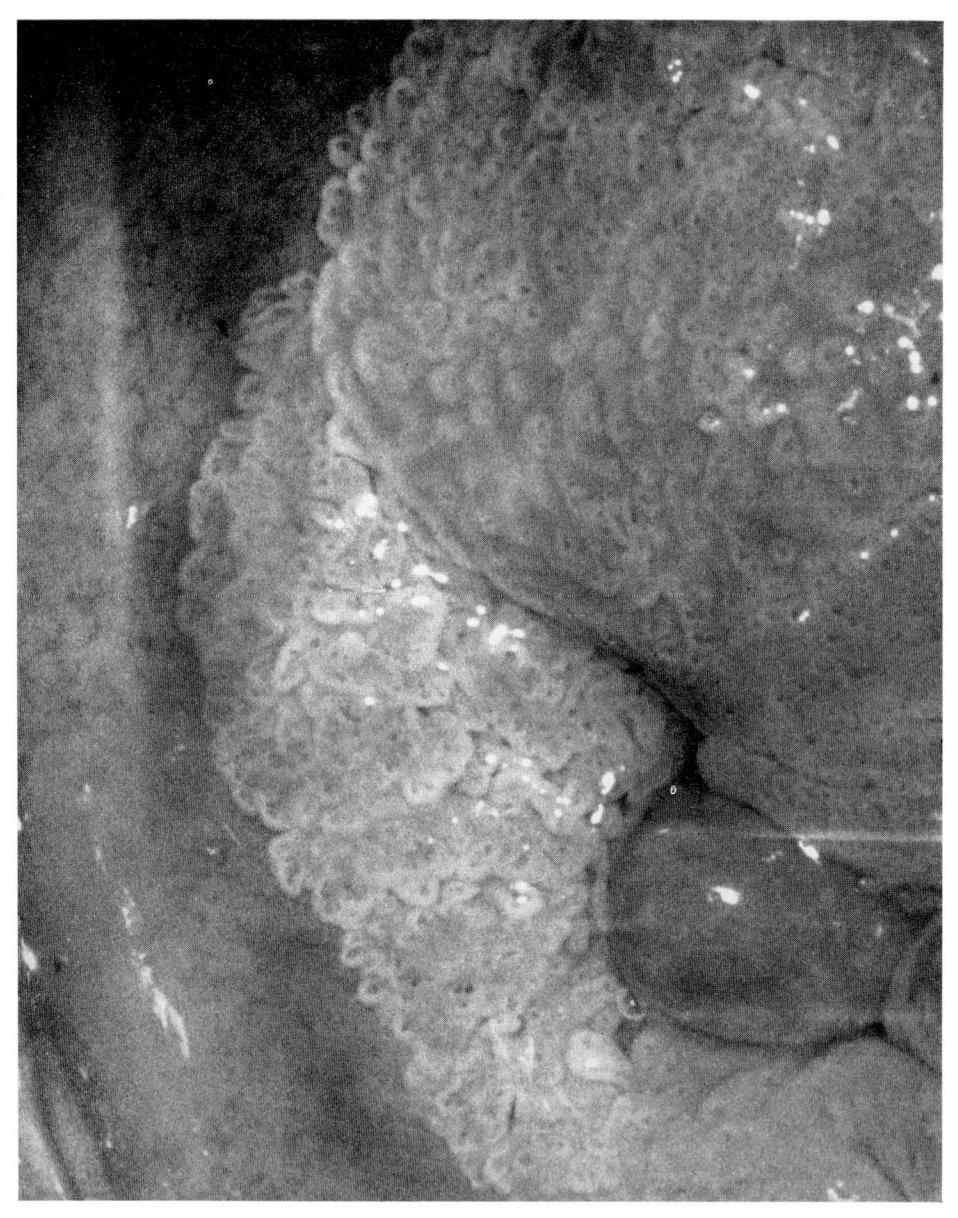

Figure 209. Condyloma. In this example, there is diffuse involvement of the transformation zone.

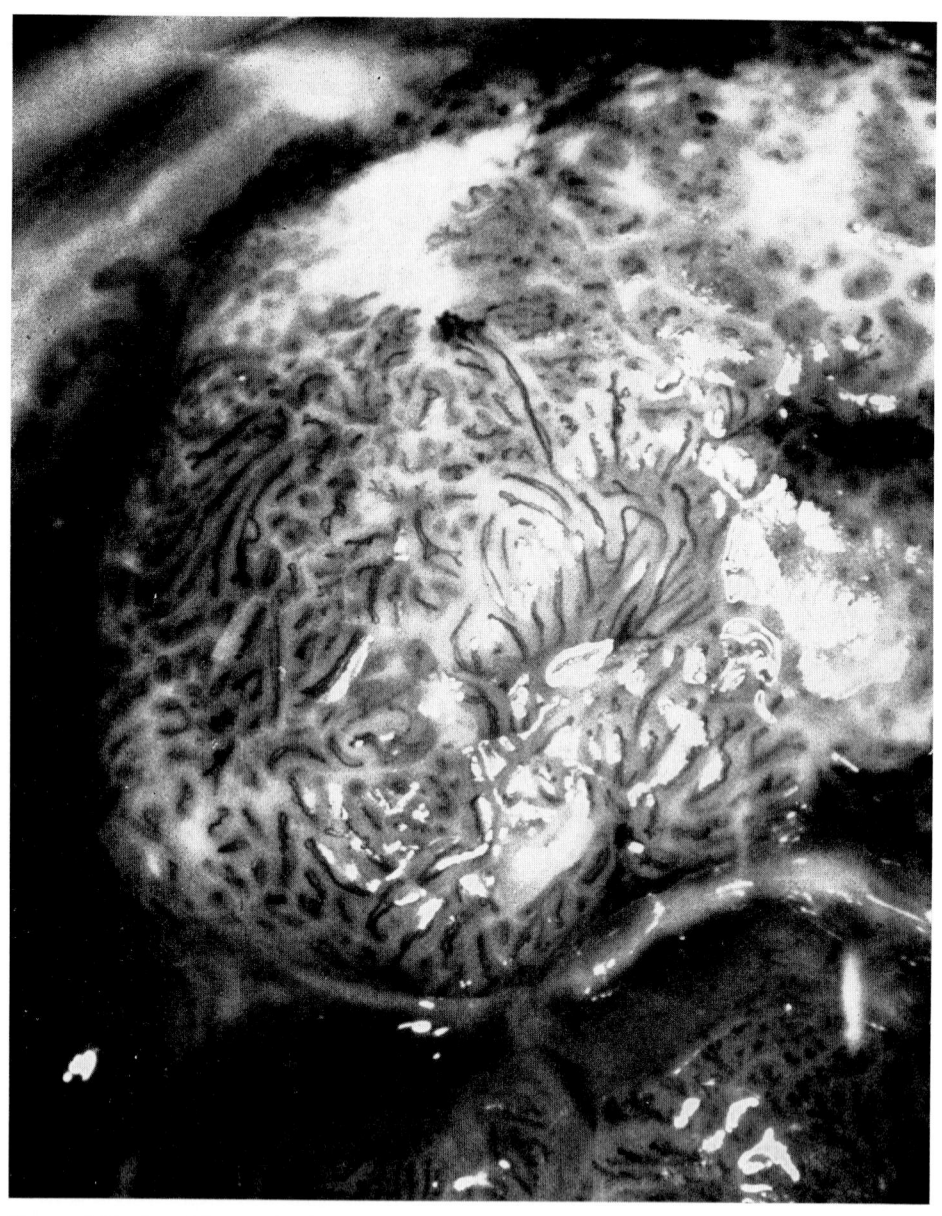

Figure 210. Condyloma. Striking terminal vascular structures that closely resemble the appearances seen in overt cancer are seen. Cytological abnormalities were present, and the histological diagnosis was condyloma.

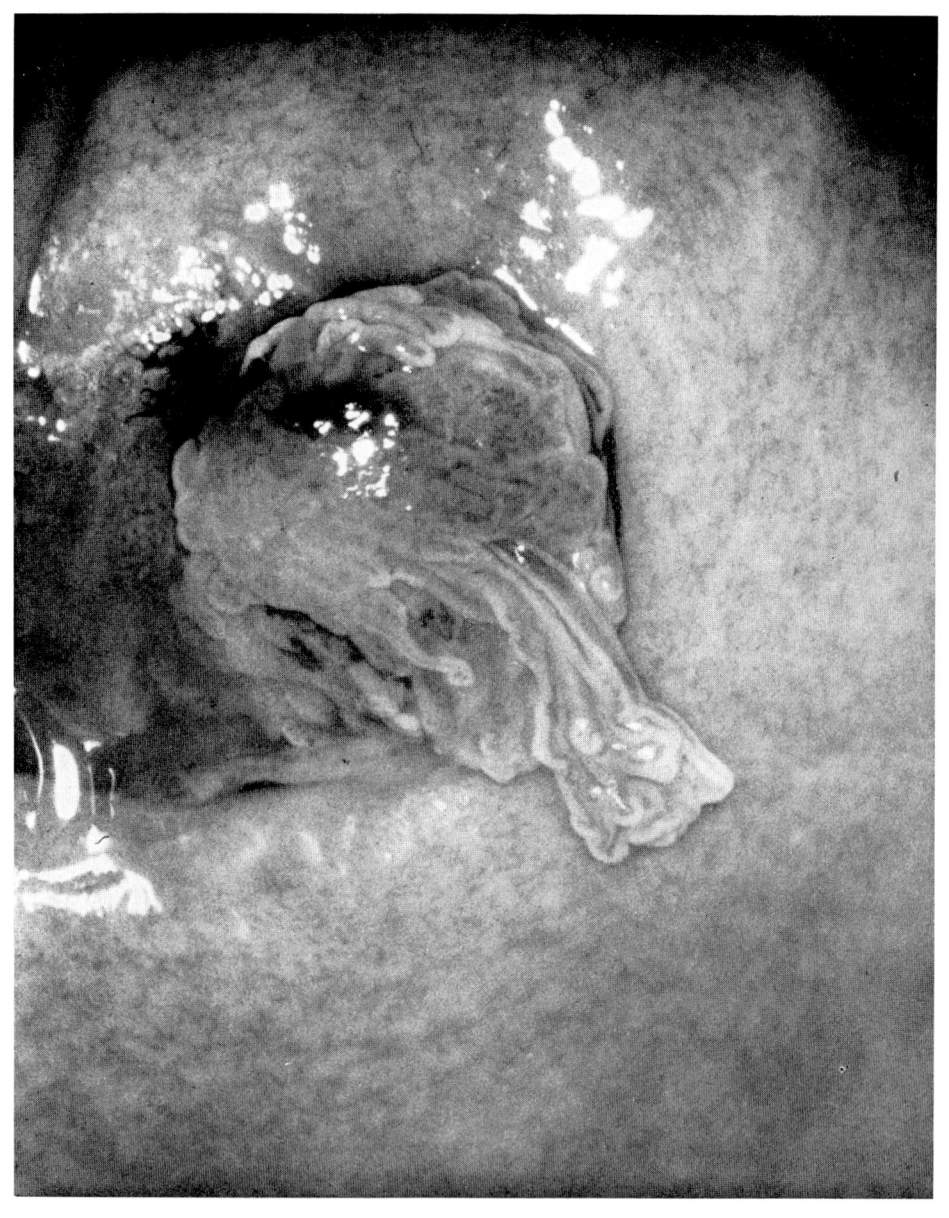

Figure 211. Condyloma. A small condylomatous polyp shows long fronds containing the characteristic terminal vessels.

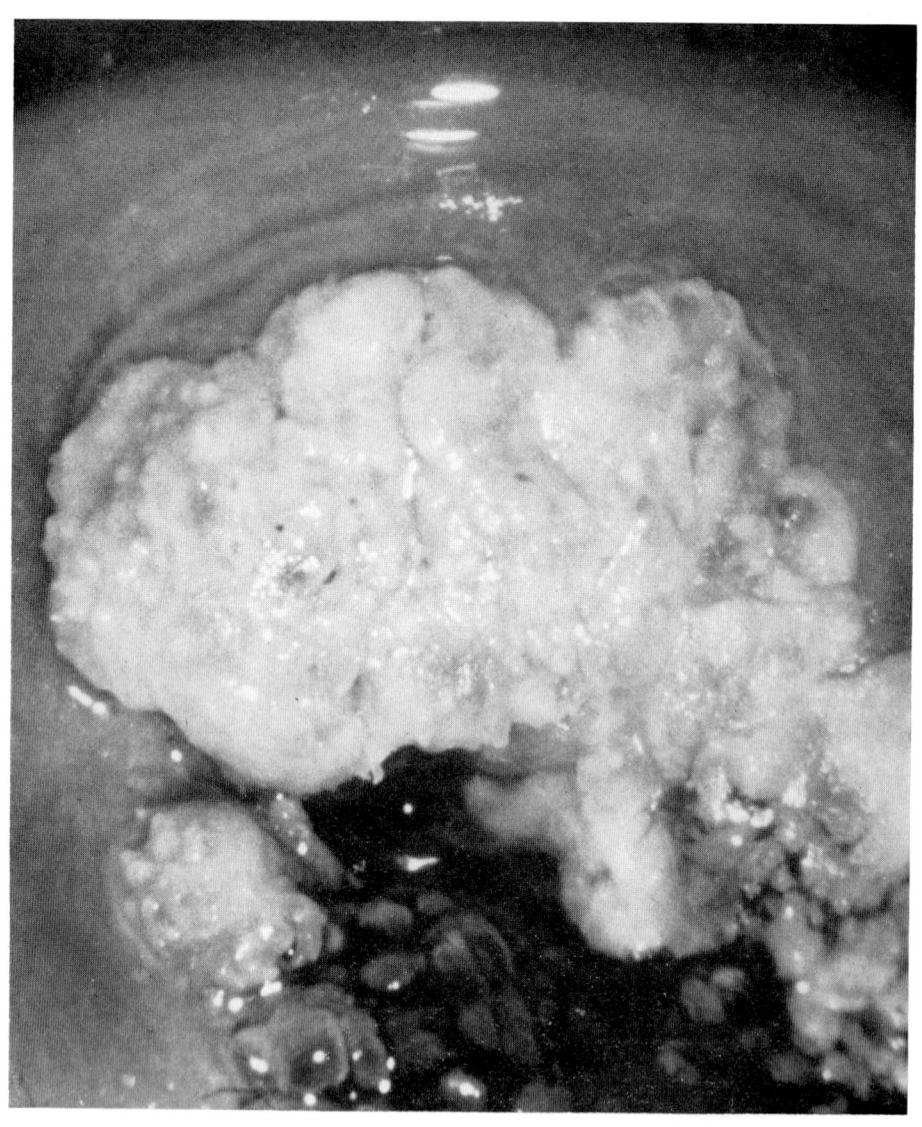

Figure 212. Condyloma. A further variant seen on the cervix produces a keratin overlay that obscures the vascular pattern and presents clinically as keratosis.

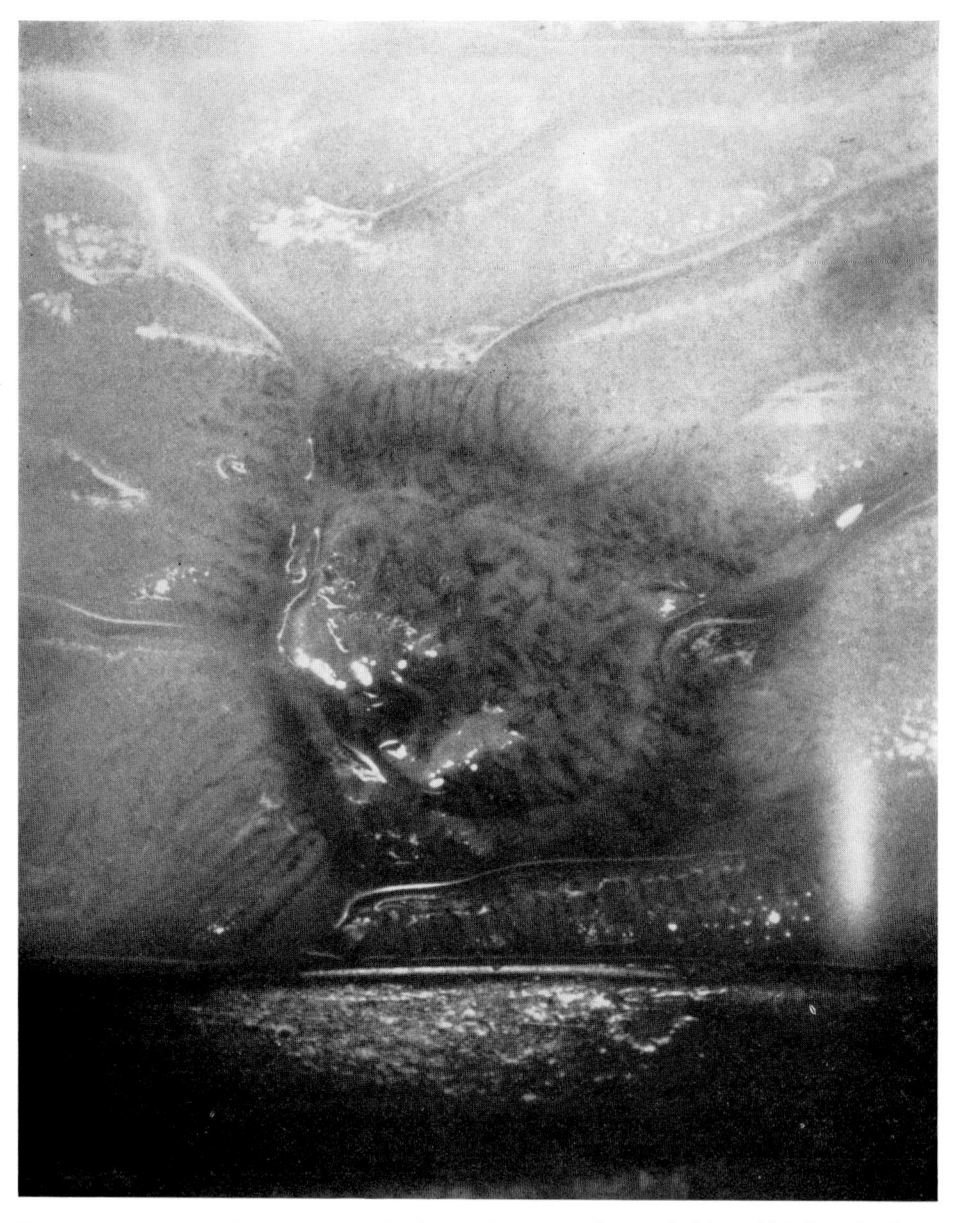

Figure 213. Non-malignant vaginal ulcer. This example, probably self-inflicted, shows a base of granulation with the vascular pattern of regeneration at the edges.

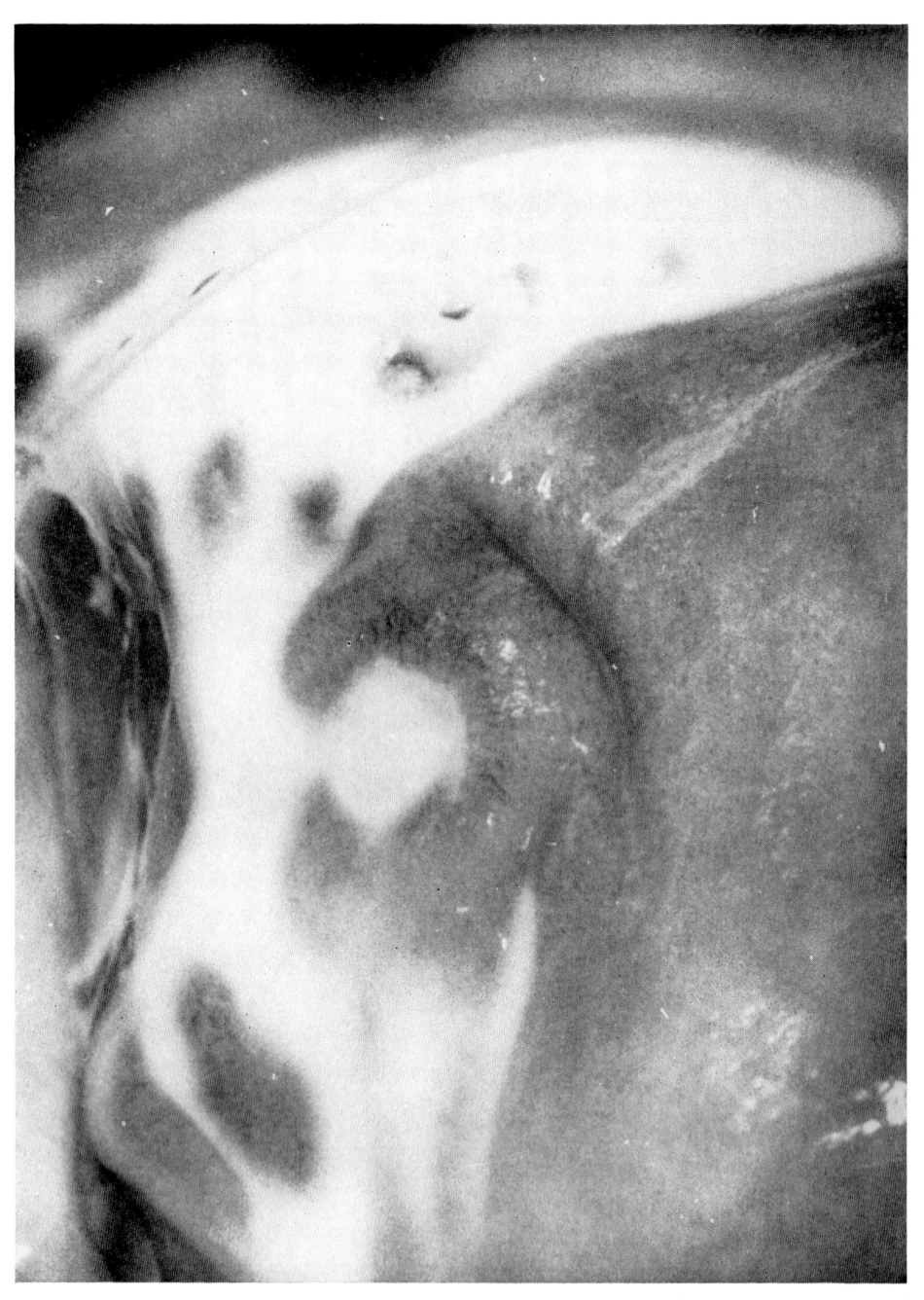

Figure 214. Herpetic ulceration. Herpes simplex virus was cultured from this small discrete ulcer on the vagina, in the centre of the photograph. Note the radial disposition of vessels generally found at sites of regeneration and the thick white discharge.

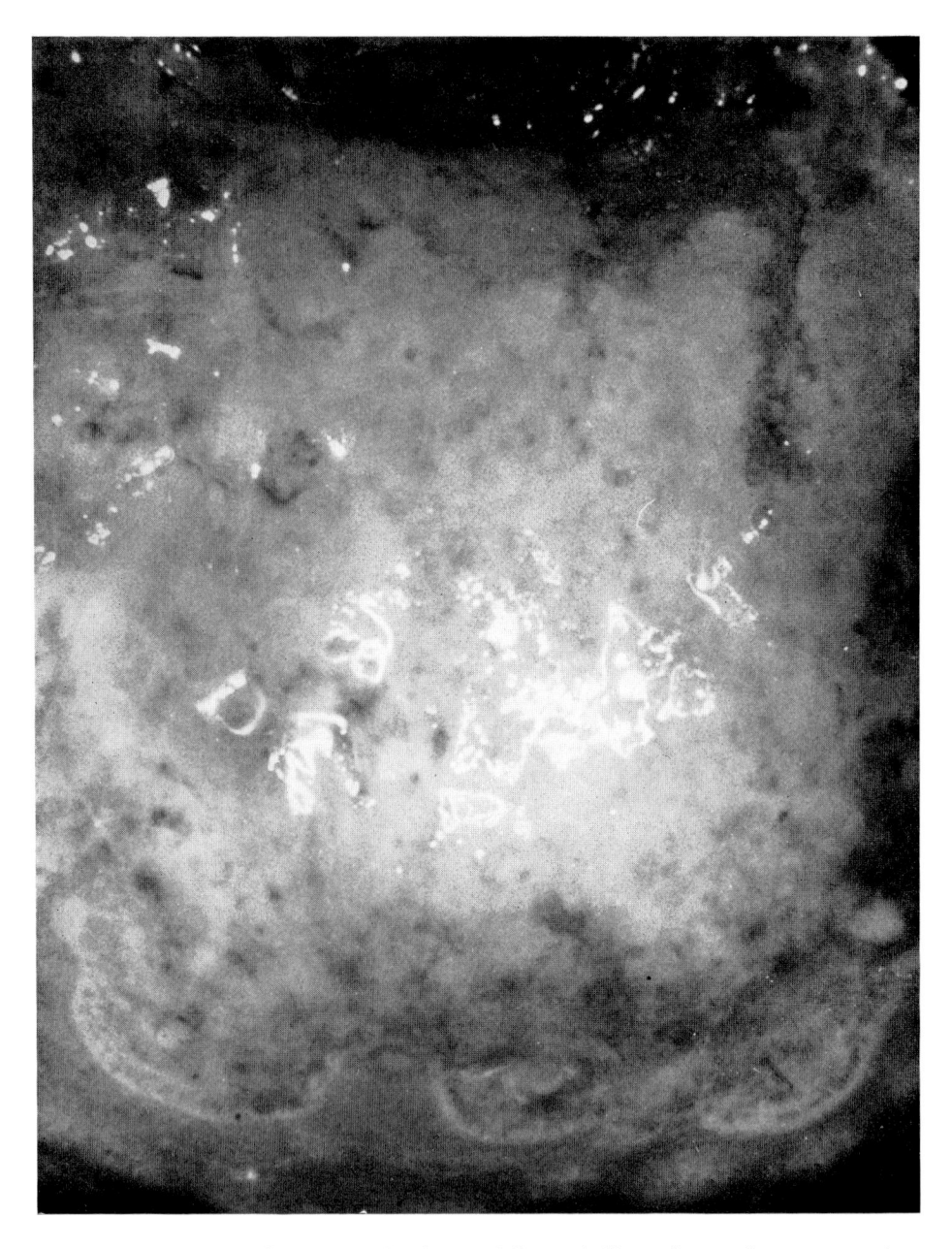

Figure 215. Herpetic ulceration. This large, diffuse, shallow ulcer with a necrotic base on the posterior cervical lip occupying most of the photograph proved to be herpetic in origin. The whole of the transformation zone appears affected.

no particular significance. The surface usually exhibits features of either columnar epithelium, typical transformation zone, or combinations of each (Fig. 216). The existence of metaplastic epithelium on the adenomatous polyp is evidence of the discrete and isolated nature of the metaplastic change. If atypical transformation zone is present elsewhere, then the polyp may have a surface covering of similar epithelium (Fig. 217). Some areas containing single or multiple inclusion cysts may be sufficiently elevated to be termed *polypoidal* (Fig. 218).

APPEARANCES FOLLOWING ELECTRODIATHERMY AND CRYOSURGERY

Following adequate cryosurgery or electrodiathermy, the original topography is permanently destroyed. The original squamocolumnar junction and the transformation zone are no longer visible. The injured area is re-epithelialized by the process of regeneration, and the new squamous epithelium is usually featureless, apart from the characteristic linear patterns of vascular structures (Fig. 219). The experienced colposcopist can usually identify these regenerate patterns when no history is available of such procedures. A newly formed squamocolumnar junction arises between the regenerate epithelium and columnar epithelium. Normal scar contraction results, in most cases, in reversion of this junction within the endocervical canal. The clinical implications of this event are discussed on page 419. Incomplete destruction results in the persistence of some of the original structures at the surface.

Colposcopic appearances suggesting an atypical epithelium, such as white epithelium, with or without punctation and/or mosaic structure, can occur after treatment of either benign or atypical histological disorders. This matter is further discussed on page 429.

APPEARANCES AFTER IRRADIATION

After irradiation of the cervix and vagina for clinically overt cancer, bizarre vessel patterns may be seen colposcopically on a white background (Fig. 220). These features can be mistaken for, or are even indistinguishable from, atypical vessels associated with malignant disease.

INCONSPICUOUS IODINE NON-STAINING AREAS

On occasion, sharply limited iodine-negative areas of small or large size, single or multiple, are seen which show no atypical features on colposcopic examination (Fig. 221). These areas may be found on any part of the ectocervix and, at times, extend to the vaginal fornix. They occur within the original transformation zone (p. 374), have no particular significance, and histologically show parakeratosis.

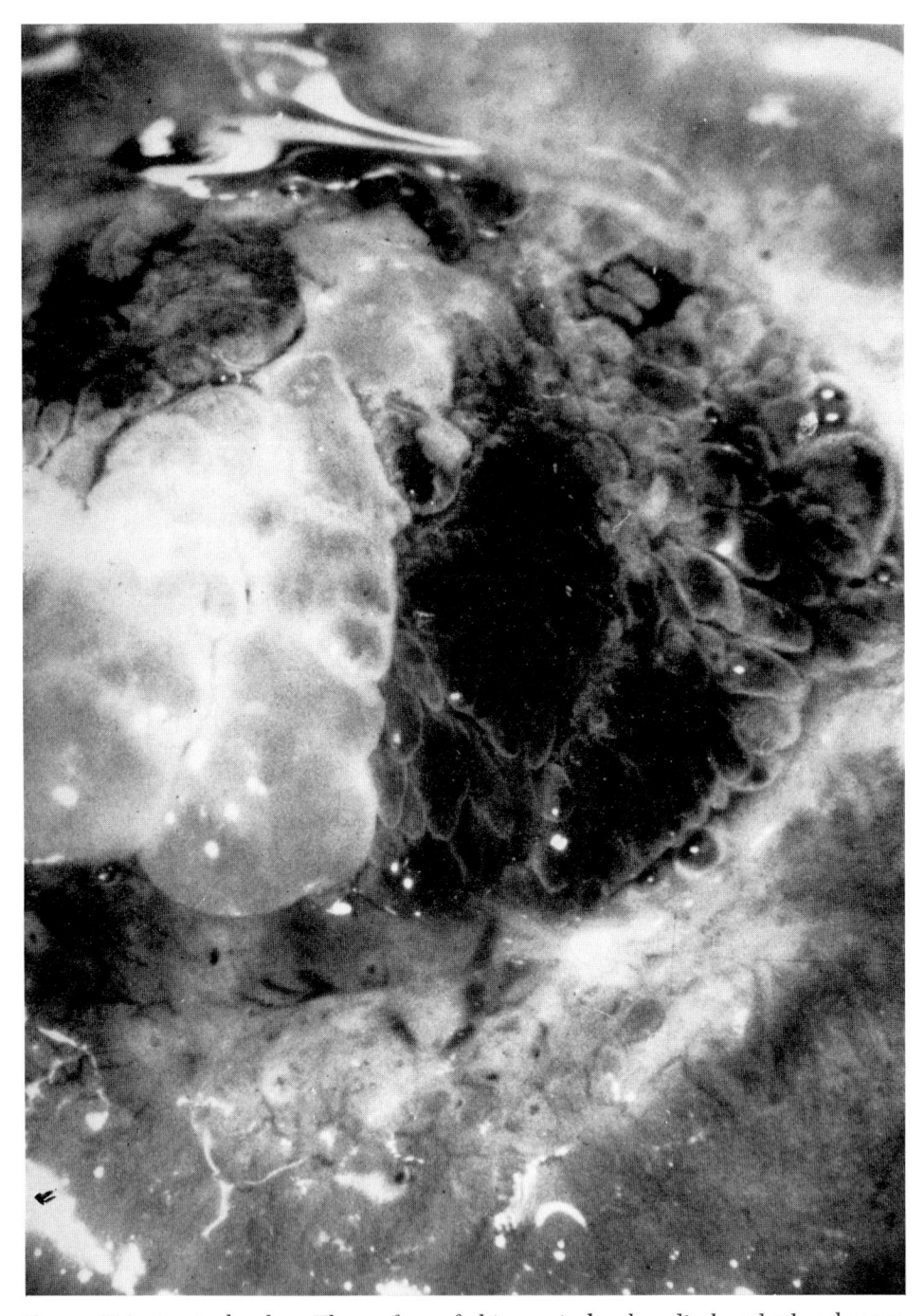

Figure 216. Cervical polyp. The surface of this cervical polyp displays both columnar epithelium on the right and patchy physiological metaplasia on the left of the photograph.

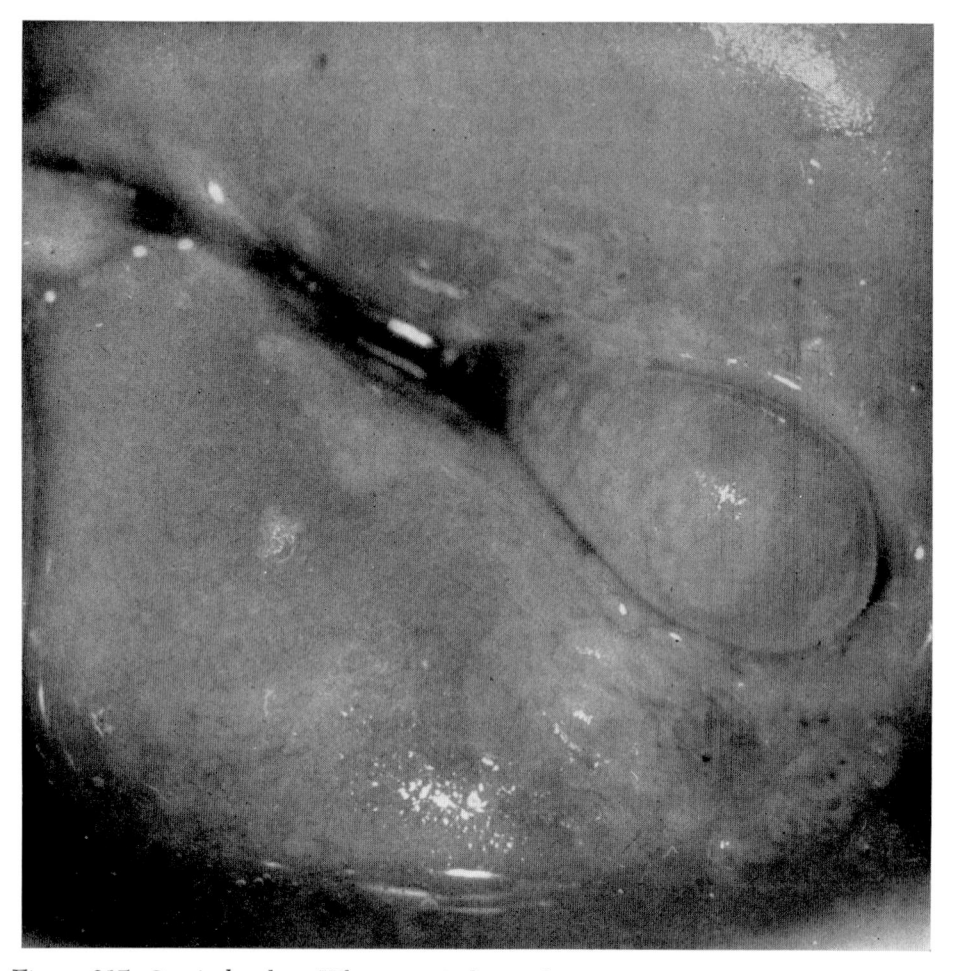

Figure 217. Cervical polyp. When atypical transformation zone is present, the polyp may also be affected by the process. Histological examination of the white epithelium with mosaic structure on the surface of this polyp showed carcinoma in situ.

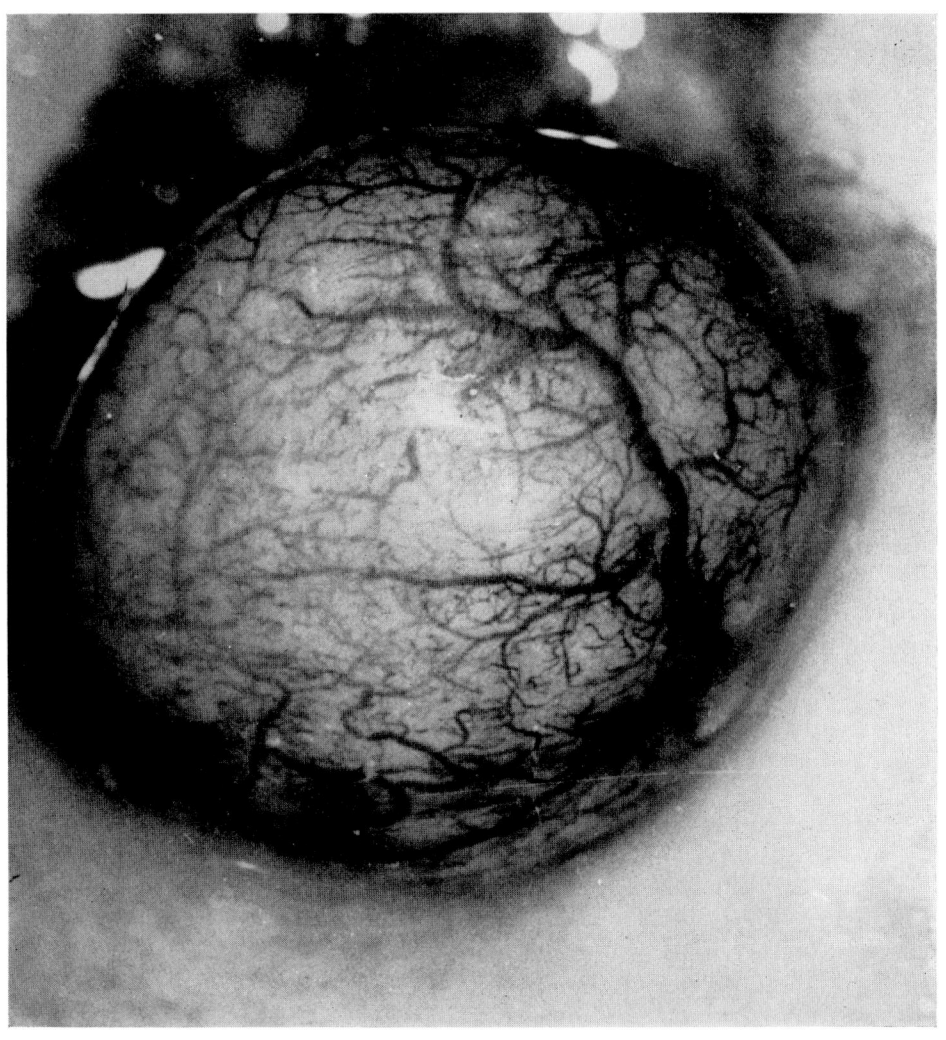

Figure 218. Cervical polyp. This retention cyst near the cervical canal clinically resembled a polyp. Colposcopy showed a nabothian cyst covered by squamous epithelium.

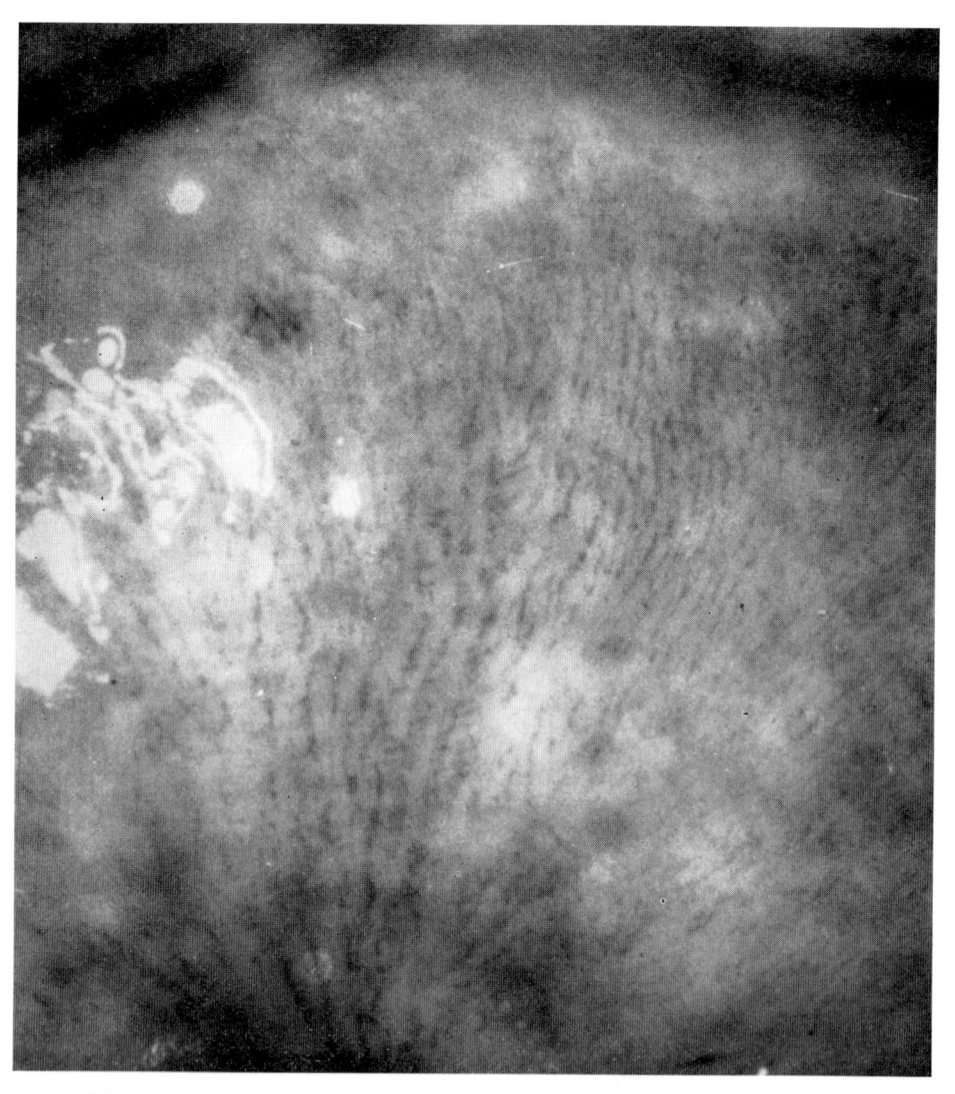

Figure 219. Regeneration after electrodiathermy. The most common end-result of electrocoagulation or cryosurgery of the cervical epithelia is a new appearance, smooth and featureless, in which fine linear vascular structures are seen.

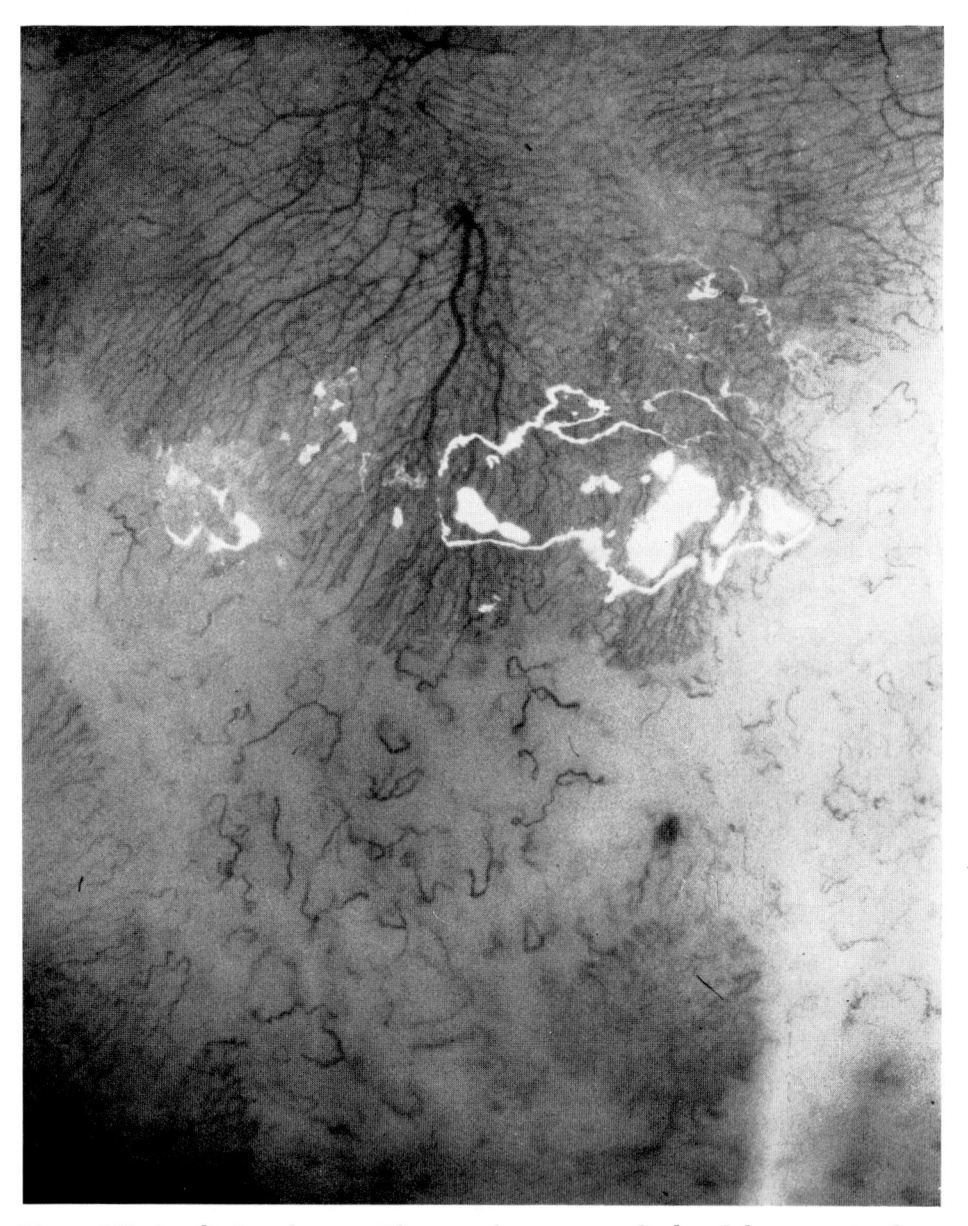

Figure 220. Irradiation changes. The vascular patterns displayed have persisted unchanged for some years after treatment. Regular branching vessels are visible in the upper half of the photograph, and atypical vessels indistinguishable from those of neoplasia are seen in the lower half.

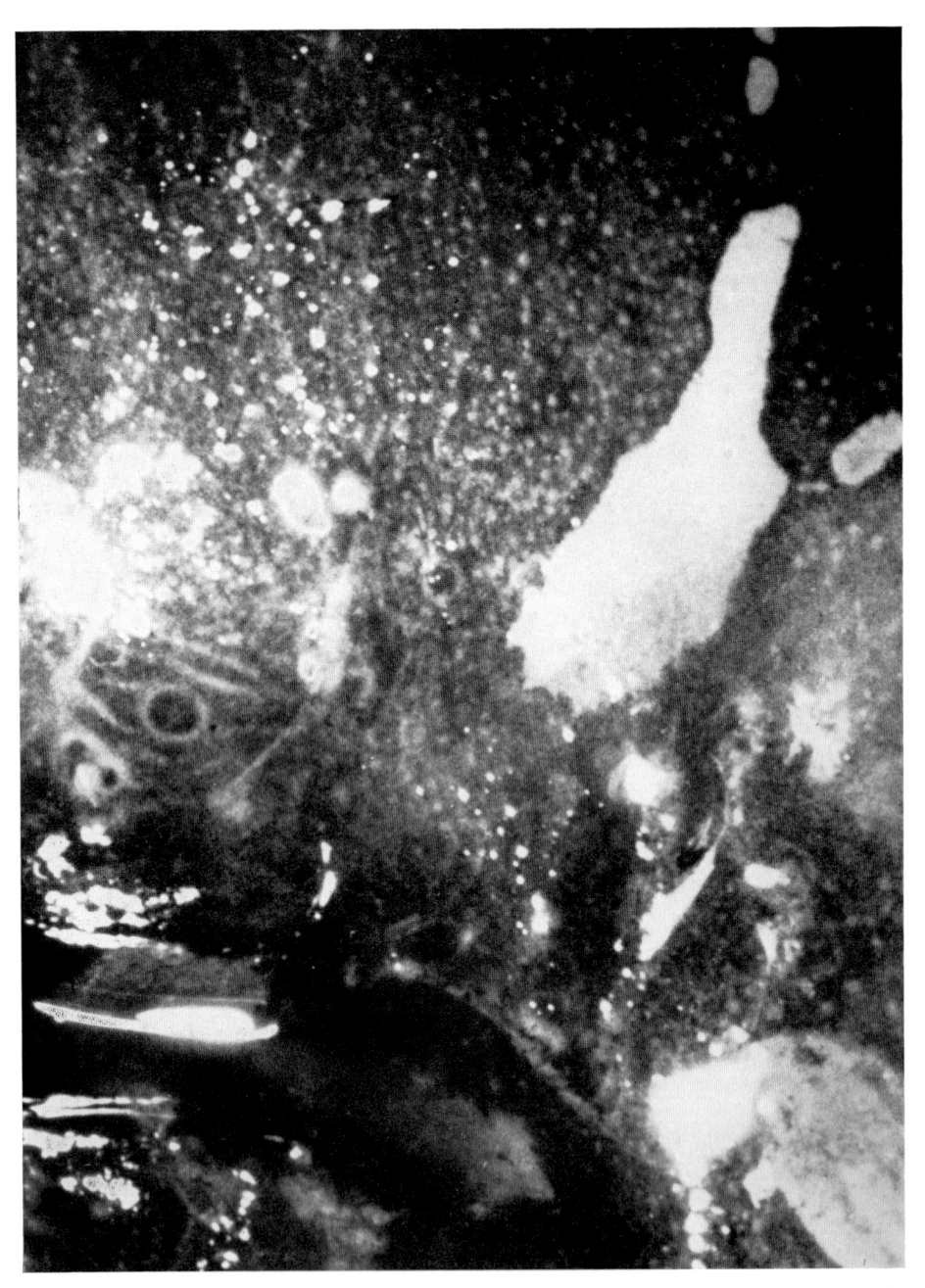

Figure 221. Inconspicuous iodine-negative areas. Small discrete areas are evident after the application of Schiller's iodine solution. Lying within original squamous epithelium, they are probably isolated areas of original transformation zone.

PART V
Recent Advances

Chapter 12

THE VAGINA

DURING THE PAST DECADE, there has been a quickening of interest in the vaginal epithelium. Awareness of the presence of a transformation zone in the upper vagina, the occurrence of intraepithelial neoplasia within the zone, and most strikingly, the recognition of the teratogenic and carcinogenic implications of exposure *in utero* to non-steroidal oestrogens has focussed anew the interest of gynaecologist and pathologist on this area.

New observations have demonstrated a need for an improved understanding and description of the various epithelial structures which may be found in the human vagina. This need has also been expressed in a revision of embryological descriptions. In this revision, the colposcopist is in a unique position, for in the course of daily clinical practice, a large, mainly unselected group of subjects in whom the cervical, vaginal, and vulval epithelia can be inspected is available. The overall view of epithelia in the living state far exceeds observations possible on necropsy material. Biopsy material can easily be obtained in the presence of features other than the normal pink, rugose, iodine-positive epithelium.

In our experience, observations of adult material have been complemented by studies of several hundred necropsy specimens of foetuses, young girls, and adolescents. The continuity of embryonic and extrauterine development has been available for examination.

EMBRYOLOGY

The derivation of the vaginal and cervical epithelia remains controversial. However, an interpretation of observations on our material supports theories of vaginal embryogenesis that show the original squamous epithelium of the vagina and cervix is derived from canalisation of the vaginal plate of the urogenital sinus and columnar epithelium is derived from canalisation of the müllerian uterovaginal rudiment. The original squamocolumnar junction represents the boundary that develops at the site where sinus and müllerian rudiments meet during embryogenesis. The metaplastic epithelium develops in epithelium of müllerian origin during the intrauterine phase of development, as well as during those eras when it can be observed postnatally.

THE EPITHELIA OF THE VAGINA

A conventional approach to the nomenclature applied to the epithelial structures of the vagina does not allow a proper description of the variations and abnormalities observable in the organ. The distribution of characteristic epithelia cannot easily be related to classical anatomical features, such as the external cervical os, vaginal fornix, hymen, or vaginal introitus. It is necessary to use the terminology of epithelial boundaries already developed in this text (see Chap. 3). These boundaries and the epithelia between them are best appreciated by tracing them from without inwards.

The *vulvovaginal boundary* is clearly seen following application of Schiller's iodine solution to the vulva. A sharp line of demarcation forms between pale vulval epithelium and dark vaginal epithelium (Fig. 222). Histological examination of tissue from the line shows an equally sharp distinction (Fig. 223).

The original squamous epithelium of the lower genital tract extends cephalad from the line of demarcation. It is histologically similar, whether covering the vaginal introitus, the vagina, or ectocervix. However, in various situations, the stroma confers upon it characteristics of surface variations. It is usually smooth at the introitus, rugose and papillary in the vagina, and again smooth on the ectocervix.

The original squamous epithelium extends cephalad to the boundary separating it from the epithelia of müllerian derivation. When it adjoins columnar epithelium, the cranial boundary is termed the *original squamocolumnar junction* (Fig. 224). This junction, which is most commonly found at some site on the ectocervix or within the endocervical canal, has already been described in Chapter 3 (p. 72). In about 4 per cent of cases, the junction is sited on the vagina beyond the boundaries of the cervix (Fig. 225). In the majority of subjects, metaplasia has occurred in most of the extent of the columnar epithelium (Fig. 226). The junction, now squamosquamous between two different forms of squamous epithelium, is still termed the *original squamocolumnar junction* (Fig. 226). Between the original and the *new squamocolumnar junction* lies the metaplastic cell population of the transformation zone of the vagina and cervix.

Conventional nomenclature also fails in using *vaginal adenosis* (see Chaps. 13 and 14) as a comprehensive term to define a variety of glandular structures found from time to time in the vaginal epithelium. An interpretation associated with the use of the term *adenosis* is that the condition is abnormal in the same way as the term *cervical erosion* was used earlier this century to cover the same condition on the cervix. The colposcope shows that most areas of adenosis are of columnar or of mixed columnar-metaplastic epithelia, lying within the transformation zone precisely as in the case of glandular epithelium on the cervix.

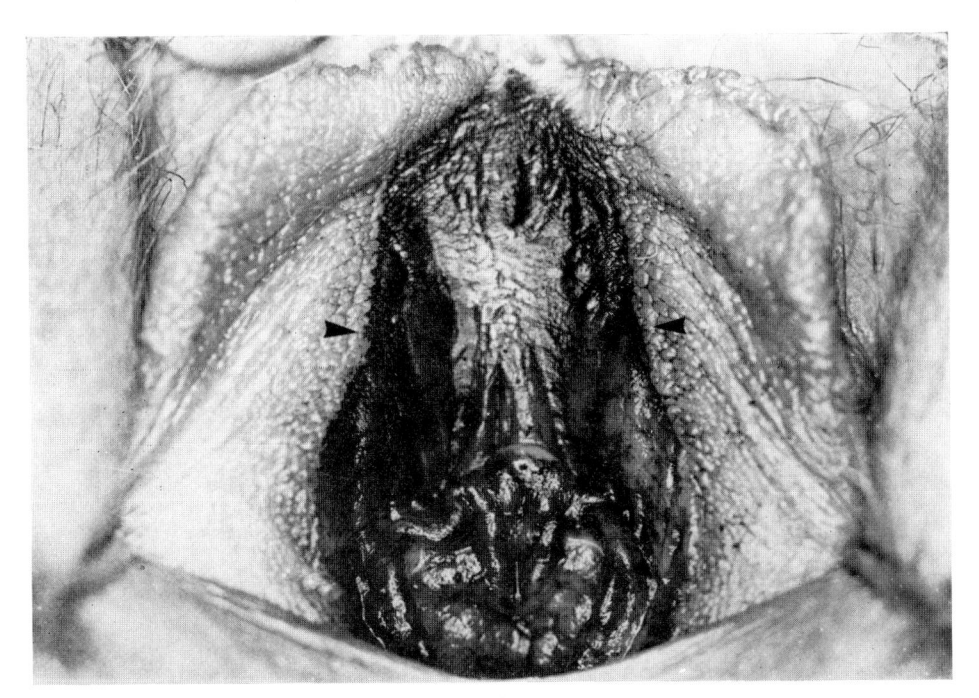

Figure 222. Vulvovaginal line. Photograph showing the labia minora separated. Schiller's iodine solution has been applied. A sharp line of demarcation circumscribes the introitus (arrows) between the iodinated vaginal and non-iodinated skin epithelia.

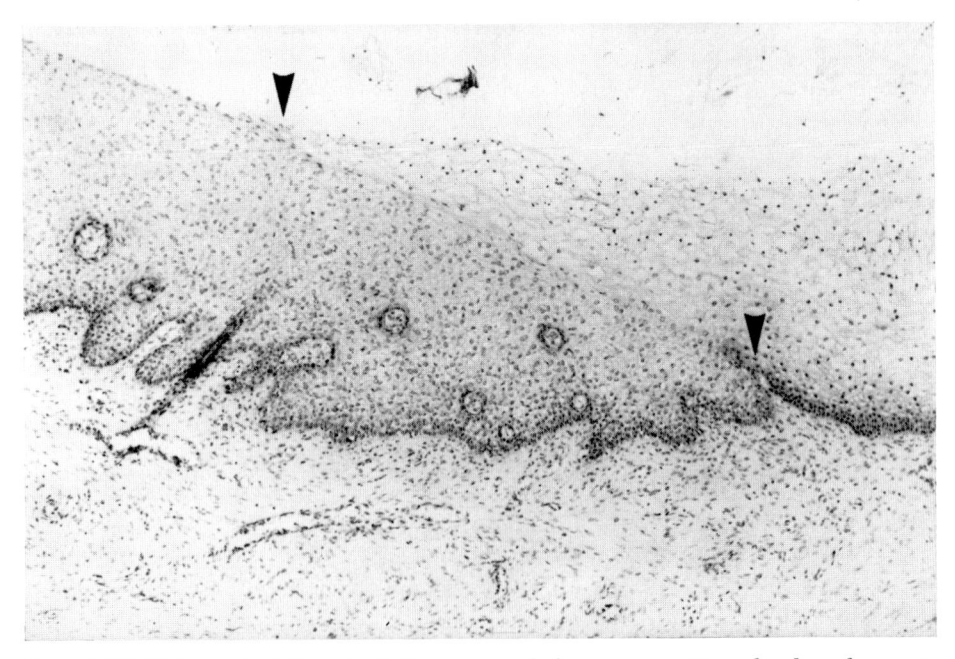

Figure 223. Vulvovaginal line. A photomicrograph from preparation of vulva of neonate. A sharp, oblique line (arrow) separates the original squamous epithelium of the vagina on the right from vulval squamous epithelium on the left.

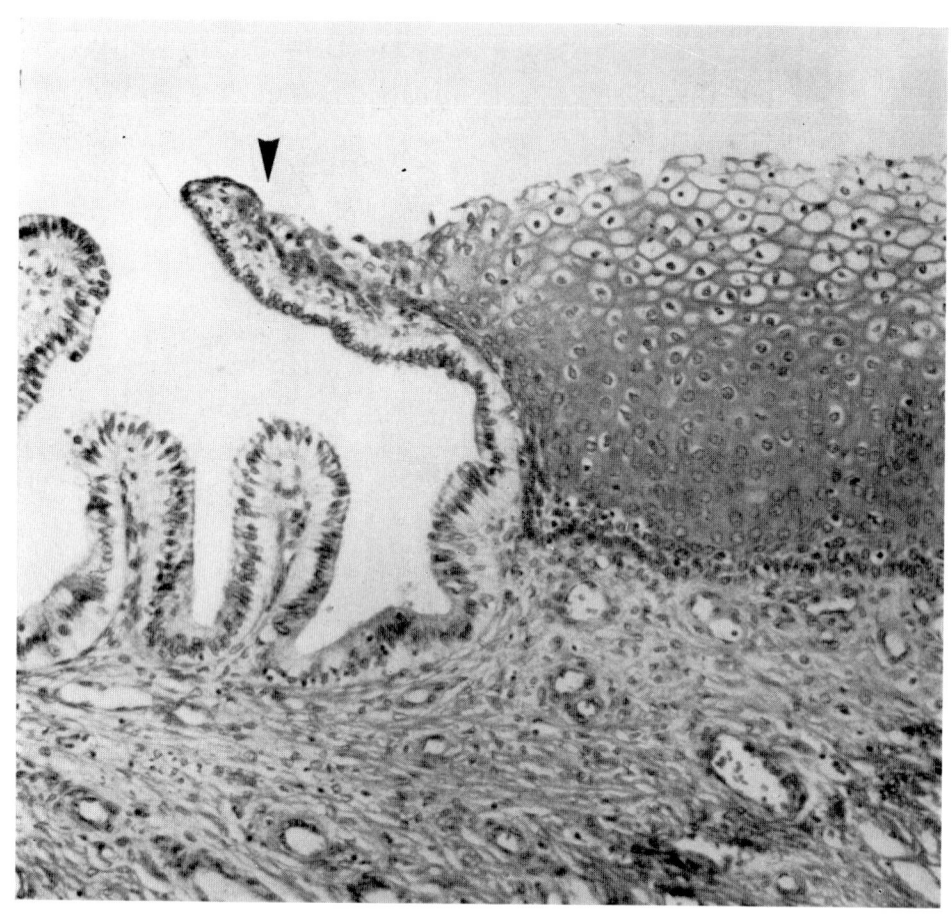

Figure 224. Original squamocolumnar junction. Photomicrograph of the original squamous epithelium on the right adjoining the columnar epithelium (arrow).

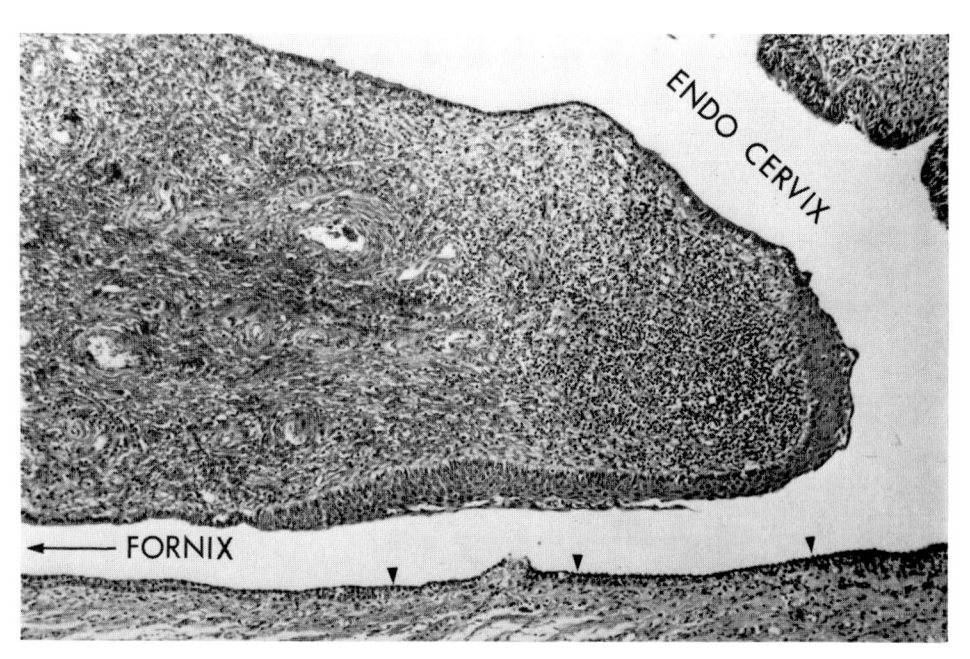

Figure 225. Müllerian epithelium on vagina of a two-year-old. Photomicrograph of posterior lip of cervix and adjoining vaginal wall seen in the bottom of the photograph. Metaplastic epithelium covers most of the ectocervix and columnar epithelium with a single row of subsurface cells and is present in the vaginal wall. These epithelia are adjudged to be müllerian in origin.

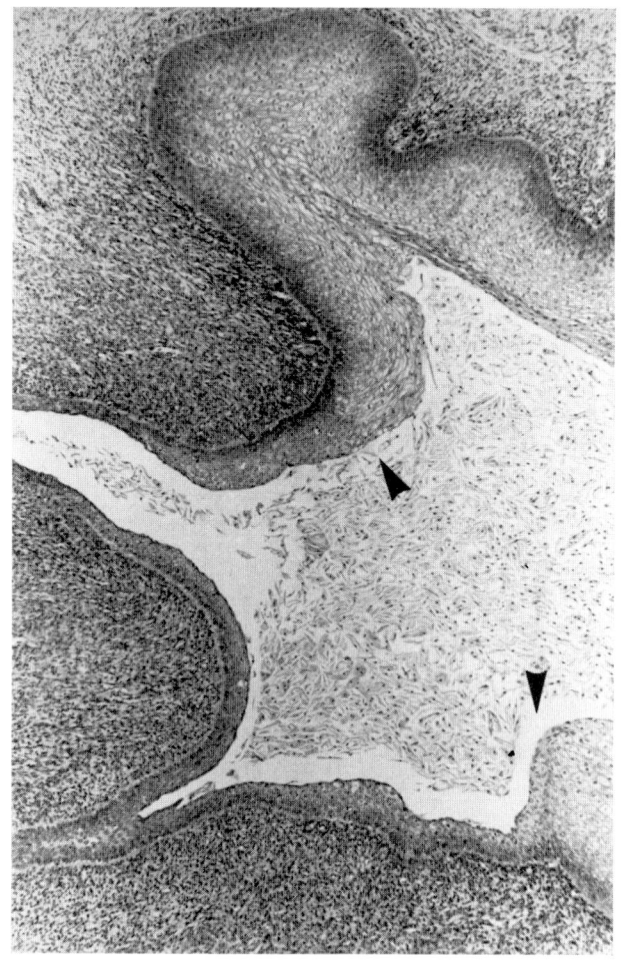

Figure 226. Müllerian epithelium on vagina of twenty-four-week-old fetus. Photomicrograph showing the original squamocolumnar junction on the ectocervix anteriorly (upper arrow) and on the vagina posteriorly (lower arrow). The stratified squamous metaplastic epithelium (to the left of the arrows) covers the upper vagina posteriorly, the ectocervix, and lower endocervix.

THE VAGINAL TRANSFORMATION ZONE

In 4 per cent of subjects examined, including foetuses, young girls, adolescents, and adults, the original squamocolumnar junction is found upon a portion of the upper vagina (Fig. 227). Such an arrangement indicates that epithelia of müllerian origin form a portion of the epithelial surface of the upper vagina. Columnar epithelium and transformation zone are, in these subjects, proper to the vagina.

The transformation zone may be typical, presenting the usual admixture of gland openings, retention cysts, residual areas of columnar epithelium, and the characteristic subepithelial vessels (Fig. 228).

In our experience, the most common müllerian derivative is atypical transformation zone of the original type (p. 374). Punctation and mosaic vascular arrangements are common. Keratosis may be evident, and glandular structures may be identified within the metaplastic area (Figs. 229-231). Schiller's iodine application has invariably shown the transformation zone to be non-glycogenated (Fig. 232). Histological studies confirm the nature of the epithelium as non-glycogenated metaplastic epithelium in which intraepithelial vascular structures are often present (Fig. 233). This variation has been a remarkably constant finding, which is not abnormal.

Atypical transformation zones of higher grades indicative of intraepithelial neoplasia show increasing irregularities of vascular patterns, as in

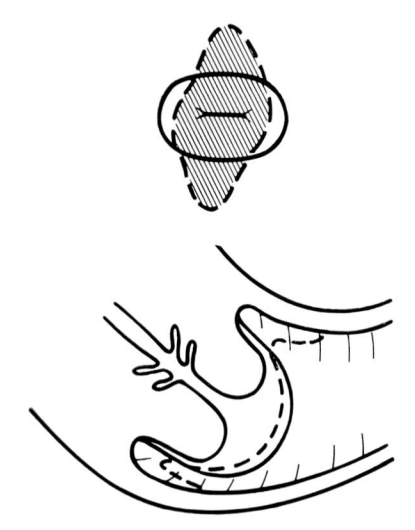

Figure 227. Schematic figure of original squamocolumnar junction. In 4 per cent of subjects, this junction is found on the vagina, müllerian-derived epithelia then forming portion of the vaginal covering.

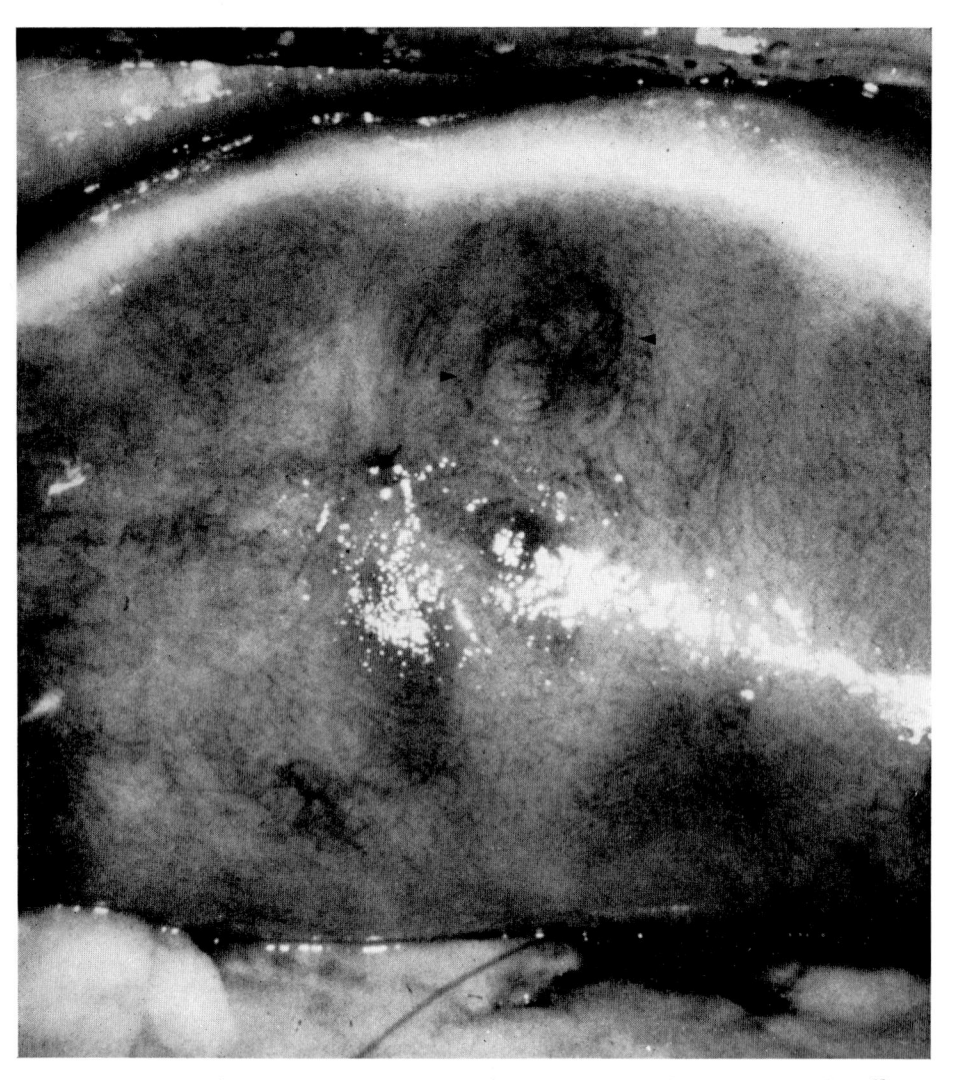

Figure 228. Vaginal transformation zone. Colpophotograph of upper vaginal wall in a forty-two-year-old subject displaying typical transformation with two small retention cysts (arrows).

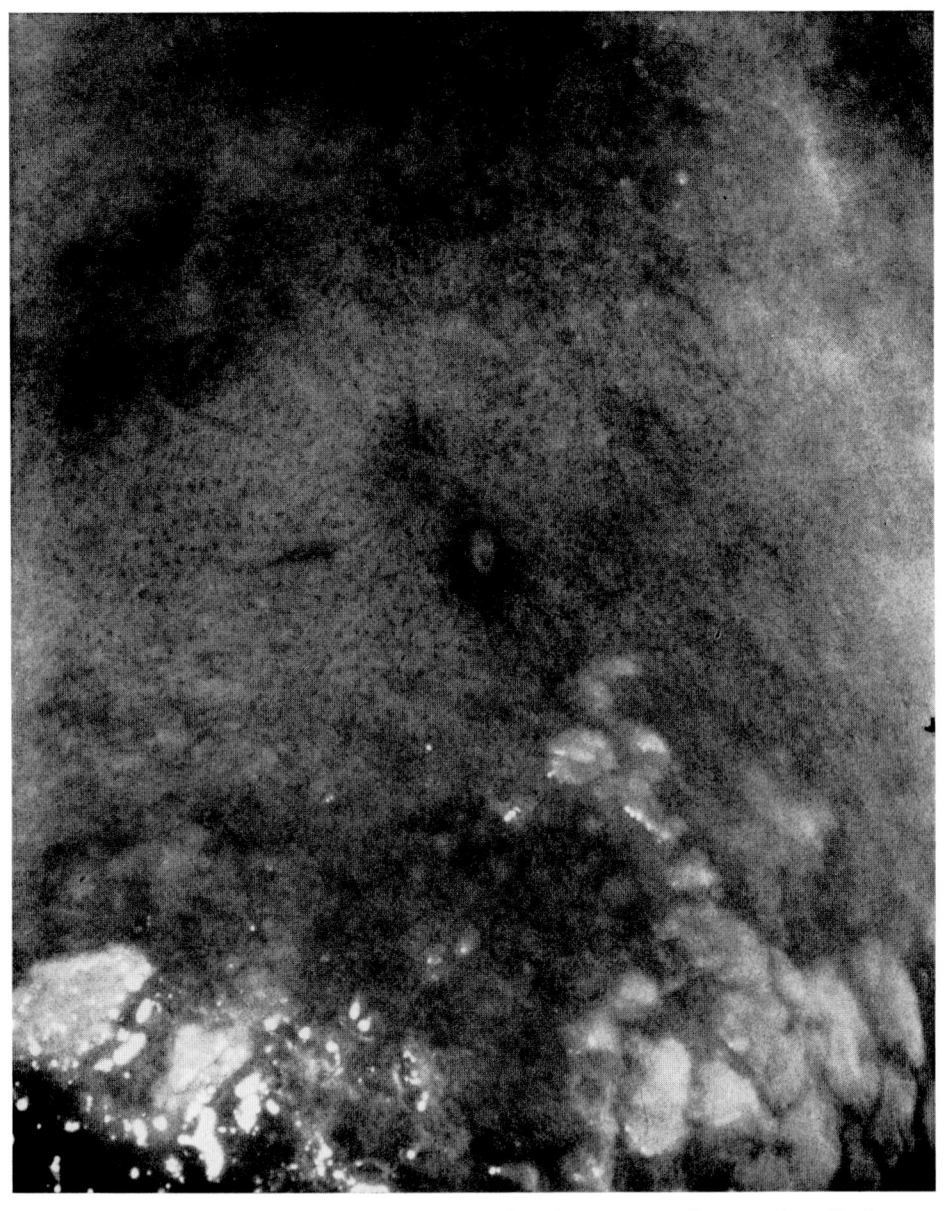

Figure 229. Vaginal transformation zone. Colpophotograph of vaginal wall showing atypical transformation zone. Punctation, keratosis in the lower third, and a glandular structure in the centre of the photograph are seen. This subject has no history of exposure to non-steroidal oestrogens.

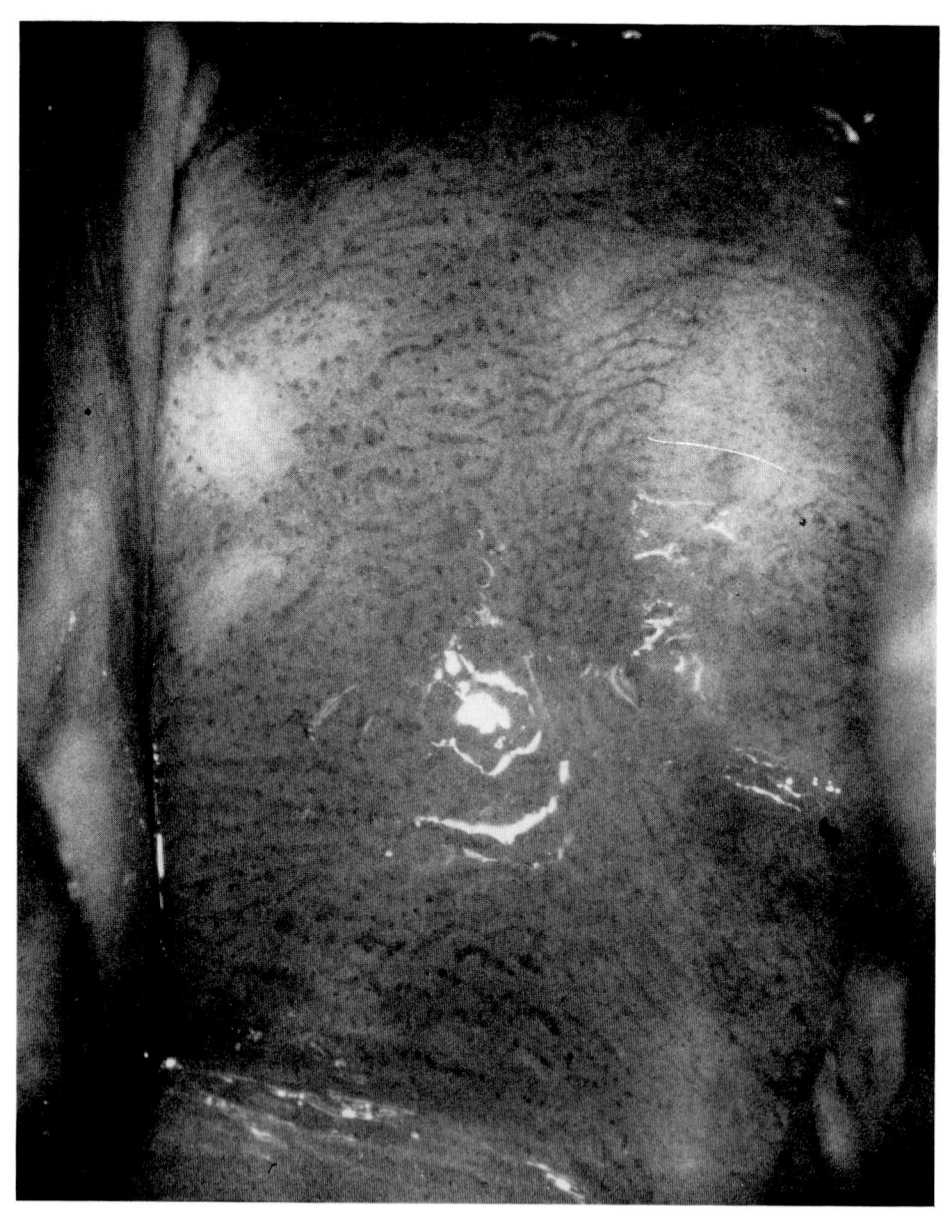

Figure 230. Vaginal transformation zone. Colpophotograph of vaginal wall showing linear punctation with a tendency to form transverse rugae.

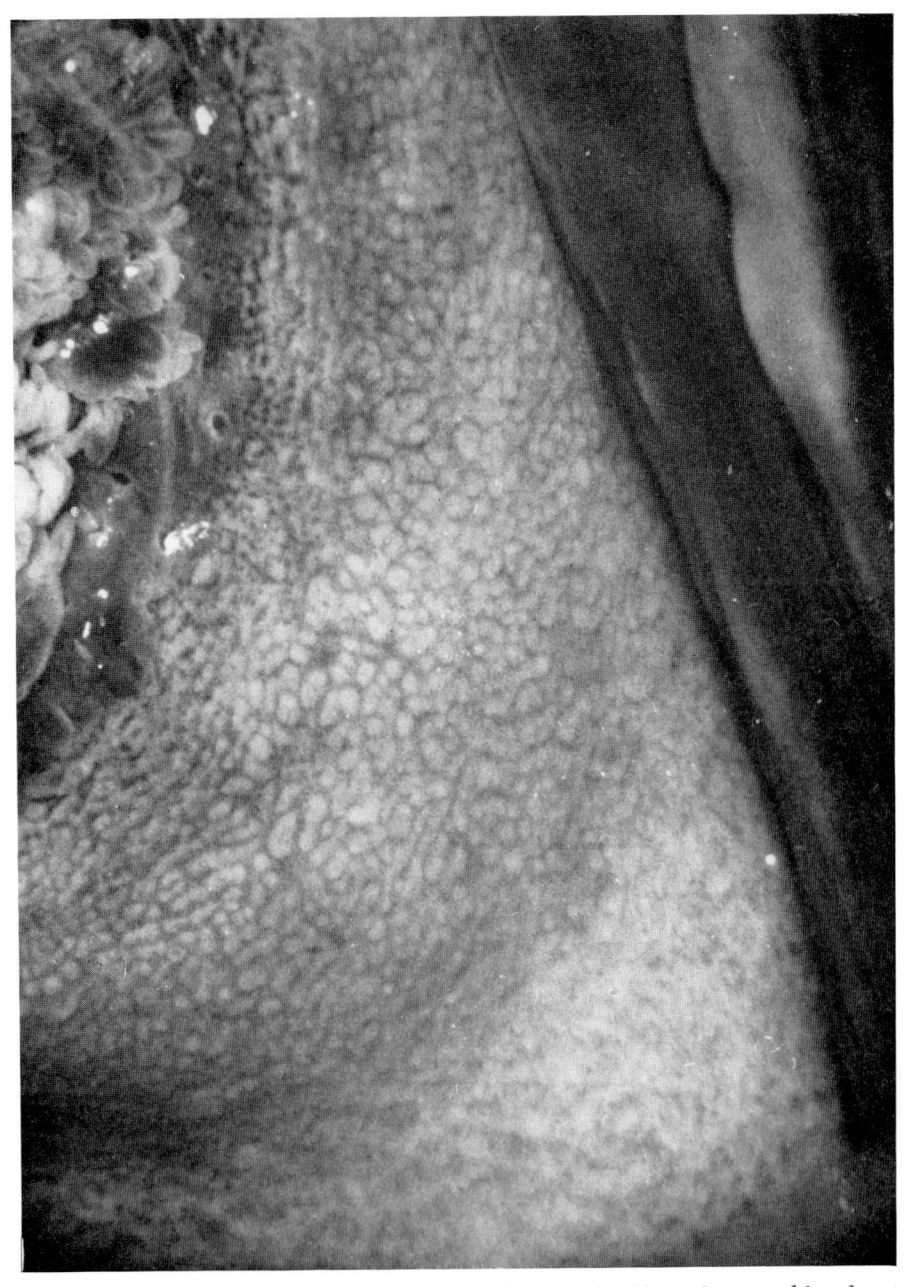

Figure 231. Vaginal transformation zone. Colpophotograph of lateral cervical lip showing fine regular mosaic extending across the fornix on to the posterior vaginal wall in the lower right quadrant of the photograph. It is evidently of the original type of transformation zone (p. 374).

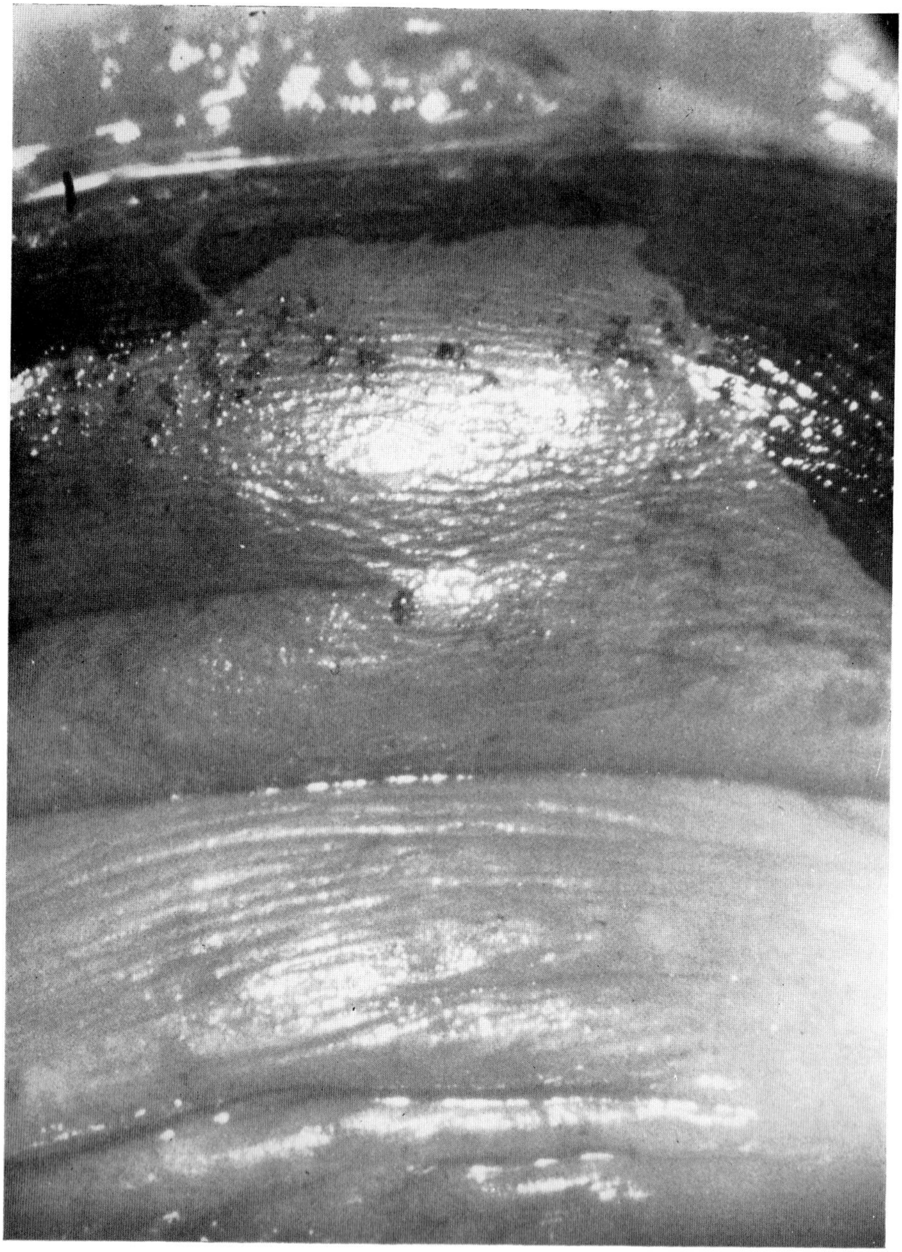

Figure 232. Vaginal transformation zone. Application of Schiller's iodine solution shows the extent of non-glycogenated epithelium both over the anterior lip of the cervix (lower one third of photograph) and onto the anterior vaginal wall (middle and upper thirds).

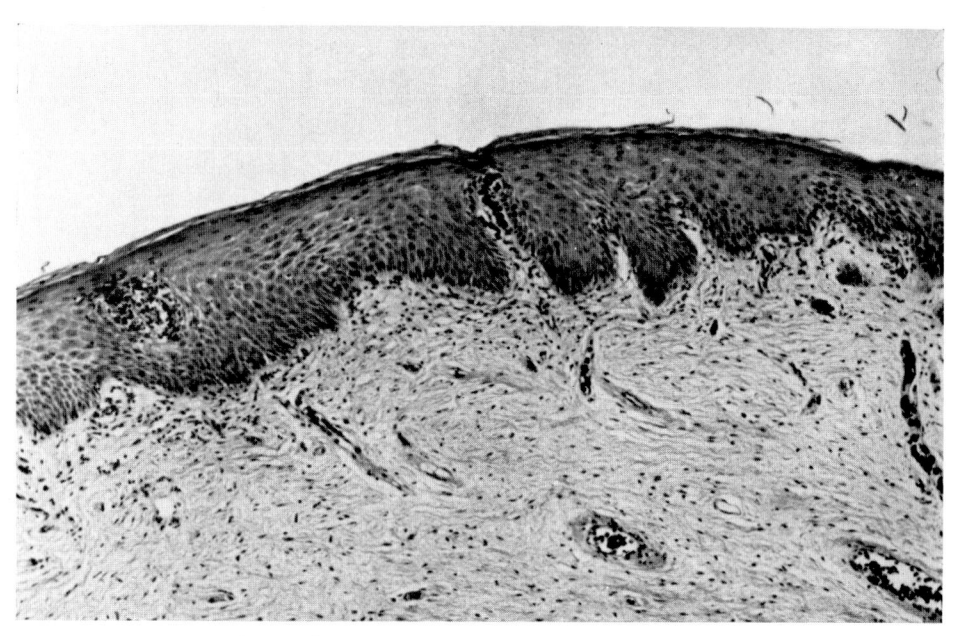

Figure 233. Vaginal transformation zone. Photomicrograph of biopsy of area of vaginal wall which failed to stain with Schiller's iodine. Non-glycogenated epithelium with intraepithelial vascular structures is present. The appearances are similar to those of original transformation zone (see Figs. 280-282).

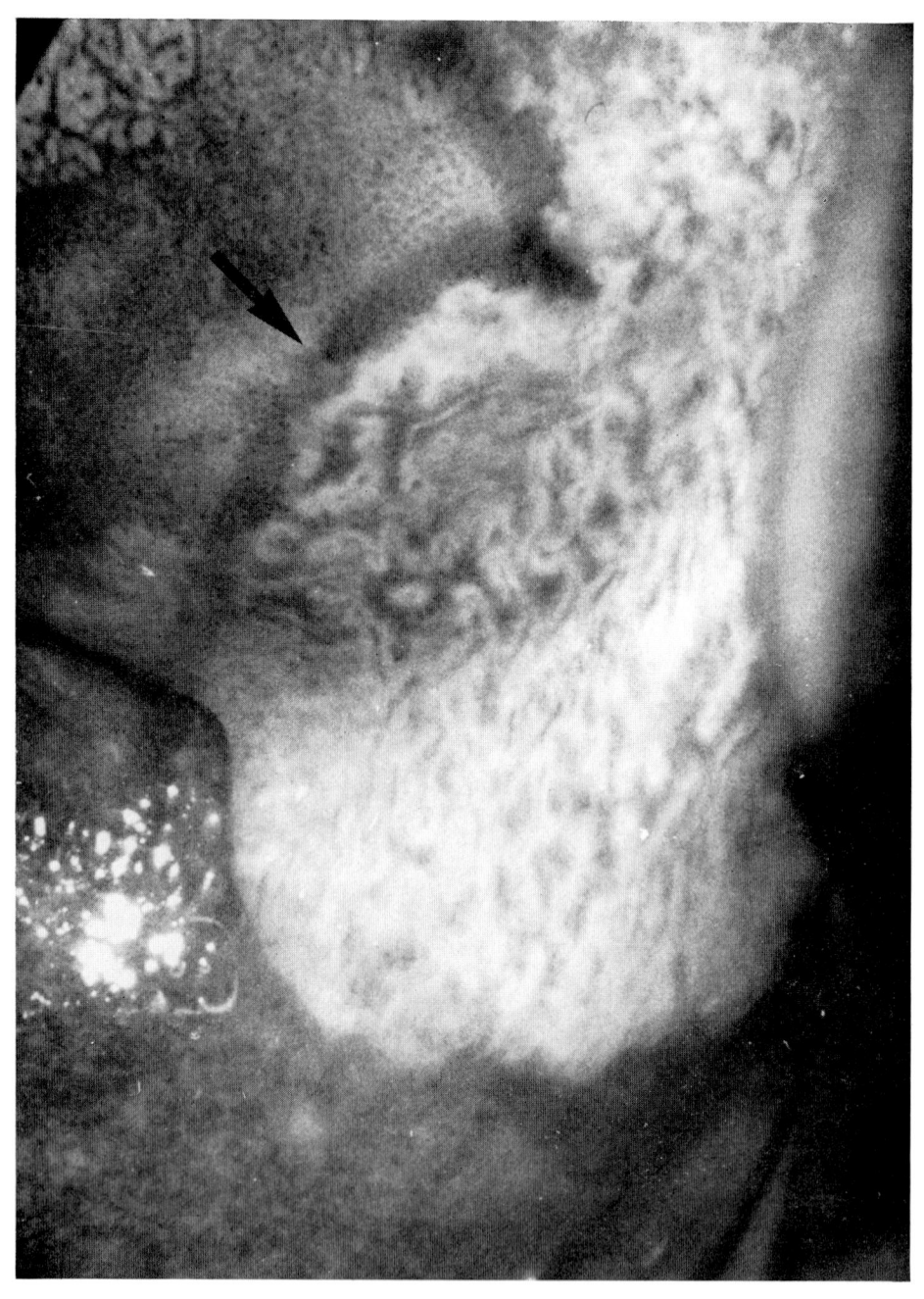

Figure 234. Vaginal transformation zone. Colpophotograph of the left cervical lip, vaginal fornix, and vaginal wall. The os is beyond the upper left corner. Carcinoma in situ was present in cervical and vaginal portions of this atypical transformation zone. On the vagina, the epithelium is whiter and the vascular structures more marked. An irregular shadow (arrow) crosses the top left corner of the photograph.

similar lesions of the cervix (Fig. 234). There is a slight tendency for significant atypical transformation zone of the vagina to display gradings based on colposcopic study which are more serious than histological appearances disclosed by biopsy. The surface configuration is more irregular, evidently due to the looser texture of the vaginal wall. These appearances can suggest invasive cancer to the inexperienced observer (*see* Fig. 301).

CLINICAL CANCER

Cancer of the vagina is most often seen as an extension from squamous cancer of the cervix. It may also represent an extension from squamous cancer of the vulva or be secondary to cancer elsewhere. Rarely, the cancer appears as a primary lesion, either squamous or adenocarcinomatous. The colposcopic appearances are similar to those seen in overt carcinoma of the cervix (Fig. 235). Clear cell adenocarcinoma arising within "vaginal adenosis" is reported in women who have no history of intrauterine exposure to non-steroidal oestrogens. The vascular response common to neoplasia will be seen at least in some cases by the experienced colposcopist.

DEVELOPMENTAL DISORDERS

Caudal displacement of the original squamocolumnar junction may result from malformations in two well-defined circumstances: vaginal atresia and exposure to transplancental non-steroidal oestrogens.

Vaginal Atresia

The epithelial distribution should be examined in all subjects in whom partial or complete occlusion is present. Most commonly, anomalies are identified; epithelia of müllerian origin are found cephalad to the level of the obstruction (Fig. 236). This is most strikingly seen when the condition of haematocolpos is relieved by incision of the obstructing membrane. Examination of this membrane shows its vaginal surface covered with columnar and metaplastic epithelia; its vulval surface is original squamous (Figs. 237 and 238). These findings support an hypothesis which recognises the original squamocolumnar junction as the site of union of the müllerian-derived epithelium with that of the urogenital sinus.

Exposure to Transplacental Non-Steroidal Oestrogens

A similar caudal displacement of the original squamocolumnar junction with some associated anatomical anomalies is found in a majority of girls whose mothers received diethylstilboestrol (DES) or other non-steroidal oestrogens in the early months of gestation (Figs. 236, 239 to 241). In such cases, the müllerian epithelia constitute an extremely variable portion of

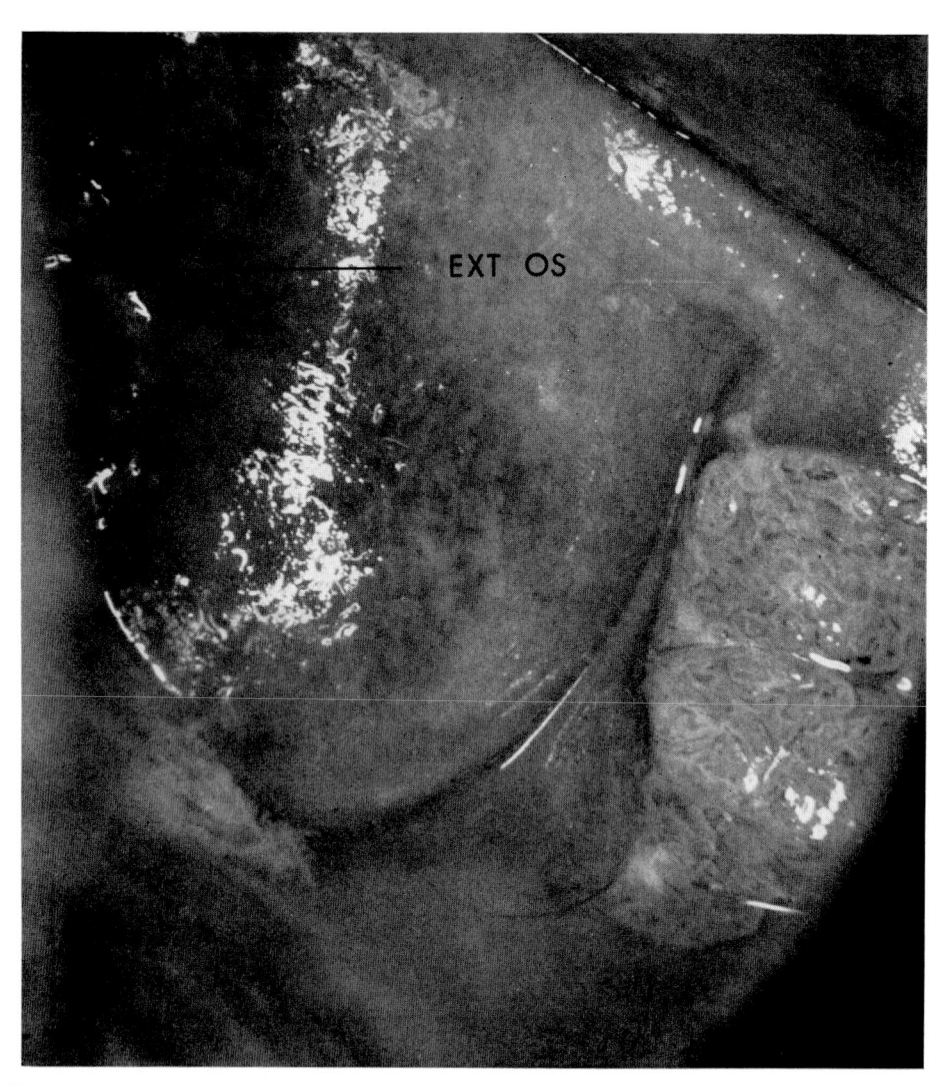

Figure 235. Squamous carcinoma of vagina. Colpophotograph of posterior lip of cervix and part of the posterior vaginal wall. The latter shows a circumscribed patch of white epithelium with bizarre surface blood vascular pattern. Subsequent histological study confirmed overt cancer. Note that the lesion shows no relationship to the small transformation zone near the cervical os.

the upper vagina as well as the cervix. Most cases of vaginal adenosis occur in this group, which is discussed in Chapters 13 and 14.

MISCELLANEOUS GLANDULAR ANOMALIES

A careful scrutiny of the vaginal surface may occasionally reveal glandular structures which do not conform in appearance to the better recognised disorders.

Vaginal Cysts

Cystic structures, single or numerous, small and large, present as obvious lesions over which the vascular structures are easily seen. They are probably of wolffian duct origin.

Endometriosis

Endometriosis can affect the vagina. When a lesion is close to the surface, it may present as a blue or red area (Fig. 242).

Minute Glandular Structures

These glands, rarely observed, open directly onto the original squamous epithelium. Their significance is unknown.

NEOPLASTIC POTENTIAL OF VAGINAL EPITHELIA

It is possible that each of the several varieties of epithelia which cover the lower genital tract generate a specific type of malignant disorder.

Most cases of *in situ* and primary invasive cancer of the vagina arise *within the transformation zone*. The occurrence of metaplasia on the vaginal wall carries the same biological significance as that on the nearby

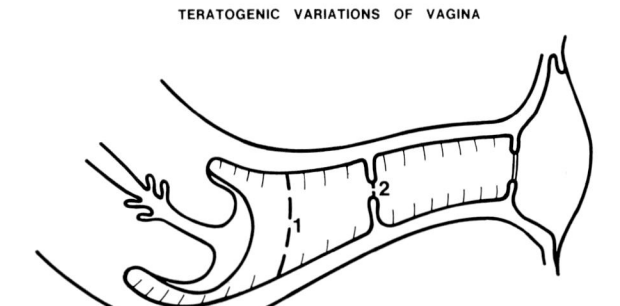

Figure 236. Vaginal abnormalities. (1) Many subjects exposed *in utero* to non-steroidal oestrogens show caudal displacement of the original squamocolumnar junction. (2) In subjects with atresia of the vagina, embryological evidence suggests that müllerian-derived epithelia lie cephalad and original squamous epithelium caudad to the obstruction.

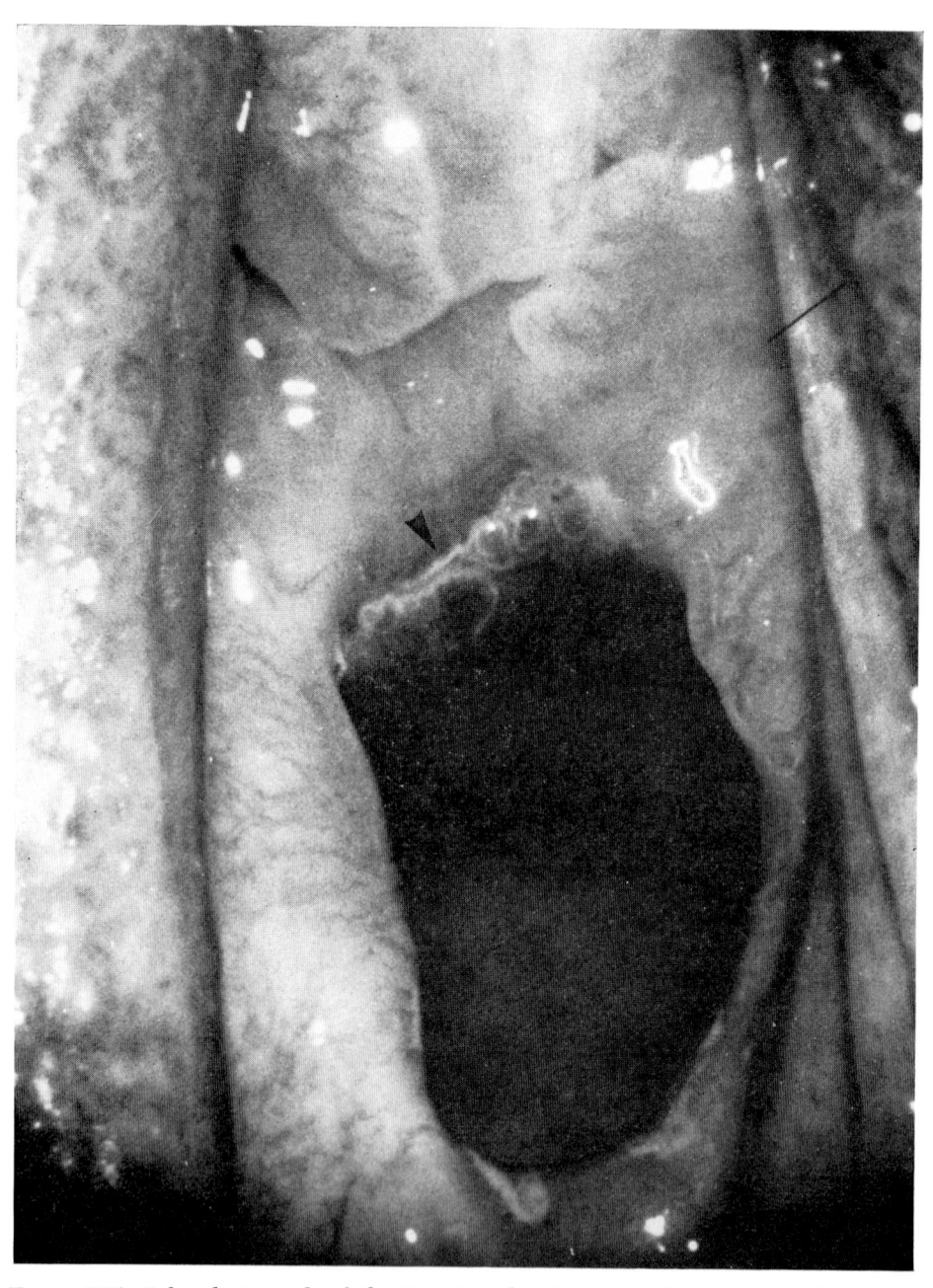

Figure 237. Colpophotograph of the introitus showing vaginal atresia. An obstructing membrane causing haematocolpos in a fourteen-year-old has been recently incised. The healed remnant shows columnar epithelium (arrow) at the level of the membrane. Columnar epithelium lines most of the vagina above.

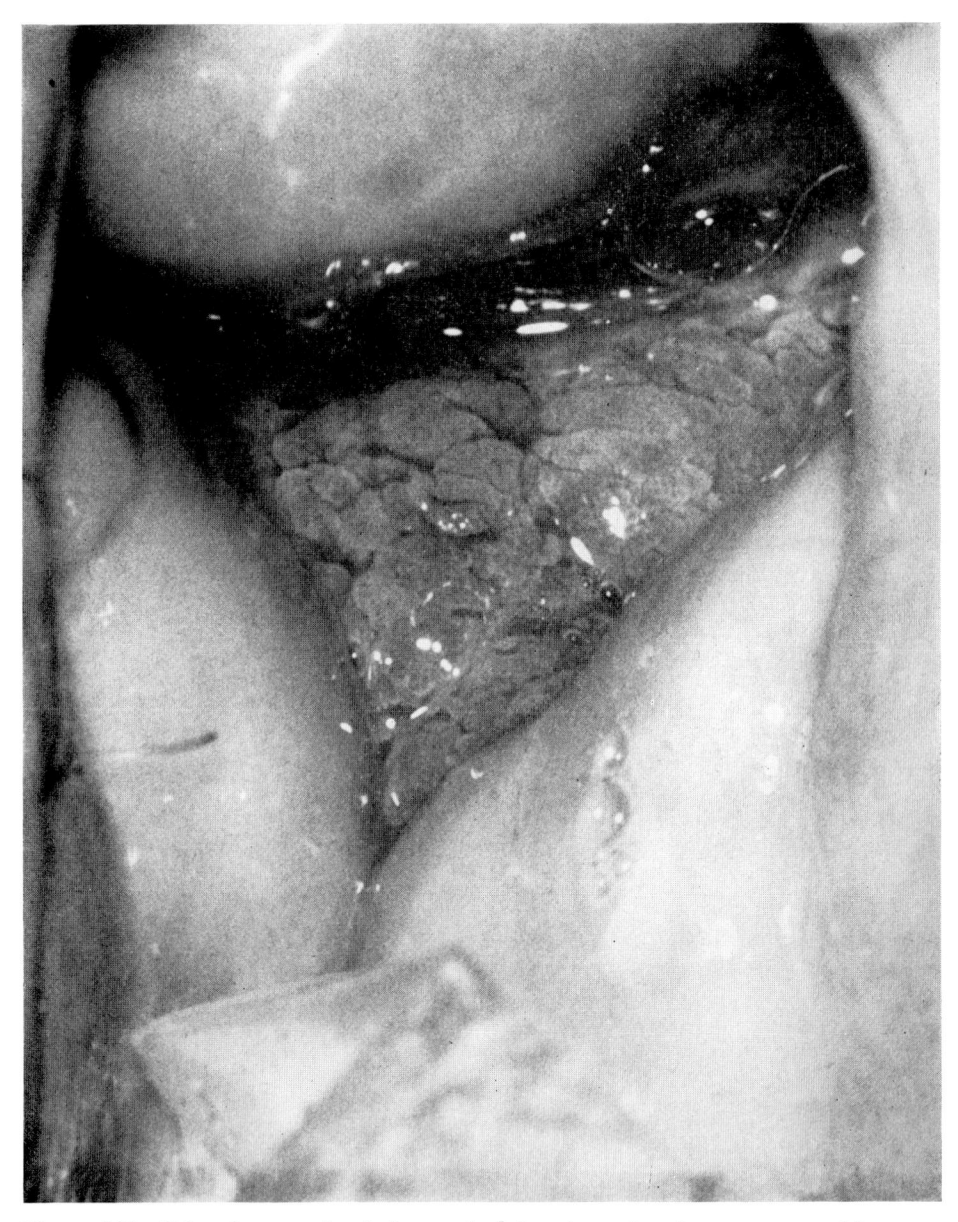

Figure 238. Colpophotograph of the vaginal introitus of a forty-two-year-old woman with a history of an operation for haematocolpos at the age of sixteen. Columnar epithelium is seen at the vaginal introitus, which has been gently retracted.

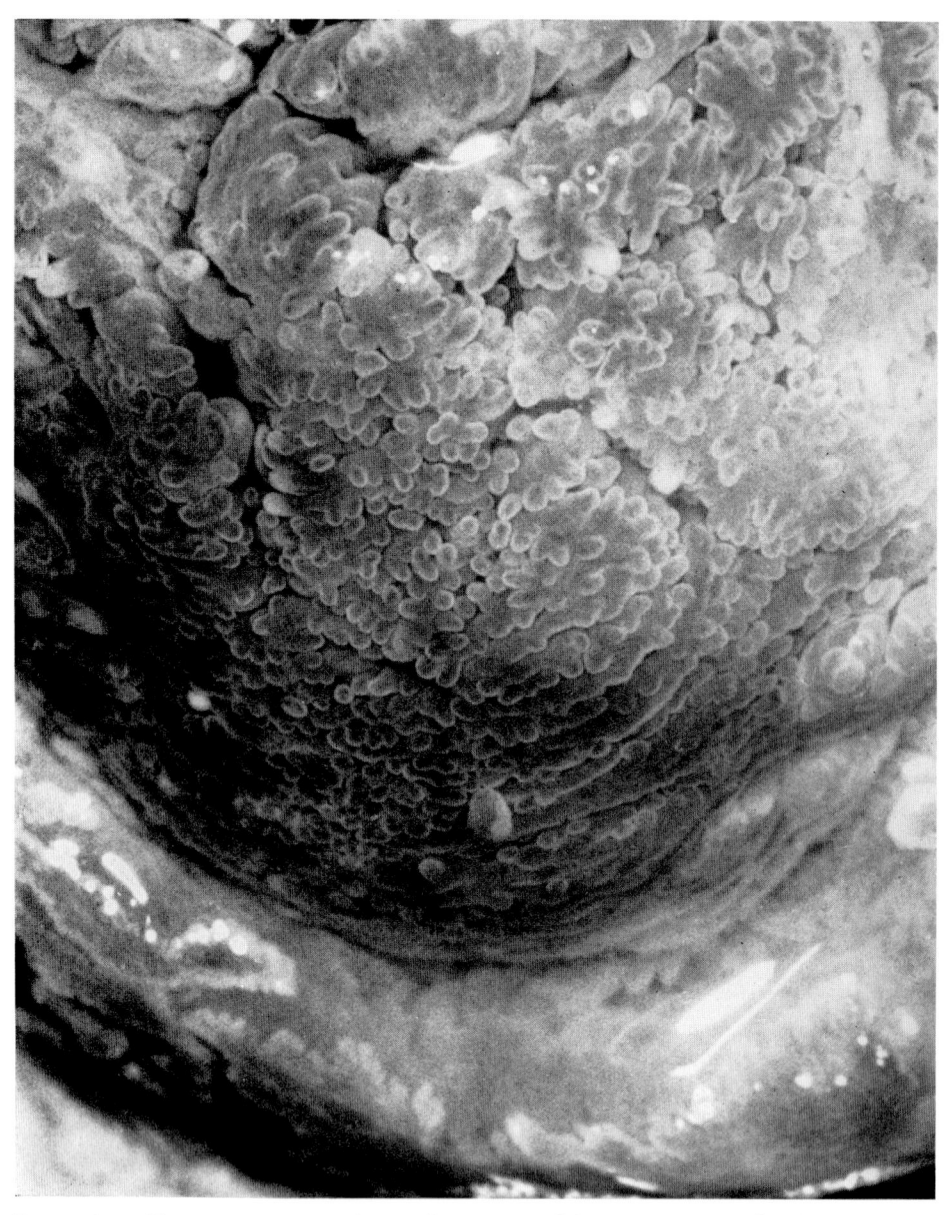

Figure 239. Exposure to transplacental non-steroidal oestrogens. Colpophotograph of posterior lip of cervix covered by columnar epithelium in this twenty-four-year-old woman with known history of maternal ingestion of diethylstilbestrol.

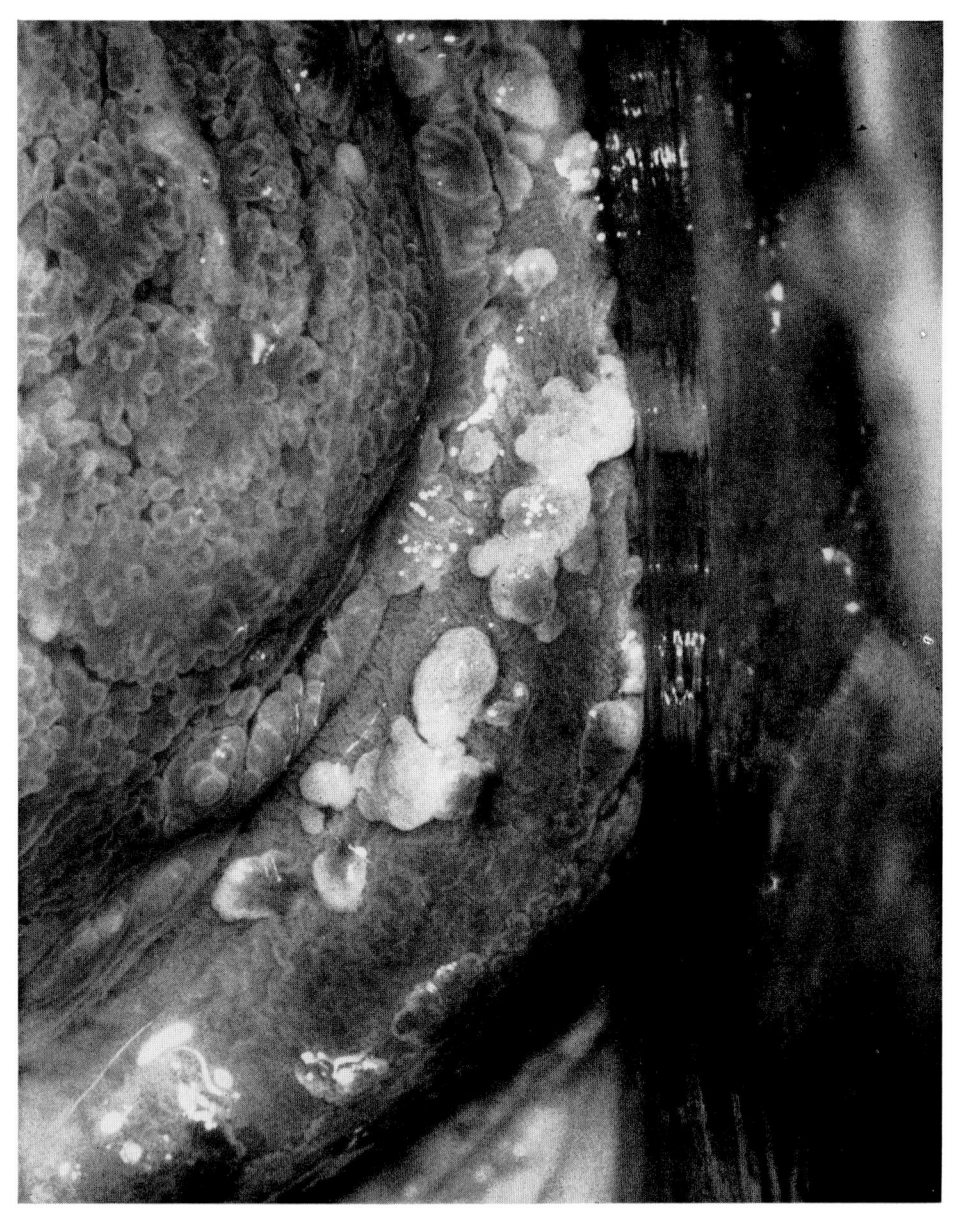

Figure 240. Same subject as Figures 239 and 241. The lateral half of the cervix occupies the upper left quadrant of the photograph. At right, a collar of the cervix shows white epithelium indicative of early metaplasia occurring in polypoidal columnar epithelium.

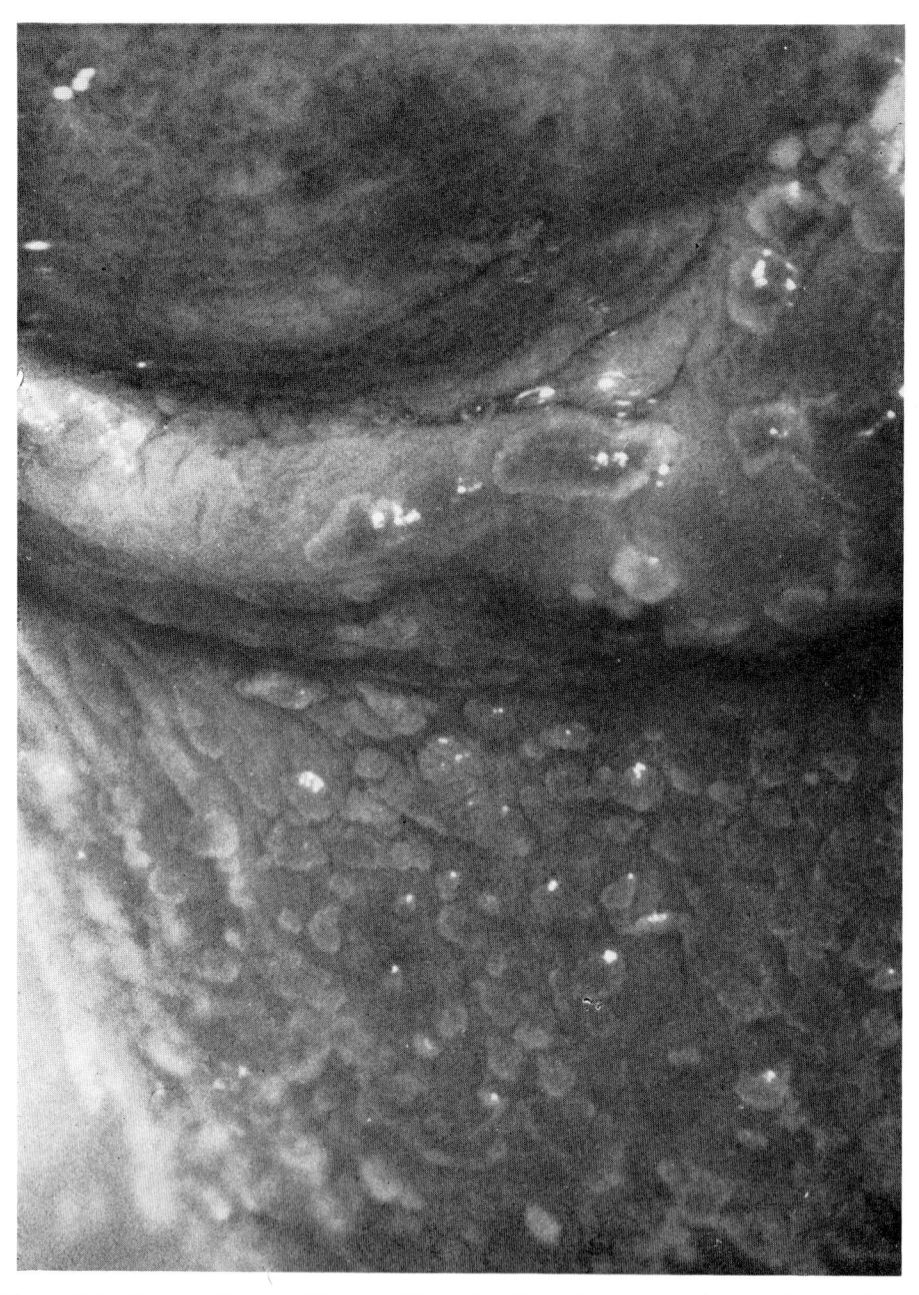

Figure 241. Same subject as Figures 239 and 240. Columnar epithelium disposed over characteristic villi is present below the collar, on the posterior vaginal wall in the lower half of the photograph.

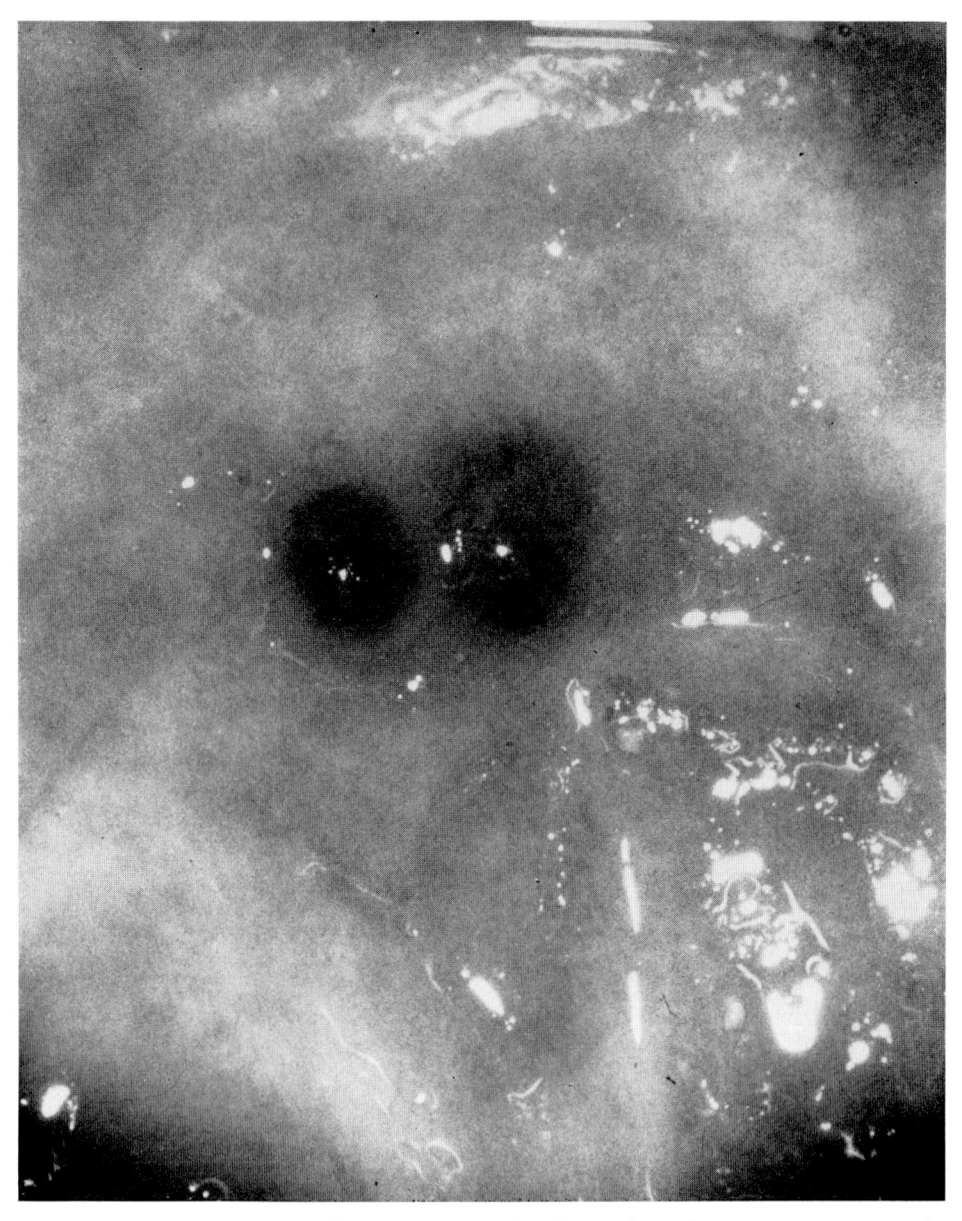

Figure 242. Endometriosis of vagina. Two chocolate-coloured cysts are seen in the wall of the vagina. A diagnosis of endometriosis was inferred from the history of minor cyclical bleeding following hysterectomy for pelvic endometriosis.

cervix. The process can become atypical, and this displays a similar natural history to that of squamous cancer of the cervix, exhibiting a spectrum of histological appearances from dysplasia to invasive cancer. Colposcopically, the atypical transformation zone may be observed to cover much of the cervix and extend onto the upper vagina. Occasionally, vaginal transformation is so extensive, parts of the vagina towards the introitus are involved. Lesions may arise from multiple foci within the transformation zone. Intraepithelial neoplasia of the vaginal portion of the transformation zone may occur independently but is more often concurrent and coextensive with cervical intraepithelial neoplasia. Failure to excise the vaginal extension results in persisting abnormality in the vaginal vault after excision, including the later emergence of invasive cancer. The interpretation in the past of lesions as "recurrent" rather than "residual" and the general question of the management of vaginal sites of preneoplasia is discussed in Chapter 16.

Neoplastic change has been reported to occur in *original squamous epithelium*. Such an occurrence is rare, and the natural history is presently obscure. When carcinoma of the vagina develops, it may be impossible to exclude a possible origin from within a transformation zone contiguous with that of the cervix. Rare reports of multicentric carcinoma of the vulva and vagina and the occurrence of lesions limited to the mid- or lower vagina support the thesis of an origin in original squamous epithelium.

Equally obscure is the occurrence of clear cell adenocarcinoma not associated with transplacental non-steroidal oestrogens.

The large amount of metaplasia involved in the vaginal wall of an individual exposed *in utero* to stilboestrol and associated oestrogens should theoretically predispose the epithelium to squamous malignant change in a manner commensurate with the cervix undergoing metaplasia. A fuller discussion of the potential of such a condition to develop squamous cancer is given in Chapters 13 to 15.

Chapter 13

VAGINAL ADENOSIS

With Special Reference to Effects of Synthetic Non-Steroidal Oestrogens

Adolf Stafl, M.D., Ph.D.

COLPOSCOPIC-HISTOLOGICAL-VASCULAR CORRELATIONS

Vaginal adenosis, by definition, is the presence of the endocervical type of columnar epithelium in the vagina. Colposcopic appearance of the columnar epithelium in vaginal adenosis is identical to the appearance of columnar epithelium on the cervix. After acetic acid application, typical grapelike structures are visible (Fig. 243). In the vagina, the columnar epithelium is much more exposed to the vaginal environment than on the cervix, and therefore, most of this columnar epithelium is replaced by metaplastic squamous epithelium. Columnar epithelium in its original form can persist only in the deeper vaginal folds where it is protected from vaginal acidity.

The histological picture of the columnar epithelium in vaginal adenosis is identical to the histological picture of columnar epithelium in the endocervix (Fig. 244). When the pathologist is not informed from where the biopsy was taken, it is impossible to distinguish between the columnar epithelium on the cervix or in the vagina. The columnar epithelium in vaginal adenosis, in some cases, shows some endometrial form of epithelium; however, we feel that these changes merely represent morphological variation of the endocervical columnar epithelium.

Studies of the terminal vascular network in columnar epithelium in vaginal adenosis demonstrate that the vascular network is identical to the vascular network in columnar epithelium on the cervix (Fig. 245). In each of the grapelike structures, there is a rich vascular network separated from the surface by a single layer of columnar cells. This explains why the areas of vaginal adenosis look intensely red.

The morphogenesis of squamous metaplasia in vaginal adenosis resembles corresponding changes on the cervix. Squamous metaplasia starts in the areas most exposed to the vaginal environment, mainly on the tops of vaginal ridges. Individual grapelike structures of the columnar epithelium are connected, and a flat surface covered with columnar epithelium develops. The coalescence of the villi is never complete, and some colum-

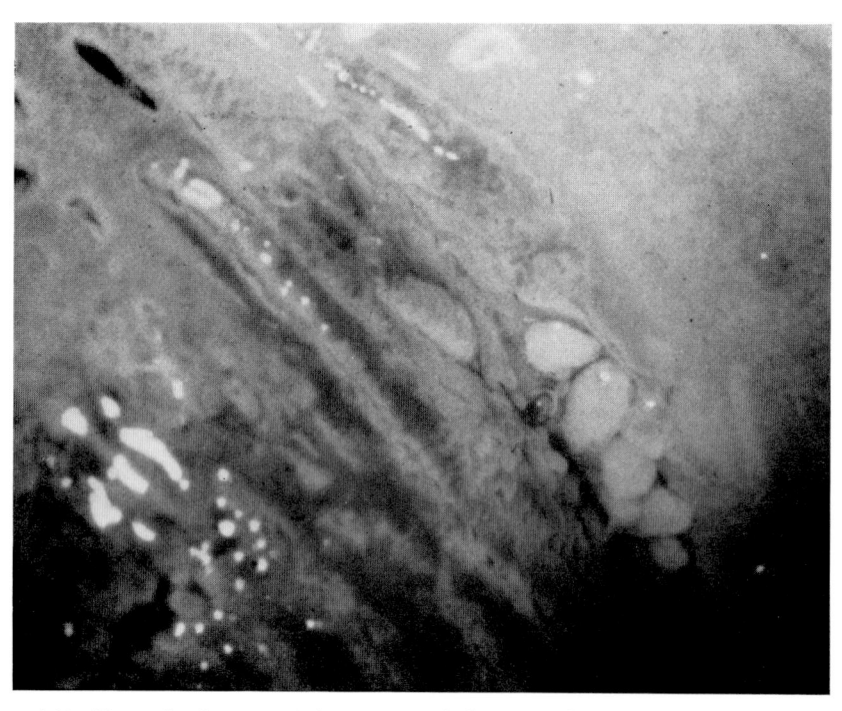

Figure 243. Vaginal adenosis. Columnar epithelium in the vagina can be recognized colposcopically because of typical grapelike structures.

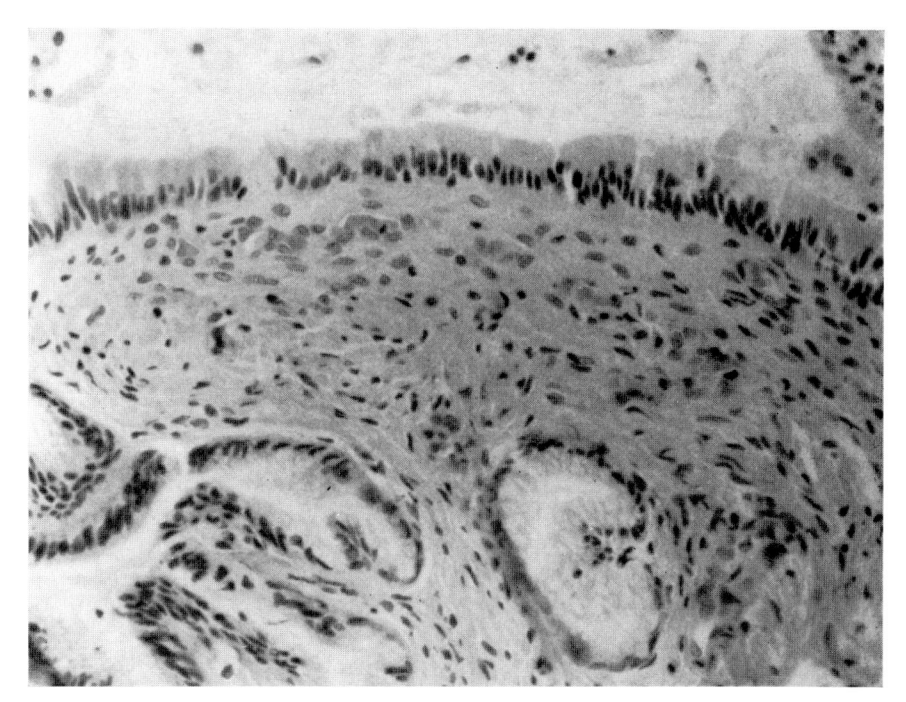

Figure 244. Histological picture of vaginal adenosis. Columnar epithelium is present on the surface of the vagina and also in the deeper clefts in the vaginal stroma.

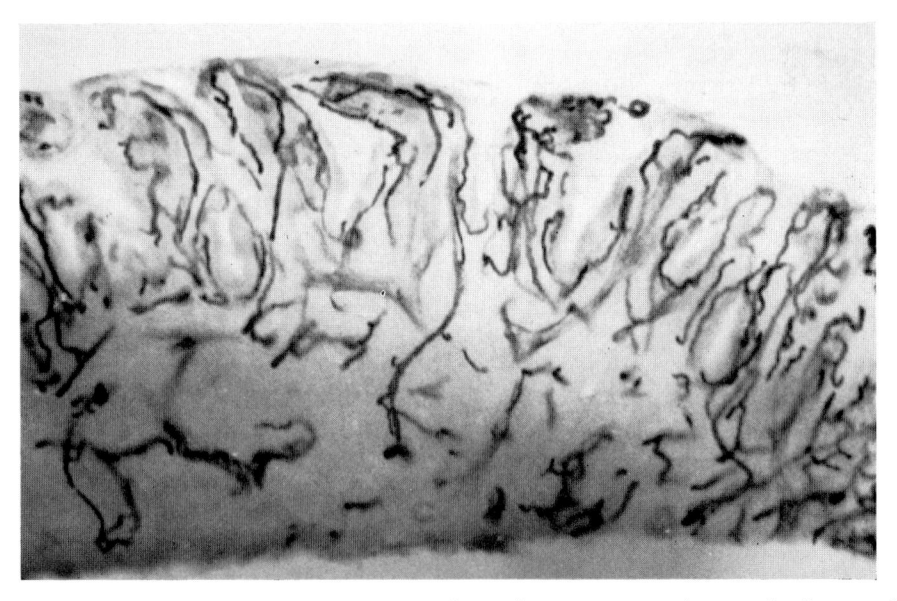

Figure 245. Histochemical demonstration of vessels in an area of vaginal adenosis. In each of the grapelike structures is a rich vascular network separated from the observer by a single layer of columnar cells.

nar epithelium therefore always remains in the stroma. Columnar epithelium on the surface is later replaced by metaplastic squamous epithelium (Figs. 246 and 247). The columnar epithelium in the stroma retains its function, which is secretion. There are two possibilities; either there is some connection with the surface, and these connections are visible in the colposcope as so-called gland openings, or the connection with the surface is lost and then small nabothian cysts develop. By the process of squamous metaplasia, the entire area of columnar epithelium in the vagina is changed to the transformation zone, which, in some cases, might involve almost the entire vagina. The components of this transformation zone are areas of squamous metaplasia, islands of columnar epithelium, gland openings, and small nabothian cysts.

After application of acetic acid, in most cases, white epithelium develops, which usually represents histologically immature squamous metaplasia (Figs. 248 and 249). An interesting observation in girls exposed to diethylstilboestrol (DES) in utero, concerns this immature metaplasia, which is often arrested for long periods of time so that the colposcopically visible white epithelium usually remains unchanged for several years. This position is different in women unexposed to DES. In these women, white epithelium representing immature squamous metaplasia usually can be seen only in the very young and changes quickly to normal metaplastic epithelium. The reason for this *arrested immature metaplasia* in DES-exposed girls is not known, nor is it known if this finding might have any relation to the future frequency of squamous neoplasia.

In DES-exposed women, squamous metaplasia often starts as isolated islands within columnar epithelium, and this supports the concept that squamous metaplasia develops *in situ* and not by overgrowth of squamous epithelium from the periphery.

Abnormal colposcopic findings (white epithelium, punctation, mosaic) in DES-exposed women with vaginal adenosis are very common (in our material in 96% of patients). The changes in colour after application of acetic acid are striking. The whiteness and sharpness of the borders of white lesions might suggest much more significant histopathological changes than those actually present. The acetic acid test in DES-exposed girls might be misleading; therefore, it is very important to use the saline technique as well and carefully study the vessels with a green filter (p. 179). It is possible to observe that in most cases of these striking white lesions, the intercapillary distance is minimal, and the morphology of the vessels is not significantly changed (Fig. 248). When the intercapillary distance is significantly increased or if there are changes in the vascular morphology, then the same type of histopathological changes as those expected in girls unexposed to DES can be predicted. A large atypical transformation zone

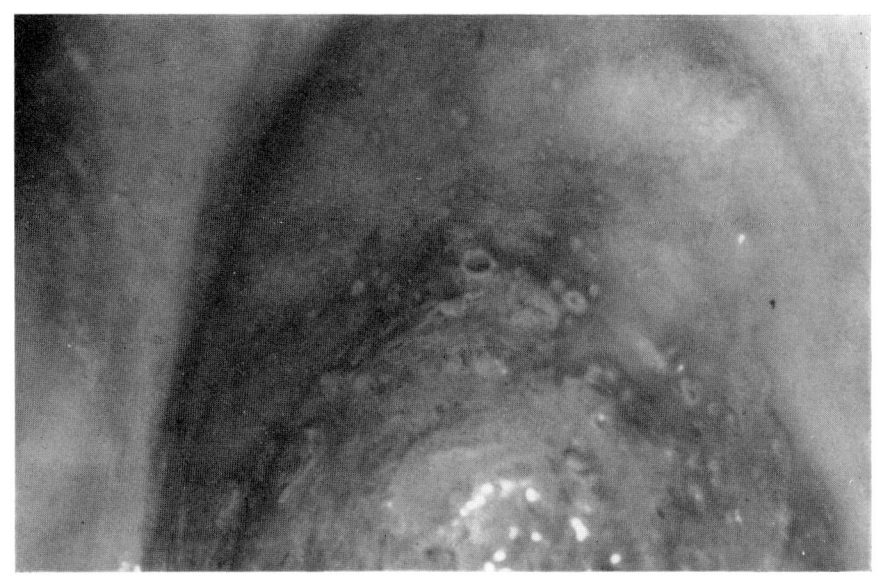

Figure 246. Colpophotograph of the upper third of the vagina. Several "gland openings" present in the vagina signify that this area, originally covered with columnar epithelium, has been almost completely replaced by well-differentiated metaplastic epithelium.

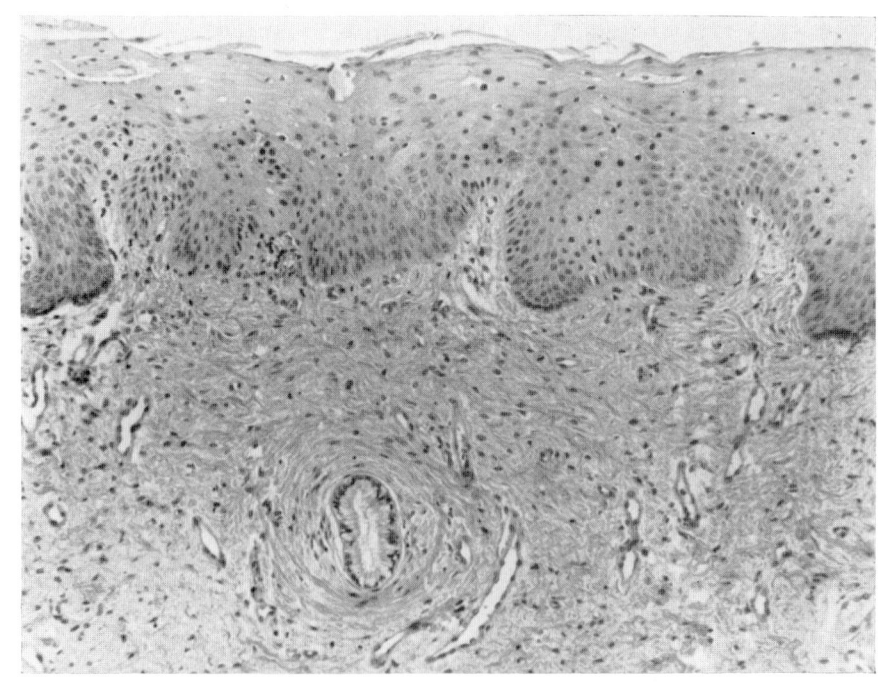

Figure 247. Corresponding histological picture to Figure 246. Well-differentiated metaplastic epithelium is present on the surface of the vagina. In the stroma an island of columnar epithelium is visible.

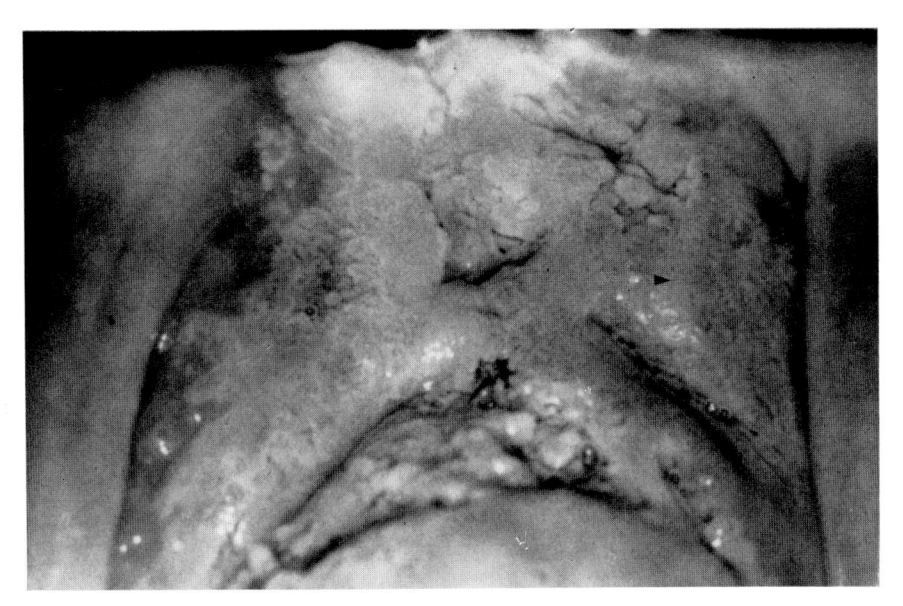

Figure 248. Colpophotograph of the anterior vaginal fornix. Most of the columnar epithelium of vaginal adenosis has been replaced by metaplastic squamous epithelium. After acetic acid test, the epithelium is strikingly white and in some areas shows punctation (arrow). However, the intercapillary distance is minimal. Histology showed immature squamous metaplasia.

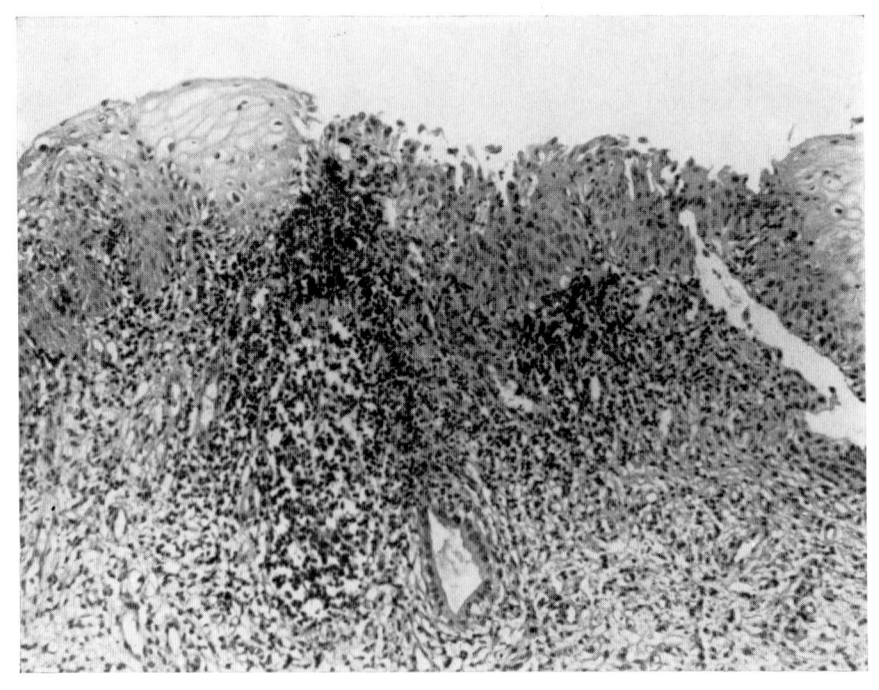

Figure 249. Histological specimen corresponding to Figure 248. Immature squamous metaplasia is seen on the surface with significant inflammatory reaction and an island of columnar epithelium deeper in the stroma.

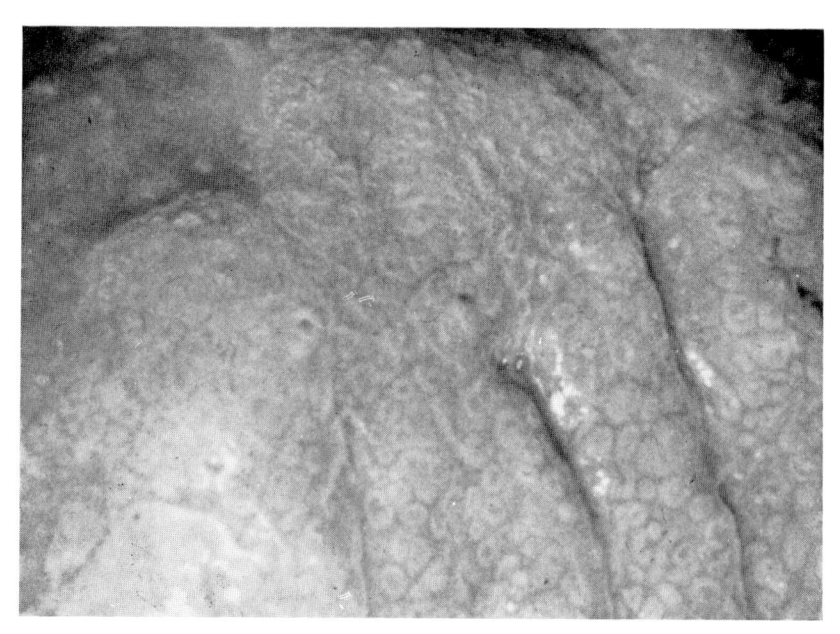

Figure 250. Colpophotograph showing gross mosaic pattern in the anterior vaginal fornix. The intercapillary distance is significantly increased. Vaginal biopsy demonstrated carcinoma in situ.

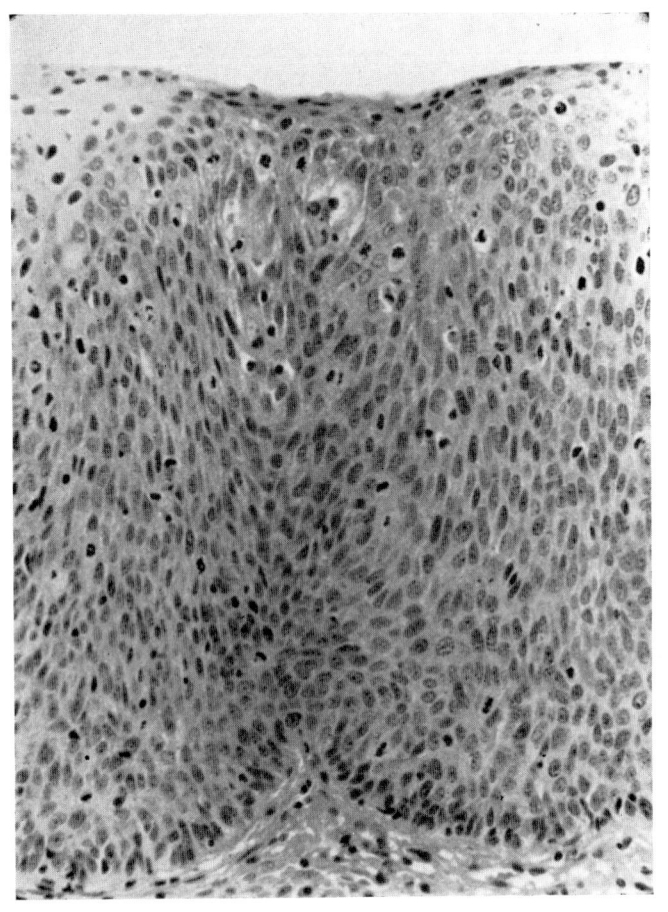

Figure 251. Corresponding histological picture to Figure 250. The appearances show vaginal carcinoma in situ with complete loss of differentiation. Some mitotic figures are present near the surface of the epithelium.

with mosaic with significantly increased intercapillary distance which extends from the cervix into the anterior vaginal fornix is illustrated in Figure 250. Because of the increased intercapillary distance, the colposcopic prediction was carcinoma in situ, which was confirmed by vaginal biopsy (Fig. 251).

In summary, colposcopic, histological and vascular changes in vaginal adenosis are almost identical to changes in the areas covered with columnar epithelium on the ectocervix in girls unexposed to DES. The only change is in the intensity of the change in colour after acetic acid test, which might lead an inexperienced colposcopist to overcalling a prediction of histopathological changes. However, by careful evaluation of other diagnostic factors involved (such as vascular pattern and intercapillary distance), the histological prediction in colposcopic changes in vaginal adenosis is identical to the prediction of changes on the ectocervix.

PROGNOSIS
Risk of Clear Cell Adenocarcinoma

With the recognition of the teratogenic effect of diethylstilboestrol on the maldevelopment of the lower genital tract, the major clinical concern has been related to the association of vaginal adenosis and clear cell adenocarcinoma in DES-exposed young women. Statistical data now available show that the frequency of clear cell adenocarcinoma is very low. The exact denominator (the number of female offspring exposed to stilboestrol) is not known, but the estimates are that between 500,000 to 2,000,000 women were exposed to stilboestrol *in utero*. To date, about 200 cases of clear cell adenocarcinoma have been reported in girls who were exposed to DES *in utero*.

Risk of Squamous Carcinoma

In 1974, Stafl and Mattingly expressed the initial concern that the major clinical risk in DES-exposed women is the development of squamous neoplasia of the vagina and cervix rather than clear cell adenocarcinoma. This concern was based on the fact that the transformation zone in DES-exposed women is more extensive than in women unexposed to DES and sometimes involves the entire vagina. Considering the potential risks in women with extensive transformation zone, the probability of neoplastic transformation by carcinogens present in the vagina is higher when the transformation zone is extensive. In this study, among the 280 patients exposed to stilboestrol *in utero,* four cases of vaginal and cervical carcinoma in situ were found, a prevalence rate of 1.4 per cent. Similar experiences were reported from the Mayo Clinic, where among 259 DES-exposed young women, the prevalence rate of carcinoma in situ was 1.4 per cent.

In this small series, the prevalence rate is almost five times higher than in a group of similarly aged patients unexposed to DES (*see* Chaps. 14 and 15).

Before final conclusions can be drawn, the incidence of intraepithelial squamous neoplasia of the lower genital tract in DES-exposed women must be particularly observed during the next decade, to determine the potential increase in the development of squamous neoplasia in this high-risk group of young women.

MANAGEMENT

Optimal management of non-malignant lesions of the cervix and vagina in DES-exposed women is uncertain. At the present time, no case has been reported in which vaginal adenosis has progressed to clear cell adenocarcinoma under direct observation.

Further management of patients with vaginal adenosis depends on the colposcopic findings and biopsy results. If the biopsy shows changes in cervicovaginal epithelium, which are less than carcinoma in situ, then the colposcopy examination is repeated after four months. If there is no change from the initial examination, no further biopsies are necessary, and the patient is followed colposcopically and cytologically in six- to twelve-month intervals, depending on the severity and extent of the lesions. The only indication for treatment is when carcinoma in situ of the cervix or vagina develops.

Chapter 14

THE CERVIX AND VAGINA OF WOMEN EXPOSED TO SYNTHETIC NON-STEROIDAL OESTROGENS

Duane E. Townsend, M.D.

Since the initial report in 1971 drawing attention to the association between *in utero* exposure to stilboestrol (DES) and the subsequent development of clear cell adenocarcinoma (Herbst, Ulfelder, and Poskanzer, 1971) and more recent reports of structural and epithelial changes of the vagina and cervix (Herbst, Kurman, and Scully, 1972; Sandberg, 1976), there has been considerable speculation concerning the risk of malignancy in individuals so exposed. Initially, radical therapy of vaginal adenosis was employed by a few gynaecologists because it was believed that it was the precursor for clear cell adenocarcinoma (Sherman et al., 1974). This immediate association to date has not been confirmed. There has been additional speculation by others that the DES-exposed offspring run a greater risk for developing squamous cell lesions of the vagina and cervix than they do for clear cell adenocarcinoma (Stafl and Mattingly, 1974; Fetherston, 1975; Bibbo et al., 1977). The answers to many other potential problems associated with the syndrome, such as infertility, pregnancy wastage, and malignant diseases in later decades of life, remain to be resolved. Progress in these matters will undoubtedly be assisted by the careful documentation of cases. Despite the relative paucity of scientific information regarding the medical risks in the DES-exposed offspring, current attitudes and opinions regarding these subjects are reviewed.

CLEAR CELL ADENOCARCINOMA

Shortly following the association of maternal ingestion of diethylstilboestrol with the subsequent development of clear cell adenocarcinoma in a few exposed female offspring, a registry was formed to collect as much information as possible about the clear cell adenocarcinomas (Herbst, Robboy, Scully, and Poskanzer, 1974). To date, over 300 clear cell adenocarcinomas of the cervix and vagina have been reported to the registry. About three fourths of these cases have a history of maternal exposure either to DES or similar synthetic non-steroidal oestrogens or to medication for high-risk pregnancy. Some of the residue may have been similarly exposed, although this assumption is speculative by reason of incomplete or missing records. Approximately two thirds of the malignancies are located primarily in the vagina and the remaining third in the cervix.

342   *Colposcopy*

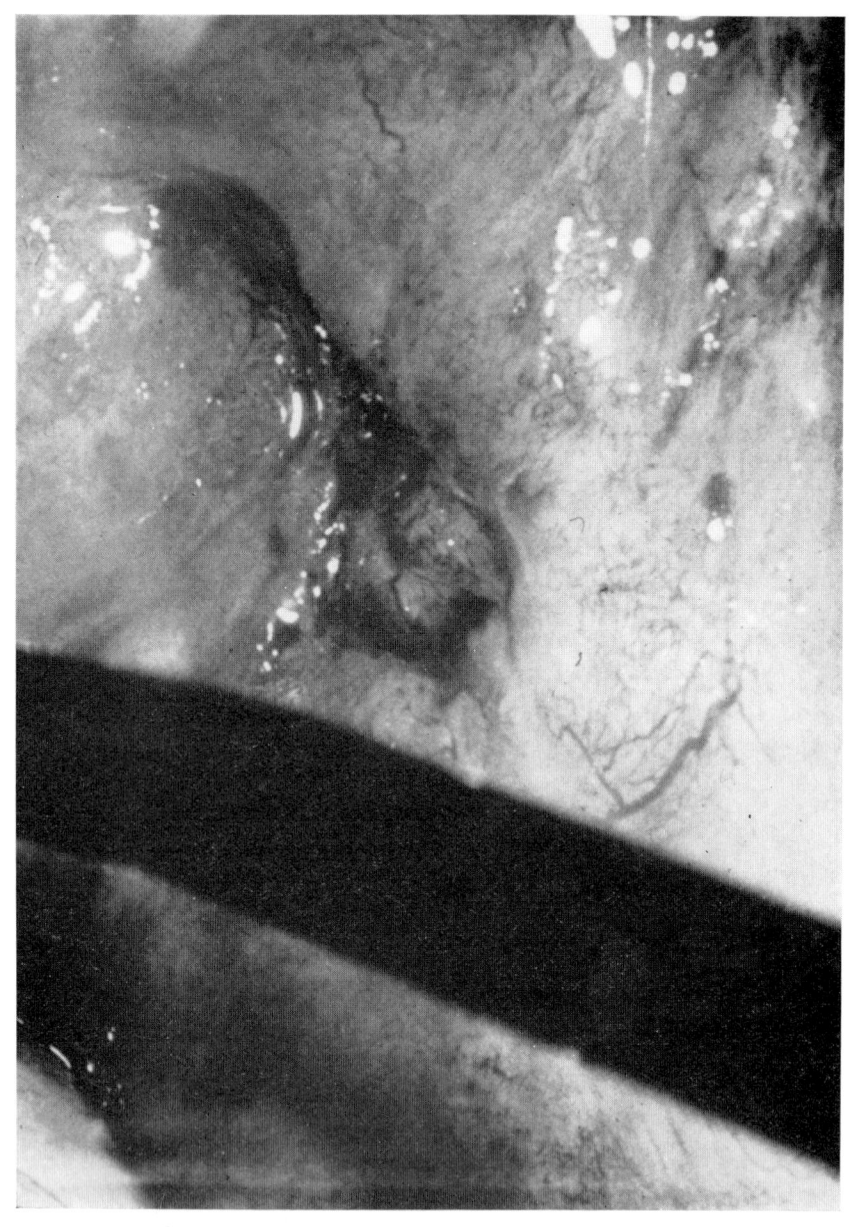

Figure 252. Colpophotograph of clear cell adenocarcinoma in twenty-two-year-old DES-exposed offspring. The posterior portion of the photograph is partially blocked by a uterine sound, which is displacing the cervix to the left. In direct centre is a small clear cell adenocarcinoma which is breaking through the squamous epithelium. Although this lesion was quite small, the entire epithelium in view was undermined by clear cell adenocarcinoma. The lesion was cytologically positive.

The youngest individual with clear cell adenocarcinoma with known exposure was seven and the oldest was twenty-nine, with the mean in the later teenage years. The first DES-related tumour was diagnosed in 1951. There was a progressive increase in the number of cases diagnosed per year, with a peak number of twenty-eight cases recorded in 1972. Since then, there has been a gradual decline in the annual incidence, suggesting that the peak years for this tumour have passed.

Initially, most of the tumours were advanced, and the results of therapy were disappointing. With the emphasis now upon early detection, a greater number of early malignancies are being noted with an anticipated higher cure rate.

The detection of clear cell adenocarcinoma of the vagina and cervix is purely clinical. The colposcope has not proved to be of any major benefit. In fact, there have been no known clear cell adenocarcinomas picked up solely by colposcopy, and there are cases in which the lesions would have gone unnoticed if colposcopy had been the sole means of detection. A small clear cell adenocarcinoma is shown in Figure 252.

Cytology was initially thought to be relatively poor in the detection of clear cell adenocarcinoma, but more recently it has been found that with proper cytological sampling, the detection rate for clear cell adenocarcinoma is highly acceptable and equals that for squamous cell lesions of the lower genital tract (Reagan, 1977).

Clear cell adenocarcinoma metastasizes with a frequency equal to that of squamous cell lesions; perhaps, according to some authors, at a slightly earlier stage. Therapy for the earlier lesions has thus usually been radical hysterectomy with removal of all or part of the vagina with or without ovarian conservation. In those patients where a substantial amount of the vagina has been removed, a vaginal graft is necessary. Occasionally, the two extremes of surgical intervention have been employed; pelvic exenteration or local excision. In some centers, radiation therapy has been found to be highly effective. Unfortunately, in almost all cases, therapy for the tumour results in sterility, although in our own institution we have one woman who has recently delivered after treatment of clear cell adenocarinoma. The individual was treated by transvaginal radiation followed by local radium needles. The overall results of treatment show that the management of early lesions is frequently successful but that the outcome of more advanced lesions is predictably poorer.

STRUCTURAL CHANGES IN CERVIX AND VAGINA

Gross structural changes in the DES-exposed offspring involve the cervix and vagina. In 20 to 30 per cent of exposed offspring, the cervix exhibits changes. The anterior cervical lip has an irregular shape, sometimes peaked

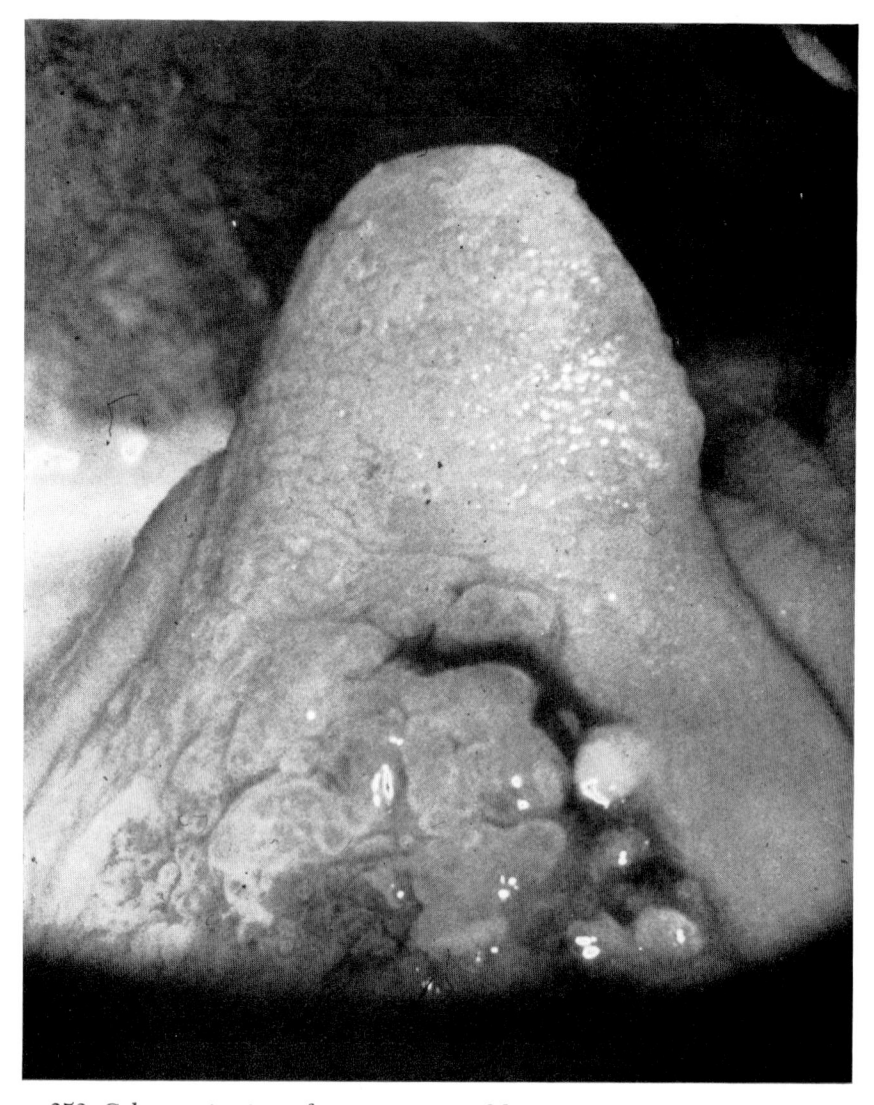

Figure 253. Colposcopic view of anterior cervical lip in eighteen-year-old DES-exposed offspring demonstrating cervical cockscomb. Note the roughness of the squamous epithelium. The large, grapelike clusters of columnar tissue are due to the patient taking oral contraceptives. This type of structural defect has no apparent effect upon fertility or pregnancy.

and other times slightly roughened. The term *cockscomb* (Fig. 253) has been applied to some of these changes. In other instances, there appears to be redundant tissue disposed in collarlike form around the cervix. There is disagreement over whether the collar should be considered part of the vagina or the cervix. In some patients, the cervix is hypoplastic (Fig. 254).

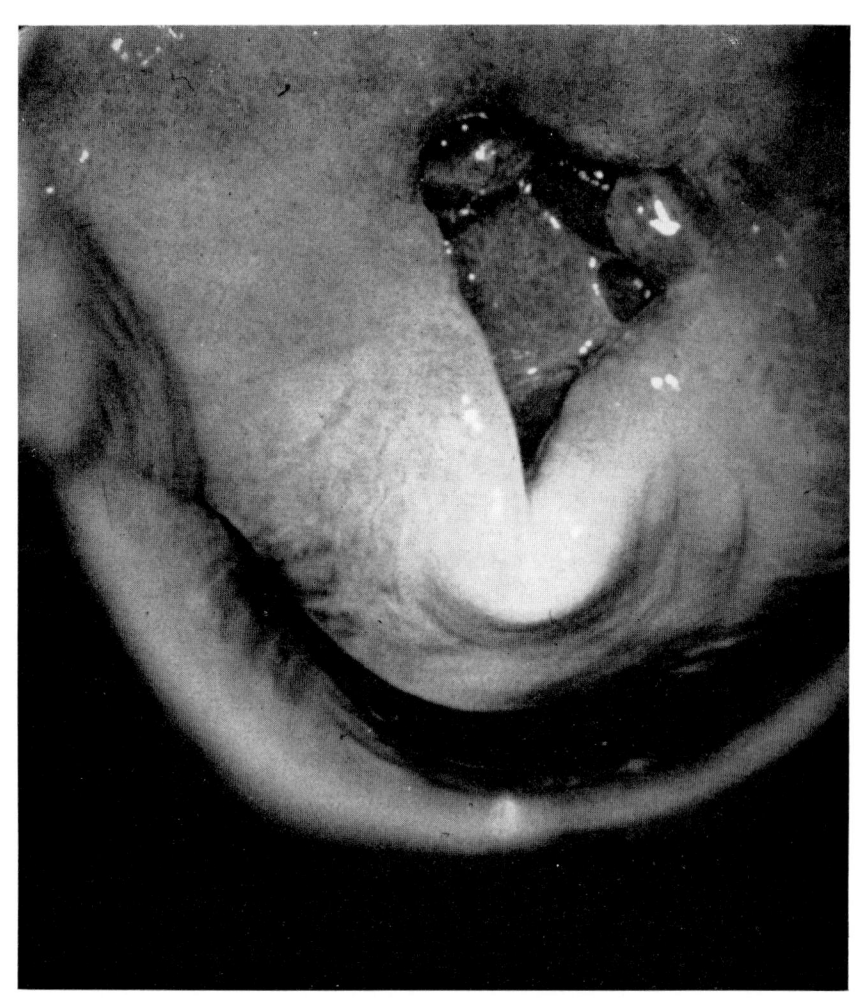

Figure 254. Colpophotograph of cervix in seventeen-year-old DES-exposed offspring demonstrating hypoplastic cervix. Note that the cervical lips are very thin. The os is triangular. The columnar-covered villi within the os are very small. The significance of such a hypoplastic cervix remains to be determined.

Although the consequences of the hypoplastic cervix are unknown, the possibility of an incompetent cervical os has not been discounted.

The vaginal structural changes, which are rare, include an absent pars vaginalis and an incomplete transverse vaginal septum. The latter occurs invariably in the upper one third of the vagina. Such a constriction may prevent the upper one third of the vagina and cervix from being thoroughly examined.

COLPOSCOPIC APPEARANCES

As well as gross or structural changes obvious to the naked eye, epithelial

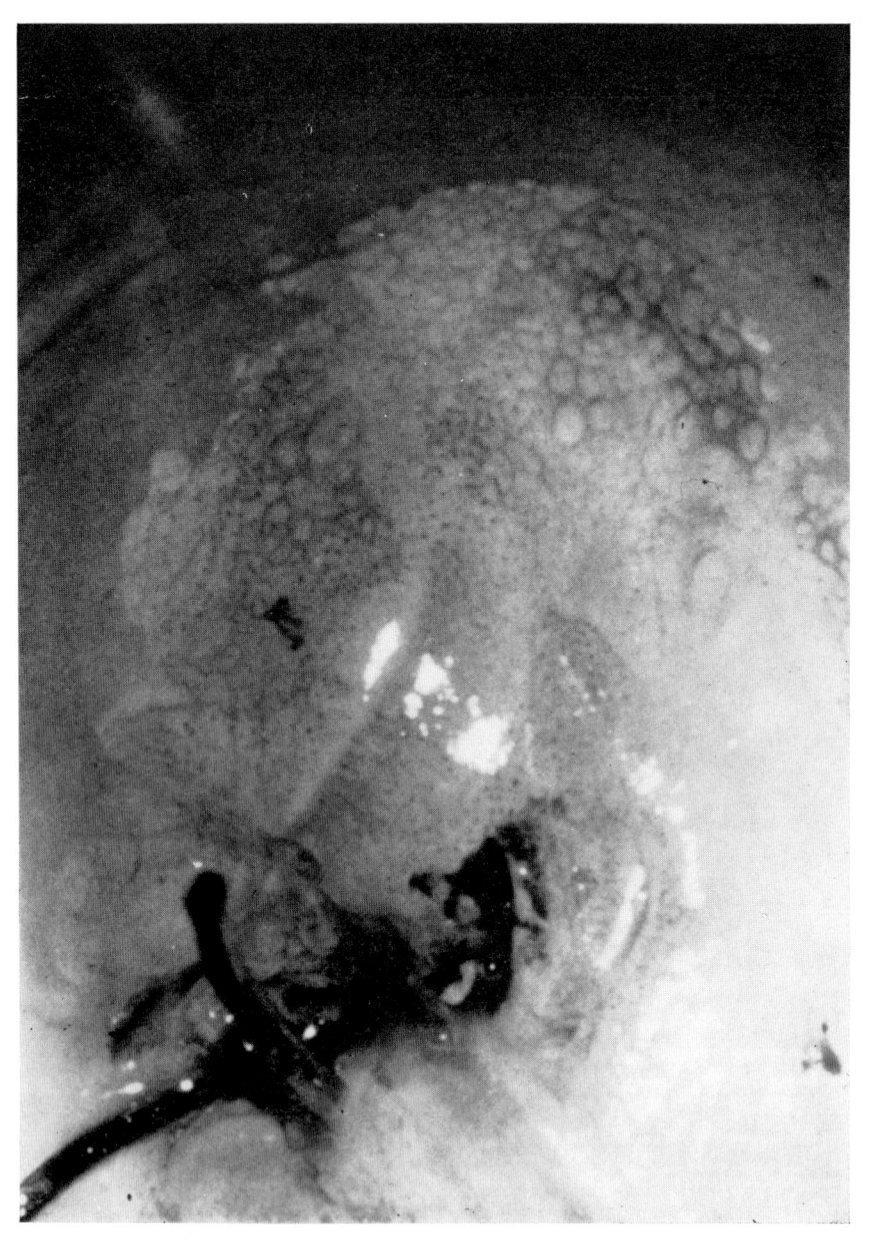

Figure 255. Colpophotograph of cervix in twenty-one-year-old DES-exposed subject. An IUD is present in the lower left. Note the heavy white epithelium, punctation, and mosaic. Although the colposcopic interpretation was that of moderate dysplasia, directed biopsy showed only squamous metaplasia.

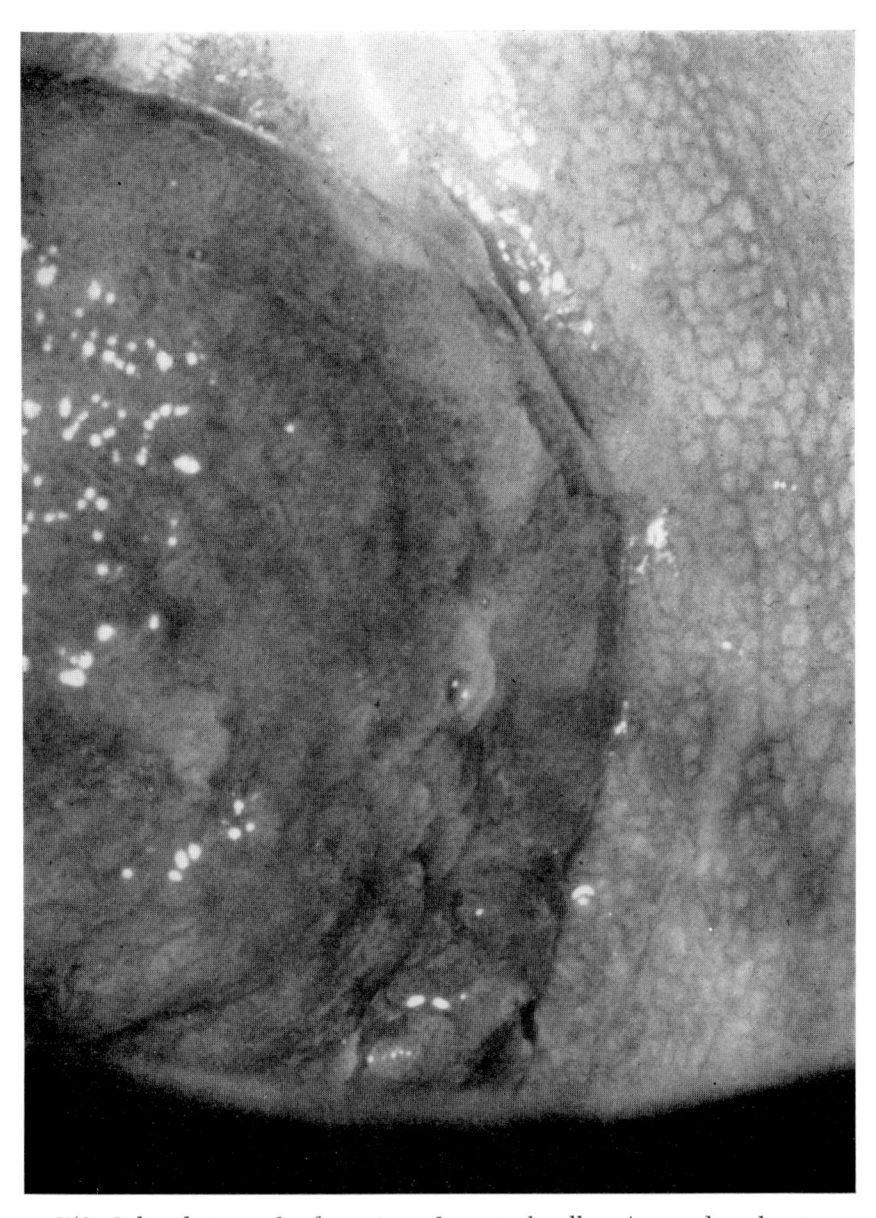

Figure 256. Colpophotograph of cervix and cervical collar. A pseudo-polyp is present occupying the left portion of the photograph. A sulcus is present on the right side between the cervical collar, covered by metaplastic epithelium with mosaic pattern and the main body of the cervix. Directed biopsy of the mosaic pattern showed only squamous metaplasia.

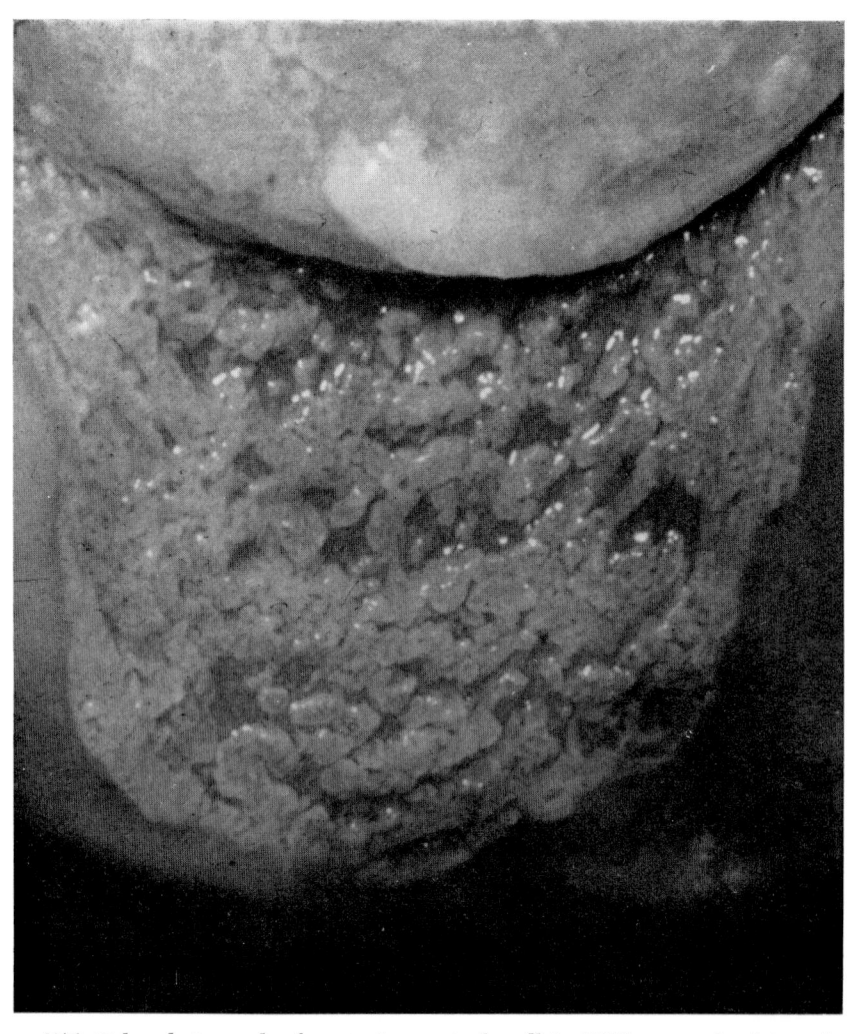

Figure 257. Colpophotograph of posterior vaginal wall in DES-exposed subject demonstrating adenosis. Note the irregular surface contour with areas of metaplasia. Directed biopsy of this area showed columnar epithelium and immature squamous metaplasia.

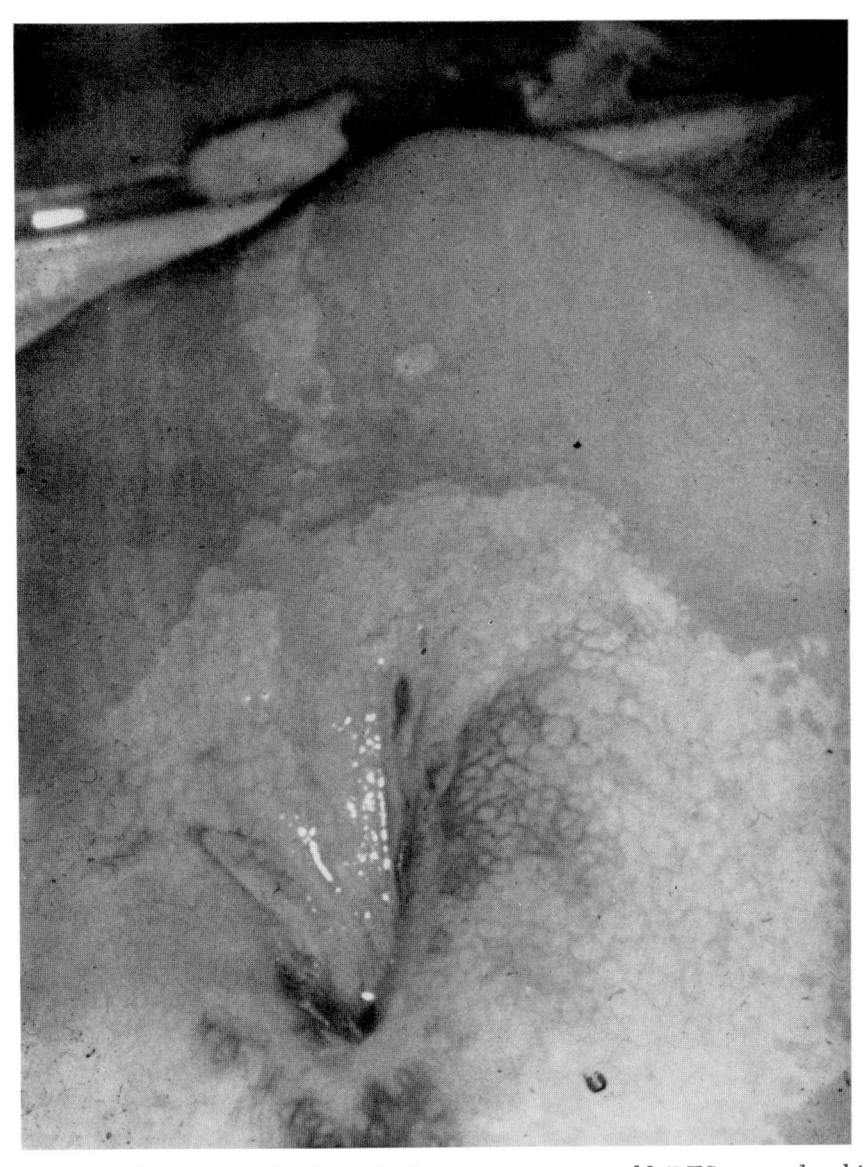

Figure 258. Colpophotograph of cervix in twenty-two-year-old DES-exposed subject. Note the anterior cervix is slightly peaked. The transformation zone is comprised of white epithelium and mosaic structure. Impression at the time of colposcopic examination was Grade II atypical transformation zone, i.e. moderate dysplasia. Directed biopsy showed squamous metaplasia.

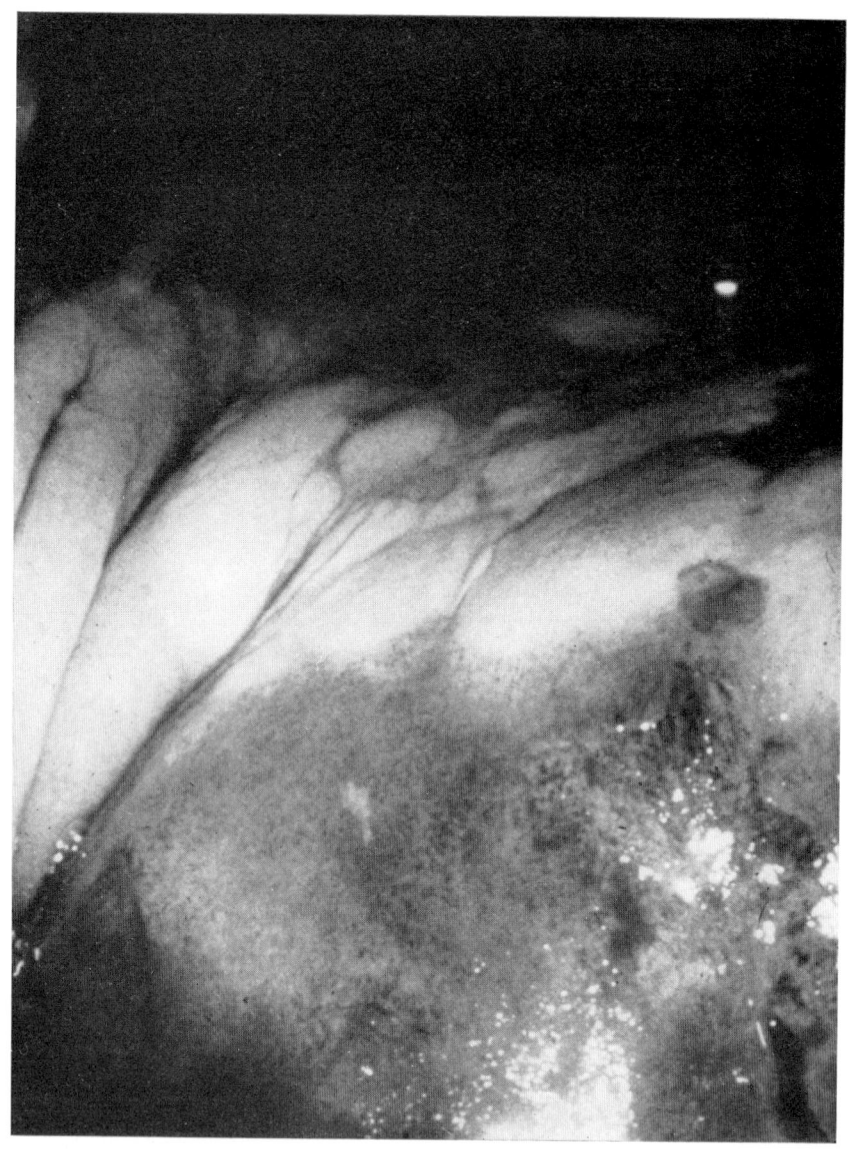

Figure 259. Colpophotograph of anterior vagina in nineteen-year-old DES-exposed offspring. Note the areas of white epithelium which were visible to the naked eye, i.e. keratosis. Hyperkeratosis is seen in approximately 20 percent of the DES-exposed offspring. The significance of such a finding remains to be determined.

changes that may be detailed with the colposcope occur. It was initially believed that colposcopy would be the ideal instrument in the evaluation of such lesions. Unfortunately, results of its use have been confusing.

The colposcopic features of the vaginal as well as cervical lesions are depicted in Figures 255 to 259. Note that the colposcopic appearance of the squamous cell lesions appear to be ominous, but the histological counterpart in all of the patients was squamous metaplasia (*see* Chaps. 13 and 15).

MANAGEMENT OF ADENOSIS

The current attitudes regarding those individuals who have been exposed *in utero* to diethylstilboestrol are positive expectation, reassurance, and a great deal of compassion and understanding for the mother and the exposed subject.

Regular examinations are recommended from either the menarche or the age of fourteen, whichever is first. This recommendation is predicated on the finding that clear cell adenocarcinoma of the cervix and/or vagina is extremely rare prior to the age of fourteen. The psychological trauma that a young adolescent may encounter when subjected to such an examination outweighs its benefits. However, a DES-exposed offspring, prior to menarche, with unusual vaginal bleeding or discharge should be examined, preferably under anaesthesia.

The current technique for examination of suspected cases is shown in Table V. If the hymen appears to be unusually tense, the patient is advised to use vaginal tampons for several menstrual periods before returning for a repeat examination. Palpation is important, and several clear cell adenocarcinomas at our institution were detected solely by this means.

Following palpation, an appropriate-sized vaginal speculum is inserted, the cervix is exposed, and the excess mucus and debris often found in the subjects is carefully removed. Cytological sampling is taken of the upper one third of the vagina, with great care being taken to avoid the lateral

TABLE V
CURRENT TECHNIQUES

1. Palpation of vagina
2. Cytology
   a. Vagina
   b. Cervix
3. Inspection
4. Colposcopy
   a. Acetic acid
   b. Iodine stain
5. Biopsies
6. Bimanual examination

walls of the cervix. If there appear to be epithelial changes in the mid- or lower third of the vagina on gross inspection, such as redness or roughness, then the speculum must be withdrawn and these areas also cytologically sampled. All vaginal samples are kept separate from the cervix. The cervical os is then aspirated, followed by an ectocervical scrape. The colposcope may be used at this point in the course of examination, although it is believed by many individuals that the colposcopic examination is not essential for the routine evaluation of these subjects. However, in the presence of an abnormal Papanicolaou test, then the colposcopic evaluation is mandatory. Any areas that appear to be grossly abnormal colposcopically are sampled. Other areas for sampling include those which are vividly red and those showing nodularity on palpation. Lugol's iodine solution is used as a stain. Non-staining areas invariably correlate with the transformation zone, which is usually seen colposcopically. After tissue sampling, hemostasis is secured, and a bimanual examination completes the procedure.

If clear cell adenocarcinoma is detected, the patient must be referred to a physician who has had experience in managing such lesions.

Since vaginal adenosis has a similar natural history to that of columnar tissue on the ectocervix and is usually resolved by physiological metaplasia, therapy is generally not necessary. However, some DES-exposed offspring do complain of a copious vaginal discharge, obviously due to the large areas of columnar tissue. Local destructive processes such as cryosurgery, electrocautery, and the CO_2 laser appear to be highly satisfactory in relieving the discomfort. Vaginal acidification to accelerate the metaplasia has been successfully employed in our own clinic. Local progesterone, initially believed to be beneficial (Herbst, Robboy, Macdonald, and Scully, 1974) is no longer recommended.

Follow-up examinations are usually dictated by the epithelial findings. Yearly examinations are recommended if only cervical changes are noted. Those with adenosis and/or squamous metaplasia of the vagina are examined every six months. If minor atypia is noted on the cervix or vagina, more frequent checkups are suggested. More severe changes, such as severe dysplasia or carcinoma in situ, usually require therapy. The squamous epithelial changes require very careful evaluation before any type of therapy is initiated, especially since present experience indicates that many of the histological atypias even though they are called carcinoma in situ may, in fact, represent the unique metaplasia of the DES subjects (*see* Chaps. 13 and 15). Careful deliberation is now the hallmark in the evaluation of squamous cell lesions in the DES-exposed subject.

Contraception

There has been no evidence that the use of oral contraceptives accelerates or precipitates clear cell adenocarcinoma or squamous cell lesions. All current data suggest that the DES-exposed offspring can use any form of contraception.

Fertility and Pregnancy

A recent report suggests that there may be some problems with fertility in the DES-exposed female, as well as an increase in pregnancy wastage (Bibbo et al., 1977). However, the number of patients in this series is relatively small, and more data is necessary before any definite conclusions can be reached.

NATURAL HISTORY OF ADENOSIS

The natural history of vaginal adenosis is similar to that of columnar epithelium, i.e. replacement by squamous epithelium through the process of metaplasia. The atypical or arrested immature metaplasia noted with colposcopy in virtually every DES-exposed subject had led to the speculation that many individuals were likely to develop squamous cell lesions of the vagina and cervix. Indeed, such lesions have been noted in a few offspring, but the predicted explosion of bona fide squamous cell lesions has fortunately not materialized.

The hypothesis was based upon the applicability of the concept of the transformation zone as applied to the cervix. It has been suggested that individuals having large areas of columnar tissue on the ectocervix are probably at greater risk for developing cervical neoplasia, because of the relatively large areas in which squamous metaplasia can occur. In at least two thirds of the DES-exposed offspring, the entire ectocervix and a portion of the vagina are initially covered by columnar epithelium. In the remaining third, most of the ectocervix is covered with columnar epithelium. Initial reports tended to confirm this hypothesis (Stafl and Mattingly, 1974; Fetherston, 1975), but more recent information suggests that tissue initially thought to be squamous neoplasia is really an unusual variant of squamous metaplasia, perhaps unique to the DES-exposed subjects (Hart et al., 1976; Ng et al., 1977) (*see* Chaps. 13 and 15).

RISK FACTOR FOR CLEAR CELL ADENOCARCINOMA

The risk factor for an exposed individual to develop clear cell adenocarcinoma remains to be determined. The current data suggests that if an individual has been exposed *in utero* after twenty weeks of intrauterine life, the risk factor is extremely small, if not zero. All of the cases in the registry to date have been associated with exposure *in utero* prior to eighteen weeks of gestation. The risk is probably around 1 : 3000 to 1 : 4000. This is based on the number of DES-related clear cell cancers, i.e. 200 to 250, and the estimated number of exposed subjects, 1 to 2 million. It is a rare disease.

PART VI

Difficulties of Colposcopic Interpretation

Chapter 15

ATYPICAL COLPOSCOPIC APPEARANCES OF DOUBTFUL OR PHYSIOLOGICAL SIGNIFICANCE

THE COLPOSCOPIC TECHNIQUE has proven as valuable as most diagnostic methods in medicine, but as with such methods, it has its anomalies. Similar colposcopic appearances may be found in conditions of very different significance. The years that have passed since the original description of the atypical transformation zone was offered have convinced us such anomalous findings deserve more thorough discussion. Originally, the atypical transformation zone was emphasised as an entity within which histologic abnormalities would be found, however minor, signifying neoplastic potential. Experience has shown that this assumption is not always warranted, and we have attempted to categorize further the atypical transformation zone and to dispose of the anomaly inherent in accepting all varieties of white epithelium with or without vascular structures as potentially abnormal.

The colour of the epithelium on colposcopic examination is basically determined by the colour reflected from the stromal blood vessels, modified by some varying characteristics of the epithelium which themselves are somehow further altered by the application of acetic acid. In general, the greater the opacity between the colposcope and the underlying stroma, the whiter the epithelium. Thus, increased cell density with an attendant increased nuclear density, increased epithelial height, and a keratin covering may all be responsible for a colposcopic white epithelium. It is well known that such factors exist in dysplasia and carcinoma in situ. On general grounds, they could also exist in other epithelial states. For example, an undifferentiated or immature epithelium early in the metaplastic process or a very thick or densely cellular epithelium can also produce a surface colour that appears white through the colposcope.

The vascular patterns of the transformation zone on colposcopy represent various remodellings of the columnar epithelial vessels. Thus, in classical terms, if the metaplastic process is normal, the capillaries within the pre-existing columnar epithelium are eventually lost, so that the new physiological epithelial sheet is not subdivided by epithelial capillaries but has a treelike branching pattern of subepithelial vessels. If the metaplastic process is atypical, the pre-existing vessels within the columnar epithelium are modified. The new atypical epithelial sheet is then frequently subdivided by epithelial capillaries, giving the classic appearances of punctation and mosaic structure. The vascular pattern is therefore the key to the

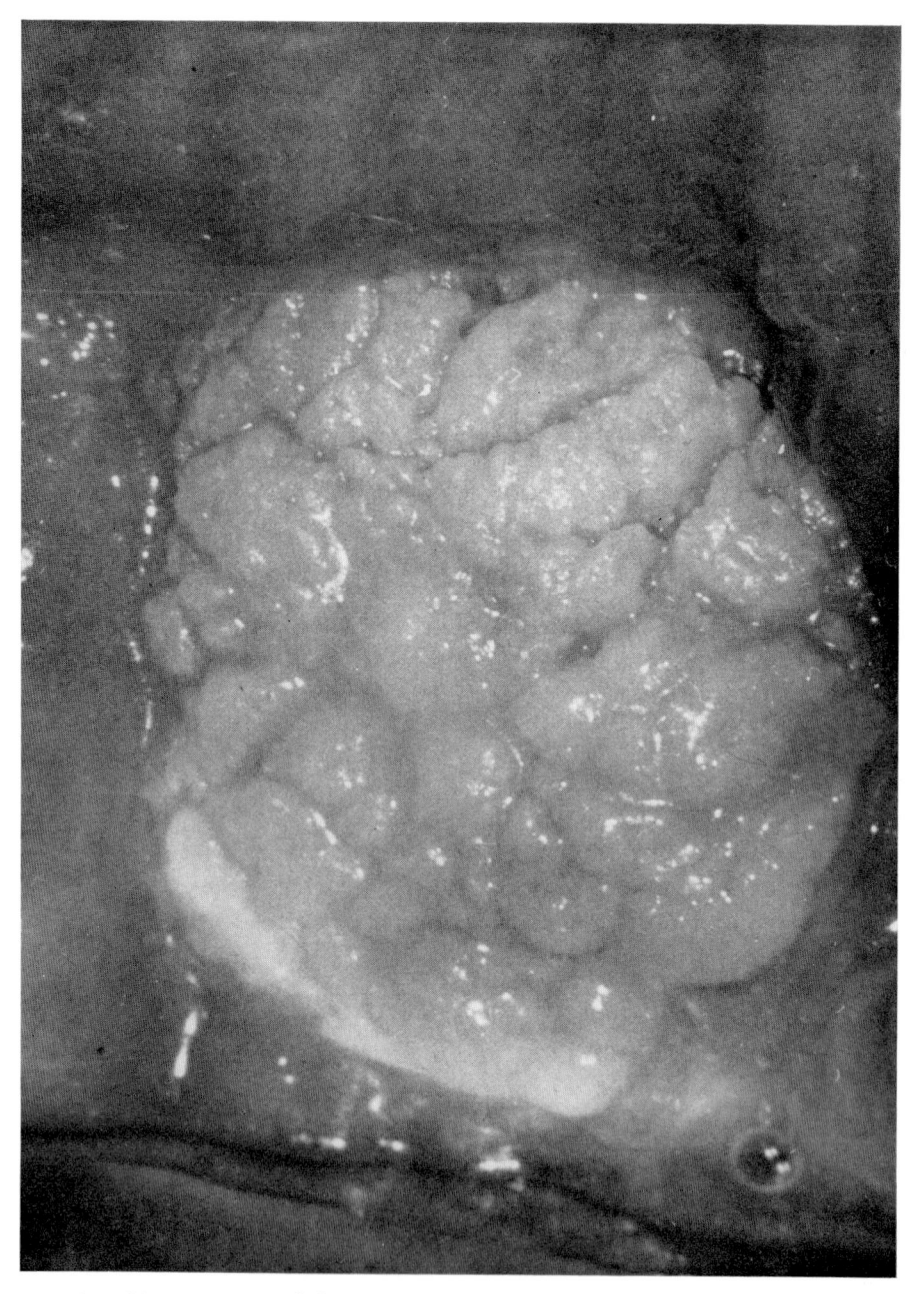

Figure 260. Keratosis. Noted during routine examination, this disorder was categorised by the pathologist as keratosis overlying original squamous epithelium.

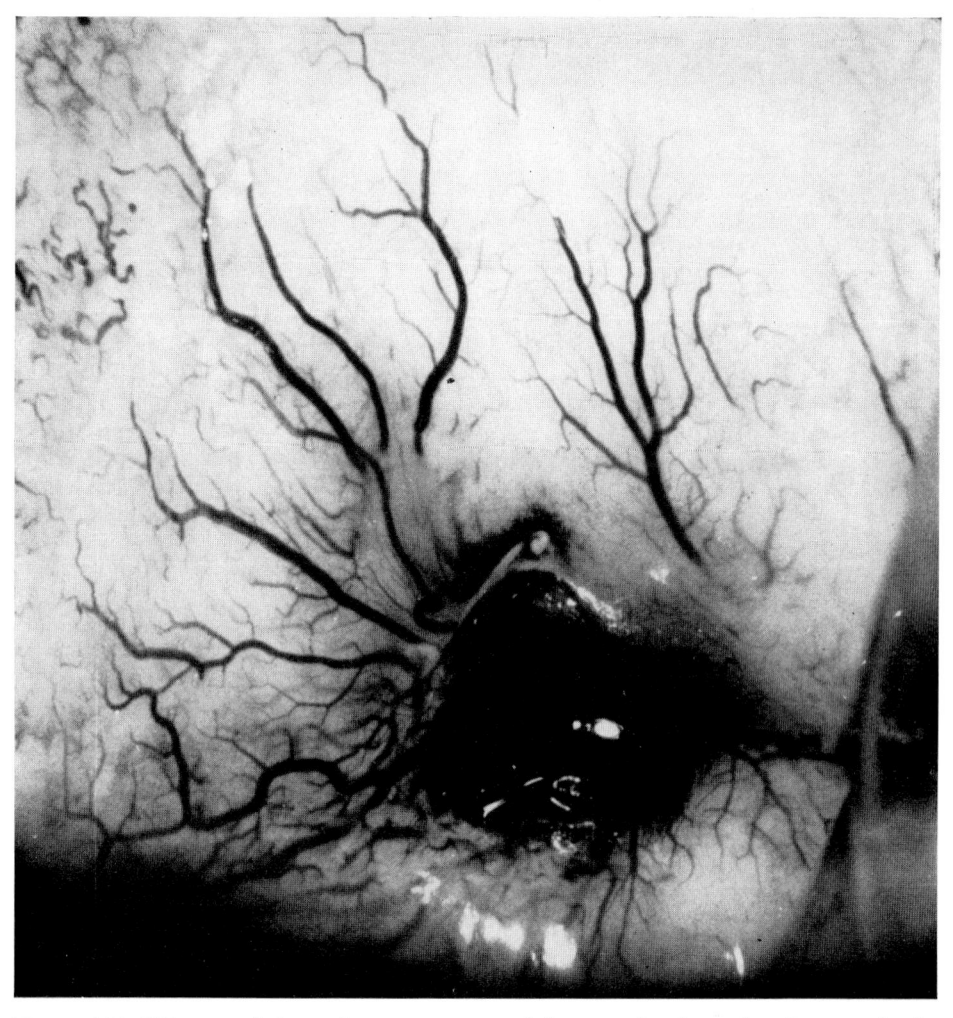

Figure 261. White epithelium due to oestrogen deficiency. In this colpophotograph of a sixty-year-old woman, treelike regular branching subepithelial vessels are starkly etched in the otherwise featureless white original squamous epithelium. The round cervical os is seen in the lower third of the photograph.

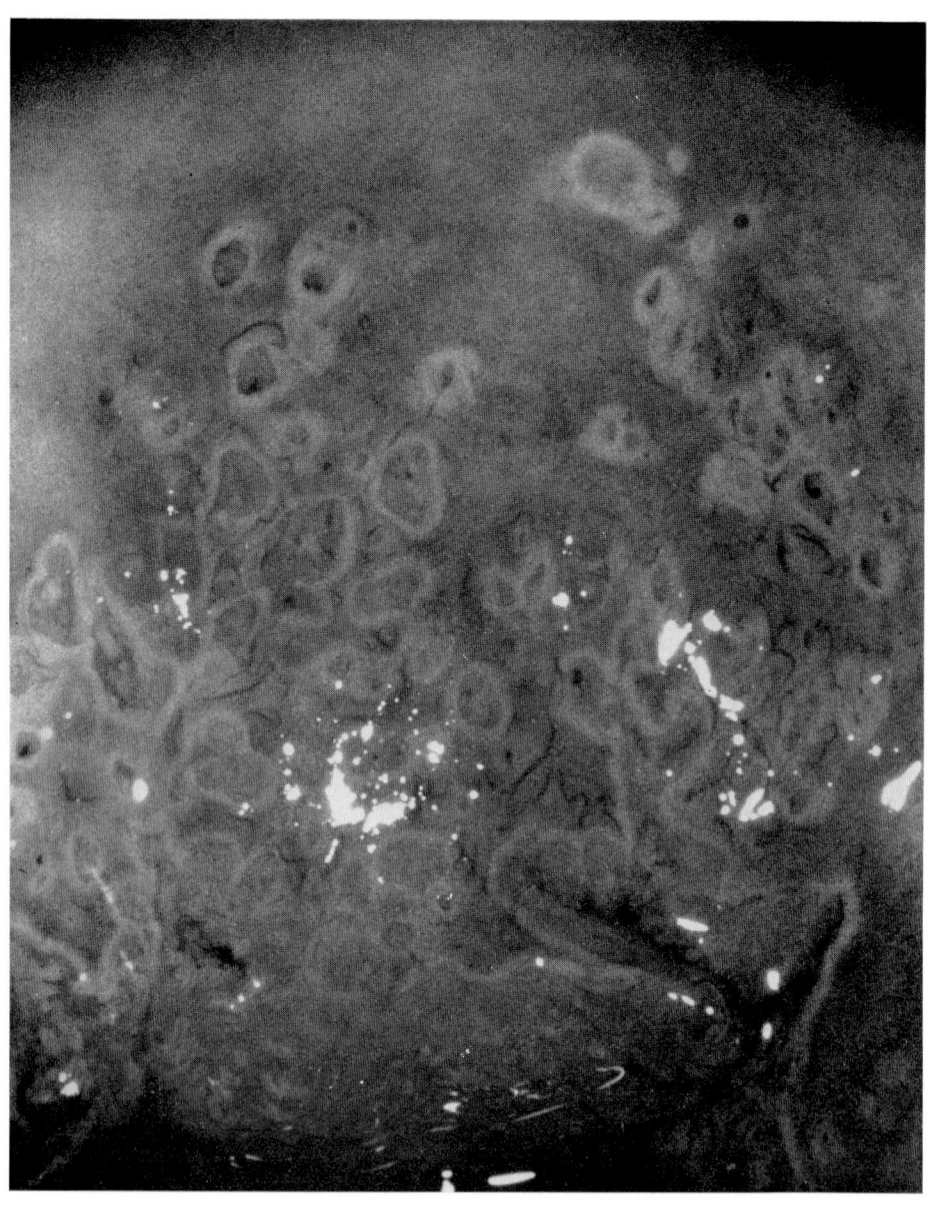

Figure 262. Colpophotograph of anterior lip of cervix featuring white rings around gland openings. The increased cell density at the margins of the opening results in a white ring.

colposcopic appearance, and it seems reasonable that at times for reasons not altogether clear, benign processes associated with the metaplastic process, a process concerned with growth, mimic those more customarily associated with preneoplastic change.

There are at least nine occasions when either colposcopic white epithelium and/or white epithelium with punctation and/or mosaic structure or keratosis can be regarded as physiological and not pathological. Their recognition is of importance in the differential diagnosis of the colposcopic atypia:

1. KERATOSIS OVERLYING ORIGINAL SQUAMOUS EPITHELIUM (Fig. 260).

2. WHITE EPITHELIUM DUE TO OESTROGEN DEFICIENCY IN THE POSTMENOPAUSAL CERVIX: The white colour is due to an avascular stroma (Fig. 261).

3. WHITE RINGS AROUND GLAND OPENINGS IN THE TRANSFORMATION ZONE: The whiteness is related to a tall and cellularly dense epithelium at the site of the ring, lining the clefts or glands (Fig. 262).

4. ATYPICAL APPEARANCES PRESENT TRANSIENTLY DURING DYNAMIC PHASES OF METAPLASIA IN ADOLESCENTS AND FIRST PREGNANCY: At its earliest appearance, the new squamous epithelium is about six to ten cells thick, and the layers of this immature metaplastic epithelium are densely packed, an arrangement which may produce an overall whiteness (Fig. 263A). As well as an overall whiteness, vascular patterns resembling punctation and mosaic may occur, but these are always modelled on the pre-existing columnar epithelial contours. The prospective significance of these changes for the individual concerned is unknown (p. 227). With subsequent differentiation, the cell content of the epithelium becomes less dense and takes on the normal colour and surface flatness of the physiological transformation zone (Fig. 263B).

5. ATYPICAL APPEARANCES PERSISTING IN PHYSIOLOGICAL TRANSFORMATION ZONE: Although patchiness of the normal metaplastic process is commonly succeeded by a uniformly pink colour of the mature transformation zone, evidence of its origin may persist as white patches for varying periods in later life and may be misinterpreted as being due to atypical metaplasia (Fig. 264). Such white epithelium is seen, often with fused villous structure (p. 88) rather than a flat surface. This arrest of the normal metaplastic process at some of its earlier phases is most frequently seen at the cephalic end of the transformation zone in the cervical canal (Fig. 265) and in other regions more remote from the vaginal environment which we believe to be the ultimate trigger to the metaplastic process (p. 88).

6. ATYPICAL APPEARANCES DURING REGENERATION AFTER CRYOSURGERY OR ELECTRODIATHERMY: The epithelial regeneration following its thera-

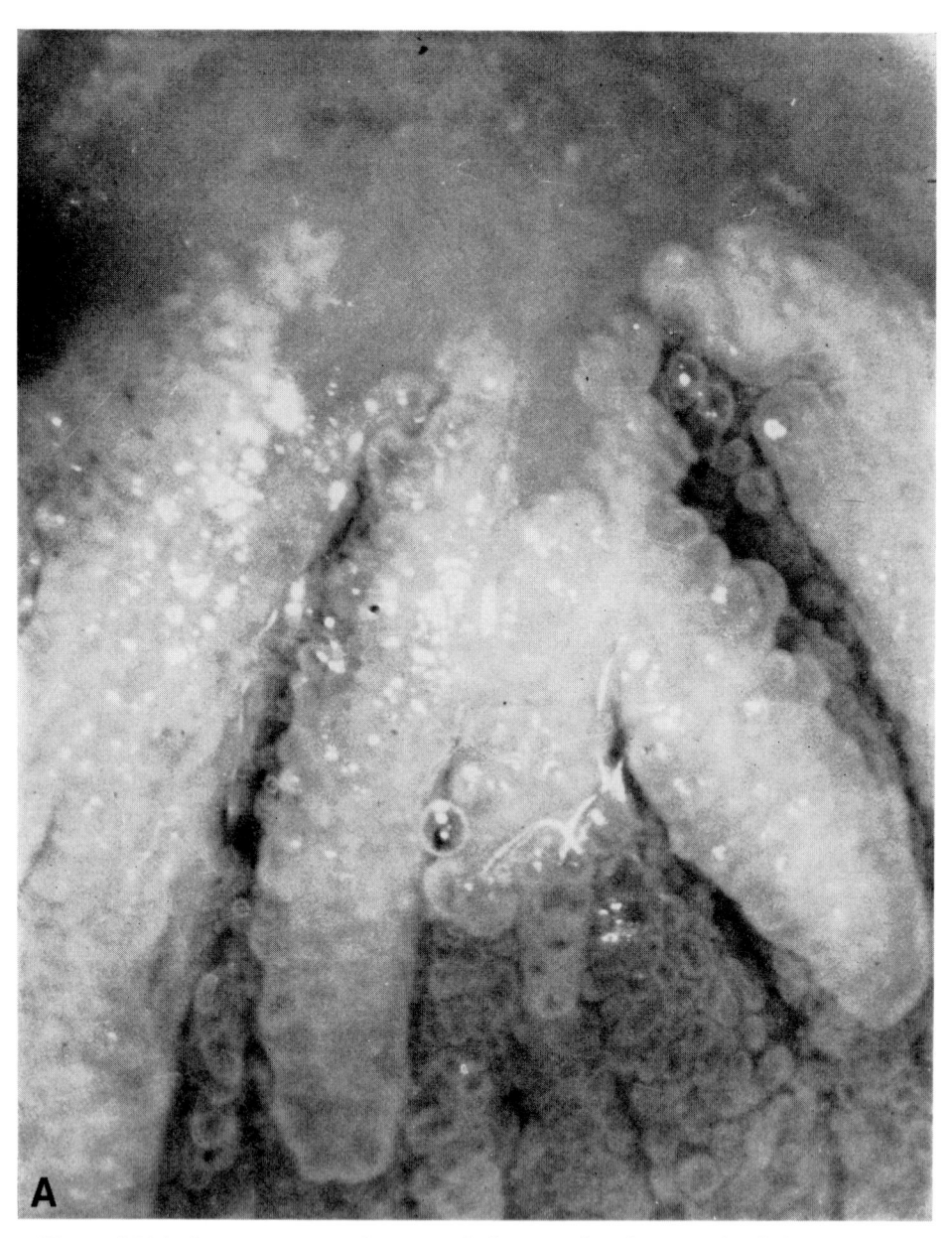

Figure 263A. Immature metaplastic epithelium. Colpophotograph of the anterior lip of the cervix in a fifteen-year-old adolescent. Note the white epithelium originating from underlying columnar cells as evidenced by persistence of villous structures.

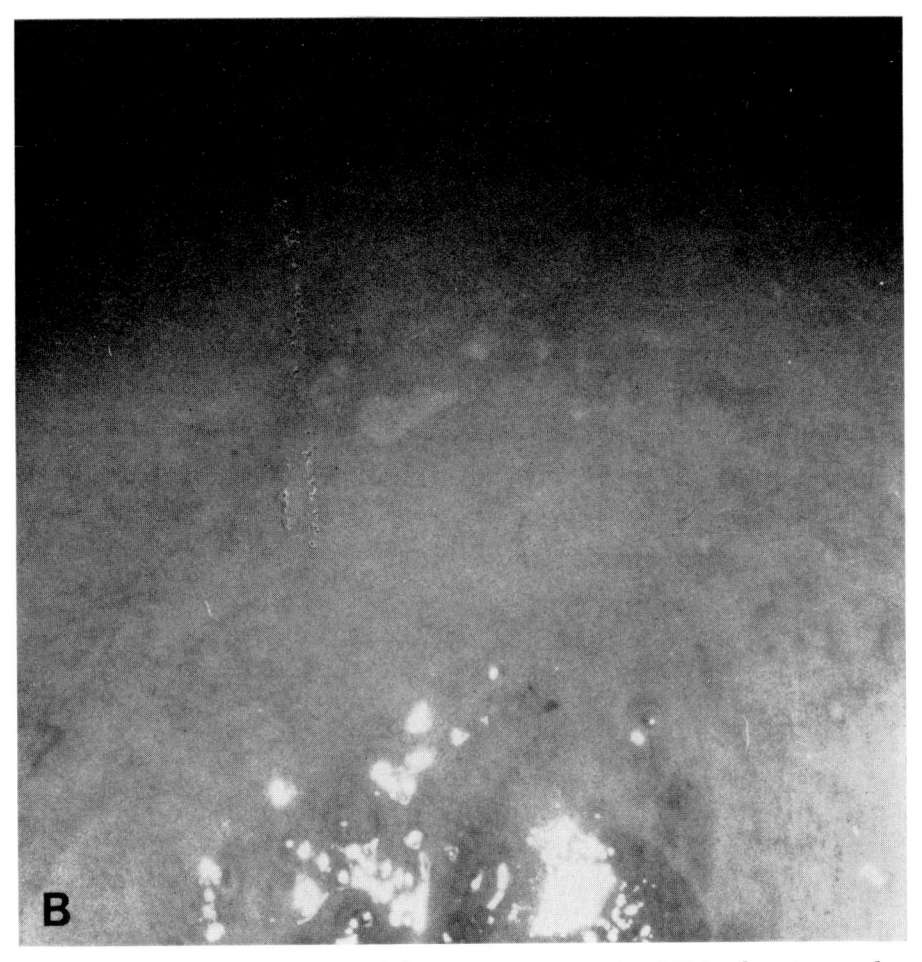

Figure 263B. Colpophotograph of the same cervix as Fig. 263A taken 8 years later. Note that the very white epithelium of this cervix has changed sometime in the interim to mature metaplastic squamous epithelium resembling original squamous epithelium, except for a patch of parakeratosis and some gland openings.

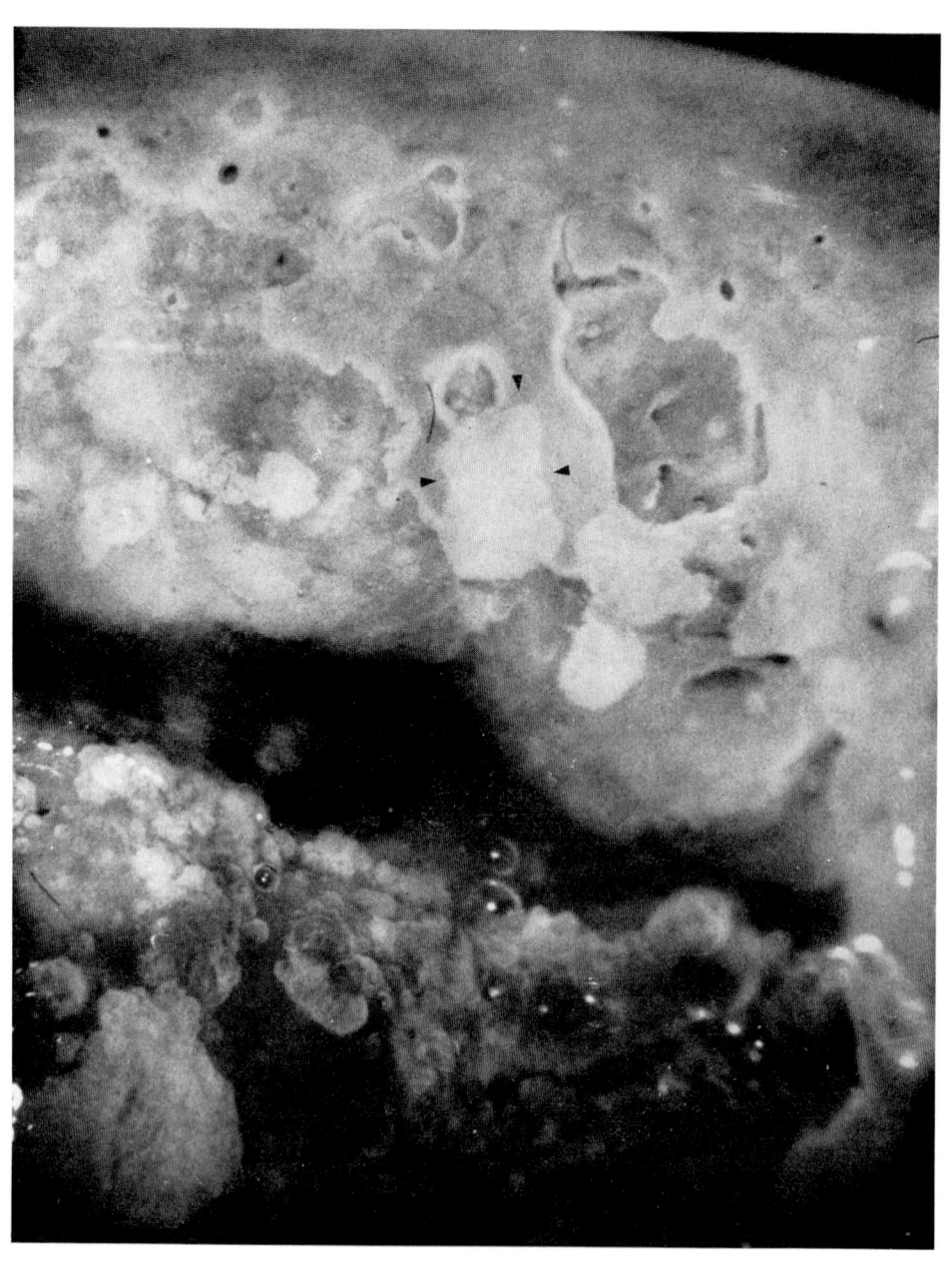

Figure 264. Colpophotograph of anterior lip and canal of a cervix showing patches of white epithelium in the transformation zone (arrows) caudad to the cervical canal. Biopsy showed immature metaplasia.

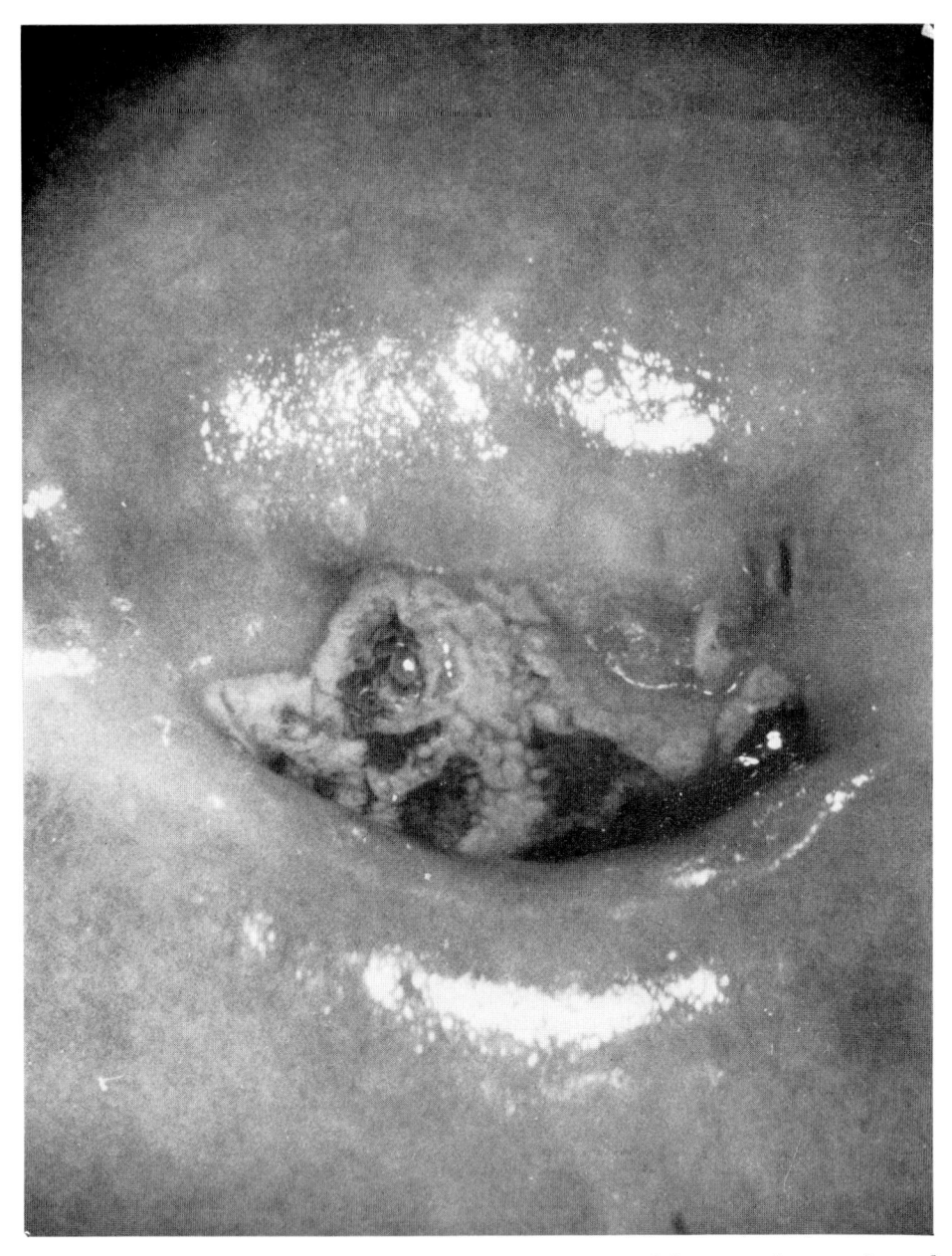

Figure 265. Colpophotograph of portion of ectocervix and lower endocervical canal. The white epithelium with fused villous structure present within the canal showed on biopsy immature metaplastic epithelium.

peutic destruction by heat or cold may at times be accompanied by similar phases to those occurring in physiological regeneration. White epithelium can appear and can be associated with punctation and/or mosaic structure. Such appearances can occur after treatment of benign cervical conditions where there seems little doubt that they represent regenerating epithelium in immature stages. Most of these abnormal colposcopic patterns regress spontaneously, but persistence for two years or more after treatment has been noted in some cases. Similar appearances may present after treatment of preneoplastic lesions. These may also have benign significance and may regress or they may represent persistence of the lesion.

7. ATYPICAL APPEARANCES IN THE ADOLESCENT: There is another period when white epithelium with or without atypical vascular changes occurs in response to the metaplastic stimulus; this is at the menarche. Insofar as this stage may be of great significance for the origin of truly neoplastic changes, the differentiation of the two metaplastic processes, physiological and atypical, is at the same time of great importance and of some difficulty. Since 1968, we have been aware that at times even the most classical atypical transformation zones with white epithelium, punctation, and mosaic structure represent the physiological process.

The evidence to be presented was obtained from studies already mentioned, including over 350 highly sexually active adolescent girls between the ages of twelve to seventeen years. A control group of forty virgins was examined colposcopically, during the course of examination under anaesthesia, for a variety of gynaecological reasons.

This study is of importance for two reasons: First, because it throws light on the association of physiological metaplasia with atypical colposcopic appearances, and second, because the two groups, sexually active and virginal, provide a convenient control for the study of groups of girls exposed to the effects of maternally administered diethylstilboestrol.

The first observation was that there was an increase of nearly five times in atypical transformation zone in the sexually active group when compared with the virgin group. Most atypical transformation zones were of the Grade I and occasionally of the Grade II variety (Figs. 266-268). At times, the colposcopic appearances of the sexually active group were similar to those which in older women are frequently associated with abnormal cytology and a histological diagnosis of some grade of cervical intraepithelial neoplasia. However, in most of these cases, the expected correlation with cytology and histology did not occur. In the absence of this correlation, this question has to be asked: Are we justified in assuming that these atypical transformation zones in this age group are necessarily precursors of cervical cancer?

The second observation in the sexually active group was that there was colposcopic evidence of the onset of metaplasia of both physiological and atypical types. Most importantly in the sexually active group, at times, atypical metaplastic epithelium could be seen, apparently in the process of formation from the underlying columnar epithelium (Fig. 269). This suggested that we were in fact seeing the beginning of the lengthy process which one day could terminate in the preneoplastic or neoplastic state.

The third observation concerns the histology of these atypical lesions. A great variety of histological appearances was encountered which can be loosely classified into four categories. The first and least common were lesions which could be fitted into conventional atypical patterns. The second showed immature squamous metaplasia. Third, in some, in addition to immature metaplasia there was a collection of round cells of lymphocytic and mononuclear type in the subepithelial and even epithelial layer (Fig. 270). The usual diagnosis returned from the pathologist for these lesions was one of "chronic cervicitis" of varying degree. Fourth, and most unexpectedly, well-differentiated metaplastic epithelium was occasionally observed. Such appearances almost certainly indicate the presence of original transformation zone (p. 374).

What are the possible reasons for the lack of histological correlation between what at times are identical atypical colposcopic appearances in the sexually active adolescent and the adult cervix? The first possibility is that the atypical appearances in the adolescent represent atypical metaplasia at an early stage of development. Later, they may readily be recognised histologically as the precursors of cervical cancer. The second possibility is that these appearances merely represent appearances generated by immature physiological metaplasia, perhaps modified by such factors as coitally transmitted infection. Support for this latter alternative is borne out by our sequential studies of areas of white epithelium developing in the adolescent which later show a normal appearance (see Fig. 263A and B). The third possibility is that the appearances represent a variety of the original transformation zone.

Studies of the virgin group give further support to the contention that some atypical transformation zones do not represent an atypical metaplastic process. While most cervices in this group showed columnar epithelium undergoing various changes associated with physiological transformation, the most striking observation was the presence of an atypical transformation zone, in 10 per cent of cases (Fig. 271). Biopsies taken from both the physiological and atypical colposcopic appearances in the virginal group showed histological patterns of immature and mature metaplastic epithelium, with an overall appearance very similar to the second and fourth categories described in the sexually active group.

In the two groups, the sexually active and virginal, the differences in

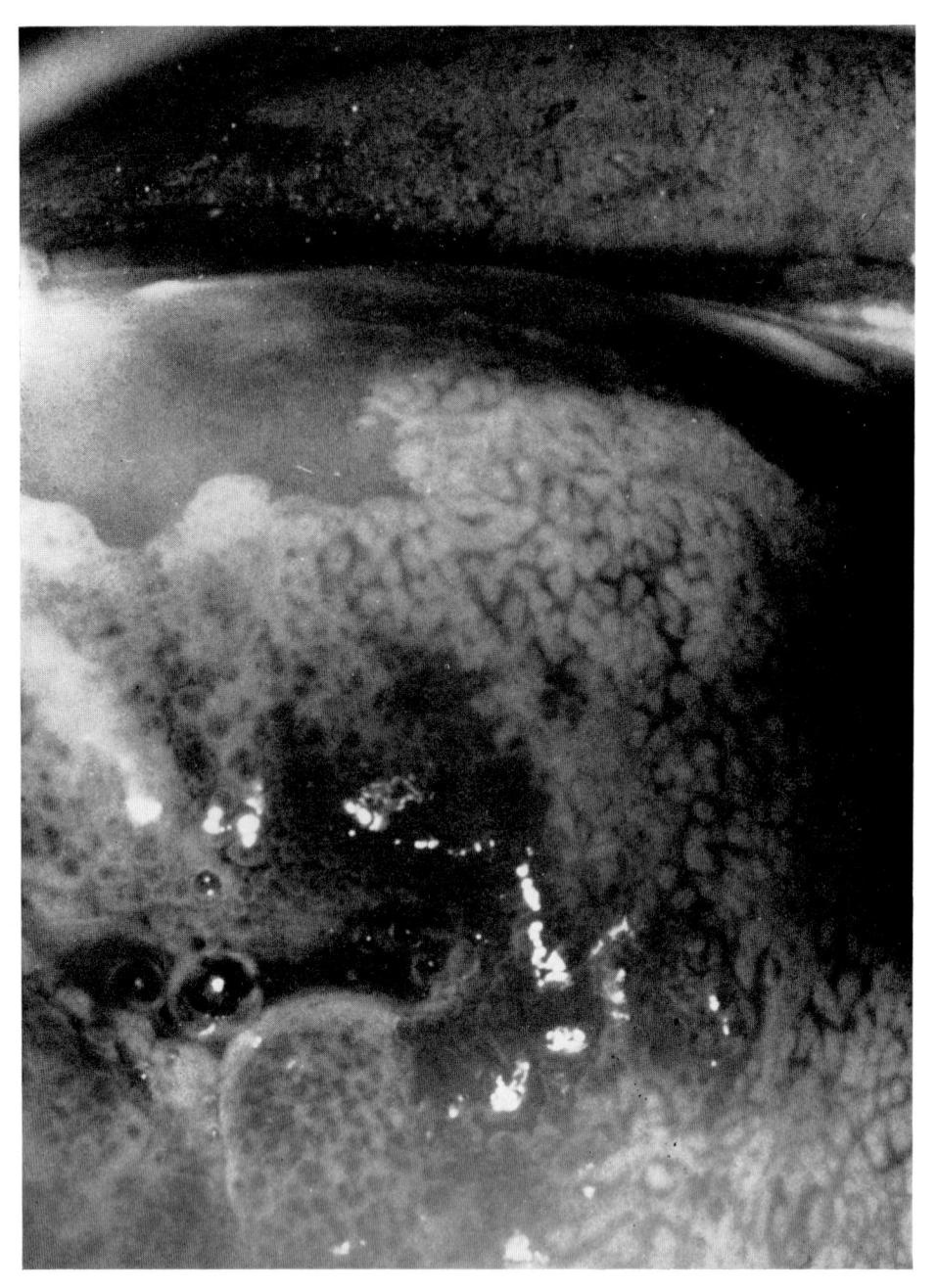

Figure 266. Adolescent cervix: sexually active subject aged seventeen years. Colpophotograph of cervix displaying an atypical transformation zone with punctation on the left of the photograph and mosaic on the right, replacing the original columnar epithelium on the ectocervix. The external os is below and left of centre.

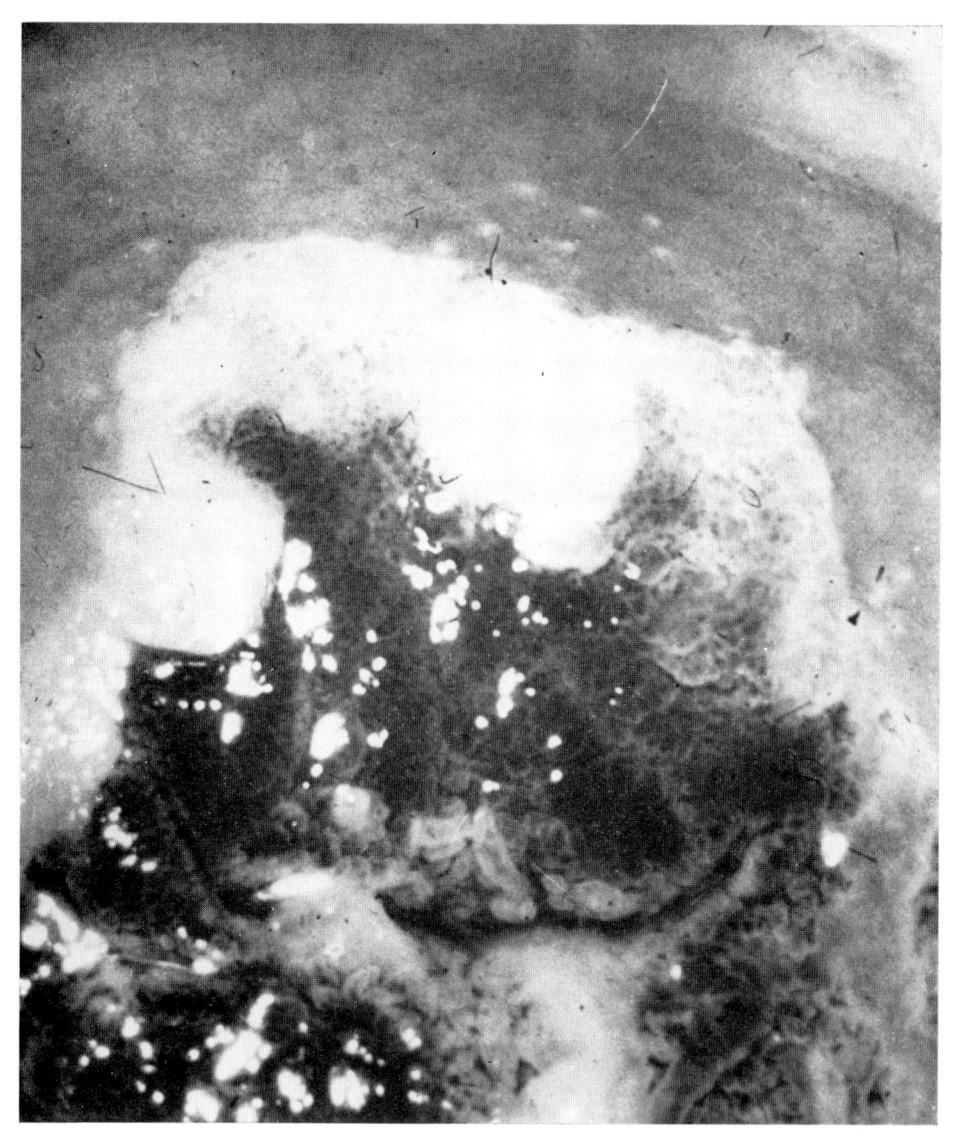

Figure 267. Adolescent cervix: sexually active subject. Colpophotograph of atypical transformation zone with an edge of keratosis especially at its central and left junctions with the original squamous epithelium in the upper quarter of the photograph.

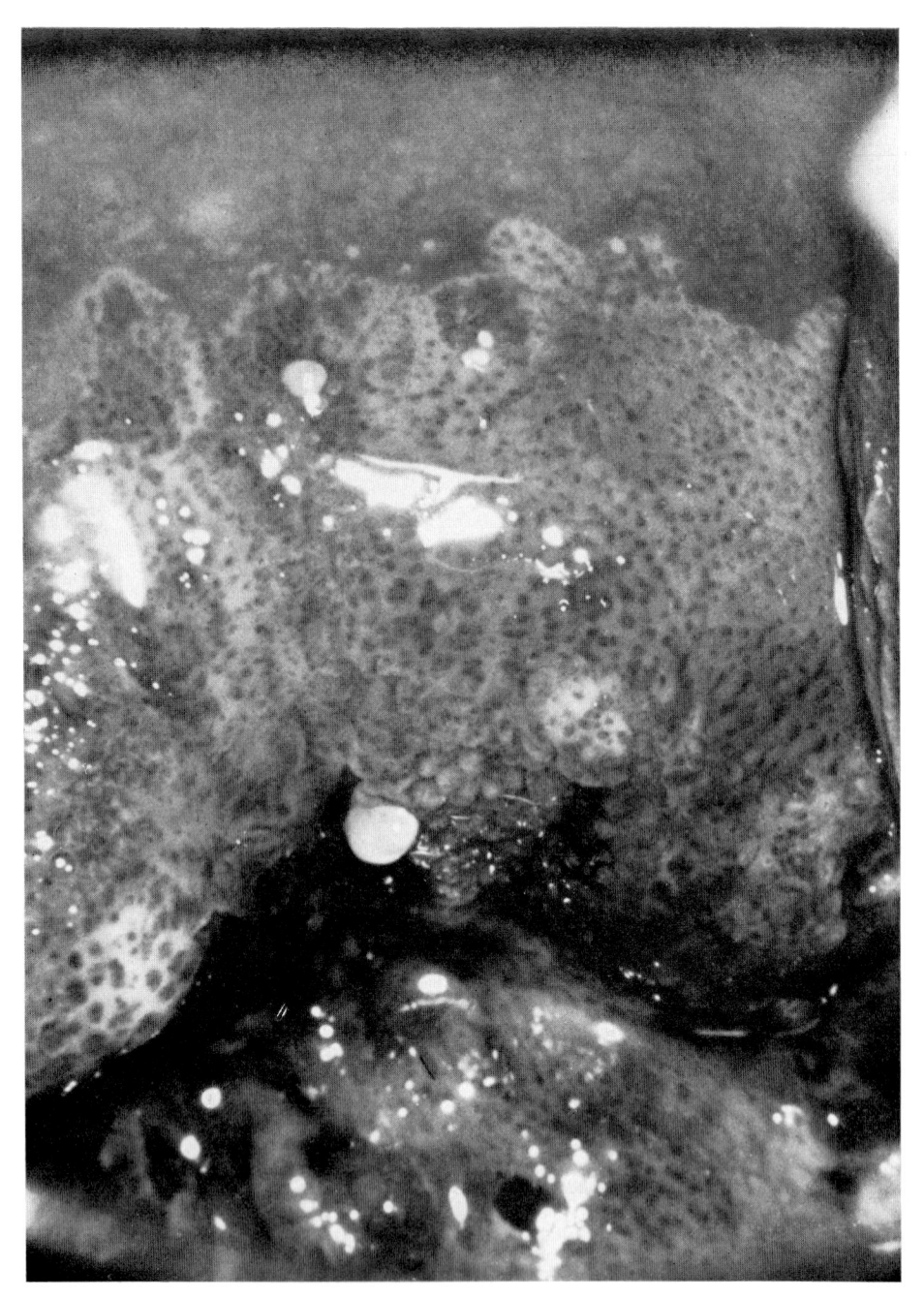

Figure 268. Adolescent cervix: sexually active subject. Colpophotograph of atypical transformation zone showing Grade II white epithelium and punctation. In this and Figures 266 and 267, there is less probability of cytological and histological abnormality than would be predicted in the presence of the same appearances in older women.

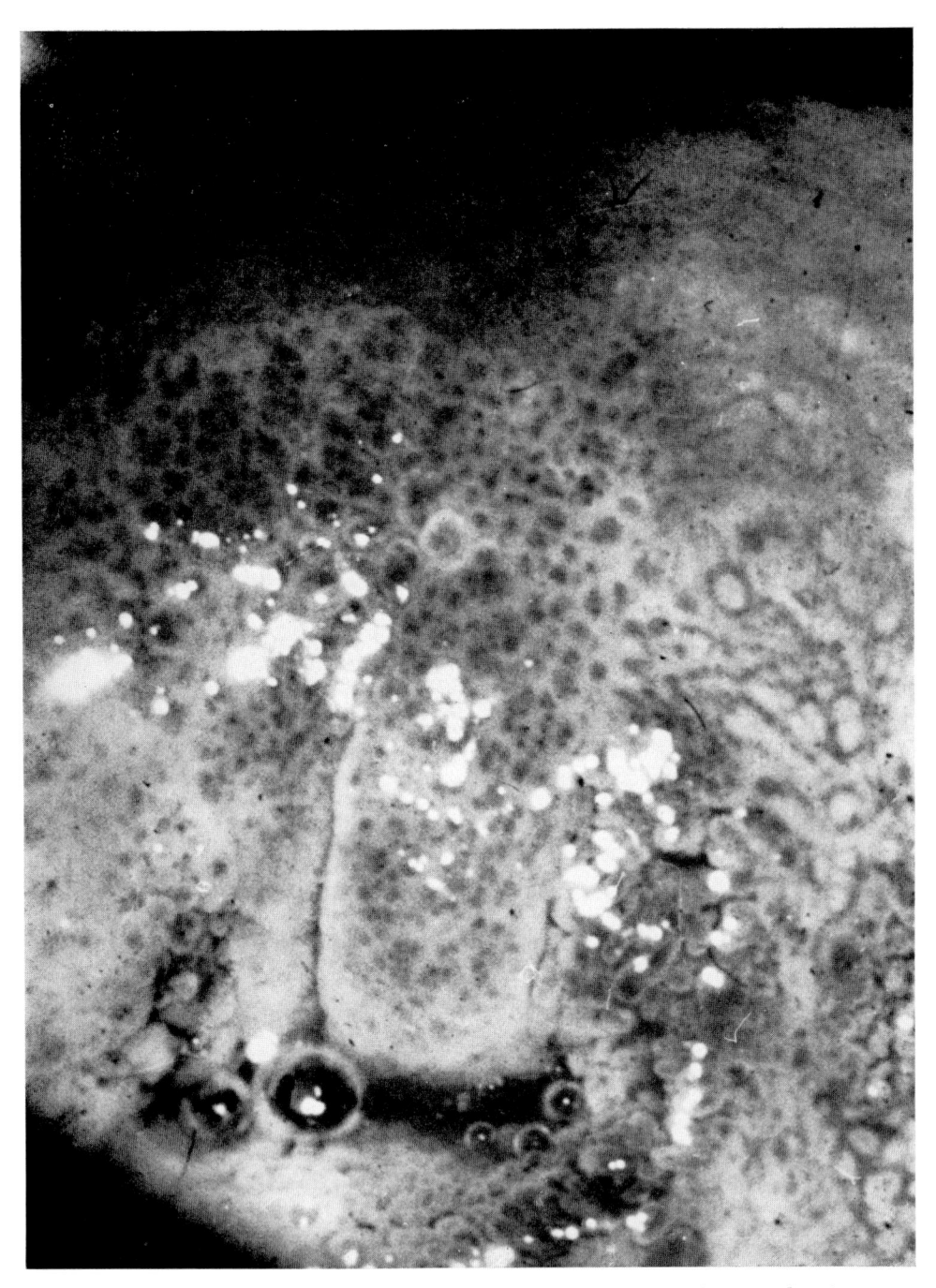

Figure 269. Adolescent cervix: sexually active subject. Colpophotograph of cervix showing punctation and mosaic in the process of formation from the underlying villous structure. Such appearances may predicate the existence of histological abnormality, although this is uncertain.

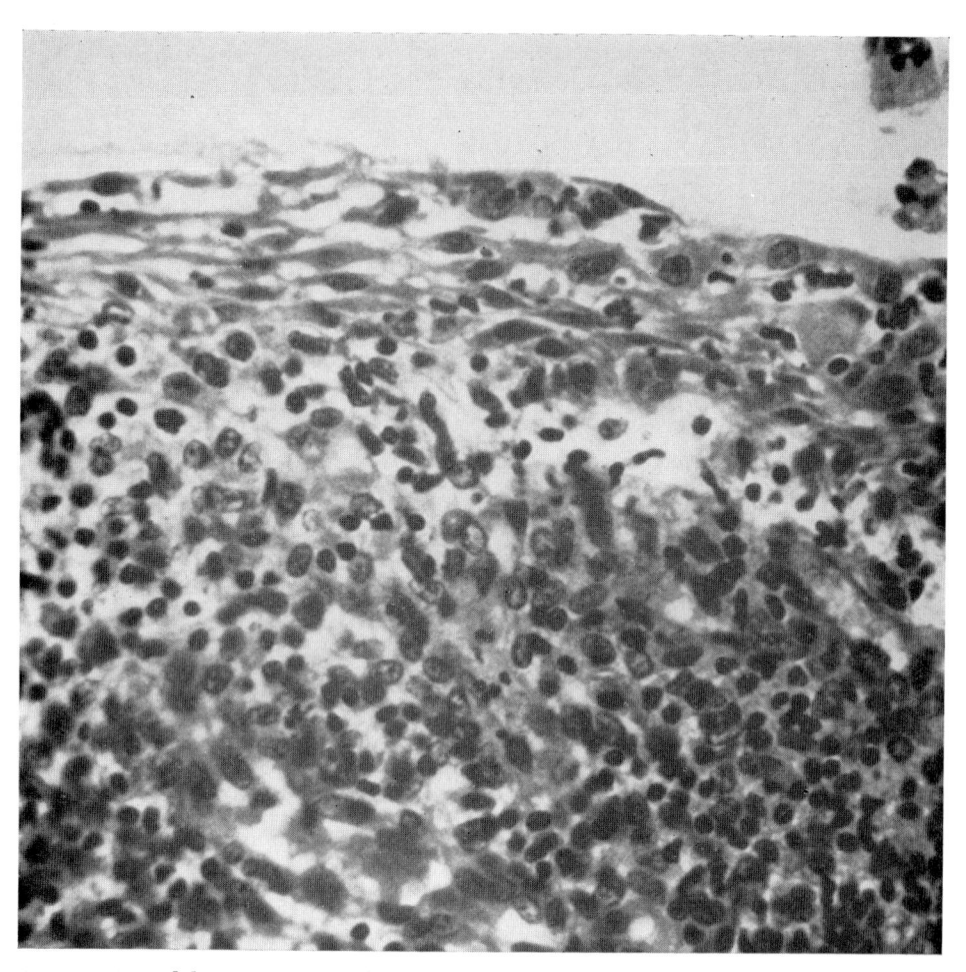

Figure 270. Adolescent cervix: photomicrograph of atypical lesion in promiscuous subject. Immature metaplastic epithelium is present, with infiltration by lymphocytic and mononuclear cells of both stroma and epithelium. The basement membrane is indiscernible.

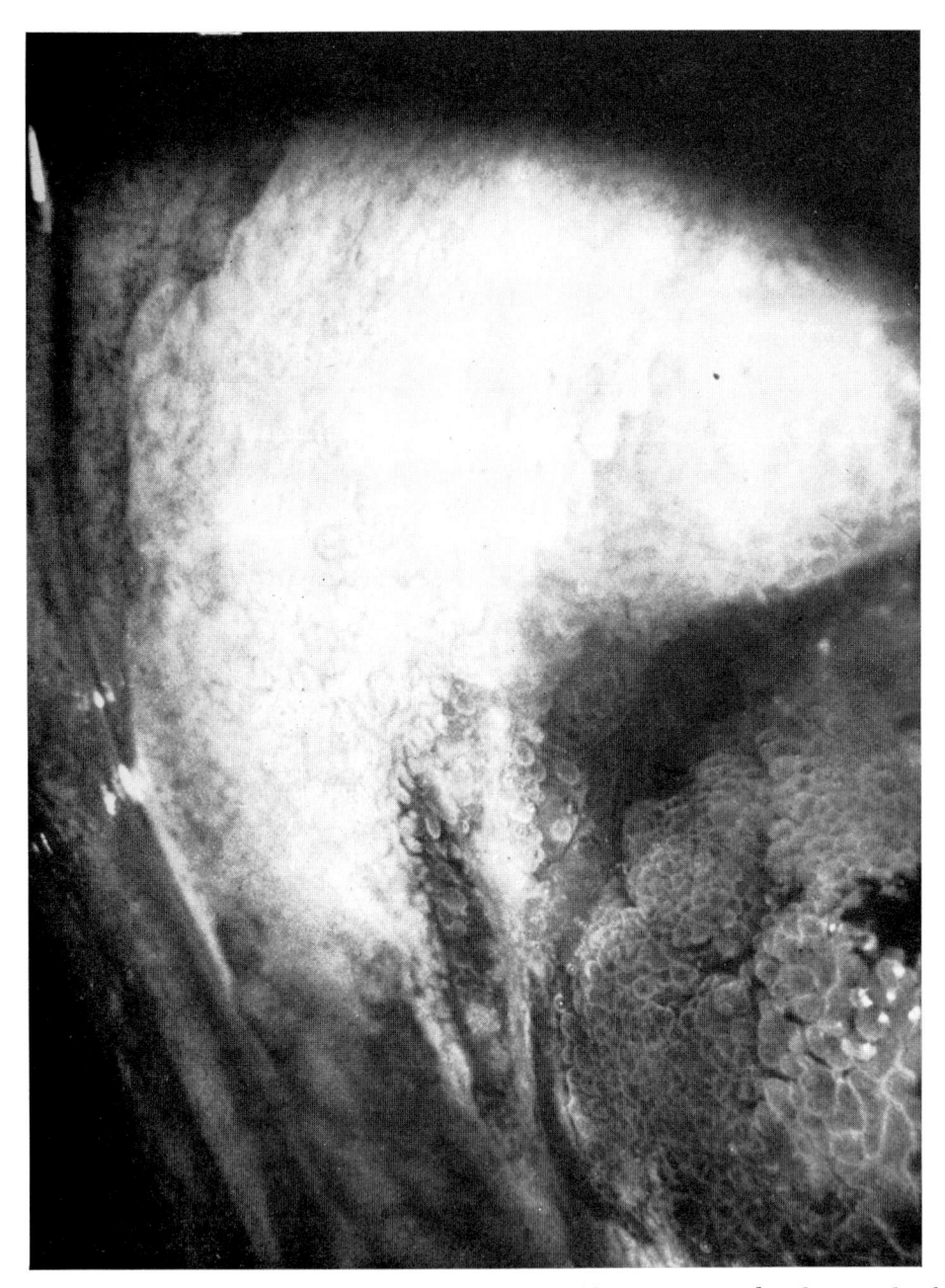

Figure 271. Adolescent cervix: virgin subject aged fifteen years. Colpophotograph of greater part of right half of cervix showing canal at centre right edge. An atypical transformation zone with white epithelium and fine mosaic is visible, probably representing original transformation zone persisting into adolescence.

colposcopic atypia were always more quantitative than qualitative: Colposcopic differentiation was usually impossible. The known absence of squamous cervical cancer in the virgin provides strong evidence for the recognition of colposcopic atypical transformation zones of benign significance and indicates that caution is necessary in regarding all atypical colposcopic appearances as possible precursors of cervical cancer, especially in this age group.

8. ATYPICAL APPEARANCES IN ADOLESCENTS FOLLOWING INTRAUTERINE EXPOSURE TO SYNTHETIC OESTROGENS: The high incidence of atypical appearances on the cervix and vagina following the use of maternally administered diethylstilboestrol has been previously discussed (see Chaps. 13 and 14). These appearances develop in the usual way by metaplastic alteration of columnar epithelium with variable expression of white epithelium, mosaic, punctation, and keratosis (see Figs. 248, 250 and 255 to 259). The development of one such lesion over a period of one year is shown in Figures 272 to 274. The significance of these changes is presently uncertain and has prompted much discussion with a proposed significance from cancer or precancer to normal metaplasia, especially when the latter is in its immature state. The real issue concerns an interpretation of the histology of those lesions which are not obviously immature metaplasia. Some authorities view the histology as indicating "an unusual variant" of metaplasia (p. 353). Others make a diagnosis of intraepithelial neoplasia for the same lesion (p. 339). Evidently, exclusive reliance on histology here is as hazardous as discussed in other contexts of this book, where an elapse of time with its accumulation of evidence and experience from other disciplines is required before the truth becomes apparent.

Our experience with the cervix of a group of adolescent girls not exposed to DES, discussed in the preceding section of this chapter and with the original transformation zone whose description follows this section, suggests that a range of conditions may be represented in the colposcopic appearances of the cervix and vagina of exposed girls. This includes the original transformation zone and varying grades of maturing metaplasia as seen in the adolescent cervix, as well as a true precursor of epithelial neoplasia. Clearly, the colposcope is not always precise in differentiating between these alternatives.

9. ATYPICAL APPEARANCES WITHIN THE ORIGINAL TRANSFORMATION ZONE: A recent review of the colposcopic and histological morphology of a large series of foetal, prepubertal, and adolescent subjects has enabled some new reflections on the results of metaplasia in these early epochs. These reflections have prompted the concept of the *original transformation zone*.

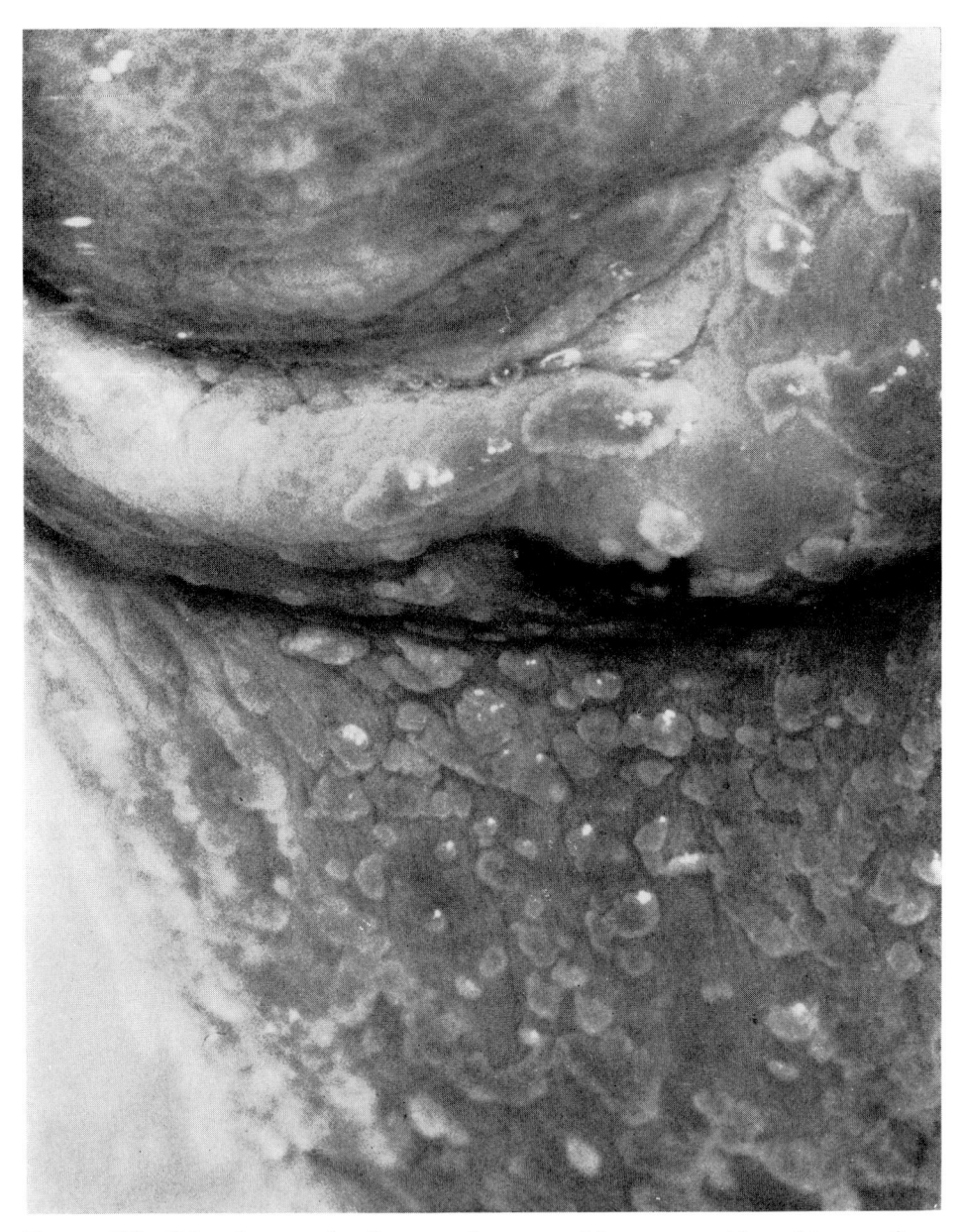

Figure 272. Colpophotograph of twenty-four-year-old woman with a history of exposure to non-steroidal oestrogens *in utero*. Columnar cell covered villi on the vagina occur below a collarlike fold of tissue surrounding the cervix seen in the upper quarter.

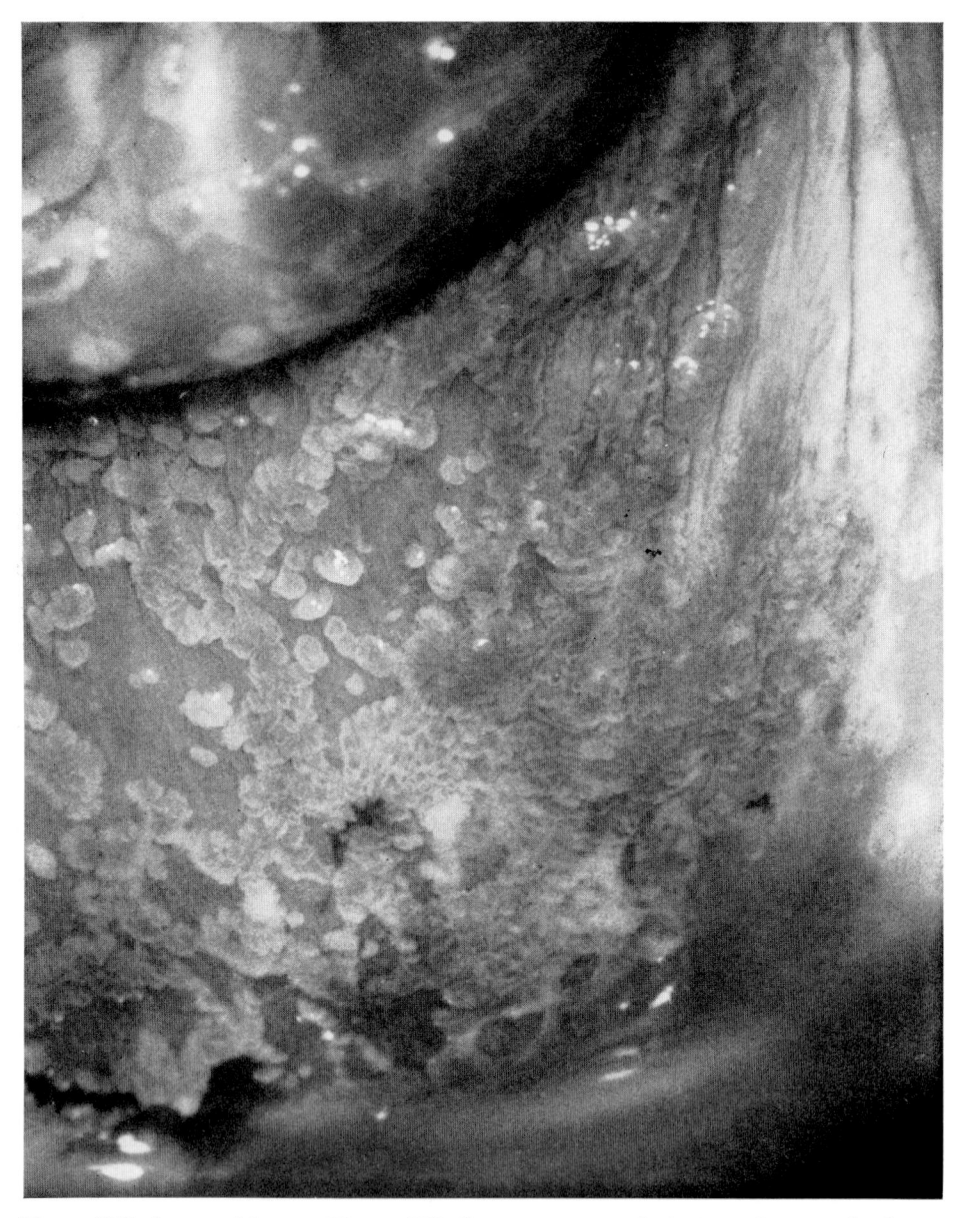

Figure 273. Same subject as Figure 272. Immature metaplasia is evident in the fusion and glazing of villi on the vaginal wall.

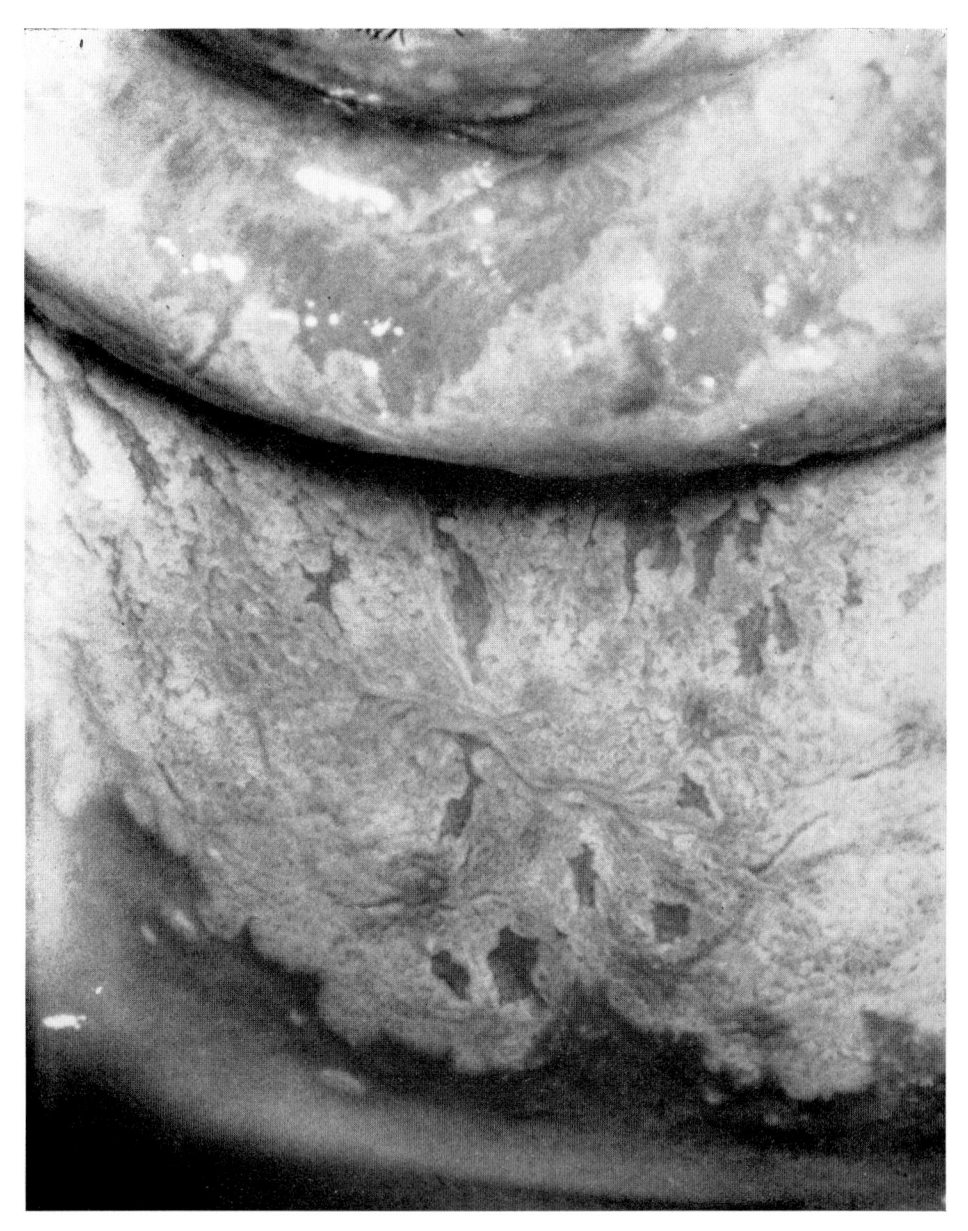

Figure 274. Same subject as Figures 272 and 273, seen at follow-up examination a year later. Atypical transformation zone has evolved. White epithelium has now replaced the original columnar epithelium on the vagina and part of the collar.

Metaplasia may be well established in foetuses at twenty-three weeks of gestation and is certainly present in the majority of subjects at birth, being then designated as original transformation zone. Metaplastic epithelium developing *in utero* persists through infancy and childhood, presenting in adolescence as a recognisable transformation zone. Such original transformation zone may present in adult life with either typical or atypical features. In its atypical form, it represents a further example of appearances of doubtful or physiological significance.

Development

The original transformation zone is best understood by consideration of those differences of metaplasia in foetal life.

The disposition of columnar epithelium at twenty-six weeks is usually flat with a few indentations (Fig. 275). Should metaplasia occur on such a scaffold during or before this early phase of organogenesis, it is probable that a simple uncomplicated sheet of original transformation zone will be laid down. It does not display intraepithelial capillaries to contribute later to the colposcopic image (Fig. 275).

Development of the original columnar epithelium during the latter weeks of gestation results in the appearance of numerous surface projections (Fig. 276). Should metaplasia then occur, it does so upon a scaffold of the new serrated stromal and surface configuration, resulting in the evolution of original transformation zone containing stromal and vascular formations, which can eventually produce a colposcopic image of punctation and mosaic (Fig. 276).

Colposcopic Appearances

The typical variety of the original transformation zone is indistinguishable from its counterpart, the typical transformation zone of the adult woman. This assertion is derived from the mature colposcopic appearance of the metaplastic epithelium of some cervices examined soon after the menarche (Fig. 277). The inference is inescapable that such epithelia have persisted from foetal to adult life.

The atypical variety is most often seen as a circumferential zone of white epithelium usually with fine mosaic and punctation (Figs. 278 and 279). Patchy keratosis is not uncommon, and glandular remnants of the original columnar epithelium are occasionally seen (*see* Fig. 229). Invariably, the area fails to stain following application of iodine solution. When transformation zone is present on the vagina, it is usually of the atypical original variety (Figs. 229 and 279).

Histological Appearances

Histological study of the original transformation zone has confirmed

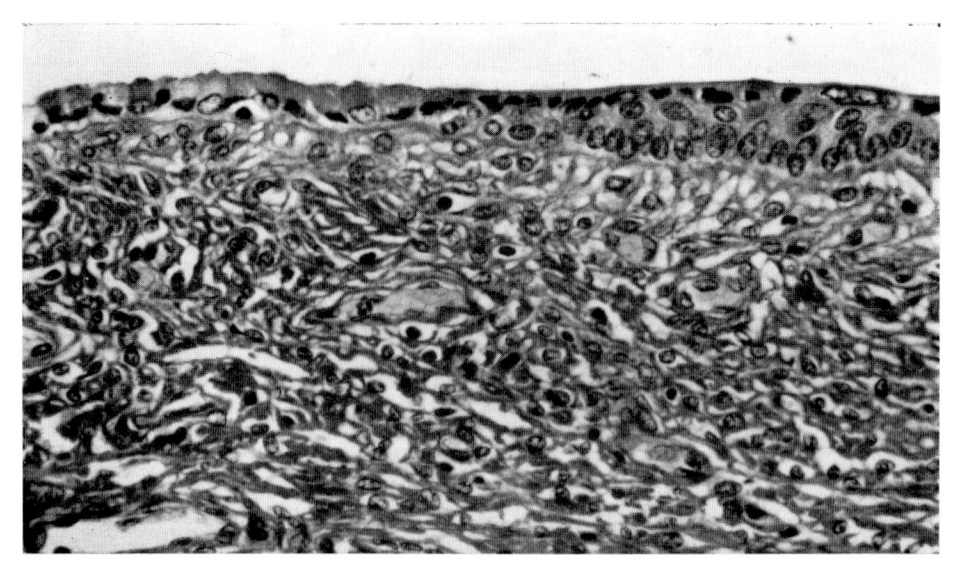

Figure 275. Photomicrograph of part of cervix of twenty-six-week-old foetus at site of original transformation zone. On the left, the columnar epithelium is flat. Developing in early foetal life, the metaplastic epithelium seen on the right has evolved without the intrusion of capillaries.

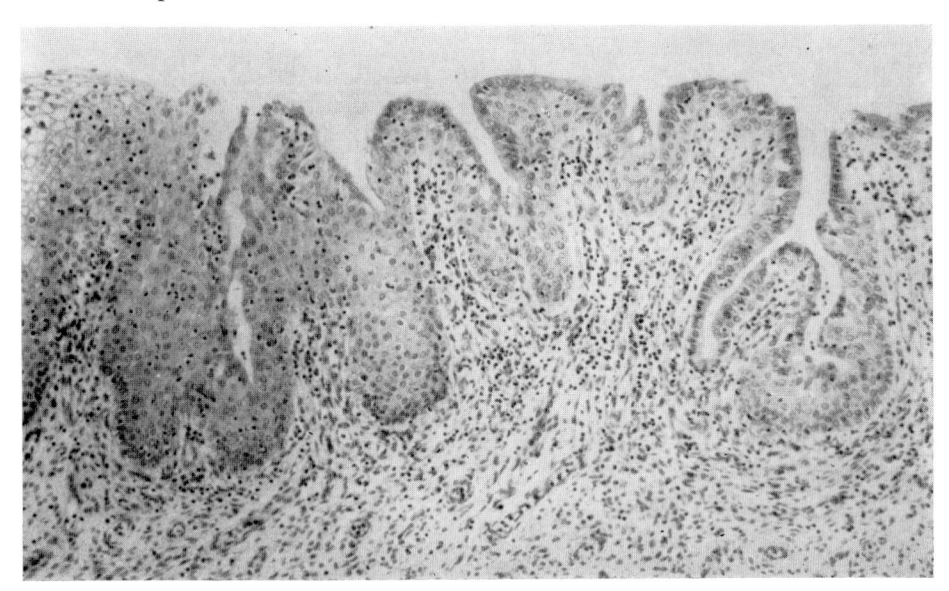

Figure 276. Photomicrograph of part of cervix of thirty-two-week-old foetus at site of original transformation zone. Developing in later foetal life and in contrast to the picture in Figure 275, the evolving transformation zone retains the stromal and vascular scaffold of the complicated columnar surface.

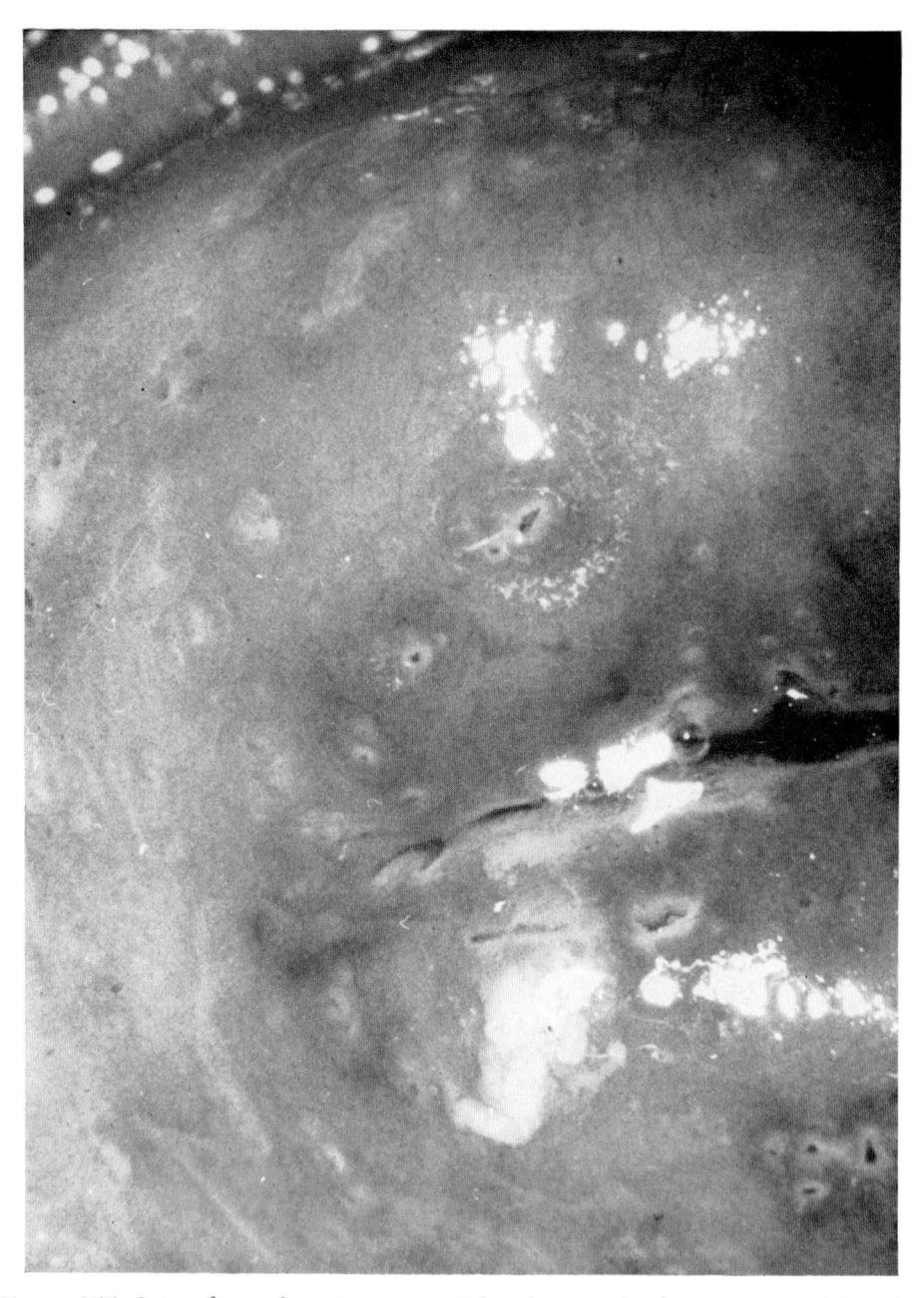

Figure 277. Original transformation zone. Colpophotograph of mature typical transformation zone in a sixteen-year-old. Note an overall similarity to original squamous epithelium, although the presence of gland openings clearly denotes a metaplastic origin. The maturity of the epithelium at this age indicates an origin in early life.

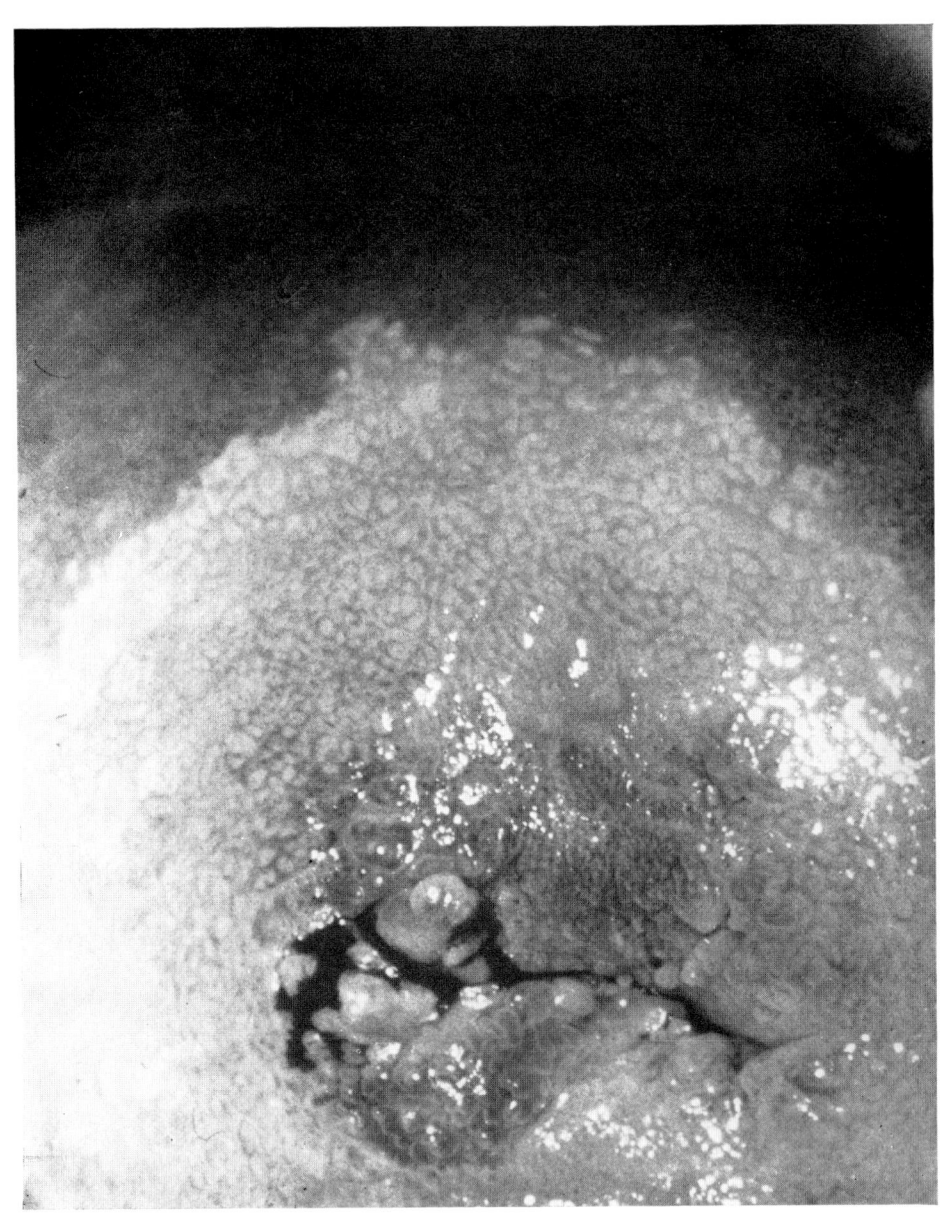

Figure 278. Original transformation zone. Colpophotograph of atypical form of original transformation zone is seen as a circumferential zone of white epithelium with fine mosaic.

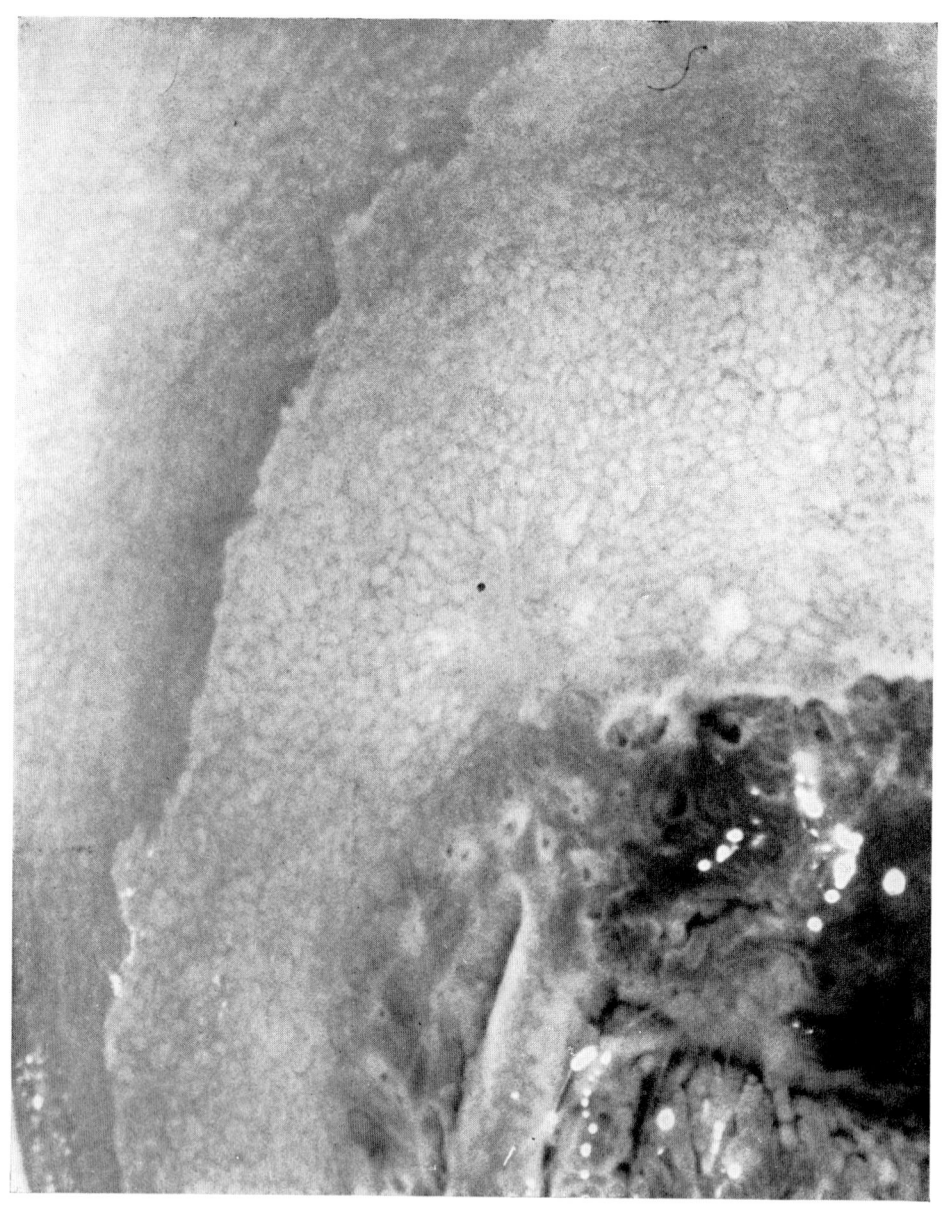

Figure 279. Original transformation zone. Colpophotograph of transformation zone with white epithelium and fine mosaic to the right and below the cervical os. At the bottom of the photograph, the zone continued onto the vaginal wall.

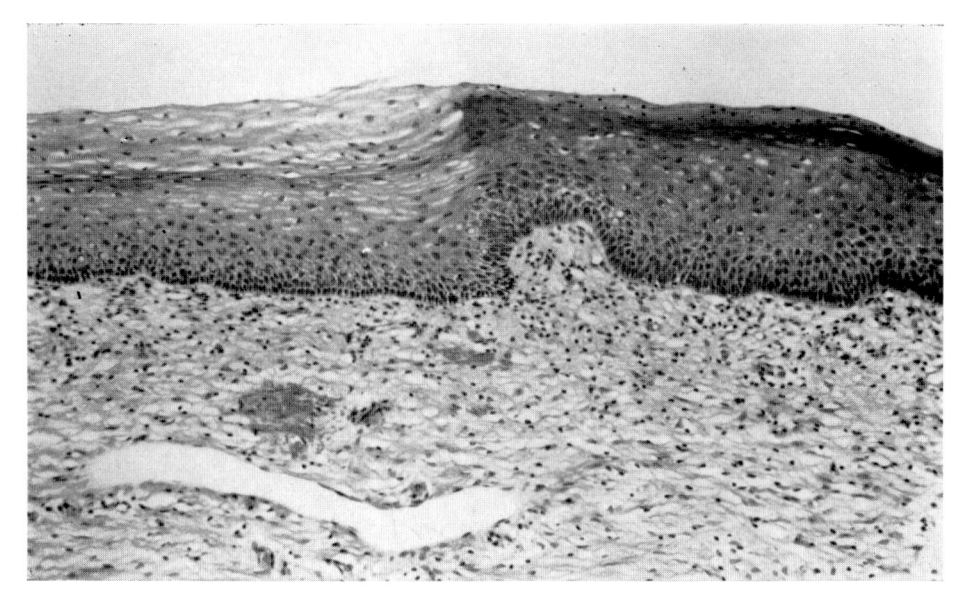

Figure 280. Photomicrograph of biopsy of original transformation zone. A biopsy at the original squamocolumnar junction shows differences in basal cell morphology, differentiation, and cell density of the metaplastic epithelium. The original squamous epithelium on the left is glycogenated, as clinically evidenced by its staining with iodine solution.

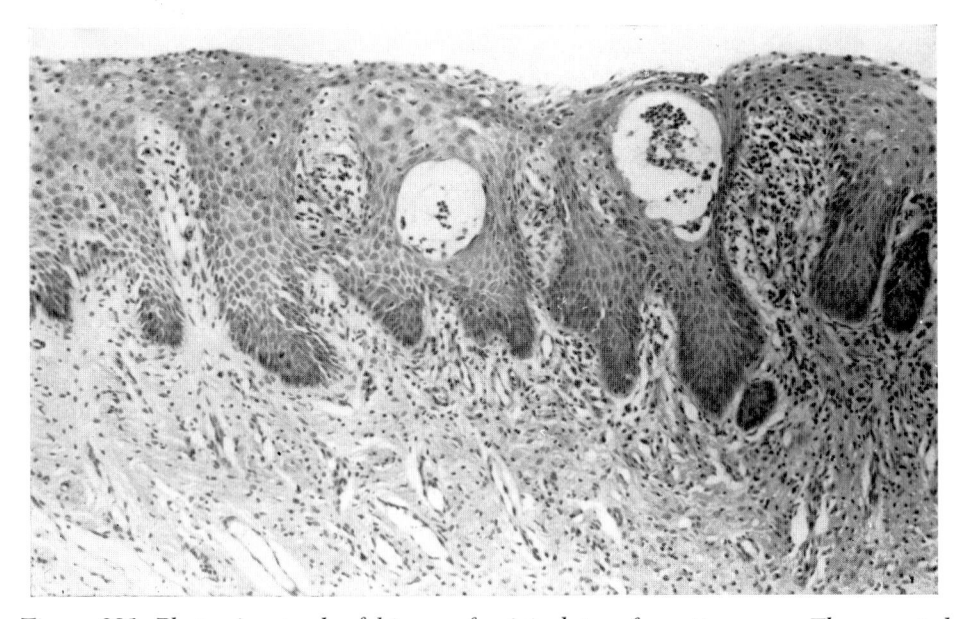

Figure 281. Photomicrograph of biopsy of original transformation zone. The crenated basal layer and intraepithelial vascular structures are remnants of the scaffold of original columnar epithelium.

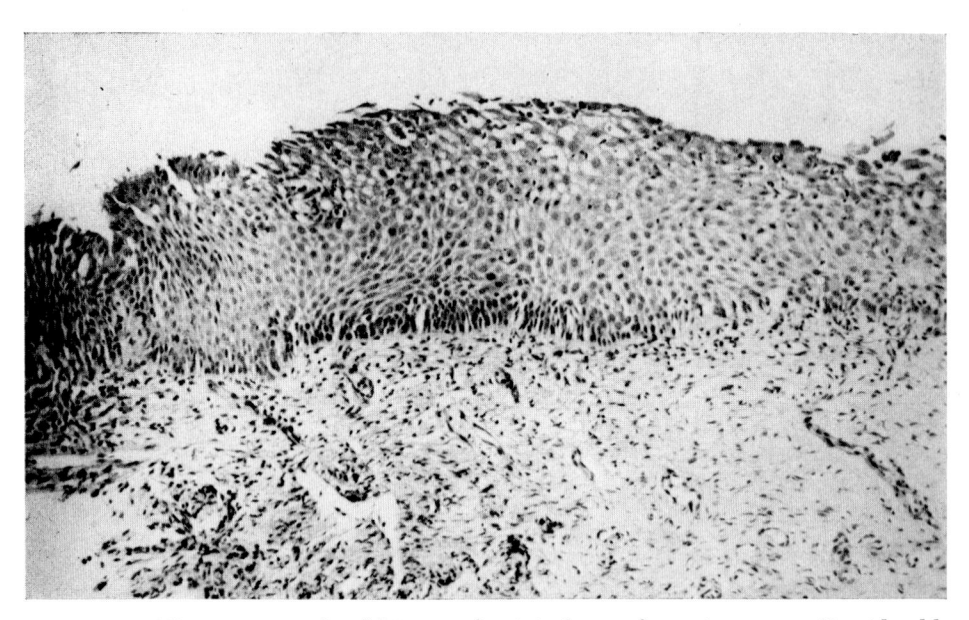

Figure 282. Photomicrograph of biopsy of original transformation zone. Considerable variation in nuclear size, differentiation, and cell density is seen.

the expected wide variety of tissue appearances that metaplasia is known to generate. This epithelial form always differs in many respects from original squamous epithelium. This difference is best seen at the original squamocolumnar junction (Fig. 280). The cells of the basal layer of the metaplastic epithelium are usually markedly different in size, shape, and nuclear characteristics.

The contour of the base is often crenated, presumably reflecting the shape of the original scaffold of the foetal stroma (Fig. 281). Intraepithelial papillae of various shapes are usually present and contain the terminal vascular structures characteristic of punctation and mosaic (Fig. 281).

There is considerable variety in the morphology of parabasal and subsequent cell types, as well as in degree of differentiation evident within the epithelium. This variation in morphological features allows many combinations to which terms of well-differentiated squamous epithelium, basal cell hyperplasia, dysplasia minor, abnormal epithelium, abnormally differentiated epithelium, and other terms might well be applied. Occasionally, the absence of differentiation is major or complete (Fig. 282). It is difficult to reconcile such appearances seen in perinatal life and their absence in biopsies of apparent original transformation zone of the atypical variety seen after puberty without assuming that the phase was evanescent and that the epithelium has differentiated.

The epithelia are invariably non-glycogenated, which is reflected later in the failure to stain with iodine. In random biopsies of a large series of original transformation zones, columnar remnants are infrequently found.

Significance

The emergence of the concept of original transformation zone helped to elucidate the general and vexatious problems of atypical colposcopic appearances associated with histology of trivial significance. Thus, it has a special place because of the clarity with which it shows that not all atypical colposcopic appearances indicate the presence of a cervical cancer precursor.

PART VII
Practical Uses of Colposcopy

Chapter 16

THE USES OF COLPOSCOPY

The use of the colposcope has revolutionized the management of preclinical cervical cancer now that the gynaecologist is afforded direct access to the display of its earliest manifestations. Historically, this display was manifest at first in tissue sections and later from suspicion provided by the use of exfoliative cytology. During the microscopic phase of their development, knowledge and therefore management of these lesions was of necessity derived from an intermediate stance between patient and gynaecologist, that of the microscopist. Bereft of an appreciation of those numerous features of the lesion which derive from their living state and effectively ignorant of the precise site on the living organ from which the tissue under study was derived, the microscopist was therefore under some limitation. The arrival of the colposcope has removed this limitation and once more involves the clinician directly in the assessment of the various stages in the development of neoplasia. By now, its use in management should be obligatory.

In this chapter, the indications for colposcopy and the specific ways in which the use of the method provides us with information of diagnostic, therapeutic, prognostic, and scientific value are laid down. Such information led us first with caution and now with confidence to dictate variable management dependent upon the individual characteristics of each case.

The management about to be recommended might at times be considered unorthodox and controversial to those new to colposcopy. Such objections appear to be theoretical only. They depend on the theory that preclinical cancer as designated by the light microscope carries the same outlook as cancer. There is, at present, no scientific basis for this assumption. Differences between results of conservative treatment of preclinical cancer of the cervix to be anticipated from the theoretical hazards and the actual practical results realised are extensive (Coppleson and Reid, 1967). With a careful selection of cases, the most conservative management seems to have the same outcome as the most radical.

It is becoming increasingly apparent that those firmly based and proven concepts on which the management of established carcinoma in the cervix and that in other organs are planned are neither valid nor proven when applied to preclinical carcinoma of the cervix. In the meantime, until firm advice and new concepts have been thoroughly established for this unique form of "cancer," the less scientific but thoroughly time-tested resort of clinical expediency should be the basis for management. However, a too-ready acceptance of regimes set out in this chapter could lead to mismanagement from inexperience, including the oversight of a frank cancer. The more conservative the management, the more expert the assessment required.

INDICATIONS FOR COLPOSCOPY

The real place of colposcopy is one of continuing debate amongst gynaecologists. Proponents exist for its routine use as a supplement to exfoliative cytology in all initial pelvic examinations, while there are others who propose a more selective role with specific indications. The school in favour of routine use points to the undoubted improvement in accuracy in the detection of precursors of cervical cancer when colposcopy and exfoliative cytology are combined, as shown in the classical reports from the European clinics of Navratil (1964), Limburg (1958), and many others. Similar results from an earlier mass screening programme in our own clinic (Coppleson and Reid, 1967) indicated that of 321 cases of preclinical carcinoma of the cervix, the percentage of positive* results were as follows: colposcopy, 92 per cent; exfoliative cytology, 93 per cent; combined, 98 per cent.

The improved accuracy in diagnosis led to an erroneous impression that the value of colposcopy depended on the effectiveness of the method to detect lesions missed by the exfoliative cytologist. This widely held impression of the exclusiveness of but one minor aspect of the value of colposcopy was also shared by us at the onset of our studies. It was subsequently abandoned as more major values become apparent. However, the studies mentioned above prove that colposcopy does detect such cases and so provides a check on the false negative smear. Furthermore, the smear fails less often if taken directly from lesions detected colposcopically. Estimates of the failure of the cervical smear to indicate the presence of cervical carcinoma in situ have varied from 2.4 to 28 per cent in nineteen different studies (Coppleson and Reid, 1967), and a more recent study (Coppleson and Brown, 1974) supports the higher rates. Without colposcopy, it is impossible to be certain of the true false negative rate, for if a patient has no suggestive symptoms and signs and the smear is negative, the cervix is not usually subjected to any further examination.

It is an ideal and was the practice in our clinic for some years to perform colposcopy *initially* in all women as a secondary screening method. The occasional case of preclinical cervical carcinoma which would have been missed by the smear is detected, and it could be argued that there is

---

* = Atypical transformation zone.
= Positive and doubtful cytology.

the additional advantage in enabling, at the outset, the identification of those dysplasias from which most carcinomas of the cervix ultimately develop.

Routine use of colposcopy is not without some disadvantage and may radically alter the number of biopsies required. Routine use has been advocated by the European sponsors of colposcopy for many years. This practice assumes that all atypical colposcopic lesions may harbour a significant lesion and should be biopsied. Biopsy of about 10 per cent of all cervices examined would, therefore, be required. In fact, atypical colposcopic appearances are frequently seen with no atypical cytological counterpart and are found on biopsy to be histologically insignificant. In this era of routine cytological screening, the extravagant biopsy rate required to assess such lesions does not convince many gynaecologists of the importance of routine colposcopy in discerning the occasional lesion overlooked by the smear, particularly when repetitive smears would probably have uncovered its presence.

A more practical policy, if routine colposcopy is employed, is to perform selective biopsy only of the colposcopic atypias. Qualitative grading of the colposcopic atypias, especially if correlated carefully with the exfoliative cytology report, allows a high degree of accuracy in predicting the histology report and this allows the effective use of selective cervical biopsy. Whereas the malignancy index of all colposcopic atypias is frequently stated to be between 6 and 14 per cent thus suggesting a high false positive rate, with the system of grading described (p. 242), a histological diagnosis of preclinical invasive carcinoma, carcinoma in situ, or major dysplasia may be correctly forecast in about 95 per cent of Grade III atypias and a benign lesion or minor dysplasia in about 95 per cent of Grade I atypias. Upon careful correlation with the exfoliative cytology report, great accuracy can also be achieved with Grade II atypias.

The decision between routine or selective use for colposcopy rests with the individual gynaecologist and is probably influenced by ancillary factors, such as time available and work schedules. In general, routine use by most gynaecologists and in most clinics seems precluded on grounds of cost and organization.

Practical Indications for Colposcopy

The practical compromise adopted is the restriction of colposcopic examinations to all women from whom positive or doubtful cervical smears have been obtained and to those women who have "relatively suspicious" or "suspicious" naked-eye cervical appearances.

Selective screening of groups of women compatible with the facilities at present available within our clinic is also undertaken. Symptom-free women attending a cancer detection clinic are all screened initially by colposcopy, and other groups are selected from time to time for colposcopic study, depending on current research projects.

For those learning the colposcopic technique, examination of females en masse is advocated to develop interpretative ability in this subjective field and to enlarge experience in the many and varied physiological and pathological colposcopic appearances.

Examination may take place in the office, the outpatient department, or the operating theatre. The establishment of a special colposcopy clinic within the hospital is an essential of organization, so that the examinations may be done speedily and separately from the initial gynaecological examination. Matters may be further expedited by the presence of another colposcope in the operating theatre, where indications exist prior to other diagnostic or therapeutic procedure and where conditions are often optimal for maximum exposure and ideal visualization.

Even with the selective use of colposcopy, in all women with positive or doubtful smear reports, it is clear that more trained personnel are required. Widespread implementation of this policy can only be achieved by increasing the number of gynaecologists expert in the method, by training programmes with basic and advanced courses of instruction, by the greater use of trained personnel as in satellite clinics (Stafl and Mattingly, 1973), and by the use of paramedical personnel as advocated by Townsend (1971).

RECOGNITION OF PRECLINICAL CARCINOMA OF THE CERVIX

Without colposcopy, the clinician has but the vaguest view of the subject of his enquiry. Preclinical carcinoma of the cervix is then a truly ghostly disease, and an accurate idea of the size, site, orientation, and quality of each individual lesion is impossible. Such imprecise ideas beget irresolute practices of management. Diagnostic and treatment schedules then tend towards inflexibility, radicality, and irrationality.

With colposcopy, the clinician can see the majority of histological preclinical carcinoma of the cervix (Table VI).

Of 321 patients with preclinical carcinoma of the cervix (Stage O and Stage 1A) all of whom had been colposcopically examined before histo-

TABLE VI

321 PATIENTS WITH PRECLINICAL CARCINOMA OF THE CERVIX

	Colposcopy (%)	*Naked Eye* (%)
Suspicious (atypical TZ)	92	14
Not suspicious	8	86

logical verification, atypical colposcopic lesions were recognised in 92 per cent (Coppleson and Reid, 1967). With the unaided eye, the clinician cannot recognise the majority of these early lesions for they have no distinctive features. In fact, of the 14 per cent with suspicious macroscopic features, colposcopy subsequently demonstrated that in some the area marked as suspicious by the gynaecologist was of benign nature and not the site of the carcinoma.

False Negative Colposcopy

As with any other technique in clinical use, false negatives do occur. The colposcope uncommonly fails to diagnose the presence of a lesion. In considering false negatives, there are three major difficulties with colposcopic interpretation which prevent adequate assessment in a small minority of women with lesions. The first of these problems, a rare occurrence in our experience, is the lesion exclusively located high in the cervical canal. The second problem, not so uncommon, is the increased vascularity often with contact bleeding, of an acute cervicitis, e.g. of *Trichomonas vaginalis* or other parasitic origin which tends to mask the true nature of the underlying epithelium (Fig. 283). The third difficulty occurs in postmenopausal women where the cervix has become rigid and inelastic; if the transformation zone has receded into the cervical canal (p. 114), a thorough survey is difficult with colposcopy (Fig. 284).

If preclinical carcinoma or dysplasia is present on the visible portion of the cervix, an atypical lesion is seen by colposcopy. As a corollary, if the colposcopic appearance is not atypical, such epithelium does not harbour a lesion, so that either the colposcopic findings have been misinterpreted, the histology should be reviewed, or the biological significance of the histological report is in doubt.

In most cases, there is a satisfactory correlation between the two techniques. In the absence of such correlation, the authority of histology is traditionally overriding, and the failure of colposcopy is always assumed. In other words, those cervices not considered by colposcopy to be suspicious but subsequently shown to have preclinical carcinoma or dysplasia on histological examination are regarded as *false negative*. While such assumption is acceptable when planning treatment, to accept the histological report as an indicator of biological potential is untenable. The predicament of the histopathologist, the subjectivity of this type of diagnosis, the causes of its errors, and its inability to determine the prognosis of these lesions have been discussed elsewhere (Coppleson and Reid, 1967; Coppleson, 1977). It is probable that an epithelium unequivocally colposcopically benign but histologically exhibiting preclinical carcinoma would, if put to the only true test, observation without treatment, never progress to undoubted clinical cancer.

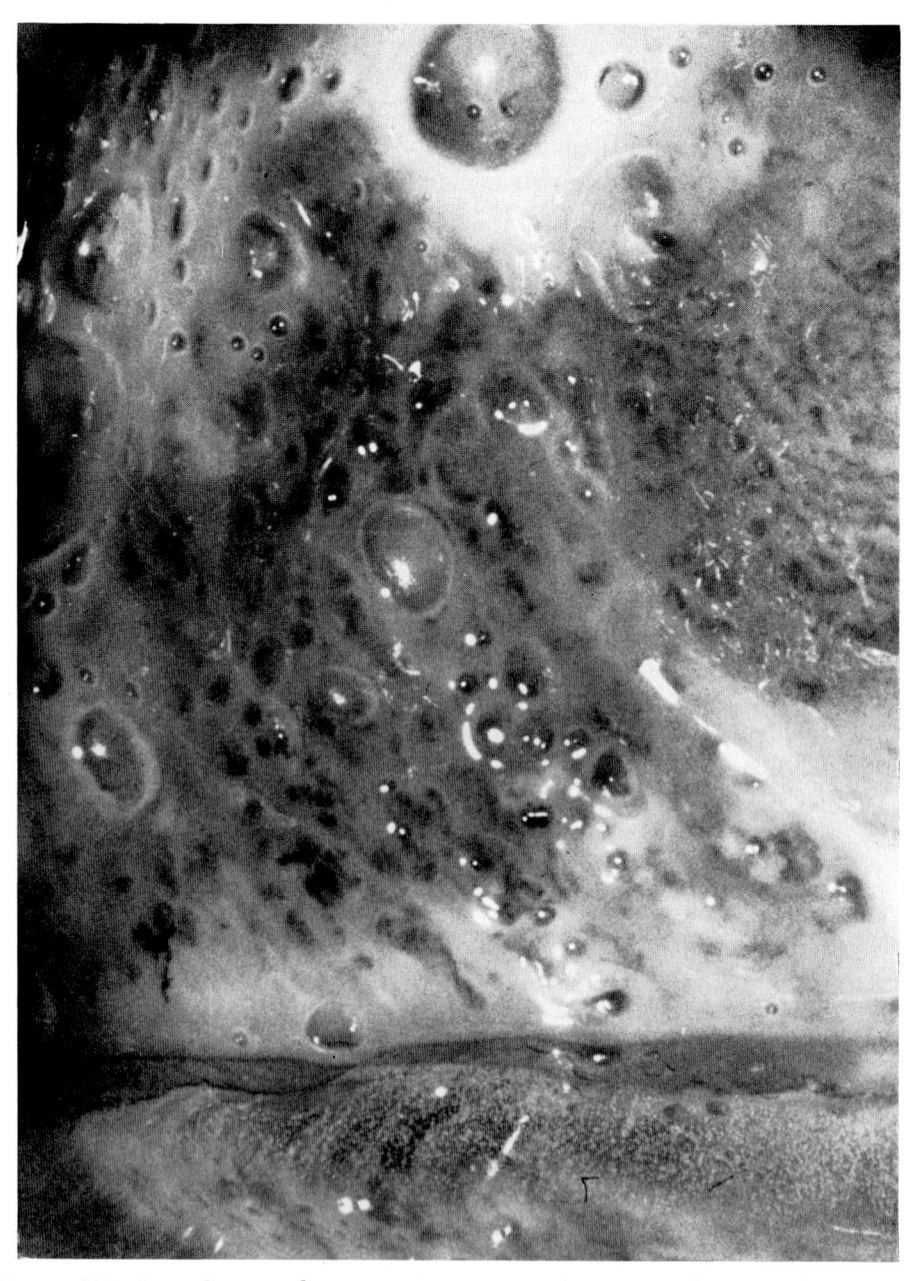

Figure 283. Inconclusive colposcopy. A severe Trichomonas infestation obscures important morphological detail. The condition must be successfully treated before adequate colposcopic opinion can be given.

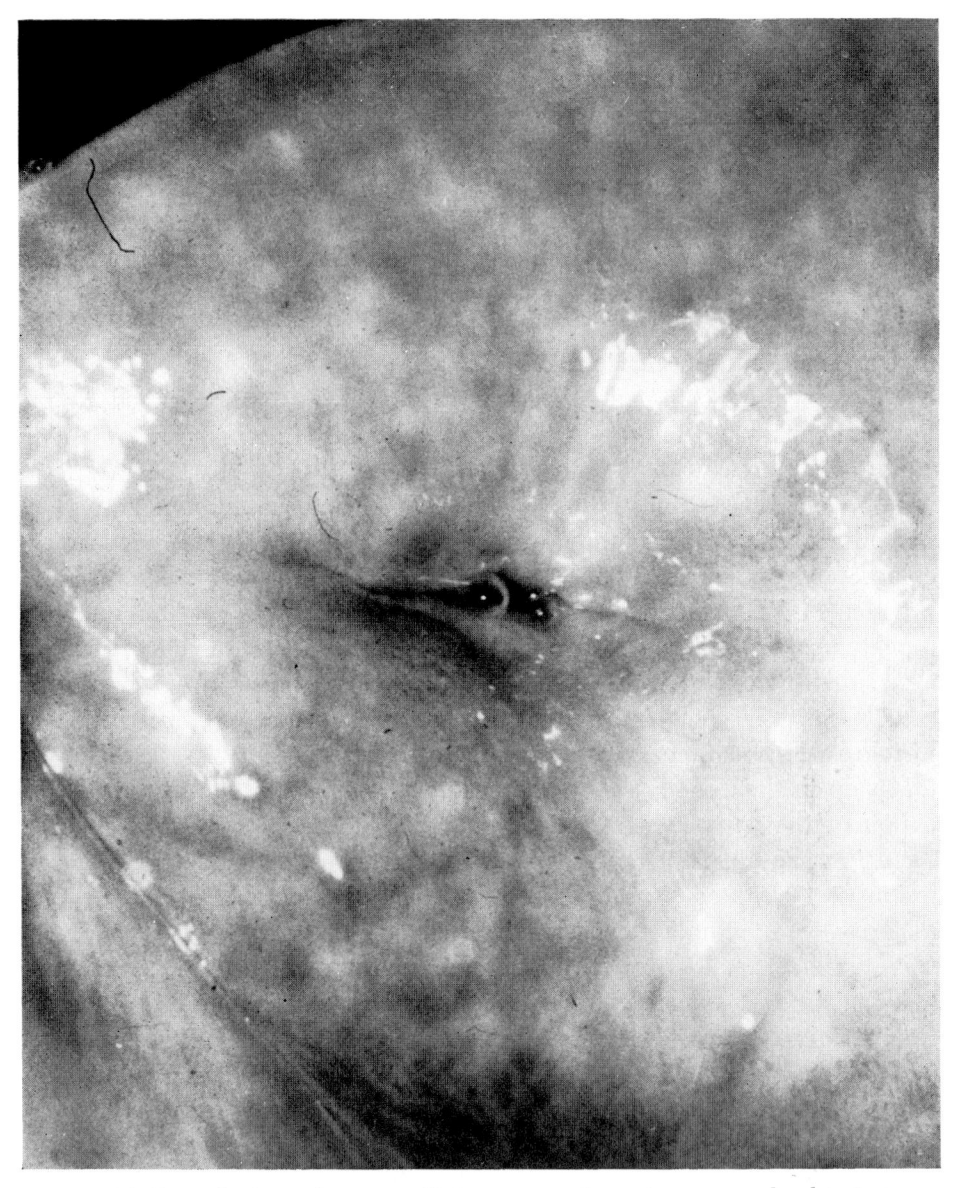

Figure 284. Inconclusive colposcopy. It is common in postmenopausal subjects to encounter the atrophic rigid cervix that does not allow examination of the endocervical canal.

AIDS EVALUATION OF ABNORMAL SMEAR

Colposcopy achieves its most valuable use in the management of a woman with an abnormal smear. Excellent as its properties for mass screening of apparently well women are, it is evident that the major purpose of the smear technique is to select women suspected of harbouring cervical lesions for more careful scrutiny by other methods. It is unfortunately true that exfoliative cytology is not a definitive test for the presence or absence of cervical cancer. The occurrence of false positive and false negative smears with a residual or "doubtful" group labelled "suspicious" or, if less significant, "atypical" or in the original numerical Papanicolaou classification, Class III, reduces the expectations of two or three decades ago that this simple test would clearly diagnose the disease. Despite some improvement from technical refinements, such as through reporting by predictive histological diagnosis, a real need has always existed for some check on the cervical smear.

Supplementary colposcopic examination fulfills just such a need, and its use is mandatory after the presence of but one abnormal smear. Such a study allows reassuring comparison of smear and appearance of lesion with histological findings on biopsy. Repeat smears should succeed and not precede colposcopic examination, if only for possible prejudice to the colposcopic opinion due to trauma from taking the smear. The common practice of following women with minor abnormalities of the smear by repeated smear taking is as irrational as it is disquieting to the patient and is no substitute for summary complete colposcopic evaluation.

A "surprise" finding of an abnormal smear is associated with a range of histological appearances, from invasive cancer to normal. The most important step in the cytological-colposcopic-histological workup is the identification of the truly invasive lesion, an uncommon entity requiring immediate intervention and radical treatment. The ready discernment of such lesions is facilitated by the colposcope. The rest of the lesions, the great majority, can be more conservatively managed after initial colposcopic survey. The broad array of appearances within this group, with which histologists are concerned, includes microinvasive carcinoma, carcinoma in situ, and major and minor dysplasias. This extensive subdivision turns out to have but limited significance from the colposcopic viewpoint. However, in general terms, *major* histological grades, such as microinvasive carcinoma, carcinoma in situ, and major dysplasia, have colposcopic pictures indicating a greater malignant potential than *minor* histological grades. The therapeutic significance of this simple subdivision will become evident.

Grading of Atypical Colposcopic Appearances as a Guide to Management and Prognosis

The existence of subtle variations in the colposcopic picture incorporating differences of colour and blood vascular patterns allows the gradation of these appearances into classes with more potent clinical and prognostic value as a supplement to the histological opinion. These different grades of atypical colposcopic appearances have already been described (p. 242).

Expert colposcopic examination of women with abnormal smears enables differentiation into five categories and allows some distinction between lesions which are important from those which are not:

1. COLPOSCOPICALLY OVERT CARCINOMA: This small but most important group signifies overt cancer, which becomes colposcopically conspicuous despite the absence of any irregularity to the naked eye. The appearances betoken a truly invasive growth requiring radical treatment (Fig. 285).

2. MAJOR ATYPICAL COLPOSCOPIC APPEARANCES (GRADE III): Indicated is a highly significant lesion requiring maximum histological study prior to the final decision regarding management to exclude the possible presence of invasive carcinoma (Fig. 286).

3. LESSER ATYPICAL COLPOSCOPIC APPEARANCES (GRADES II AND I): This category is comprised of the majority of cases derived from the pool resulting from abnormal exfoliative cytology and associated with a histological diagnosis of dysplasia or carcinoma in situ (Figs. 287 and 288). Rarely, the histology reveals minimal areas of breach of the basement membrane. Such striking histological stigmata of invasion are not to be reconciled with the less striking colposcopic picture and are certainly not indicative of that radical management which the microscopic appearance alone might encourage.

In this category, minor interference only is generally required both for diagnosis and treatment.

4. INCONCLUSIVE FINDINGS: This category includes those cases where the junction between the squamous epithelium (either original or metaplastic) and columnar epithelium cannot be seen in its entirety. Lesions may therefore exist in the endocervical canal beyond the scope of the instrument (Fig. 286). Colposcopic findings are then inconclusive, and thorough evaluation is not possible without the devices of either endocervical curettage or cone biopsy. The colposcopic appearance is also compromised by the concurrent presence of cervical hyperaemia due to the presence of acute cervicitis of trichomonad, gonococcal, or other origin. Reassessment is necessary following appropriate therapy (Fig. 283).

5. NORMAL COLPOSCOPIC APPEARANCES: In this group, where the whole of the transformation zone is on view and evidently physiological and columnar epithelium is visible surrounding the cervical canal, the smear is probably false positive (Fig. 289).

Grading of atypical colposcopic appearances, in addition to their practical importance, may also have a prognostic significance.

Despite other more complicated and refined techniques existing for the study of cervical epithelium, it is possible that colposcopy may, for example, distinguish carcinomas in situ or dysplasias which are truly premalig-

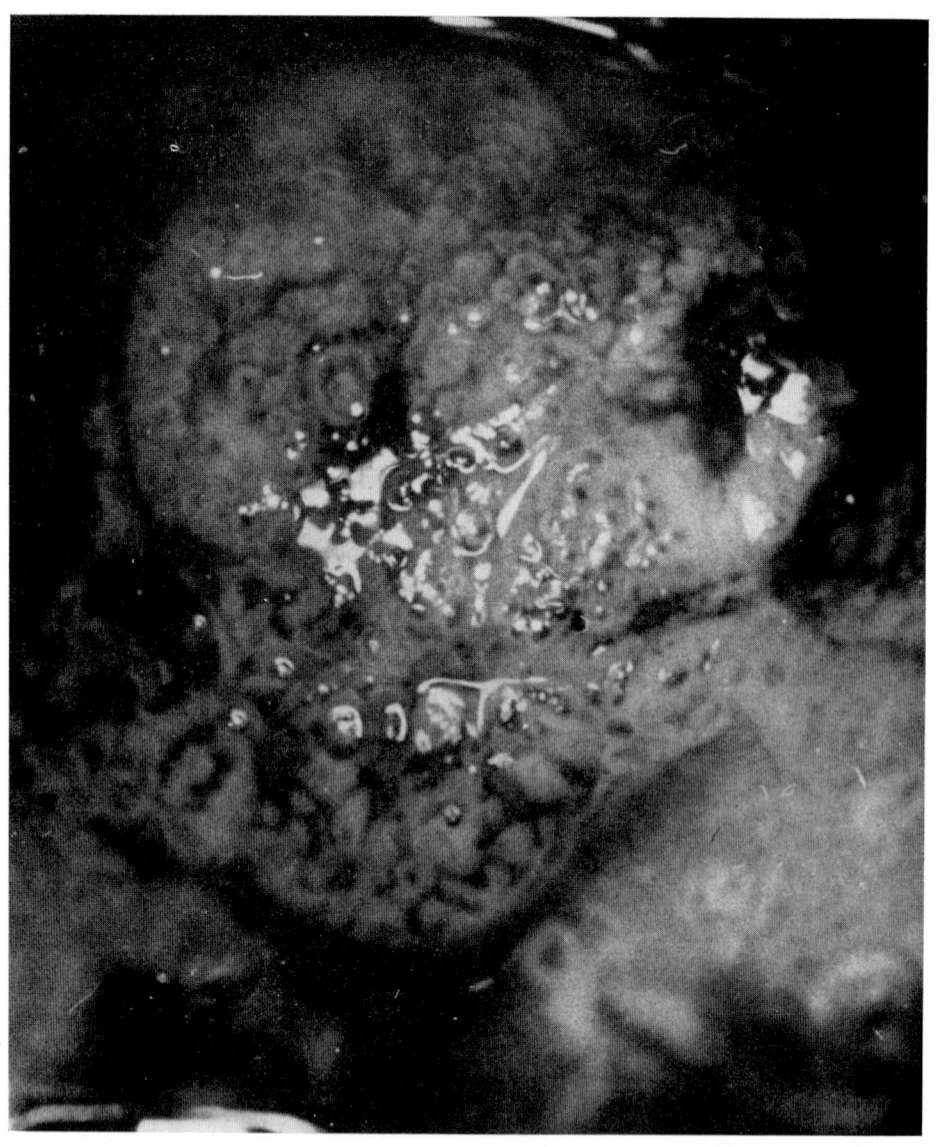

Figure 285. Colposcopically overt cancer. The surface configuration and vascular structures indicate overt cancer. Diagnosis is best established by wedge biopsy, and radical methods of treatment are indicated as for clinically overt cancer.

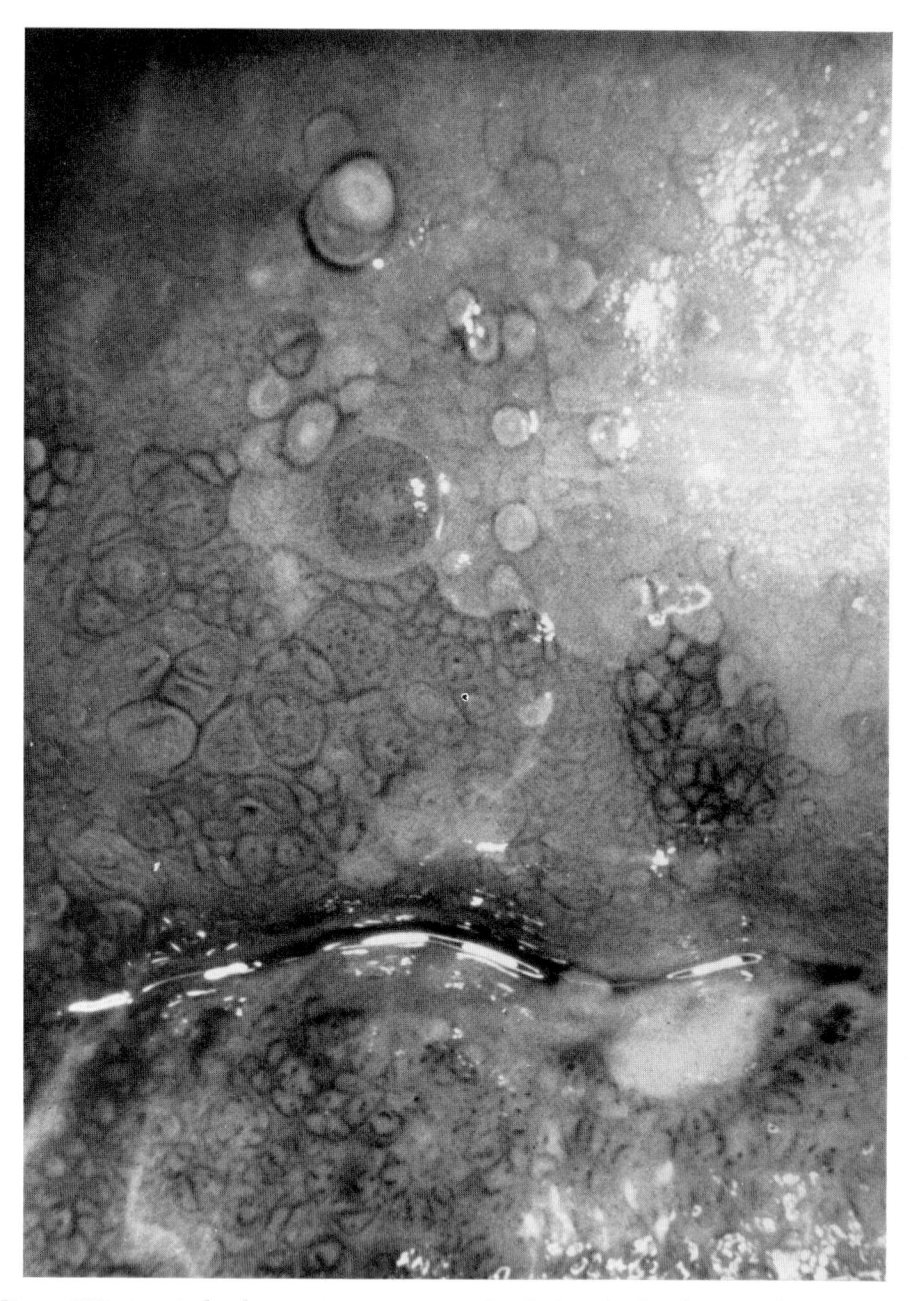

Figure 286. Atypical colposcopic appearance. Grade III. Such a lesion indicates serious potential for invasive behaviour. The mosaic structure is extensive and displays grossly irregular fields surrounded by vessels that are often superficial and dilated. The cervical os appears as a transverse slit in the lower quarter. The lesion extends beyond the endocervical limit of vision and a large cone biopsy is required to exclude the presence of invasive carcinoma.

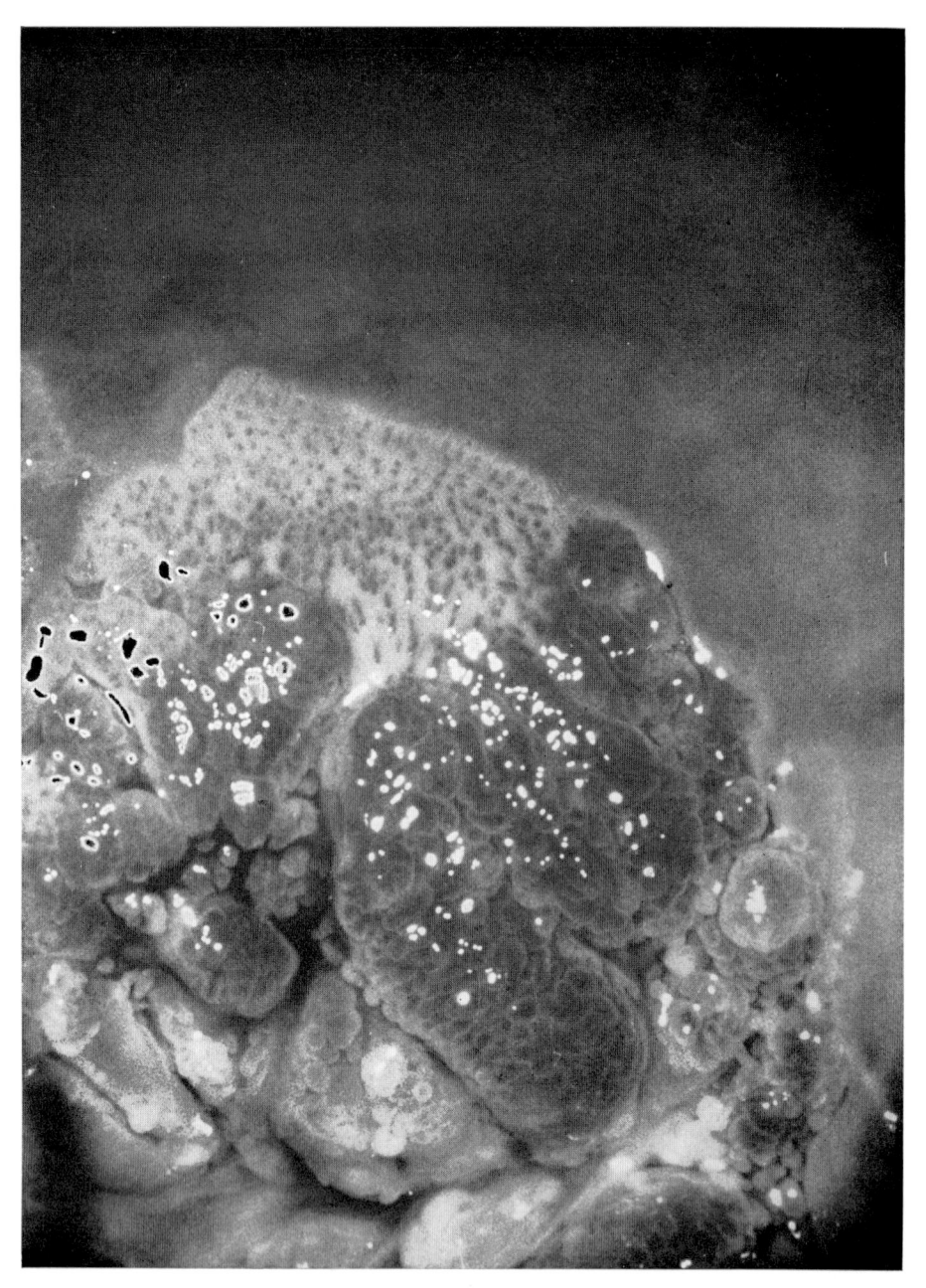

Figure 287. Atypical colposcopic appearance Grade II. This lesion displays no immediate potential for neoplastic behaviour. There is a coarse punctation within a small focal area of white epithelium situated at the peripheral extent of the transformation zone on the anterior lip. A confident prediction of major dysplasia or carcinoma in situ can be made. The new squamocolumnar junction is readily seen, and the lesion is eminently suitable for management by colposcopically directed punch biopsy and physical destruction by electrocoagulation, cryosurgery, or CO_2 laser.

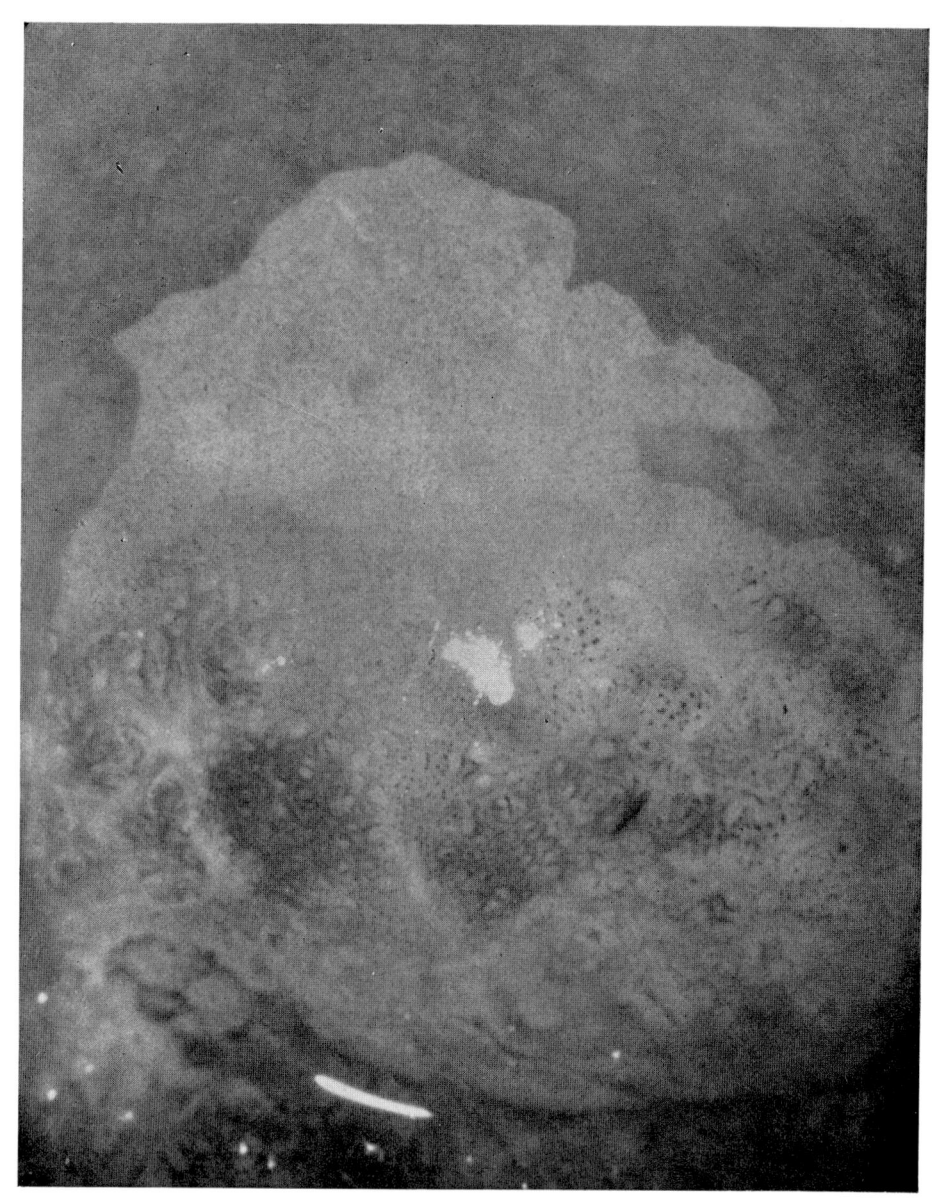

Figure 288. Atypical transformation zone. Grade I. This lesion indicates minimal potential for invasive behaviour. A large area of white epithelium is seen on the anterior lip. The terminal capillaries are small and closely spaced within the areas of punctation and mosaic. At most, a minor histological disorder is predicted.

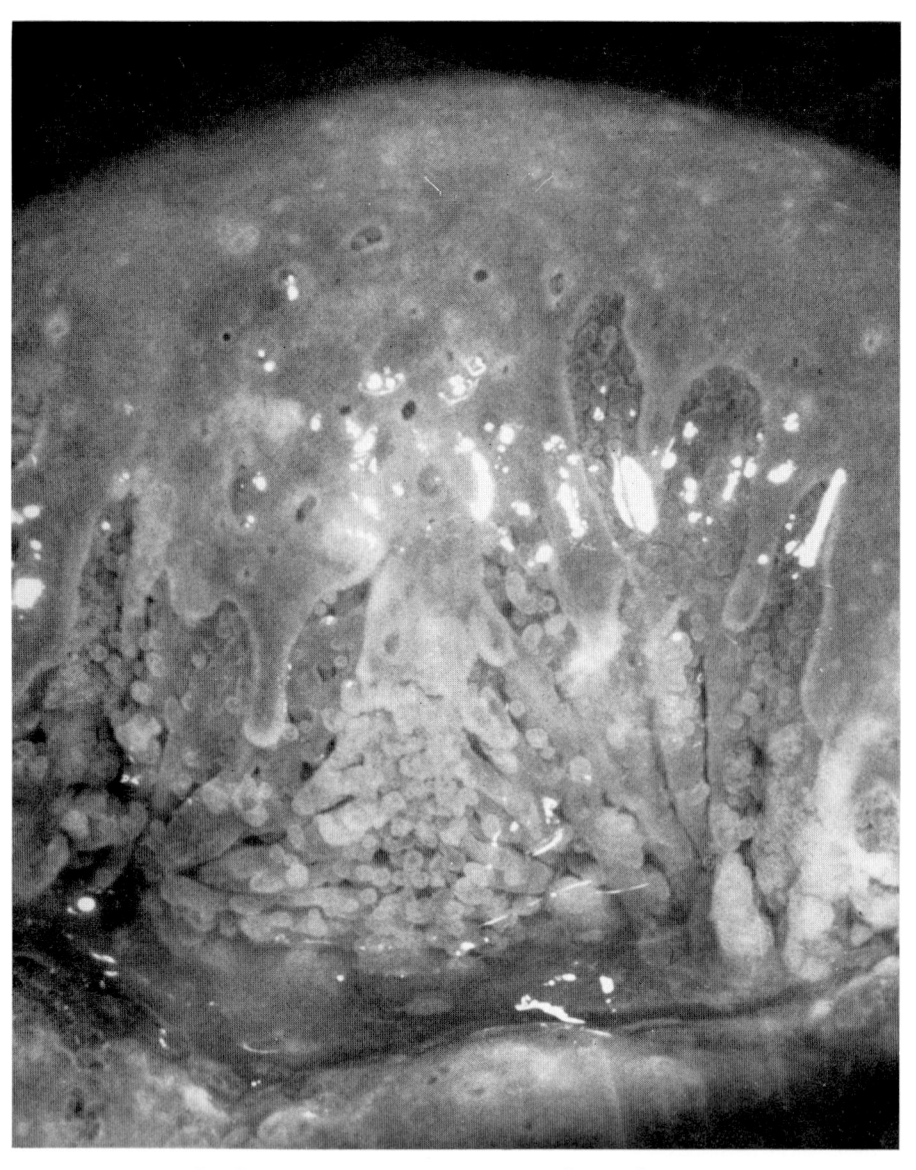

Figure 289. Normal colposcopic appearances. Typical transformation zone is present, and columnar epithelium is seen anteriorly. By gently everting the posterior lip in the lower tenth of the photograph, the new squamocolumnar junction was visible with columnar epithelium surrounding the canal. With such appearances, even in the presence of a positive smear, a confident conclusion can be reached that no preclinical carcinoma or dysplasia is present.

nant from those which, despite their similar histology, are either not truly premalignant or at least are early in the life cycle and years, if ever, from invasion.

While accepting that proof of this theory could only be forthcoming from prospective studies, supporting circumstantial evidence is available. By examination of the histologically preinvasive areas adjacent to or in association with undoubted invasive squamous carcinoma of the cervix, colposcopic appearances are seen which, when present in a purely preinvasive lesion, lead us to infer that such a lesion has a serious potential for invasion. As a corollary, when such appearances are absent in a purely preinvasive lesion, as is more often the case, then our inference is less serious.

Other evidence of various kinds has also been accumulating which indicates differing malignant potential of these lesions. These findings are consonant with the many opinions held that over half (possibly 90% or more) of histologically diagnosed cervical carcinomas in situ would never have become invasive even if untreated (Graham, Sotto, and Paloucek, 1962; Coppleson and Reid, 1967; Coppleson and Brown, 1975).

In summary, the findings within the area surveyed by the colposcope permits a reassuring grouping of cervical conditions into the following categories:

1. Those where there is already clinical invasion (the colposcopically overt carcinoma) (Fig. 285)
2. Those where there is probable imminent danger of clinical invasion (the atypical transformation zone, Grade III) (Fig. 286)
3. Those where there is no immediate danger; the most common group (the atypical transformation zone, Grade II) (Fig. 287)
4. Those where invasion is likely to be years off, if ever (the atypical transformation zone, Grade I) (Fig. 288)
5. Those where there is no danger at all; some of these will prove to be histological fallacies (no atypical transformation zone) (Fig. 289)
6. Those where the colposcopist can make no prediction, e.g. acute cervicitis (Fig. 283)

Location of the Lesion

The majority of preclinical carcinomas and dysplasias occur within view of the colposcope. The transformation zone, wherein these disorders lie, is usually visible in its entirety, either naturally or following the insertion and opening of the bivalve speculum, which everts the canal and allows easy survey of the endocervical segment. Gland openings and retention cysts, representing pre-existing columnar epithelium, are common throughout the transformation zone and cannot be regarded as occurring exclusively within the cervical canal, a limitation often presumed by pathol-

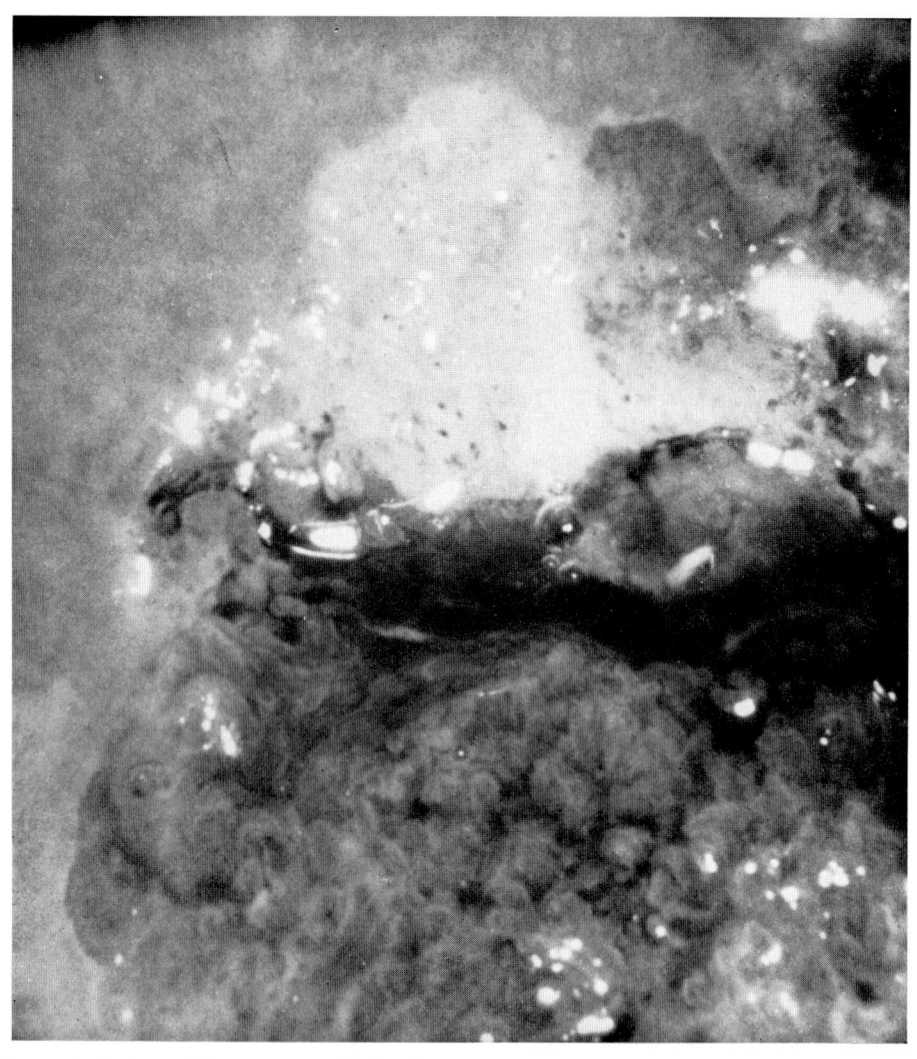

Figure 290. Site of lesion. A small focal lesion is present on the anterior lip displaying white epithelium. Columnar epithelium lines the cervical canal, and a lesion cephalad to this focus is thus excluded.

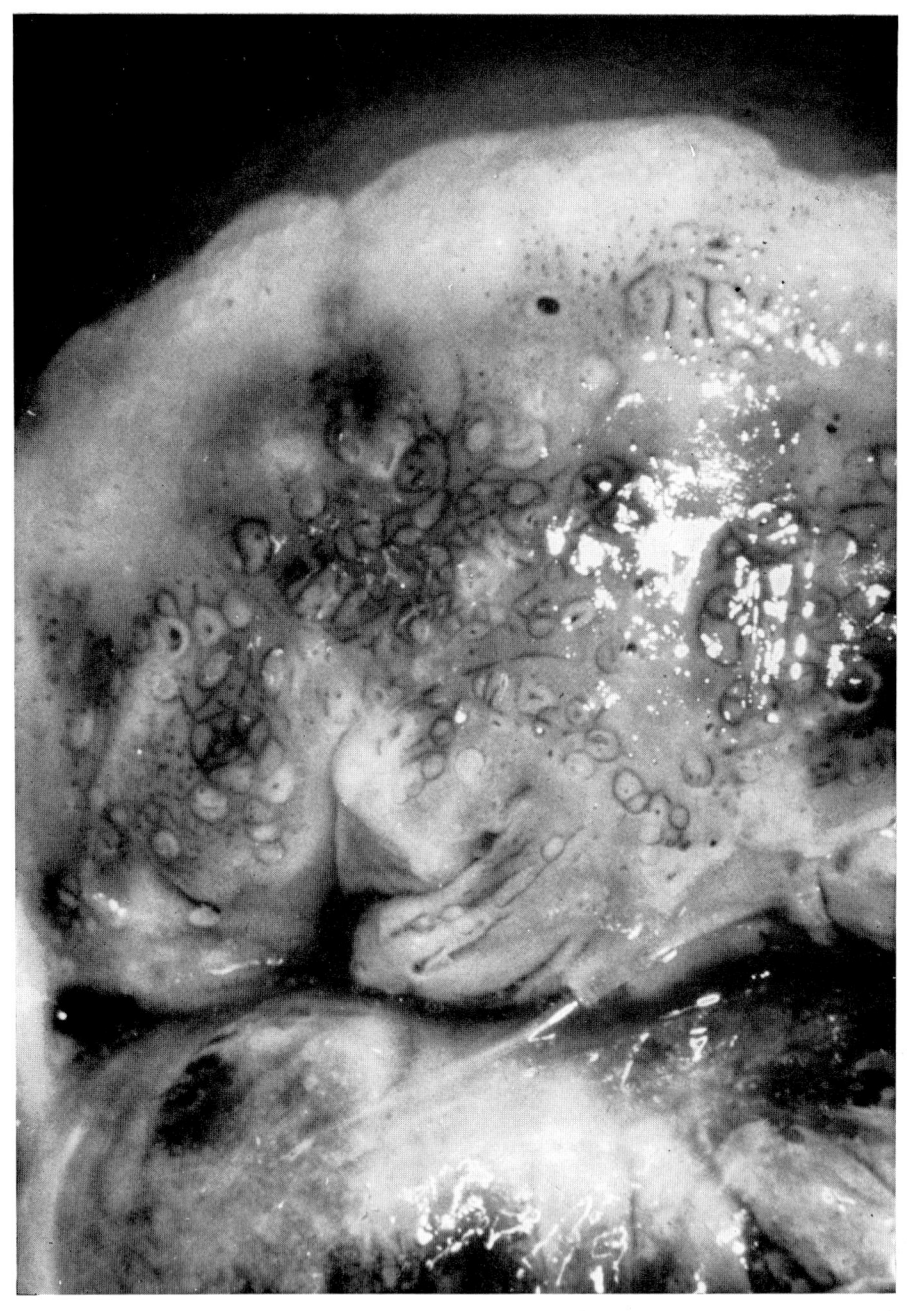

Figure 291. Site of lesion. An extensive atypical transformation zone containing white epithelium, coarse mosaic, and punctation extends into the cervical canal shown in the lower quarter of the photograph. A cone biopsy is mandatory for adequate assessment of this Grade III lesion.

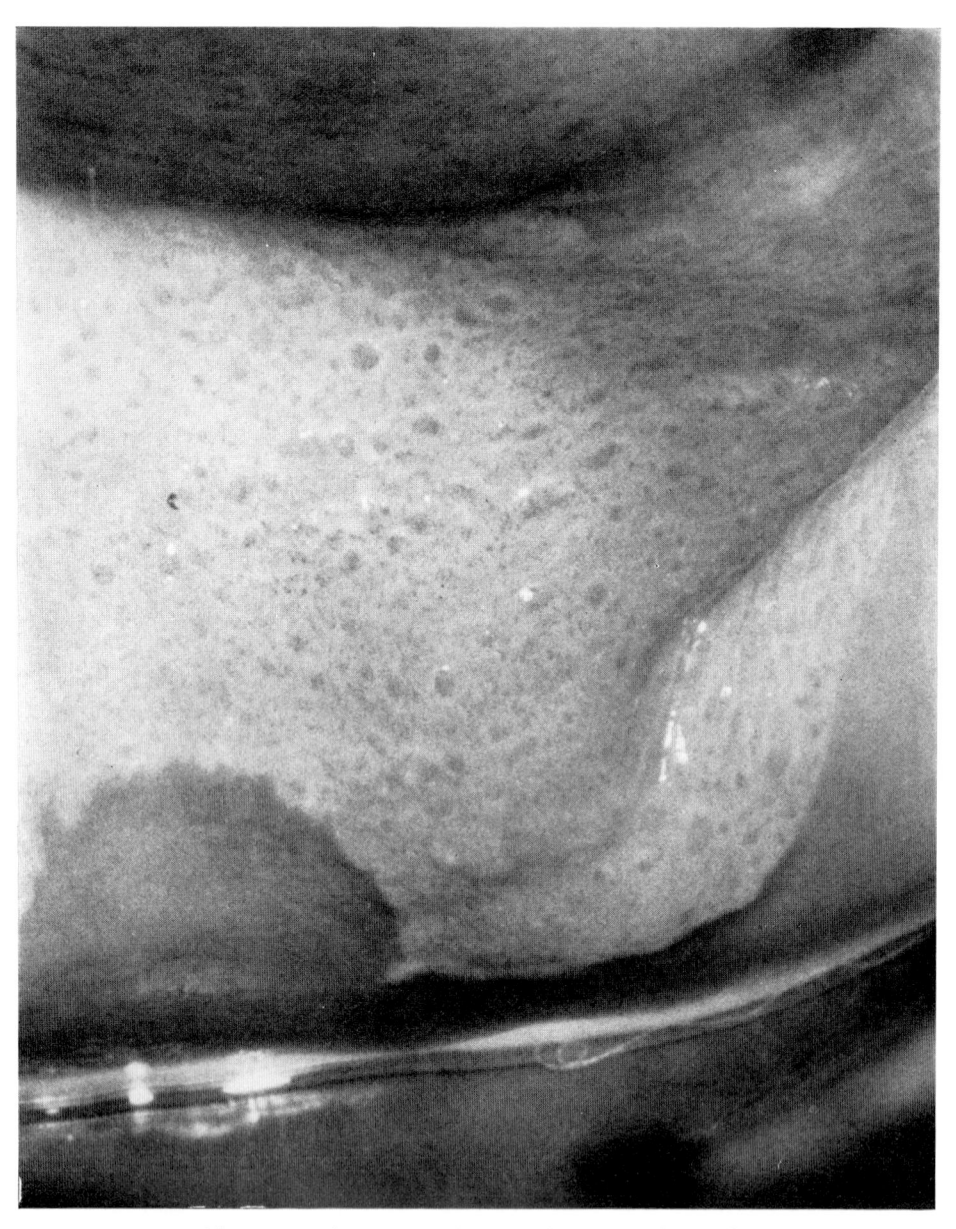

Figure 292. Site of lesion. In this retracted view, the atypical transformation zone continues across the fornix to involve the upper vagina. Present in the occasional case of preclinical cervical carcinoma, it creates practical problems.

ogists and resulting in the widely held but incorrect belief that most cervical cancer precursors are located within the cervical canal (p. 74).

Four states are possible in colposcopic assessment of an abnormal smear report:

1. The lesion is focal and can be seen in its entirety (Fig. 290).
2. The upper limit of the lesion may be out of sight in the cervical canal (Fig. 291).
3. In about 4 per cent of cases, the atypical transformation zone extends to the vagina, and this distribution is of significance when planning the complete excision of lesions (Fig. 292). Failure to note such an excursion is a probable cause of the entity "recurrence" of lesions following treatment.
4. There is no visible lesion. Either the lesion is high in the cervical canal beyond vision with the colposcope, or especially if columnar epithelium can be seen concentrically in the cervical canal, a diagnosis of a false positive smear may be warranted (Fig. 289).

Aids in Selection of Type, Size, and Site of Biopsy

By its ability to define precisely the size, site, and quality of most atypical cervical lesions, colposcopy identifies the source of cellular abnormality and allows a safe selection of the type of biopsy to be made.

In the absence of a colposcopy service, it appears that biopsy procedures tend to fall into two rigidly proscribed routines; on one hand, a majority group who favour the exclusive use of cone biopsy at all times, even in pregnancy, for investigation of both positive and doubtful smears, and on the other, those who favour the occasional use of cone biopsy. Here the fear that the random entry of the scalpel or punch biopsy instrument may have missed small, early invasive or endocervical carcinoma is only partially alleviated by the use of Schiller's test with iodine.

Neither of these routines can replace the adaptation of the biopsy type to the size and shape of the lesion as revealed by direct observation with the instrument. With this flexibility comes the assurance of dealing directly with the critical site. In this way, cone, wedge, or colposcopically directed punch biopsy may all be used, often in combination.

The overall effect of the existence of a colposcopy service is a reduction in the rate of cone biopsy and in the use of serial sectioning of the cone biopsy for histological assessment. The implications of foregoing a more serious procedure for the patient and a more costly one for both patient and state, are considerable. At the same time, there is a corresponding increase in the rate of the smaller and simpler colposcopically directed punch biopsy.

It is possible to rapidly resolve the majority of problems in diagnosis by

TABLE VII
ABNORMAL CYTOLOGY
CORRELATION OF COLPOSCOPY, EXPECTED HISTOLOGY AND RECOMMENDED BIOPSY

Patient	Colposcopy	Expected Histology	Recommended Biopsy
No. 1	Colpo overt cancer	Invasive cancer	Wedge biopsy
No. 2	Atypical TZ +++	CIS Invasive cancer	Cone
No. 3	Atypical TZ ++	CIS Major dysplasia	Punch or Cone (occas.)
No. 4	Atypical TZ +	Minor dysplasia Metaplasia	Punch (if any)
No. 5	Typical TZ	Metaplasia	None
No. 6	Original squamous epithelium	Original squamous epithelium	None

(*Note*: Patients 5 and 6 may have an "acute vaginocervicitis," complicating the picture and providing the source of the doubtful cell.)

reference to the following routine (Table VII). As previously discussed, a reassuring correlation between colposcopic and histological findings in the event of an abnormal smear provides the basis for selection of the preferred method of biopsy. The higher the grade of atypical colposcopic appearances, the higher the expected grade of histological abnormality.

Confirmation of the colposcopically suspect overt cancer is generally made by wedge biopsy. Grade III atypical colposcopic appearances, where maximum histological study is desirable, indicate hospitalization for cone biopsy. Lesser grades of colposcopic atypicality, which are much more common, generally require colposcopically directed punch biopsy as an office or outpatient procedure. Occasionally, especially with the less abnormal smear, no biopsy or other interference is required. In the latter cases colposcopy often reveals the source of abnormality in the smear to be an infection, or condyloma or oestrogen-deficient cervicitis. The ectocervix and lower endocervix can be quickly assessed as benign.

The indications for *cone biopsy* have been sharply reduced. There are several outstanding examples wherein colposcopic survey can justify the summary use of definitive management procedures thereby bypassing traditional diagnostic cone biopsy. These include the following circumstances:

1. On the rare occasion that a colposcopically suspect overt carcinoma (p. 273) is evident on examination, a lesser biopsy than the cone is required and is desirable to confirm the diagnosis.

2. In women with benign gynaecological abnormalities scheduled for hysterectomy, from whom a surprise positive smear is obtained, punch biopsy suffices if the atypical colposcopic lesion is focal and of the Grade

I or Grade II variety. Fractional curettage is also performed to exclude frank endocervical or endometrial carcinoma. The criticism may be levelled that such a limited diagnostic study may not satisfactorily exclude invasive carcinoma, so that the patient might be undertreated. The situation is purely hypothetical since total hysterectomy is also our preferred treatment for preclinical invasive carcinoma provided that colposcopically the presence of frank or obvious carcinoma has been excluded.

3. In the large group of women with abnormal smears, to be defined more accurately later, where eradication of lesions by either cryosurgery, electrodiathermy, or laser application is appropriate, diagnosis can be made by colposcopically directed biopsy.

4. When physiological colposcopic findings are evident in the ectocervix and columnar epithelium is visible concentrically in the lower endocervix, the smear is probably a false positive or false doubtful and should be reviewed and repeated, especially in premenopausal women, before any form of biopsy is undertaken.

The indications for cone biopsy, as a diagnostic or therapeutic procedure, are generally limited to the following cases:

1. Major lesions extending into the cervical canal
2. Major lesions, focal but extensive in area
3. Abnormal but inconclusive findings from endocervical curettage
4. Repeated abnormal smears in the absence of a colposcopic lesion

Whenever performed, cone biopsy should be radical enough to act as definitive treatment if required. The use of colposcopy allows variation in the size of the cone biopsy. To be able to select accurately those women in whom a small conisation is safe is of obvious advantage to those who wish to become pregnant and helps avoid the possible complication of cervical incompetence. For example, when a tiny lesion is identified on the ectocervix, it seems unrealistic to contemplate an extensive conisation (Fig. 293). On the other hand, with lesions involving a wide area, more extensive conisations are indicated (Fig. 294). In general, the ectocervical incision for the cone is made well outside the limits of the atypical area, which has been best defined beforehand by colposcopy. The cones may have wide variations both in terms of the size and form of the base and in their length, as determined by the colposcopic examination.

The lesion is first defined by Schiller's iodine stain (*see* Fig. 128) and the vasoconstrictor POR8® injected into the surrounding tissue. The dark staining area is incised by a scalpel (Bard-Parker size 11 blade) and the incision deepened to fashion the cone. Anterior and posterior Sturmdorf sutures, tied by the method of Bielecki (Fig. 295) are used, supplemented by one or two interrupted sutures as necessary.

Cone biopsy is associated with a significant percentage of complications.

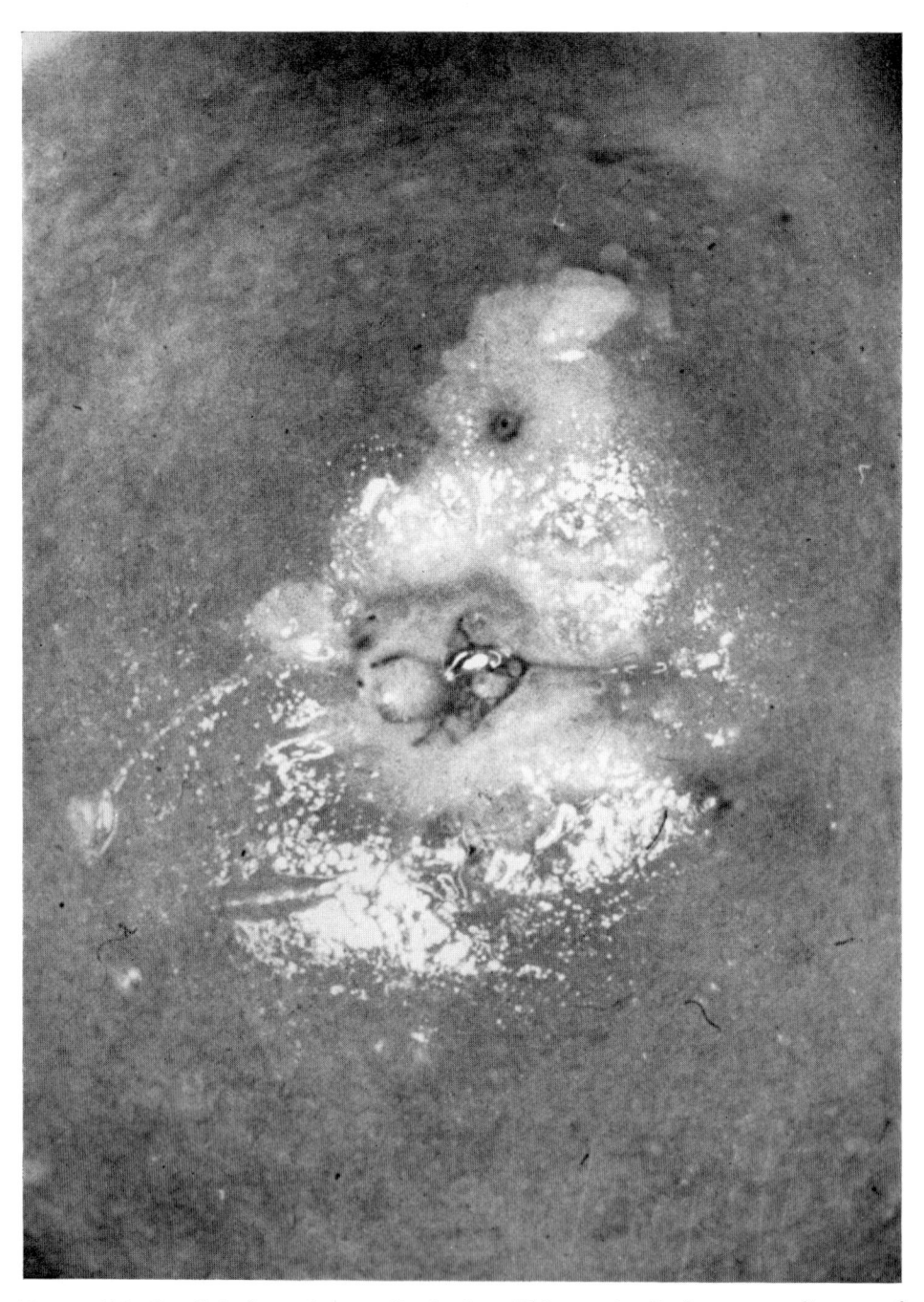

Figure 293. Preclinical carcinoma. Conisation. This cervix displays a small area of atypical transformation zone with white epithelium and keratosis on anterior and posterior cervical lips extending into the canal. The ectocervical incision for cone biopsy may be made close to the cervical os just beyond the limit of the lesion.

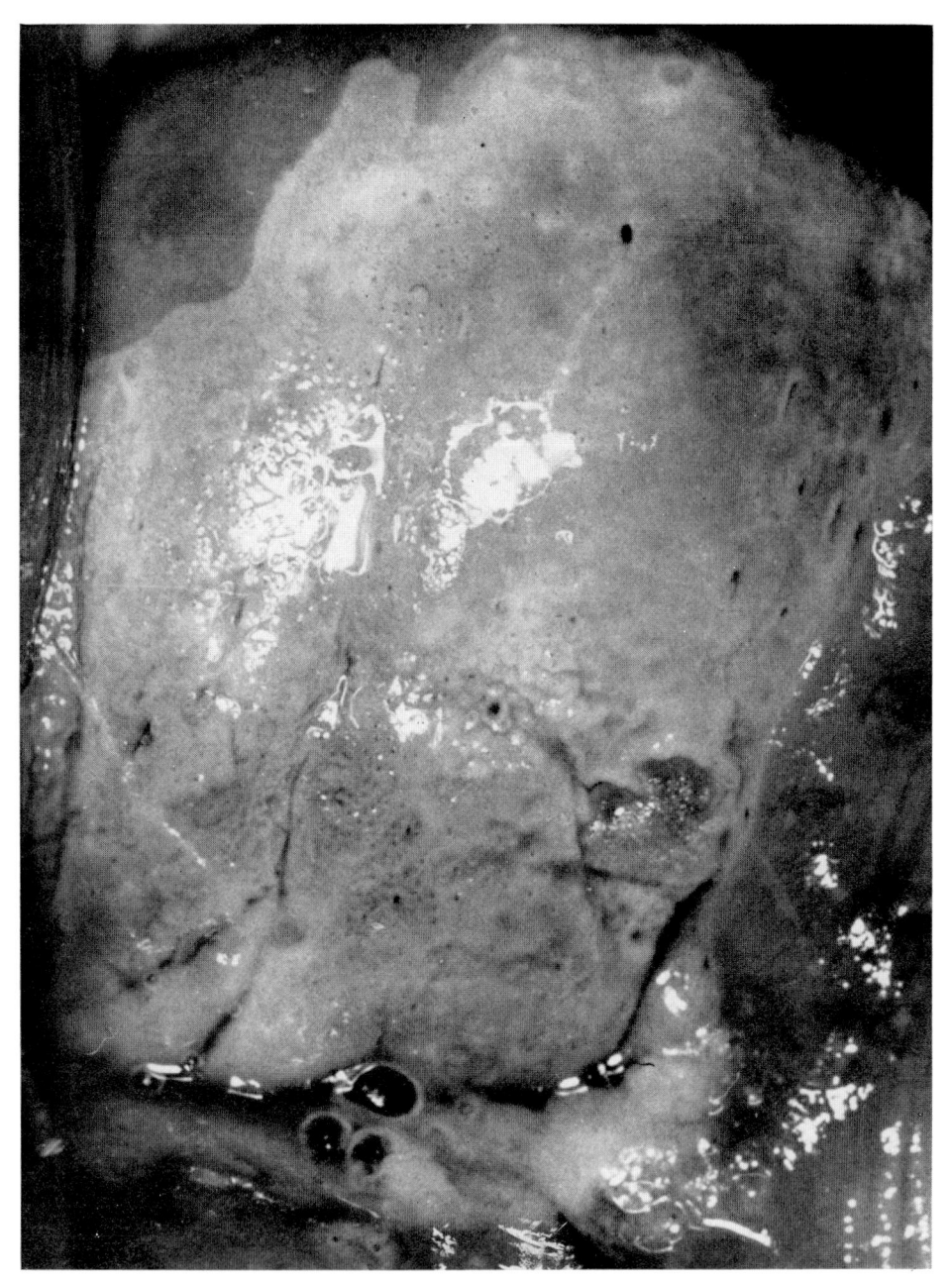

Figure 294. Preclinical carcinoma. Conisation. This cervix, by contrast with Figure 293, displays a large lesion whose limits extend almost to the vagina and into the cervical canal. Conisation is indicated and the ectocervical incision is required almost at the vaginal reflection.

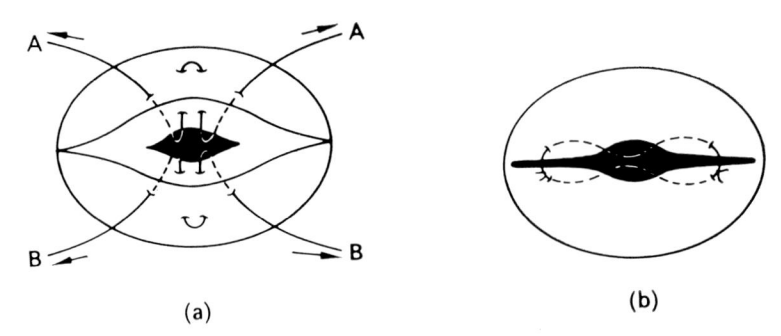

Figure 295. Modification of conisation technique—Bielecki method—Sturmdorf sutures are placed anteriorly and posteriorly (A and B). The ends of the sutures lying laterally are tied. Additional sutures are often required to ensure haemostasis.

Major complications, such as secondary haemorrhage, pelvic infection, cervical stenosis, and infertility and subsequent pregnancy complications, have been reported in from 13 to 22 per cent of cases, an incidence somewhat higher than local experience.

The *wedge biopsy* performed by cold knife excision, with or without suturing, in the anaesthetised patient has a small place in the management of the abnormal smear and should be considered in the case of the colposcopically suspect overt carcinoma when one can be confident of estab-

TABLE VIII

ASSESSMENT OF CERVICAL CANAL IN PRESENCE OF ABNORMAL CYTOLOGY

Patient	Colposcopy	Lesion	Method
No. 1	Atypical TZ +++	Extending into canal Focal	Cone biopsy Shallow cone biopsy
No. 2	Atypical TZ ++ consistent with CIS or major dysplasia	Extending into canal*	Cone biopsy
No. 3	Atypical TZ ++	Focal	Curettage under anaesthetic
No. 4	Atypical TZ + consistent with minor dysplasia	Extending into canal*	Outpatient endocervical curettage
No. 5	Atypical TZ +	Focal	None or outpatient endocervical curettage
No. 6	No lesion seen. Repeated smears indicative of major abnormality	Not seen	Cone biopsy (following gentle curettage)
No. 7	No lesion seen. Repeated smears indicative of minor abnormality	Not seen	Endocervical curettage

* Beyond vision available with bivalve speculum eversion and endocervical speculum.

lishing the diagnosis. As already discussed, cone biopsy performed immediately prior to radical methods of management required for invasive cancer is undesirable and may complicate treatment, while the small colposcopically directed punch biopsy may give insufficient material for the histologist adequately to confirm the more serious diagnosis. A generous wedge of tissue, both in terms of diameter and depth, should be excised.

The *colposcopically directed punch biopsy* is the main instrument of diagnosis of the more conservative management procedures. The punch may be single or multiple, resecting those areas most colposcopically abnormal. Slippage over the precise site selected is a problem reduced by the use of a sharp instrument and the presence of an iris hook (p. 177). Discomfort is minimal, and bleeding is most easily controlled by one or two vaginal tampons pressed hard against the cervix and removed twelve hours later. Monsel's solution (ferric subsulphate) applied directly to the biopsy site is also of value as an astringent. The minuteness of the fragment may initially cause minor technical problems for the histologist.

Aids Evaluation of the Cervical Canal

The subject of the cervical canal is of especial significance in any text on colposcopy. Historically, the inability to visualise the canal has been regarded as a stumbling block by opponents of the method. These objections are largely unfounded, provided the approach recommended is followed (Table VIII). The alternatives in further evaluation are cone biopsy, curettage of the canal under anaesthesia, curettage of the canal without anaesthesia, or no intervention. The basis for a decision between the alternatives rests on the visibility of the lesion in part or as a whole and its colposcopic grading by appearance. The use of an endocervical speculum to display better the canal has already been described (p. 180).

In summary, the major colposcopic gradings warrant cone biopsy where the lesion extends into the canal beyond visibility either with or without the aid of the endocervical speculum. A shallower cone biopsy is warranted, with curettage of the canal using a normal curette, when a focal lesion is present surrounded by columnar epithelium on its uterine side.

With atypical colposcopic lesions of minor grades consistent with histologically minor epithelial abnormalities extending into the endocervix beyond the sight of the colposcope and endocervical speculum, a more limited endocervical curettage with a special endocervical curette is indicated prior to eradication of the lesion by cryosurgery or electrodiathermy (Fig. 288). With minor focal lesions where columnar epithelium can be seen in the canal above the lesion, it is our opinion that "skip" lesions do not occur, so that the routine employment of endocervical curettage is not indicated. In our experience, the danger of missing an invasive cancer high in the canal in such cases is negligible.

For those gynaecologists not familiar with conservative methods of management presently recommended, the use of routine endocervical curettage, even with such minor focal lesions, provides additional reassurance. A supportive argument maintains that the occasional asymptomatic endocervical adenocarcinoma will be detected by such means. Endocervical curettage, if thorough, is not always painless. The instrument has already been described (p. 180). Short, sharp strokes are used, and the material is collected as recommended by Townsend et al. (1970) into a small mound on absorbent paper. Both paper and tissue are placed in a fixative, and the cell button so created is sectioned.

When repeated abnormal smears indicate the presence of a significant lesion, possibly preclinical invasive cancer, in the absence of any colposcopic abnormality, cone biopsy must be contemplated. It is generally recommended that diagnostic curettage should follow the cone biopsy, so that there is minimal interference with the endocervical epithelium prior to histological examination. However, it is our opinion that, especially in postmenopausal women, gentle curettage of the endocervical canal should be performed prior to the planned cone biopsy to facilitate the recognition of an obvious clinical endocervical cancer.

Before performing cone biopsy, one should be almost certain of establishing a diagnosis of preclinical carcinoma. For example, in a young woman with repeated abnormal smears suggestive only of minor dysplasia and without a visible colposcopic lesion, we would be reluctant to perform cone biopsy unless preliminary endocervical curettage indicated the existence of a significant lesion.

AIDS IN SELECTION OF TREATMENT FOR PRECLINICAL INVASIVE CARCINOMA

Perhaps the most important function of the colposcope is its potential for defining the management of those cases whose histopathology study shows an invasive lesion in the absence of clinical signs of overt invasion. The so-called preclinical invasive carcinoma is a real entity; the by-product of exfoliative cytology and its existence creates an immediate problem of the degree of surgical intervention. Colposcopic study provides par excellence a ready demarcation of those lesions requiring radical treatment from those which can be managed more conservatively.

Preclinical invasive carcinoma of the cervix does not present the same problems of cure as does an obvious or clinically overt carcinoma of the cervix, and results indicate that it can be safely managed by more conservative measures than have been adopted generally. Experience of two hundred women treated for preclinical invasive carcinoma in this clinic shows only two recurrences, both following the Wertheim operation. Our early approach to the management of this condition was radical. These results have been reported elsewhere (Coppleson, 1976), but it is relevant to this discussion to note that of ninety women undergoing Wertheim's radical hysterectomy, the lymph nodes were found to be involved in only one case. Colposcopically, this cervix was a suspect overt carcinoma. By comparison, the lymph node involvement in Stage 1B or clinically overt carcinoma of the cervix with the same technique of lymphadenectomy was 22 per cent (Stening, 1964). There are other reports in the literature, uncommon but factual, of either lymph node involvement or death from metastatic carcinoma (Coppleson, 1976).

To identify these rare cases of preclinical invasive carcinoma which either have node involvement or are likely to develop metastatic carcinoma would be of obvious advantage. This minority group could then be radically treated in the first instance, while all other cases could be treated more conservatively (Table IX).

Current practice throughout the world leaves the demarcation of grades of preclinical invasive cancer in an exclusive way to its histopathological features. Such a monopoly encourages a closer study of the basis for such authority. The student is confronted with a great complexity of terminology of the type associated with ultraspecialism. From this maze of terminology is derived an equally specialised format for use in prognosis, so that different specialists and their schools cite different parameters or cutoff points in defining the depth of invasive tissue beneath the basement membrane (*see* Table I, p. 43). Each places varying significance on the presence of confluent pegs of invasive tissue, the involvement of venous, lymphatic channels, and so forth (Coppleson, 1976, 1977). Extending beyond an academic dissertation between specialists, such prognostic proscriptions beget management programmes that tend to equate the degree of intervention precisely with the histological picture. Unfortunately, from retrospective studies, there is little correlation between the opinion of the histologist and the demonstrable presence of invasive tissue in the regional lymph nodes or of metastatic spread. As a bystander in the confusion amongst the histological pictures, the gynaecologist has understandably tended to overtreat the lesions.

The real problem, of course, is that the true biological nature of the

TABLE IX

OPTIONS IN TREATMENT OF PRECLINICAL INVASIVE CARCINOMA

1. Radical Therapy
　　as for Stage 1B cancer
2. Conservative Hysterectomy
3. Therapeutic Conisation

oncogenic process is yet to be defined. In its absence, a compromise between the views of pathologist and colposcopist seems appropriate embracing as they do details of state of the capillary bed, surface contour through to microscopic detail from sectioned material removed from a selected site.

As has been previously stressed, the detection of colposcopically suspect overt cancer is a valuable aid in planning management of preclinical invasive cancer. This is the cervix which, when submitted to colposcopic examination, displays overt qualities with all the characteristics of an obvious cancer, which were not in evidence on naked-eye examination (Figs. 30, 196 to 198, and 285). The condition is distinct from the varying grades of atypical transformation zone described previously, which are the usual findings in the presence of most Stage 1A and Stage O carcinoma of the cervix and is a specific appearance which characterises overt carcinoma. No matter how carefully this type of lesion is assessed by naked-eye examination or palpation, the diagnosis of an overt lesion cannot be made. This is the lesion most likely to have either a lymph node metastasis or to develop a recurrence and to require radical treatment as for Stage 1B cancer. Such treatment in our clinic involves preoperative intracavitary radium followed six weeks later by Wertheim's panhysterectomy. If the pelvic lymph nodes contain metastases, external irradiation is given postoperatively (Coppleson, 1976). In young women, preoperative radium is frequently dispensed with, and ovarian function is conserved.

In the majority of cases of preclinical invasive cancer, one can proceed confidently to therapeutic measures less radical than those used for established Stage 1B carcinoma of the cervix. The following four criteria must be observed:

1. The lesion is not colposcopically overt or conspicuous. Most frankly invasive squamous cell carcinomas are within the area of the cervix visualised by colposcopy.
2. A Grade III atypical lesion with atypical vessels suggestive of invasive cancer and histologically showing confluency and deep depth of penetration is not present.
3. By curettage, the occasional obvious cancer higher in the cervical canal is excluded. In most such instances, the woman is postmenopausal, the cervix is expanded, and atypical colposcopic appearances are seen at the external os below the advanced lesion in the canal.
4. To the experienced eye, the biopsy and curettage material is not suspicious of carcinoma.

The less radical therapeutic measures employed in such cases are conservative hysterectomy in most cases and therapeutic conisation in selected cases.

It is evident that, finally, even with this combined colposcopic-histological assessment of lesions, the decision making is necessarily subjective. Nevertheless, all our evidence suggests that the increased perspective enabled by the combined approach allows one to select a greater number of women who can be treated in more conservative fashion, with complete safety, than is possible by the exclusive reliance on histology.

AIDS IN SELECTION OF TREATMENT FOR STAGE O CARCINOMA AND DYSPLASIA (CIN)

It is unusual for an invasive cancer to be revealed after a colposcopic-histological survey of women who present with an abnormal cervical smear report. Much more commonly, an *in situ* cancer or some degree of dysplasia is revealed. The choice of optimal management of these conditions is neither critical nor urgent and certainly does not rest on precise histological definition. The frequent dilemma of the histologist in attempting to evaluate the gravity of the lesion by arbitrary criteria can be largely overlooked once a distinction between major and minor lesions is made.

Bereft of the urgency of intervention, the clinician can consider more peripheral features of the case in the choice of treatment. The ultimate choice of treatment thus depends not only on histology but on colposcopic topography and other factors such as age, parity, desire for children, desire for sterilization, pregnancy, and concurrent gynaecological and socioeconomic conditions. A broad range of techniques is currently available ranging from minimal interference in local destruction of the lesion, through wider excisions such as therapeutic cone biopsy, to the most radical, hysterectomy (Table X). Such a range ensures a true flexibility of approach.

The consensus of current opinion from most clinics not employing colposcopy in evaluation still favours total hysterectomy as the preferred treatment for lesions such as carcinoma in situ, restricting the use of therapeutic conisation to younger patients who desire further pregnancies. The view that conisation, and thus also the more conservative methods of management, is inadequate definitive therapy is largely the result of hysterec-

TABLE X

OPTIONS IN TREATMENT OF CIS AND DYSPLASIA OF CERVIX

1. Physical Destruction
    a. Electrodiathermy under anaesthesia
    b. Electrodiathermy without anaesthesia
    c. Cryosurgery without anaesthesia
    d. CO_2 laser application
2. Local Excision
    a. Therapeutic conisation
    b. Amputation of cervix
    c. Wedge biopsy
    d. Multiple-punch biopsy
3. Hysterectomy

tomy studies after conisation which occasionally show residual preclinical invasive carcinoma and often show residual carcinoma in situ. The theoretical view is that these areas are potentially dangerous and could become frankly invasive. The actual incidence of persistence of carcinoma in situ varies from 12 to 40 per cent in different series (Coppleson and Reid, 1967). It is apparent that a similar percentage of residual carcinoma should still be present in the cervices of those women who have been treated by conisation as definitive treatment. It is a striking fact, therefore, that recurrence of frank, clinically invasive carcinoma after conisation seldom, if ever, occurs. A review and possible explanation of this paradox is discussed elsewhere (Coppleson and Reid, 1967; Coppleson, 1976).

The use of colposcopy permits an efficient selection, prior to cervical biopsy, of women who can be safely treated by conservative methods. Such a practice aids the present trend towards conservatism in the management of preclinical lesions; a trend which meets with widespread approval amongst gynaecologists uneasy about the immediate use of radical measures, which was commonplace when reliance rested solely on the histological diagnosis. Testimony as to the safety of these conservative methods of management, in the presence of an expert assessment, is presented elsewhere (Coppleson, 1976. 1977).

Physical Destruction of the Lesion

Four methods are available for destroying a lesion: either electrodiathermy under anaesthesia, or electrocautery, cryosurgery, or CO_2 laser as outpatient or office procedures.

The ideal indication for the most conservative method of management is the young woman, with prospects of pregnancy, with a focal lesion of minor colposcopic grade, and with columnar epithelium visible concentrically in the lower cervical canal above the lesion (Figs. 287, 290, and 296). Expert colposcopy is essential for thorough evaluation and for correct execution of the method. The optimal arrangements for such measures are provided by a colposcopy service manned by experienced clinicians working with large numbers of patients, such as those found in large hospitals or universities. The apparent simplicity of the method requires continuing vigilance in follow-up procedures, especially the necessity of ensuring by colposcopic survey that the lesion has been replaced by normal squamous epithelium (Figs. 296 and 297). The occasional difficulty encountered in colposcopic evaluation of regenerating epithelium is mentioned later (p. 429). Evidence indicates that 90 to 95 per cent of lesions can be effectively dealt with by these methods. In the uncommon event of regeneration of an atypical epithelium, rediathermy, refreezing, or conisation can be performed. Once the whole ectocervix and lower endocervix is completely covered by mature fully differentiated squamous epithelium, staining deeply with Schiller's iodine solution, the woman may be regarded as in the lowest-risk category of developing squamous cancer of the cervix (Fig. 298).

Most authorities believe that the destruction of normal columnar epithelium in the cervical canal, concurrent with physical destruction of the cervical lesion, may produce a new squamocolumnar junction out of sight within the canal and thus make follow-up colposcopic assessment in the presence of abnormal cytology incomplete. In contrast to this view, it is our intention always to destroy, in addition to the focal lesion, the remainder of the transformation zone and the columnar epithelium in the lower canal. It is our belief that the replacement of this entire area by normal squamous epithelium is the best prophylaxis for cervical cancer and overrides prospective difficulty to be encountered in subsequent colposcopic evaluation.

After physical destruction of lesions by any method, the woman is advised not to have intercourse for three weeks and to use an acidifying cream intravaginally each night for two weeks. This cream accelerates healing by squamous rather than columnar epithelium, possibly because of its acidity.

Complications following treatment by electrodiathermy, electrocautery, or cryosurgery are minimal. Bleeding or infection requiring hospitalization are rare. Bleeding can be intermittent or continuous for three to four weeks, especially after electrodiathermy. Cervical stenosis is rare. There is little if any impairment of future fertility.

Electrodiathermy Under Anaesthesia

Electrodiathermy under anaesthesia has been used with increasing frequency in King George V Hospital in Sydney since 1966 and is now most commonly employed in the treatment of focal lesions of carcinoma in situ or dysplasia (Figs. 296 to 298). The whole of the lesion is outlined by colposcopy or, if the colposcope is not available in the theatre, by Schiller's iodine solution. The transformation zone and the columnar epithelium in the lower canal is thoroughly charred, using standard electrocoagulation machines. A pointed probe is recommended.

The great variation in the number and arrangement of clefts and glands in the individual cervix requires corresponding variation in the duration and depth of application of the heat source. Continued application of the probe until mucus production ceases is a precise indicator of total glandular destruction. Attention to this detail of the technique overcomes a theoretical objection to this method of management, namely, that inadequate depth of destruction may allow a lesion to persist and develop

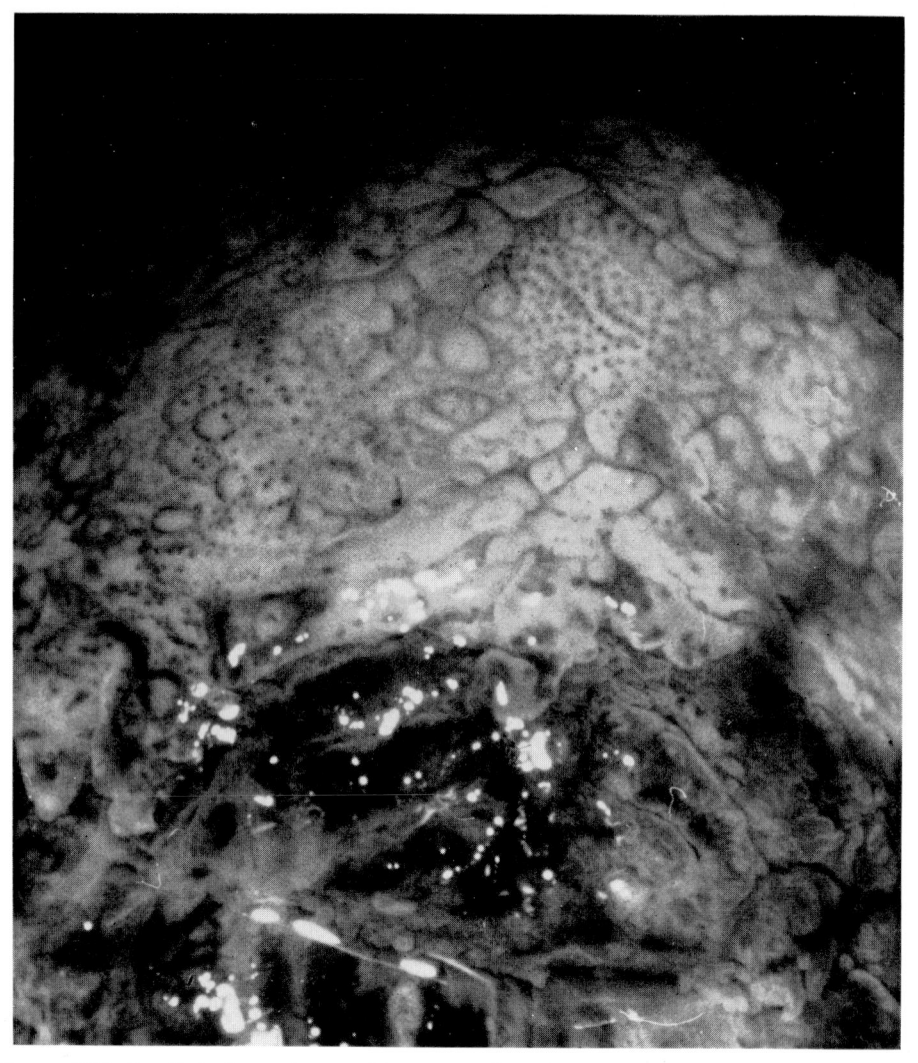

Figure 296. Preclinical carcinoma. Treatment by physical destruction. A focal lesion, Grade II atypical transformation zone, is visible with columnar epithelium surrounding the lower cervical canal in the lower third of the photograph. The diagnosis of carcinoma in situ was confirmed by colposcopically directed biopsy and the lesion eradicated by electrodiathermy under anaesthesia. The whole transformation zone and lower canal epithelium was similarly destroyed.

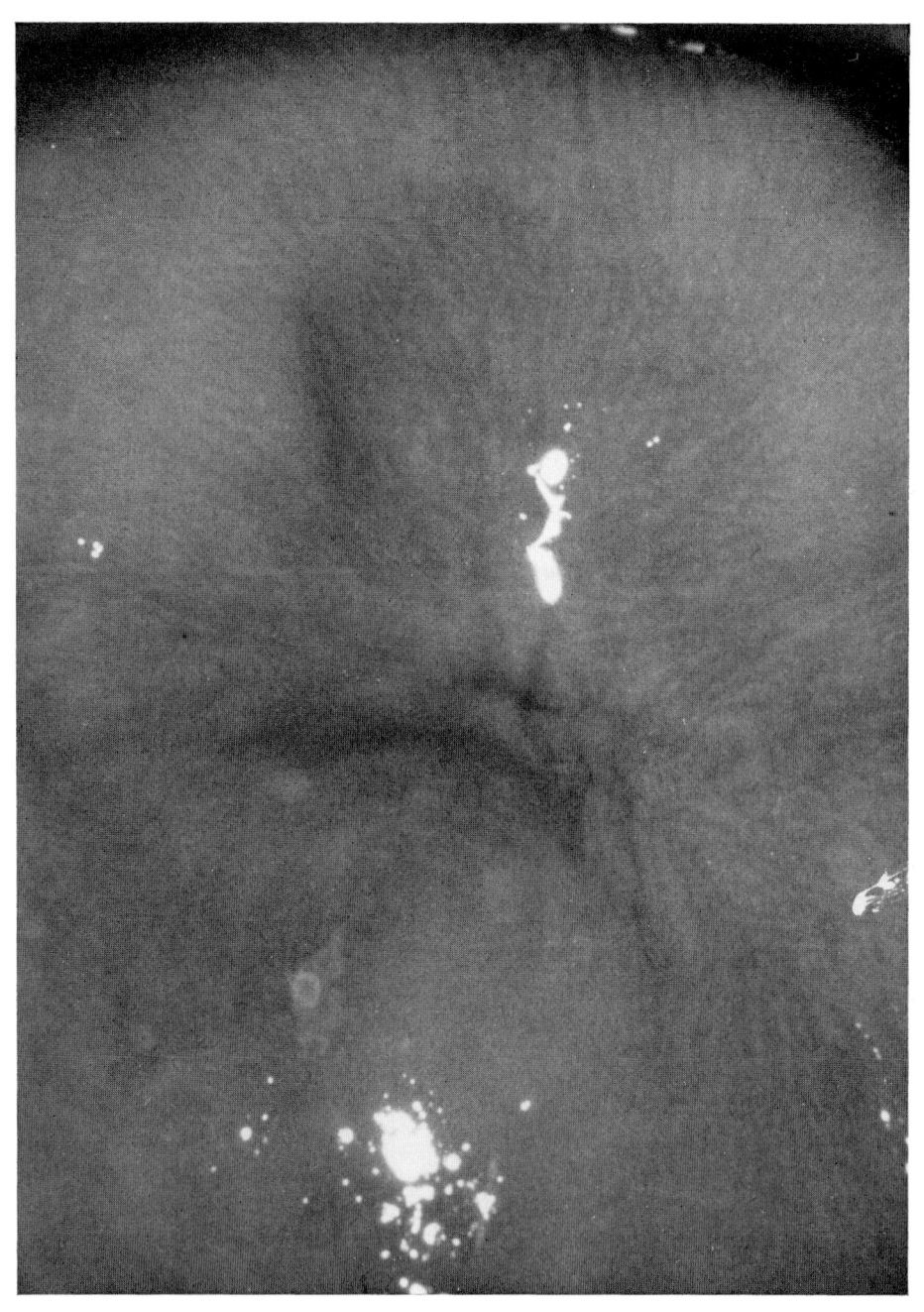

Figure 297. Preclinical carcinoma. Cervix of same subject, seen eight weeks after operation. The whole lesion has been eradicated.

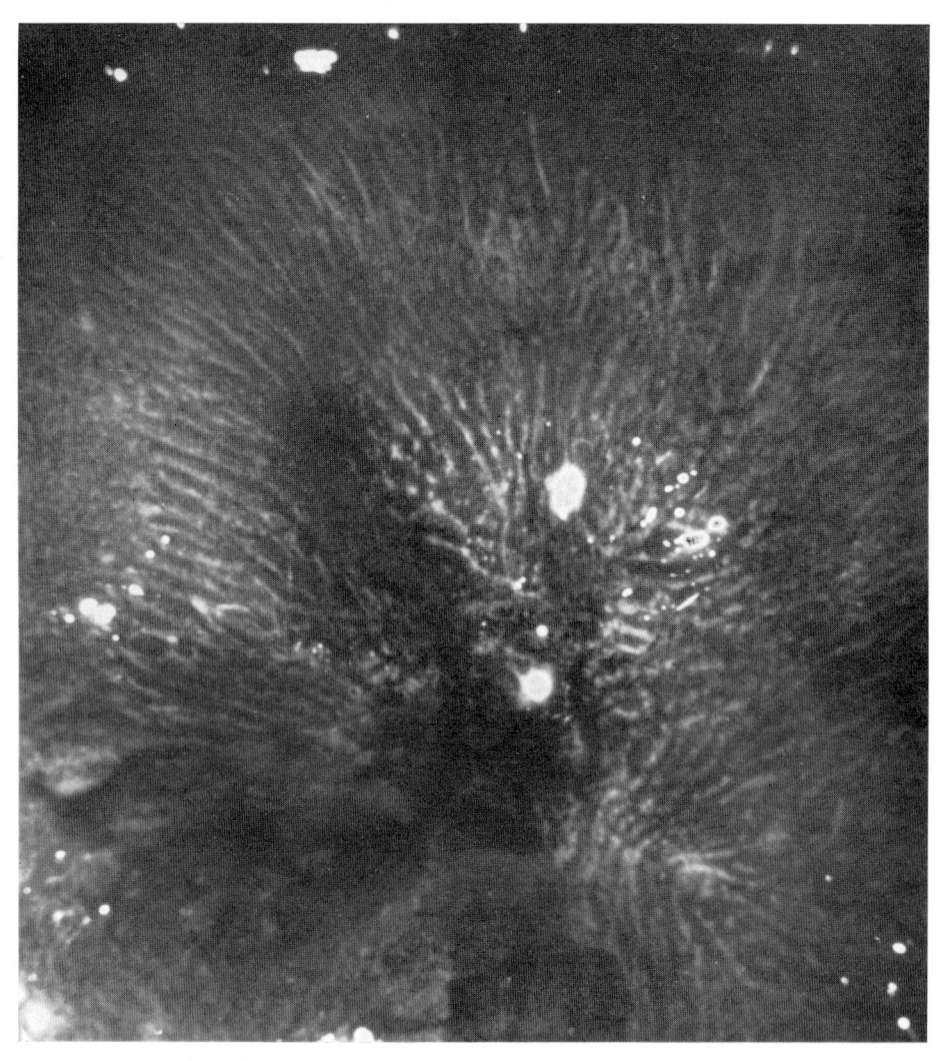

Figure 298. Preclinical carcinoma. Cervix of same subject. After treatment iodine application shows the ideal result. The ectocervix is covered by normal regenerate epithelium, deeply staining with iodine extending well into the canal. Note the characteristic radial pattern following physical destruction. The subject is now at least risk of developing cervical squamous cancer.

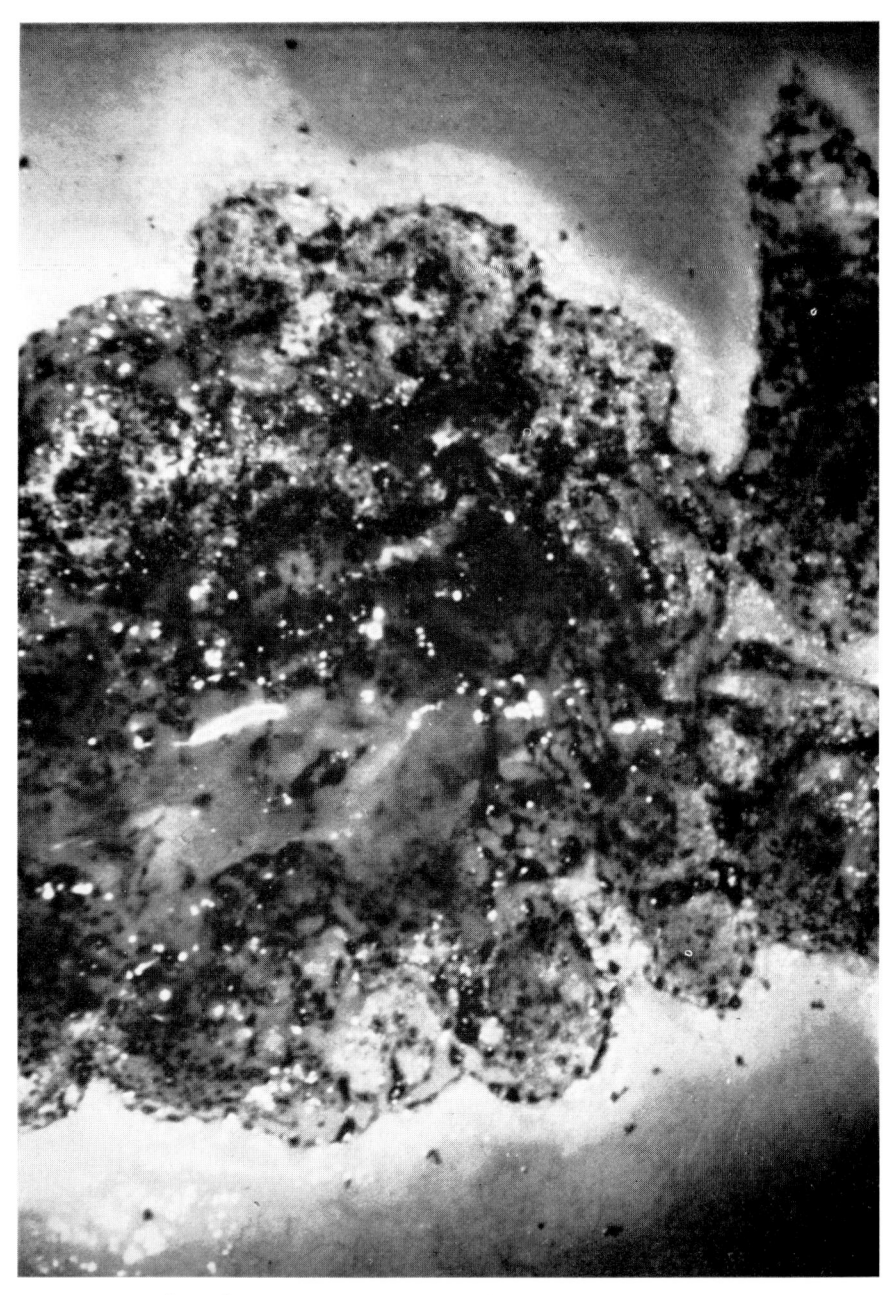

Figure 299. Preclinical carcinoma. Treatment by CO_2 laser therapy. The colpophotograph was taken immediately on completion of the vaporisation. Each pulse destroyed a roughly circular area which is surrounded by a precise edge and more peripherally by a characteristic ischemic white rim. Reepithelialization took place within 14 days. With laser therapy the end result is usually achieved earlier than after electrodiathermy or cryosurgery possibly by reason of the minimal damage to tissue at the edge of the circle.

unnoticed, perhaps without exfoliation of abnormal cells, deep in the regenerate epithelium.

Electrocautery Without Anaesthesia

Electrocautery without anaesthesia does not allow the same depth of destruction of tissue as radical diathermy under anaesthesia and is less acceptable to the patient than cryosurgery. Although there are several reports attesting to the satisfactory eradication of lesions (Coppleson, 1976), the procedure is not recommended.

Cryosurgery Without Anaesthesia

Cryosurgery without anaesthesia, currently popular in the United States, has the advantage over electrodiathermy under anaesthesia in that it is effective as an outpatient and office procedure. However, we remain unconvinced that it is more effective in eradicating lesions than the electrodiathermy method. We believe electrodiathermy provides more accuracy in determining the depth of tissue destruction so vital in ensuring eradication of those lesions with glandular involvement. With nitrous oxide as the freezing agent, we use a continuous freezing technique, reapplying the probe if freezing seems inadequate, and insuring that the ice ball extends at least 3 mm beyond the edge of the lesion. The instrumentation and technique is described in detail by Townsend (1976).

CO_2 Laser

The energy of the laser beam emitted through carbon dioxide is the most recent method available for physical destruction of lesions. The instrument requires only a conventional electrical power outlet and water circulation, and the laser head attaches to standard colposcopes. Its invisible beam, which is traced by a coaxial beam of visible light is directed with the aid of an arm with mirrors and a focussing lens onto the site with the colposcope. The aiming beam produces a small luminous spot which persists throughout the procedure and may be shifted by a micromanipulator attached to the colposcope. The laser shutter is activated by a foot switch. The illuminated cells are then vaporised (Fig. 299). The exposure may be electively continuous or timed. Precision of destruction of the lesion is controllable from the power source. Contiguous tissues may not be damaged and may be one reason for the notably faster repair of the destroyed area. Haemostasis of smaller vessels is instantaneous.

Therapeutic Conisation and Cervical Amputation

Conisation as definitive treatment is safe treatment at any age, provided the whole lesion can be colposcopically defined and columnar epithelium

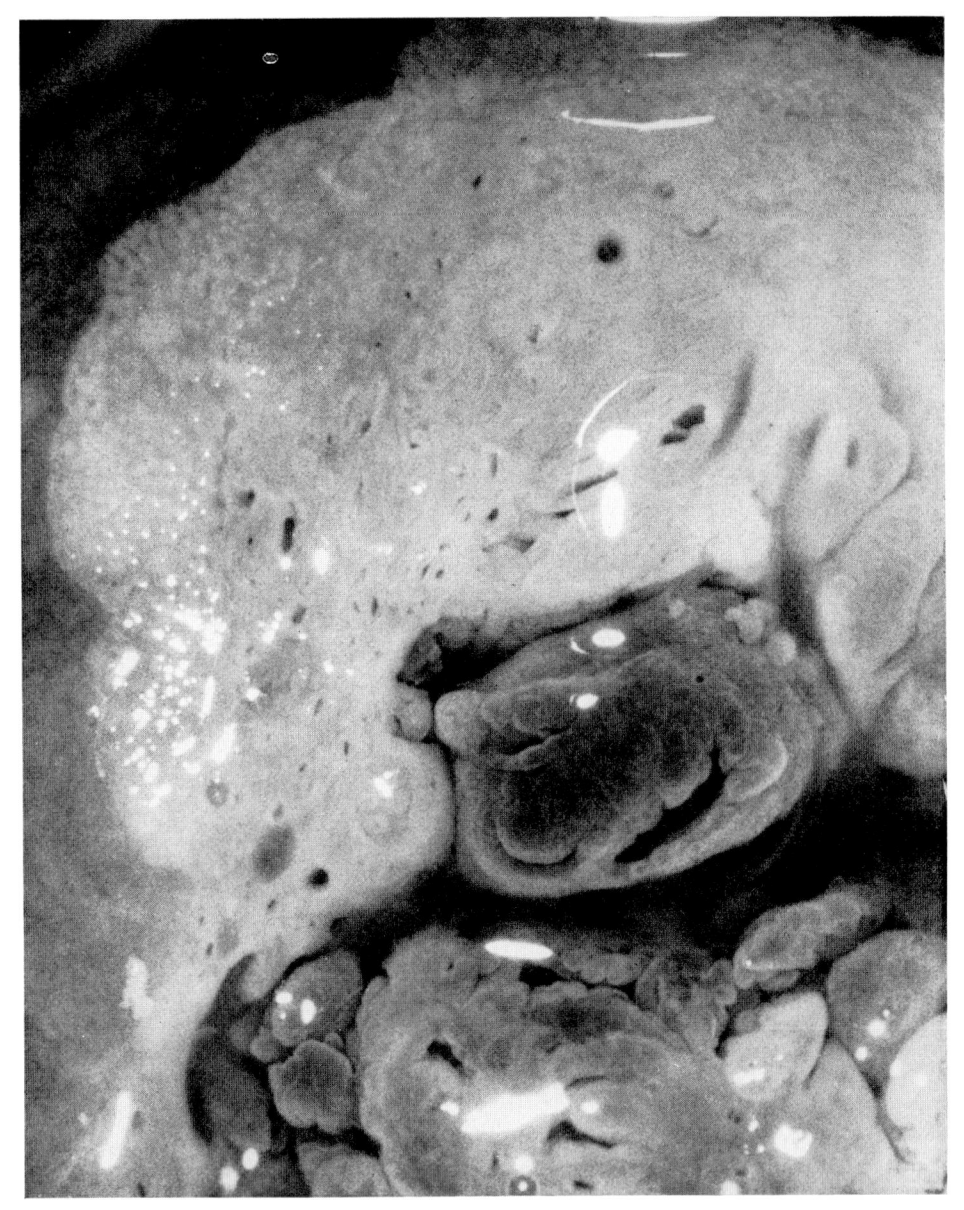

Figure 300. Preclinical carcinoma. Treatment by conisation. The full extent of this atypical transformation zone on the anterior lip can be seen. The cervical columnar epithelium of the lower canal adjoins directly below in the bottom right corner of the photograph so that conisation is adequate treatment.

can be seen surrounding the lower cervical canal above the atypical colposcopic lesion (Fig. 300). The majority of women with cervical carcinoma in situ are in this category.

In the less common case where the lesion is seen by colposcopy to be disappearing higher in the cervical canal or when no atypical colposcopic lesion has been seen, the status of the epithelium in the histological sections at the upper limit of the cone is a useful indicator. If the epithelium at the lines of excision is normal, conisation is sufficient treatment. If the marginal epithelium is CIN, one must assume there is involvement above but experience has shown a conservative policy may still be safely adopted. Since the introduction of the endocervical speculum, lesions whose upper limits are not visible are few. The upper limit of the lesion is often coincident with the line of maximum eversion produced by the open vaginal speculum. Frequent follow-up smears and occasionally further investigation at a later date may be required.

The technique used for therapeutic cone biopsy is no different from that of diagnostic cone biopsy (p. 409).

Biopsy Excision

Multiple colposcopically directed punch biopsies or a wedge biopsy by scalpel is of value in eliminating small lesions, either primary lesions or those persisting after electrodiathermy or cryosurgery.

Hysterectomy

The indications for hysterectomy become more stringent in the presence of a colposcopy service. Hysterectomy is rarely indicated in the absence of some other indication. These are, as follows:
1. Intraepithelial lesions at the histological limits of the cone biopsy: This is not an absolute indication in younger women, provided careful follow-up is assured.
2. Other gynecological disorders requiring hysterectomy: These include prolapse, dysfunctional uterine bleeding, or fibromyomata.
3. Sterilization hysterectomy: This procedure may constitute an acceptable alternative to other methods of sterilization.
4. Fear of conservative treatment: This is a rare indication, provided the gynaecological advice is confident and well based.
5. Less reliable patients unlikely to return for follow-up examinations: Therapeutic conisation is a reasonable option in most of these cases.

AIDS IDENTIFICATION AND MANAGEMENT OF VAGINAL LESIONS

In about 4 per cent of cases, the atypical colposcopic lesion can be observed to extend beyond the cervix to the vaginal wall (Fig. 301). Irrespective of the method of ablation employed for the cervical lesion, whether it is cryosurgery, electrodiathermy, conisation, or hysterectomy, these vaginal extensions must be eradicated, since they carry the same neoplastic significance of a more central lesion. On the other hand, routine excision of a vaginal cuff at the time of hysterectomy as recommended by most au-

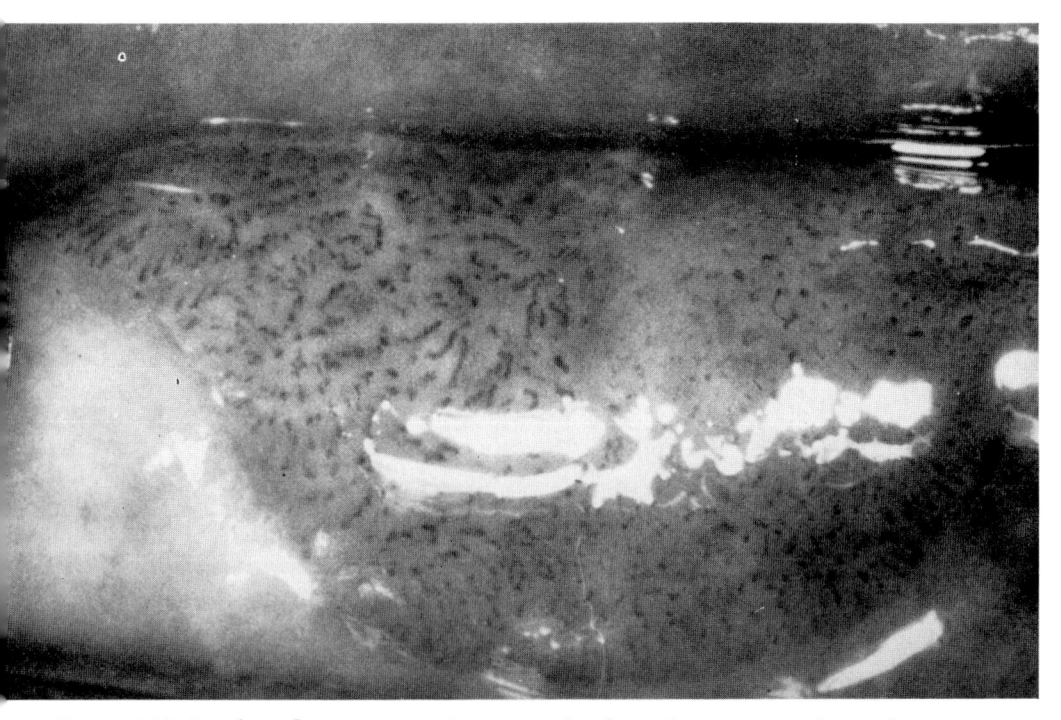

Figure 301. Preclinical carcinoma. Treatment. In this subject, atypical transformation zone is seen well down the posterior vaginal wall as the speculum is withdrawn. The cervix has receded from view. This lesion requires a special approach to diagnosis and treatment.

thorities is, in our opinion, unnecessary and is only indicated in these rare cases.

In the absence of colposcopy, vaginal extensions are often overlooked where they doubtless contribute to the problems after treatment of the positive smear and the so-called recurrent carcinoma, both of which invariably indicate persistence of the field of neoplastic potential as a result of inadequate excision or destruction.

The management of the woman with the uncommon primary carcinoma

TABLE XI

OPTIONS IN TREATMENT OF CIS AND DYSPLASIA OF VAGINA

1. Careful follow-up
2. Cryosurgery
3. Shallow electrodiathermy
4. CO_2 laser application
5. Local excision
6. Local application of 5-fluorouracil
7. Intravaginal radium or radon
8. Partial vaginectomy
9. Total vaginectomy

in situ or dysplasias of the vagina, or the more common vaginal extensions of cervical lesions, or "recurrent lesions" after treatment present the gynaecologist with similar problems (Table XI). The colposcope aids in recognising the site of the lesion or lesions, which at times can be so extensive as to involve most of the vaginal epithelium. The choice of therapy after establishing the preinvasive nature of the lesion by punch biopsy lies between the more desirable conservative methods of either cryosurgery, shallow electrodiathermy, CO_2 laser, local excision or application of the cytotoxic agent, 5-fluorouracil cream* to the most radical, partial, or complete vaginectomy followed by split-thickness skin graft. Application of intravaginal radium either in ovoids or cylinder or radon is common practice. Occasionally, in younger women with minor histological abnormalities, close follow-up by regular colposcopy, cytology, and selective biopsy may be justifiable.

AIDS IN ASSESSMENT OF ABNORMAL SMEAR DURING PREGNANCY

The use of colposcopy further enhances the safety of a conservative diagnostic approach during pregnancy. The recognition of the rare colposcopically overt carcinoma as illustrated previously is the basis for our management (Figs. 30, 196 to 198, and 285). Immediate biopsy and radical management is indicated in such cases. In nearly all cases, however, no overt carcinoma is seen on colposcopy, and normal columnar epithelium exists in the canal above any intraepithelial lesion which might be present. Thorough investigation and selection of treatment is then delayed until after the six weeks postnatal check, although frequently a punch biopsy is taken from any obvious atypical transformation zone to establish a diagnosis, and colposcopic examination is repeated later in the pregnancy.

It is difficult to understand the approach to diagnosis by conisation during pregnancy adopted in so many clinics. When performed in pregnancy, conisation may produce troublesome haemorrhage, abortion, or premature labour. As conditions are not ideal for this procedure in pregnancy, the cone is probably less satisfactory and, therefore, less likely to be effective as a definitive method of treatment than if performed some weeks after delivery.

The motive prompting the use of diagnostic conisation in pregnancy is the exclusion with as much assurance as possible of the presence of histologically invasive carcinoma, a condition presumably in need of urgent treatment. The frank undoubted clinical invasive carcinoma is an obvious

---

* Efudex® (Roche). The cream is inserted by standard vaginal applicator after preliminary test application to determine sensitivity. Application is daily for two weeks. The epithelium excoriates and then regenerates. Vulvovaginitis may occur.

danger if neglected in pregnancy. It seems reasonable to suggest, however, that clinics, including our own, not employing diagnostic conisation must fail to detect an occasional case of preclinical invasive carcinoma. Yet, the published reports from these clinics do not differ significantly in the final analysis.

AID IN THE FOLLOW-UP OF WOMEN TREATED FOR PRECLINICAL CERVICAL CARCINOMA AND DYSPLASIA

Recurrent preclinical carcinoma of the vaginal vault following treatment by total hysterectomy should be readily observed by colposcopic examination (Fig. 302). *In situ* lesions frequently have an irregular surface configuration suggestive to the inexperienced colposcopist of invasive cancer and can lead to an error in initial assessment. This difference in configuration compared to cervical lesions is the result of the different texture of the vaginal epithelium. However, provided the initial pretreatment assessment of lesions has been adequate and included colposcopy, any such vaginal extension should have been recognised and dealt with so that "recurrence" in this area will seldom occur. It is, therefore, not present policy to use colposcopy in follow-up, except for further investigation of positive or doubtful smear reports.

Colposcopy is also of limited value in the follow-up of women treated by conisation as definitive treatment. Colposcopic control at the time of conisation allows the incision always to be made distal to the atypical area on the ectocervix, so that no recurrent or persistent ectocervical lesion should be seen. Any residual or new disease then would be high in the cervical canal and beyond vision with the colposcope. Colposcopy is used initially in the first year of follow-up of these patients but then only in the presence of doubtful or positive smears. In the absence of preoperative colposcopic control, residual lesions on the ectocervix and lower endocervix after conisation are not uncommon, and extension of an inadequately excised lesion to the vaginal vault is occasionally seen.

Colposcopy is essential in the follow-up of women with lesions treated by methods involving physical destruction. The first examination should be performed six to twelve weeks after treatment. Frequently, the whole of the ectocervix and lower endocervix is covered by fully differentiated regenerate squamous epithelium which stains deeply with iodine. Less commonly, white epithelium almost certainly indicative of immature regenerate epithelium has replaced the area, and least commonly, atypical colposcopic appearances with vascular abnormalities resembling punctation and mosaic can be seen (Fig. 303). Reference has already been made to the atypical colposcopic appearances which seem to occur more frequently and persist longer following cryosurgery than after electrodiathermy (p. 361).

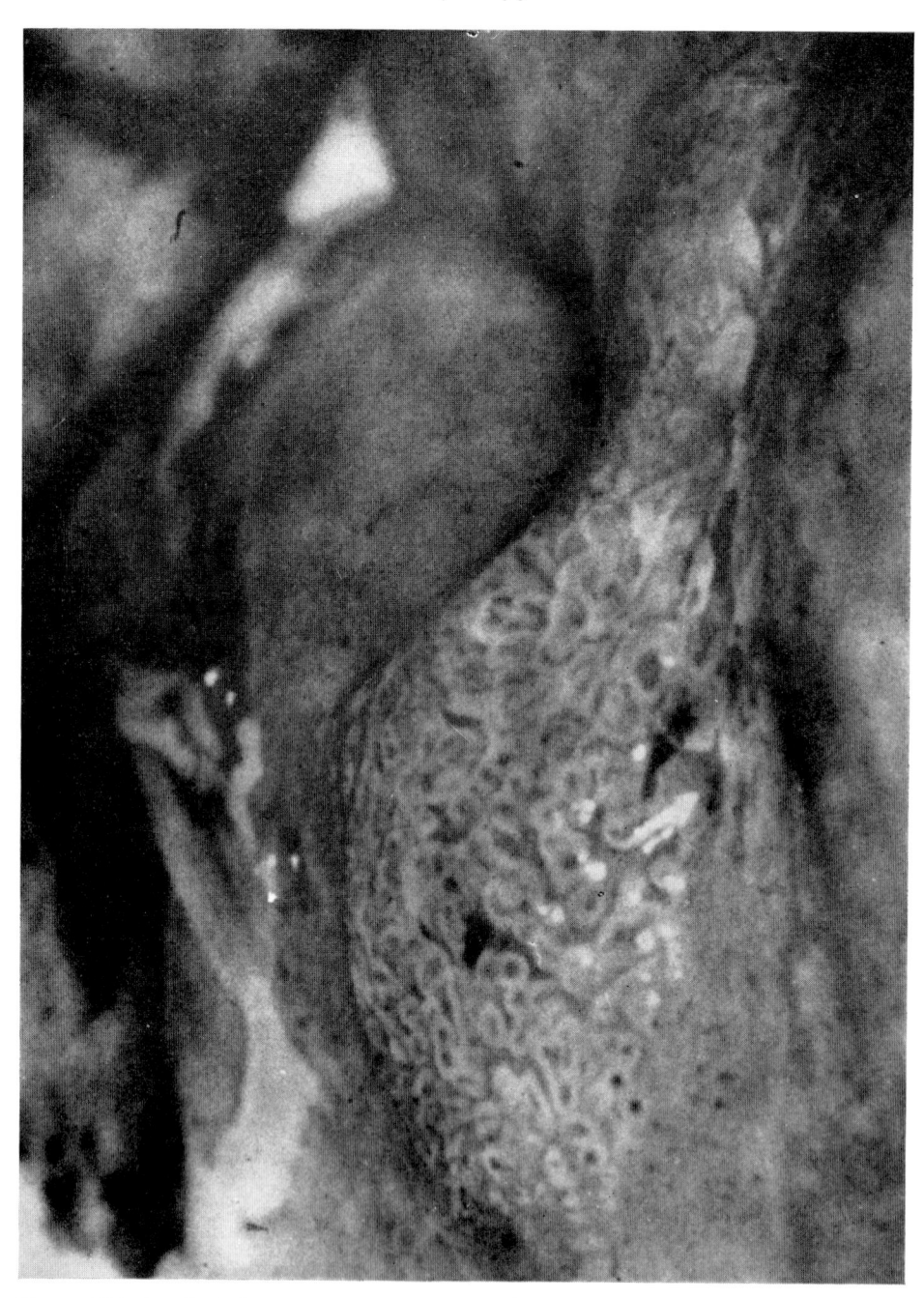

Figure 302. Preclinical carcinoma. Treatment. This atypical transformation zone, histologically shown to be carcinoma in situ lies at the vaginal vault. The lesion was discovered several months after total hysterectomy performed for carcinoma in situ and is probably not a true recurrence but represents inadequate excision of a lesion of the type shown in Figure 301.

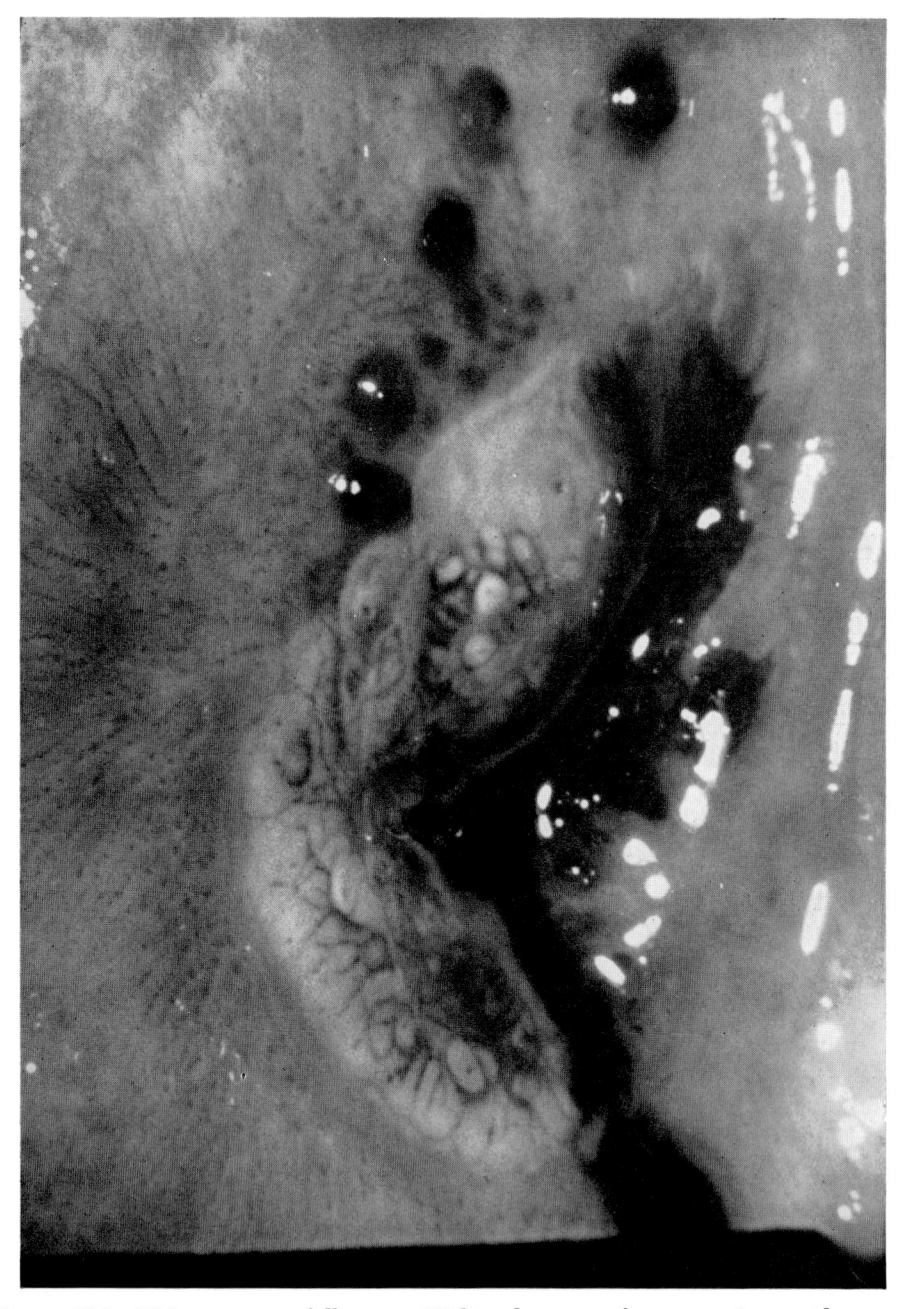

Figure 303. CIN treatment: follow-up. Within the area of regeneration, evident as a crescent at the left side of the photograph with characteristic radial distribution of vessels, a residual lesion is present closer to the canal, signifying inadequate destruction by physical methods. The finding emphasises the need for expert use of conservative methods involving physical destruction and for careful follow-up.

If persistent for six months, the lesion should be further biopsied and eradicated either by repeat cryosurgery, diathermy, or conisation.

MANAGEMENT AND FOLLOW-UP OF ATYPICAL TRANSFORMATION ZONES OF DOUBTFUL SIGNIFICANCE

When women attend for routine colposcopic examination or for evaluation of minor cytological abnormalities, a proportion display an atypical transformation zone of doubtful significance (*see* Chap. 15). Frequently, histological studies show one of the many varieties of normal metaplastic epithelium or minor abnormalities of atypical metaplastic epithelium. These patients pose problems relating to therapy or follow-up.

If there is a cytological disorder or if the patient is a poor prospect for follow-up, the situation is ideal for cryosurgical destruction in the office.

When no cytological disorder is present and the patient is able to attend on a regular basis, then such doubtful areas can be safely observed for long periods. In one of our clinics, regular examination of such subjects for up to twenty years has rarely resulted in the observed evolution of significant disorder. We are convinced that significant changes are heralded by the expected change in the grade of atypical transformation zone present and in alteration of the smear.

Perhaps the most striking finding in this follow-up study was that most, if not all, atypical transformation zones do not alter significantly in shape or size from year to year, unless biopsied or diathermied. A subsequent labour (other than the first) generally does not alter the area. They neither increase in size nor apparently spontaneously disappear. These lesions have never been observed to extend in an outwards direction to replace contiguous original squamous epithelium.

AID IN MANAGEMENT OF VAGINAL ADENOSIS

Although the value of colposcopy in the overall screening of vaginal adenosis is controversial (p. 352), its capacity to select sites for biopsy especially in the presence of an abnormal exfoliative cytological report is acceptable. There is general agreement that carcinoma in situ lesions are a possible sequel to the disturbed epithelial states in such women, although there is disagreement as to the frequency. We have discussed elsewhere difficulties for the clinician who must rely solely on histological diagnosis, and these discussions have particular relevance to the differential diagnosis of some of the lesions appearing in metaplastic phases of the cervix and vagina following exposure to non-steroidal oestrogens *in utero* (p. 374).

Most authors, in the absence of cervical intraepithelial neoplasia, do not treat vaginal adenosis, although some have advocated removal of the area as a type of prophylaxis. Thus, the chance of prolonged embryonic phases

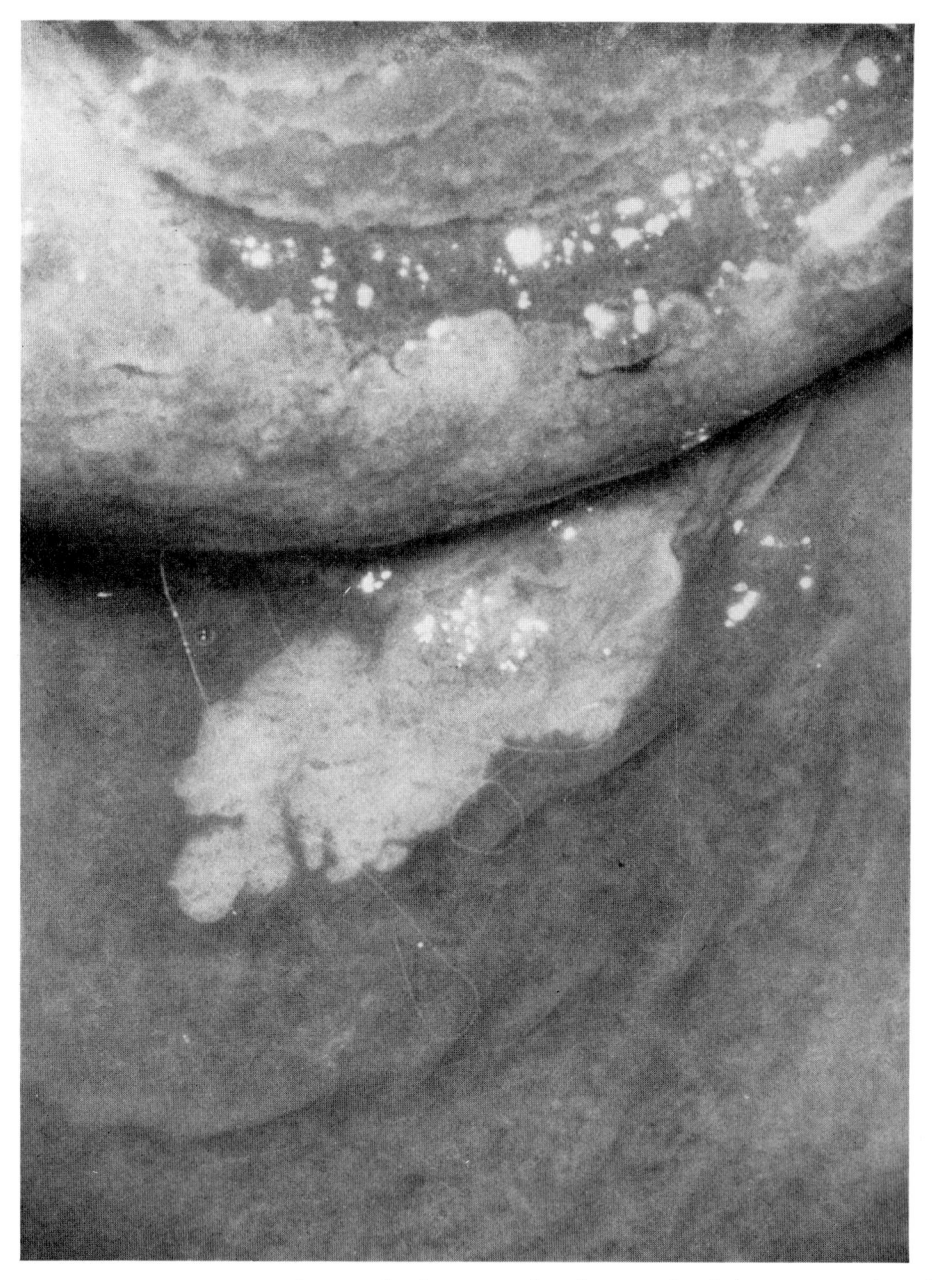

Figure 304. Management of vaginal adenosis. Colpophotograph of the posterior lip of cervix and posterior fornix showing a small circumscribed area of white epithelium on the vaginal wall. Although the conservative approach with regular observation is advised, some clinicians may use the colposcope to identify and eradicate such small areas of adenosis.

with their risk of developing glandular or squamous cancer is minimised by such ablation and its rapid regeneration to well-differentiated squamous epithelium.

As a result of more reliance on colposcopy to support the conventional histological diagnosis, two aspects can be emphasised. First, screening of women with vaginal adenosis by expert colposcopy is valuable, and second, a greater individualization of management is possible. An election within the range of ablation of the small lesion (Fig. 304) to surveillance of the large is simple. Modalities for ablation, whether for prophylaxis or for treatment of cervical intraepithelial neoplasia, include cryosurgery, electrodiathermy, and CO_2 laser vaporization. The CO_2 laser has prospectively the most merit.

AID IN ERADICATION OF CONDYLOMATA

Cervical, vaginal, and vulval condylomata seem to be increasing in incidence. Extensive and gross examples are being seen (*see* Figs. 207 to 212). The colposcope is a valuable aid in identifying all lesions present so that none are left to emerge in the post-treatment phase. Eradication may be achieved by cryosurgery or electrodiathermy under anaesthesia. Surgical laser is being used with increasing frequency, and the precision of both the colposcopic direction of its focus and the extent of its destructive ability allows virtual eradication of all lesions.

ALLOWS UNDERSTANDING OF *CERVICAL EROSION, CHRONIC CERVICITIS*, AND OTHER BENIGN CONDITIONS

The persistent attempts at macroscopic descriptions of the cervix and the preoccupation of clinicians with such ill-defined conditions as *cervical erosion* and *chronic cervicitis* serve only to underline the inadequacy of the naked eye as a means of studying the organ. Many simple and even physiological states of the cervix appear to the naked eye as vivid red patches. The commonest example is normal columnar epithelium of ectocervical distribution which takes on a plush red aspect often with contact bleeding and a mucous discharge which may resemble pus (Fig. 305). The diagnosis of "chronic cervicitis" is frequently made and there are often suspicious overtones of the presence of more serious conditions. The critical examination of epithelial surface structure available through the colposcope allows a rapid and specific diagnosis to be made.

The terms cervical erosion and chronic cervicitis are outdated and should be eliminated from the gynaecologist's vocabulary (p. 15). They are seen immediately to be entities in which variable proportions of columnar and metaplastic epithelium are seen. In a few instances, however, there is colposcopic evidence of dysplasia or carcinoma. These common, frequently troublesome naked-eye cervical appearances are so easily re-

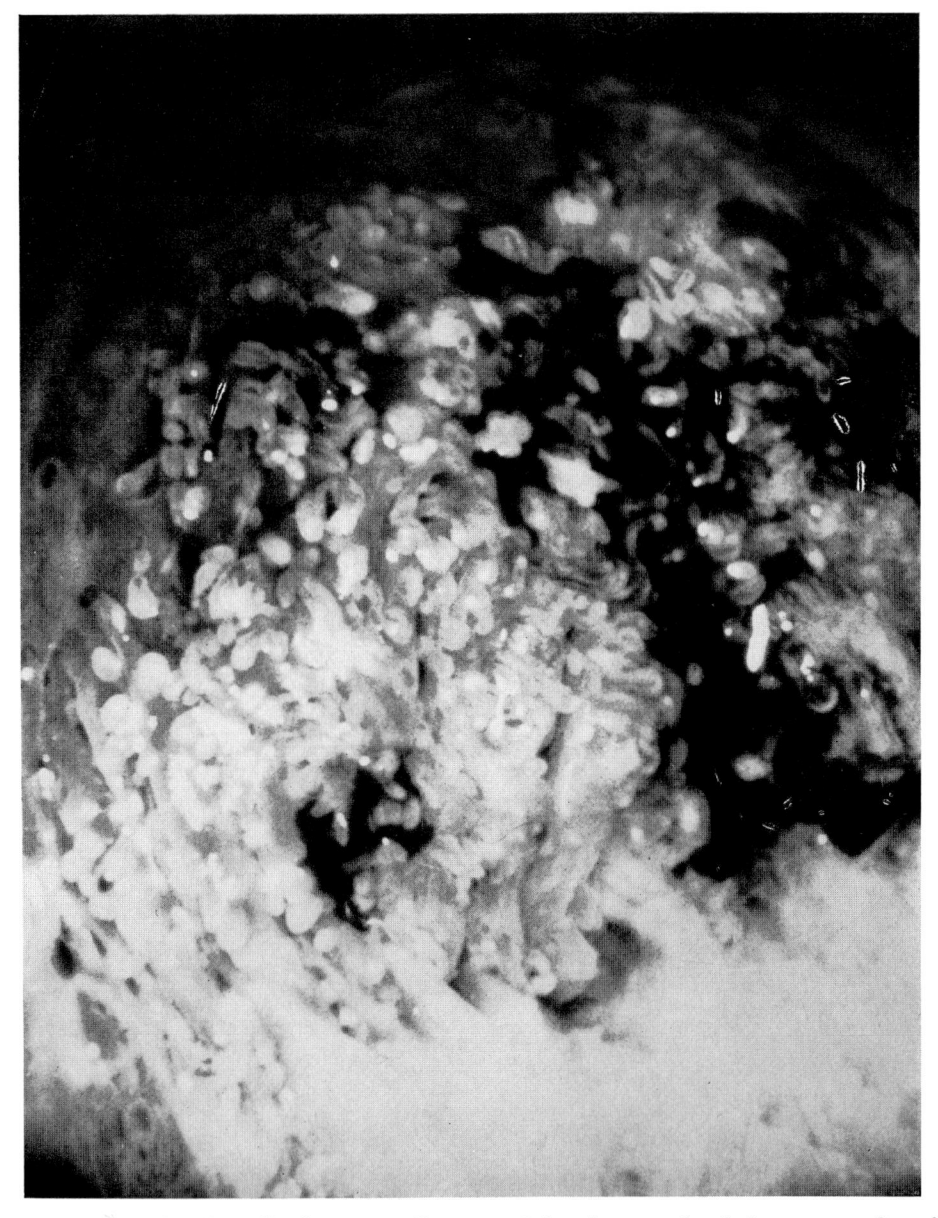

Figure 305. The clinically "suspicious" cervix. Colpophotograph of the anterior lip of the cervix showing normal villi, contact bleeding, and normal cervical mucus in the lower quarter of the photograph. To the naked eye, such appearances may be suspect of early cancer.

solved by colposcopy as to strengthen our conviction that no adequate description of the cervix is possible in its absence.

Older gynaecologists frequently claim that the routine practice of electrocautery destruction of these states present on the cervix effectively prevents cancer of the cervix. We believe this may be true, provided that the physical destruction of the transformation zone is complete in depth and extent. Such a program involves a large proportion of women and is not recommended. Nevertheless, some women persistently complain of discomfort and embarrassment obviously due to the secretion produced in the glandular structures of the cervix. Physical destruction of the mucous-secreting area by cryosurgery, electrocautery, electrodiathermy, or CO_2 laser vaporization effectively relieves symptoms. Other women requiring similar therapy are those with troublesome postcoital bleeding resulting from exposed and often oedematous columnar epithelium on the ectocervix.

SAVES UNNECESSARY BIOPSIES

The occurrence of a *red erosion*, often with contact bleeding in the consulting room or in the operating theatre prior to cryosurgery, electrodiathermy, vaginal repair, or total hysterectomy, often finds the clinician anxious for more rapidly available information as to the gravity of the appearance, especially as false negative smears can occur in the presence of frank cancer. Most often, such appearances are summarily and satisfyingly resolved as physiological columnar epithelium through the colposcope so that unnecessary biopsy is avoided (Fig. 305). Occasionally, atypical colposcopic lesions worthy of biopsy or even frank cancer are evident.

AID TO RESEARCH

Despite the need for the establishment of colposcopy as an aid to clinical affairs, there can be little doubt of its unique and established value to the medical scientist. The living organ at serial examination provides a life story highlighting periods of change that can be singled out for further study. From the precision allowed in the selection of sites for biopsy comes the distinct advantage of being able to harness the most potent tools of modern scientific enquiry, such as electron microscopy, tissue culture, and autoradiography, to any particular aspect of this life-history study. It is difficult to forsee the limits of such unison. At least, it renders woman herself an experimental animal as readily available as the usual laboratory animals. At best, it may place the pathogenesis of squamous cancer of the cervix amongst the first of all human cancers to be unravelled.

REFERENCES

A.C.O.G. Technical Bulletin No. 38. (1976). *Management of Abnormal Cytology by Colposcopy and/or Conization.* Chicago, American College of Obstetricians and Gynecologists.
Bendich, A., Borenfreund, E., and Sternberg, S. S. (1974). Penetration of somatic mammalian cells by sperm. *Science 183*:857.
Bibbo, M., Gill, W. B., Friedoon, A., Blough, R., Fang, V. S., Rosenfield, R. L., Schumacher, G. F. B., Sleeper, K., Sonek, M. G., and Wied, G. L. (1977). Follow-up study of male and female offspring of DES exposed mothers. *Obstet Gynecol, 49*:1.
Boutselis, J. G., Ullery, J. C., and Charme, L. (1971). Diagnosis and management of Stage 1A microinvasive carcinoma of the cervix. *Am J Obstet Gynecol, 110*:984.
Boyes, D. A., Worth, J. A., and Fidler, H. K. (1970). The results of treatment of 4389 cases of preclinical cervical squamous carcinoma. *J Obstet Gynaecol Br Commonw, 77*:769.
Coppleson, L. W. and Brown, B. (1974). Estimation of the screening error rate from the observed detection rates in repeated cervical cytology. *Am J Obstet Gynecol, 119*:953.
―――. (1975). Observation on a model of the biology of carcinoma of the cervix. A poor fit between observation and theory. *Am J Obstet Gynecol, 122*:127.
Coppleson, M. (1964). Colposcopy, cervical carcinoma in situ and the gynaecologist. Based on experience with the method in 200 cases of carcinoma in situ. *J Obstet Gynaecol Br Commonw, 71*:854.
―――. (1976). Management of premalignant carcinoma of the cervix. In Jordan, J. A. and Singer, A. (Eds.): *The Cervix Uteri.* London, Saunders.
―――. (1977). Colposcopy. In Stallworthy, J. and Bourne G. (Eds.): *Recent Advances in Obstetrics and Gynaecology.* London, Churchill.
Coppleson, M. and Reid, B. L. (1967). *Preclinical Carcinoma of the Cervix Uteri: Its Origin, Nature and Management.* Oxford, Pergamon.
―――. (1975). Origin of premalignant lesions of cervix uteri. In Taymor, M. L. and Green T. H. (Eds.): *Progress in Gynecology.* New York, Grune, vol. 6.
DiSaia, P. J., Morrow, C. P., and Townsend, D. E. (1975). *Synopsis of Gynecologic Oncology.* New York, Wiley.
Fetherston, W. C. (1975). Squamous neoplasia of vagina related to DES syndrome. *Am J Obstet Gynecol, 122*:176.
Graham, J. B., Sotto, L. S., and Paloucek, F. P. (1962). *Carcinoma of the Cervix.* Philadelphia, Saunders.
Gray, L. A. (Ed.). (1964). *Dysplasia, Carcinoma In Situ and Micro-invasive Carcinoma of the Cervix Uteri.* Springfield, Thomas, p. 424.
Hart, W. R., Townsend, D. E., Aldrich, J. O., Henderson, B. E., Roy, M., and Benton, B. (1976). Histopathologic spectrum of vaginal adenosis and related changes in stilbestrol-exposed females. *Cancer, 37*:763.
Herbst, A. L., Kurman, R. J., and Scully, R. E. (1972). Vaginal and cervical abnormalities after exposure to stilbestrol in utero. *Obstet Gynecol, 40*:287.
Herbst, A. L., Robboy, S. J., Macdonald, G. J., and Scully, R. E. (1974). The effects of local progesterone on stilbestrol-associated vaginal adenosis. *Am J Obstet Gynecol, 118*:607.

Herbst, A. L., Robboy, S. J., Scully, R. E., and Poskanzer, D. C. (1974). Clear cell adenocarcinoma of the vagina and cervix in girls: Analysis of 170 registry cases. *Am J Obstet Gynecol, 119*:713.

Herbst, A. L., Ulfelder, H., and Poskanzer, D. C. (1971). Adenocarcinoma of the vagina. Association of maternal stilbestrol therapy with tumor appearance in young

Hinselmann, H. (1955). *Colposcopy.* (With a section on colpophotography by A. Schmitt) Girardet, Wuppertal-Elberfeld.

International Federation of Gynecology and Obstetrics. (1976). In Kottmeier, H. L. (Ed.). *Annual Report on the Results of Treatment in Carcinoma of the Uterus, Vagina and Ovary.*

Koller, O. (1963). *The Vascular Patterns of the Uterine Cervix.* Oslo, Universitetsforlaget.

Kolstad, P. (1964). *Vascularisation, Oxygen Tension and Radiocurability in Cancer of the Cervix.* Oslo, Universitetsforlaget.

Kolstad, P. and Stafl, A. (1977). *Atlas of Colposcopy,* 2nd ed. Baltimore, Univ Park.

Kos, J. (1960). Distribution of the vessels in the portiovaginalis cervix uteri under the normal non-diseased pavement epithelium. *Zentralbl Gynaekol, 82*:1849.

———. (1962). Demonstration of capillaries in excised tissue from the cervix uteri by histochemical methods. *Zentralbl Gynaekol, 84*:538.

Limburg, H. (1958). Comparison between cytology and colposcopy in the diagnosis of early cervical carcinoma. *Am J Obstet Gynecol, 75*:1298.

Mussey, E., Soule, E. H., and Welch, J. S. (1969). Microinvasive carcinoma of the cervix. *Am J Obstet Gynecol, 104*:738.

Navratil, E. (1964). Colposcopy. In Gray, L. A. (Ed.): *Dysplasia, Carcinoma In Situ and Micro-invasive Carcinoma of the Cervix Uteri.* Springfield, Thomas, p. 273.

Nelson, J. H., Averette, H. E., and Richart, R. M. (1975). *Dyplasia and Early Cervical Cancer.* New York, Professional Education Publication, American Cancer Society.

Ng, A. B. P. and Reagan, J. W. (1969). Microinvasion of the uterine cervix. *Am J Clin Pathol, 52*:511.

Ng, A. B. P., Reagan, J. W., Nadji, M., and Greening, S. (1977). Natural history of vaginal adenosis in women exposed to diethylstilbestrol in utero. *J Reprod Med, 18*:1.

Poulsen, H. E. Taylor C. W. and Sobin, L. H. (1975). *Histological Typing of Female Genital Tumours.* Geneva, World Health Organization.

Reagan, J. W. (1977). Personal communication with the author.

Reid, B. L. and Coppleson, M. (1976). Natural history. Recent advances. In Jordan, J. A., and Singer, A. (Eds.): *The Cervix Uteri.* London, Saunders, p. 317.

Roche, W. and Norris, H. J. (1975). Microinvasive carcinoma of the cervix. The significance of lymphatic invasion and confluent patterns of stromal growth. *Cancer, 36*:180.

Sandberg, E. C. (1976). Benign cervical and vaginal changes associated with exposure to stilbestrol in utero. *Am J Obstet Gynecol, 125*:777.

Sherman, A. I., Goldrath, M., Berlin, A., Vakhariya, V., Banooni, F., Michaels, W., Goodman, P., and Brown, S. (1974). Cervical-vaginal adenosis after *in utero* exposure to synthetic estrogens. *Obstet Gynecol, 44*:531.

Stafl, A. (1962). Use of the azocoupling method for identification of alkaline phosphatase in study of the capillary network of the cervix uteri. *Cesk Morf, 10*:336.

———. (1976). New nomenclature for colposcopy. Report of the Committee on Terminology. *Obstet Gynecol, 48*:124.

Stafl, A. and Mattingly, R. F. (1973). Colposcopic diagnosis of cervical neoplasia. *Obstet Gynecol, 41*:168.

———: Vaginal adenosis: A precancerous lesion? *Am J Obstet Gynecol, 120*:666.
Stening, M. (1964). The surgical treatment of carcinoma of the cervix. *J Coll Radiol Aust, 8*:113.
Townsend, D. E. (1971). A cancer detection clinic in the United States. (Letter) *Med J Aust, 2*:113.
———: (1976). The management of cervical lesions by cryosurgery. In Jordan, J. A. and Singer, A. (Eds.): *The Cervix Uteri*. London, Saunders, p. 305.
Townsend, D. E., Ostergard, D. R., Mishell, D. R., and Hirose, F. M. (1970). Abnormal Papanicolaou smears—Evaluation by colposcopy, biopsies and endocervical curettage. *Am J Obstet Gynecol, 108*:429.
Way, S. (1968). Management of cervical carcinoma in situ. *Lancet, 2*:637.

BIBLIOGRAPHY

A.C.O.G. Technical Bulletin No. 38. (1976). *Management of Abnormal Cytology by Colposcopy and/or Conization.* Chicago, American College of Obstetricians and Gynecologists.

Adam, E., Kaufman, R. M., Melnick, J. L., Levy, A. H., and Rawls, W. E. (1974). Sero-epidemiologic studies of herpes virus type 2 and carcinoma of the cervix IV. *Am J Epidemiol,* 98:77.

Adelman, H. C. and Hadju, S. I. (1967). Role of conisation in the treatment of cervical carcinoma in situ. *Am J Obstet Gynecol,* 98:173.

Ahlgren, M., Ingemarsson, I., Lindberg, L. F., and Nordquist, S. R. B. (1975). Conisation as treatment of carcinoma in situ of the uterine cervix. *Obstet Gynecol,* 46:135.

Alexander, R. E. (1973). Possible etiologies of cancer of the cervix other than herpes virus. *Cancer Res,* 33:1485.

Almendral, A. C., Szalmay, G., Jochum, L., and Muller, H. (1974). Vor-und Fruhstadien des Zervixkarzinoms. *Fortschr Med,* 92:1007.

Anderson, A. F. 1962. New inventions: The Vann-Watson colposcope. *Lancet,* 2:813.

———. 1965). Treatment and follow-up of non-invasive cancer of the uterine cervix—Report on 205 cases (1948-57). *J Obstet Gynaecol Br Commonw,* 72:172.

Anderson, M. C. (1976). The aetiology and pathology of cancer of the cervix. *Clin Obstet Gynaecol,* 3:317.

Anderson, S. G. and Linton, E. B. (1977). The diagnostic accuracy of cervical biopsy and cervical conisation. *Am J Obstet Gynecol,* 99:113.

Andrys, J., Vacha, K., Rosol, M., and Kopecny, J. (1974). Prakanzerosen der Cervix uteri in der Schwangerschaft. *Zentralbl Gynaekol,* 96:1012.

Antoine, T. (1964). Colpomicroscopy. In Gray, L. A. (Ed.): *Dysplasia, Carcinoma In Situ and Micro-invasive Carcinoma of the Cervix Uteri.* Springfield, Thomas.

Antoine, T., Boyes, D. A., Fidler, H. K., and Schuller, E. (1962). May one treat the "early invasive carcinoma (microcarcinoma) less radically than the more extensive, invasive carcinoma?" (Symposium). *Acta Cytol,* 6:173.

Antoine, T. and Grunberger, V. (1956). *Atlas der Kolpomikroskopie.* Stuttgart, Thieme.

Aruta, J. (1967). Colposcopy contribution to the early diagnosis of cancer of the uterine cervix. *Rev Chile Obstet Ginecol,* 32:286.

Ashley, C., Kirkland, J. A., and Stanley, M. A. (1974). Antigenic deletion in cervical neoplasia. *Pathology,* 6:329.

Ashley, D. J. B. (1966). Evidence for the existence of two forms of cervical carcinoma. *J Obstet Gynaecol Br Commonw,* 73:382.

Atkin, N. B. (1976). Chromosonal changes in cervical neoplasia. In Jordan, J. A. and Singer, A. (Eds.): *The Cervix Uteri.* London, Saunders, p. 385.

Attwood, H. D. (1966). Carcinoma in situ: Fact and fiction. *Aust NZ J Obstet Gynaecol,* 6:11.

Attwood, M. E. (1966). Cytology and the contraceptive pill. *J Obstet Gynaecol Br Commonw,* 73:662.

———. (1976). The cytological recognition of physiological and neoplastic epithelium. In Jordan, J. A. and Singer, A. (Eds.): *The Cervix Uteri.* London, Saunders, p. 393.

Aurelian, L., Strandberg, J. D., and Davis, H. J. (1972). HSV2 antigens absent from biopsied cervical tumour cells; A model consistent with latency. *Proc Soc Exp Biol Med,* 140:404.

Averette, H. E. (1971). What is the effective method of therapy for stage 1A carcinoma of the cervix? *Med Opin Rev*, 7:73.

Averette, H. E., Nasser, N., Yankow, S. L., and Little, W. A. (1970). Cervical conisation in pregnancy. *Am J Obstet Gynecol*, 106:543.

Averette, H. E., Nelson, J. H., Jr., Ng, A. B. P., Hoskins, W. J., Boyce, J. G., and Ford, J. H., Jr. (1976). Diagnosis and management of microinvasive (State 1A) carcinoma of the uterine cervix. *Cancer [Suppl. 1]*, 38:414.

Ayre, J. E., Hillemanns, H. G., and Le Guerrier, J. (1966). Influence of norethynodrel and mestranol upon cervical dysplasia and carcinoma in situ. *Obstet Gynecol*, 28:90.

Bajardi, F. (1972). Spontanregression des pathologischen Gebarmutterhalsepithels im Histologischen. *Bild Ost Z Erforsch Bekampf Krebskrh*, 27:1.

Bajardi, F., Bret, J. A., and Coupez, F. J. (1959). Symposium on diagnostic accuracy of colposcopy as compared to cytology in the detection of cervical carcinoma during pregnancy. Discussion: A. Alvarez-Bravo, C. I. do Amaral Ferreira, J. W. Jenny, H. I. Wyss, W. R. Lang, and H. Mutch. *Acta Cytol*, 3:107.

Bajardi, F., Bret, J. A., Coupez, F. J., Lang, W. R., and Walz, W. (1961). Symposium on colposcopy of leukoplakia. Discussion: J. Berger, H. Janisch, M. Stucin, E. Vasquez Ferro, and H. I. Wyss. *Acta Cytol*, 5:115.

Bajardi, F., Burghardt, E., Kern, H., and Kroemer, H. (1959). Nouveaux résultats de la cytologie et de la colposcopie systématiques dans le diagnostic précoce du cancer du col de l'utérus. *Gynecol Prat*, 5:315.

Bajardi, F., Lang, W. R., de Moraes, A., and Rieper, J. P. (1959). Symposium on colposcopy of the irradiated cervix. Discussion: E. H. Kruger and O. Nyklicek. *Acta Cytol*, 3:369.

Barron, B. A. and Richart, R. M. (1968). A statistical model of the natural history of cervical carcinoma based on a prospective study of 557 cases. *J Natl Cancer Inst*, 41:1343.

Barter, R. A. (1966). Histomorphology of minimally invasive cervical squamous cancer. *Aust NZ J Obstet Gynaeccol*, 6:25.

Bauer, H. (1968). Uber den gegenwartigen Stand der Diagnostik und Therapie des weiblichen Genitalkarzinoms. *Hess Aerztebl*, 29:552.

———. (1970). Die Bedeutung der Kolposkopie bei der Fruhdiagnostik des Kollumkarzinoms in der taglichen Praxis. *Frauenarzt*, 11:200.

———. (1971). Zur problematik falsch negativer zytologischer Befunde. *Geburtshilfe Frauenheilkd*, 31:572.

———. (1976a). *Farbatlas der Kolposkopie*. Stuttgart, Schattauer.

———. (1976b). Kolposkopische Kriterien der atypischen Umwandlungszone. Vortrag gehalten auf der 3. Arbeitstagung der Arbeitsgemeinschaft "Cervix uteri." Wiesbaden, vom 1.-5. Mai, 1976.

Beard, R. W. (1964). Diathermy coning and cautery in the treatment of the eroded cervix. *J Obstet Gynaecol Br Commonw*, 71:287.

Beecham, C. T. (1975). The management of microcarcinoma (Stage 1A) of the cervix. In Taymor, M. L. and Green, T. H., Jr. (Eds.): *Progress in Gynecology*. New York, Grune, vol. 6, p. 599.

Beecham, C. T. and Andros, G. J. (1960). Cervical conisation in pregnancy. *Obstet Gynecol*, 16:521.

Beecham, C. T. and Carlin, E. S. (1962). The management of cervical carcinoma in situ. *Ann NY Acad Sci*, 97:814.

Beller, F. K. and Khatamee, M. (1966). Evaluation of punch biopsy of the cervix

under direct colposcopic observation. *Obstet Gynecol, 28*:622.
Bellina, J. (1974). Gynecology and the laser. *Contemporary Ob-Gyn, 4*:24.
Bendich, A., Borenfreund, E., and Sternberg, S. S. (1974). Penetration of somatic mammalian cells by sperm. *Science, 183*:857.
Benedet, J. L., Boyes, D. A., Nichols, T. M., and Millner, A. (1976). Colposcopic evaluation of patients with abnormal cervical cytology. *Brit J Obstet Gynaecol, 83*: 177.
Beral, V. (1974). Cancer of the cervix: A sexually transmitted infection. *Lancet, 1*:1037.
Bergleiter, R. and Bettzieche, H. (1975). Klinische und kolposkopische Befunde bei Prakanzerosen der Zervix uteri—Ein Beitrag zur Wertigkeit einer Auswahlzytologie. *Zentralbl Gynaekol, 97*:12.
Bibbo, M., Gill, W. B., Friedoon, A., Blough, R., Fang, V. S., Rosenfield, R. L., Schumacher, G. F. B., Sleeper, K., Sonek, M. G. and Wied, G. L. (1977). Follow-up study of male and female offspring of DES exposed mothers. *Obstet Gynecol, 49*:1.
Bickenbach, W., Soost, H. J., Boyes, D. A., Fidler, H. K., Jordan, M. J., Day, E., Bader, G. M., and Koss, L. (1962). Advantages and disadvantages of conservative management of carcinoma in situ. (Symposium.) *Acta Cytol, 6*:163.
Blunt, V. A. and Lang, L. P. (1967). A review of 307 cone biopsy examinations of the cervix. *Med J Aust, 2*:64.
Boddington, M. M., Spriggs, A. E., and Wolfendale, M. R. (1965). Cytogenic abnormalities in carcinoma in situ and dysplasia of the uterine cervix. *Br Med J, 1*: 154.
Boelter, W. C. and Newman, R. L. (1975). The correlation between colposcopic grading, directed punch biopsy and conization. *Am J Obstet Gynecol, 122*:945.
Bolten, K. A. (1967). Practical colposcopy in early cervical and vaginal cancer. *Clin Obstet Gynecol, 10*:808.
Bolten, K. A. and Jacques, W. E. (1960). *Introduction to Colposcopy*. New York, Grune.
Bonfiglio, T. A. and Patten, S. F. (1976). Histopathologic spectrum of benign proliferative and intraepithelial neoplastic reactions of the uterine cervix. *J Reprod Med, 16*:253.
Bonilla-Musoles, F. (1969). *Microscopía Electrónica Del Cervix Uterino*. Valencia, Facta.
Borja, M. M. (1962). The diagnosis of early cervical carcinoma by colposcopy. *Philippine J Cancer, 4*:283.
Boutselis, J. G. (1972). Intraepithelial carcinoma of the cervix associated with pregnancy. *Obstet Gynecol, 40*:657.
Boutselis, J. G., Ullery, J. C., and Charme, L. (1971). Diagnosis and management of stage 1A microinvasive carcinoma of the cervix. *Am J Obstet Gynecol, 110*:984.
Bowen-Simpkins, P. and Hull, G. R. (1975). Intraepithelial vaginal neoplasia following immunosuppressive therapy treated with topical 5FU. *Obstet Gynecol, 46*:360.
Boyce, J. G., Lu, T., Nelson, J. H., and Joyce, D. (1972). Cervical carcinoma and oral contraception. *Obstet Gynecol, 40*:139.
Boyd, J. R., Royle, D., Fidler, H. K., and Boyes, D. A. (1963). Conservative management of in situ carcinoma of the cervix. *Am J Obstet Gynecol, 85*:322.
Boyes, D. A. and Worth, J. A. (1976). Cytological screening for cervical carcinoma. In Jordan, J. A. and Singer, A. (Eds.): *The Cervix Uteri*. London, Saunders, p. 404.
Boyes, D. A., Worth, J. A., and Fidler, H. K. (1970). The results of treatment of 4389 cases of preclinical cervical squamous carcinoma. *J Obstet Gynaecol Br Commonw, 77*:769.

Breinl, H., Denhard, F., and Wilhelm, J. (1971). Intensivierte Fruhdiagnostik des Gebarmutterhalskarzinoms. Ergebnisse und Folgerungen. *Minerva Ginecol,* 23:86.

Bret, A. J. and Coupez, F. J. (1960). *Colposcopie.* Paris, Masson.

―――. (1963). Four cases of vaginal recurrences of invasive or intraepithelial carcinoma of the uterine cervix. *Acta Cytol,* 7:277.

Bret, A. J., Coupez, F. J., Ganse, R., Nyklicek, O., and Zinser, H. K. (1961). Symposium on colposcopy of ectopy, ectropion, and epidermization. Discussion: J. Berger, H. Janisch, W. Korte, E. H. Kruger, W. R. Lang, and E. Vasquez Ferro. *Acta Cytol,* 5:83.

Bret, A. J., Coupez, F. J., and Lang, W. R. (1959). Symposium on colposcopy of normal and abnormal cervices during pregnancy and the post-partum period. Discussion: F. Bajardi, O. Nyklicek, and H. I. Wyss. *Acta Cytol,* 3:61.

Brown, G. R., Fletcher, G. H., and Rutledge, F. N. (1971). Irradiation of in situ and invasive squamous cell carcinomas of the vagina. *Cancer,* 28:1278.

Brudenell, M., Cox, B. S., and Taylor, C. W. (1973). The management of dysplasia, carcinoma in situ and microcarcinoma of the cervix. The results of a survey organised by the Royal College of Obstetricians and Gynaecologists. *J Obstet Gynaecol Br Commonw,* 80:673.

Burghardt, E. (1959). Uber die atypische Umwandlungszone. *Geburtshilfe Frauenheilkd,* 19:676.

―――. (1963). Die diagnostische Konisation der Portio vaginalis uteri. *Gerburtshilfe Frauenheilkd,* 23:1.

―――. (1966). Zur Frage der Dysplasien des Portioepithels. *Wien Med Wochenschr,* 116:839.

―――. (1970). Latest aspects of precancerous lesions in squamous and columnar epithelium of the cervix. *Int J Obstet Gynecol,* 8:573.

―――. (1973). *Early Histological Diagnosis of Cervical Cancer. Textbook and Atlas.* E. A. Friedman, trans. Stuttgart, Thieme.

―――. (1976). Premalignant conditions of the cervix. *Clin Obstet Gynecol,* 3:257.

Burghardt, E. and Albeggar, H. (1969). Local infiltration for cone biopsy. *Geburtshilfe Frauenheilkd,* 29:1.

Burghardt, E. and Bajardi, F. (1956). Ergebnisse der Fruherfassung des Collumcarcinoms mittels Cytologie und Kolposkopie an der Universitats-Frauenklinik Graz. *Arch Gynaekol,* 1987:621.

―――. (1958). Simultaneous colposcopy and cytology used in screening for carcinoma of the cervix. *Am J Obstet Gynecol,* 75:1292.

Burghardt, E. and Holzer, E. (1970). Die Lokalisation des pathologischen Zervixepithels. I. Carcinoma in situ, Dysplasien und abnormes Plattenepithel. *Arch Gynaekol,* 209:305.

―――. (1972). Die Lokalisation des pathologischen Zervixepithels. IV. Epithelgrenzen. Letzte Zervixdrüse. Schussfolgerungen. *Arch Gynaekol,* 212:130.

Burke, L. and Antonioli, D. (1976). Vaginal adenosis. Factors influencing detection in a colposcopic evaluation. *Obstet Gynecol,* 48:413.

Burke, L., Antonioli, D., Knapp, R. C., and Friedman, E. A. (1974). Vaginal adenosis. Correlation of colposcopic and pathologic findings. *Obstet Gynecol,* 44:257.

Burke, L. and Mathews, B. (1977). *Colposcopy in Clinical Practice.* Philadelphia, Davis. cases of preclinical cervical squamous carcinoma. *J Obstet Gynaecol Br Commonw,* 6:266.

Canales Perez, E. S., Loria Mendez, L. M., and Mendez Gonzalez, S. (1965). Cyto-

logical and histopathological correlation of colposcopically atypical epithelia. *Ginecol Obstet Mex, 20*:1001.
Carmichael, R. and Jeaffreson, B. L. (1939). Basal cells in the epithelium of the human cervical canal. *J Pathol Bacteriol, 49*:63.
———. (1942). Squamous metaplasia of the columnar epithelium in the human cervix. *J Pathol Bacteriol, 52*:173.
Carrera, J. M. and Dexeus, S., Jr. (1971). Estudio colposcópico de los cambrios cervicales inducidos por anovulatórios orales. *Prog Obstet Ginecol, 14*:1.
Carrera, J. M., Dexeus, S., Jr. and Coupez, F. (1973). *Tratado y Atlas de Colposcopia*. Barcelona, Salvat Editores.
Cartier, R. (1974). *Atlas d'endoscopie. Colposcopie.* Paris—Editions prescript.
Catalano, W. L. and Johnson, L. D. (1971). Herpes virus antibody and carcinoma in situ of the cervix. *JAMA, 217*:447.
Cavanagh, D. and Rutledge, F. (1960). The cervical cone biopsy-hysterectomy sequence and factors affecting the febrile morbidity. *Am J Obstet Gynecol, 80*:53.
Chanen, W. and Hollyock, V. E. (1971). Colposcopy and electrocoagulation diathermy for cervical dysplasia and carcinoma in situ. *Obstet Gynecol, 37*:623.
———. (1974). Colposcopy and the conservative management of cervical dysplasia and carcinoma in situ. *Obstet Gynecol, 43*:527.
Chao, S., McCaffrey, R. M., Todd, W. D., and Moore, J. G. (1969). Conisation in evaluation and management of cervical neoplasia. *Am J Obstet Gynecol, 103*:574.
Christopherson, W. M. (1969). Concepts of genesis and development in early cervical neoplasia. *Obstet Gynecol Surv, 24*:842.
Christopherson, W. M. and Broghamer, W. L., Jr. (1961). A study of the reversibility of dysplasia of the uterine cervix. *Proceedings of the First International Congress of Exfoliative Cytology.* Philadelphia, Lippincott, p. 269.
Christopherson, W. M., Gray, L. A., and Parker, J. E. (1967). Role of punch biopsy in subclinical lesions of the uterine cervix. *Obstet Gynecol, 30*:806.
———. (1976). Microinvasive carcinoma of the uterine cervix—A long-term follow-up study of 80 cases. *Cancer, 38*:629.
Christopherson, W. M. and Parker, J. E. (1964a). Carcinoma in situ. In Gray, L. A. (Ed.): *Dysplasia, Carcinoma in Situ and Micro-invasive Carcinoma of the Cervix Uteri.* Springfield, Thomas, pp. 309-342.
———. (1964b). Microinvasive carcinoma of the uterine cervix. A clinical-pathological study. *Cancer, 17*:1123.
Collins, C. G., Roman-Lopez, J. J., and Lee, F. Y. L. (1970). Intraepithelial carcinoma of the vagina. *Am J Obstet Gynecol, 108*:1187.
Collins, R. J. and Pappas, H. J. (1972). Cryosurgery for benign cervicitis: Follow up of six and one half years. *Am J Obstet Gynecol, 113*:744.
Collins, R. J., Pappas, H. J., and Way, T. M. (1971). Cryosurgery in the treatment of abnormal cervical lesions. An invitational symposium. *J Reprod Med, 7*:147.
Conner, J. S. and Kaufman, R. H. (1970). Treatment of dysplasia of the cervix uteri by electrocauterisation. *Surg Gynecol Obstet, 131*:726.
Cope, I. (1961). The place of colposcopy in cancer detection. *Med J Aust, 48*:164.
———. (1964). The colposcopic appearances with adenocarcinoma of the cervix. *Aust NZ J Obstet Gynaecol, 4*:73.
———. (1966). The place of colposcopy in the detection and diagnosis of carcinoma in situ of the cervix. *Aust NZ J Obstet Gynaecol, 6*:1.
Copenhaver, E. H. and Bahner, D. (1963). Positive cytology registry. *Am J Obstet Gynecol, 86*:937.

Coppleson, L. W. and Brown, B. (1974). Estimation of the screening error rate from the observed detection rates in repeated cervical cytology. *Am J Obstet Gynecol, 119*:953.

———. (1975). Observation on a model of the biology of carcinoma of the cervix. A poor fit between observation and theory. *Am J Obstet Gynecol, 122*:127.

———. (1976). The prevention of carcinoma of the cervix. *Am J Obstet Gynecol, 125*: 153.

Coppleson, M. (1959). The use of colposcopy in the early detection of carcinoma of the cervix. *Med J Aust, 46*:64.

———. (1960). The value of colposcopy in the detection of preclinical carcinoma of the cervix. *J Obstet Gynaecol Br Emp, 67*:11.

Coppleson, M. (1964). Colposcopy, cervical carcinoma in situ and the gynaecologist. Based on experience with the method in 200 cases of carcinoma in situ. *J Obstet Gynaecol Br Commonw, 71*:854.

———. (1966a). *A Colposcopic Study of the Human Cervix Uteri in Health and Disease.* Unpublished dissertation. University of Sydney, Australia.

———. (1966b). Colposcopy in controversial problems associated with cervical carcinoma in situ. *Aust NZ J Obstet Gynaecol, 6*:5.

———. (1967a). Colposcopy in the early detection of carcinoma of the cervix. *Postgrad Med J, 23*:70.

———. (1967b). Treatment of preclinical invasive carcinoma of the cervix. *Proceedings of the Fifth World Congress of Obstetrics and Gynaecology.* London, Butterworths, p. 856.

———. (1968a). Cervical conisation. *Mod Med Aust, 10*:119.

———. (1968b). Treatment of Stage O carcinoma of the cervix. *Med J Aust [Supp. 6], 1*:61.

———. (1969). Carcinoma of the cervix. Epidemiology and aetiology. *Br J Hosp Med, 2*:961.

———. (1970). Origin and nature of premalignant lesions of the cervix uteri. Proceedings of the Sixth World Congress of Obstetrics and Gynaecology. *J Int Fed Gynecol Obstet, 8*:539.

———. (1972a). La iniciación del carcinoma pavimentoso del cuello. In Jakob, C. A. and Franco, M. A. (Eds.): *Proceedings of the First World Congress of Colposcopy and Cervical Pathology.* Rosario, Argentina, Molachino Establecimiento Gráfico, p. 39.

———. (1972b). La zona de transformación. Un nuevo concepto en colposcopía. In Jakob, C. A. and Franco, M. A. (Eds.): *Proceedings of First World Congress of Colposcopy and Cervical Pathology.* Rosario, Argentina, Molachino Establecimiento Gráfico, p. 125.

———. (1974a). Cervical cytology. *Ob-Gyn. Collected Letters, Series XV.* Lakeland, Florida, Ob. Gyn. Letters, Inc., p. 179.

———. (1974b). Treatment of preclinical carcinoma of the uterine cervix. *Oxford Med Gazette, 26*:20.

———. (1976a). The new colposcopic terminology. *J Reprod Med, 16*:214.

———. (1976b). Management of premalignant carcinoma of the cervix. In Jordan, J. A. and Singer, A. (Eds.): *The Cervix Uteri.* London, Saunders.

———. (1977a). Colposcopy. In Stallworthy, J. and Bourne, G. (Eds.): *Recent Advances in Obstetrics and Gynaecology.* London, Churchill.

———. (1977b). Epidemiology and etiology of carcinoma of the cervix. In Chamberlain, G. G. (Ed.): *Contemporary Obstetrics and Gynaecology.* London, Northwood.

Coppleson, M., Pixley, E. C., and Reid, B. L. (1974). *Colposcopía.* Barcelona, Ediciones Toray.
Coppleson, M., Pixley, E. C., Singer, A., and Reid, B. L. (1967). Etiology of carcinoma of the cervix. *Scientific Exhibition of the Fifth World Congress in Obstetrics and Gynaecology.* Basel, Sandoz.
Coppleson, M. and Reid, B. L. (1966). A colposcopic study of the cervix during pregnancy and in the puerperium. *J Obstet Gynaecol Br Commonw,* 73:575.
———. (1967a). *Preclinical Carcinoma of the Cervix Uteri: Its Origin, Nature and Management.* Oxford, Pergamon.
———. (1967b). Aetiology of squamous carcinoma of the cervix. *Proceedings of the Fifth World Congress of Obstetrics and Gynaecology.* London, Butterworths, p. 854.
———. (1968). Aetiology of squamous carcinoma of the cervix. *Obstet Gynecol,* 32:432.
———. (1969). Interpretation of changes in the uterine cervix. *Lancet,* 2:216.
———. (1975a). Observations on the initiation of squamous cancer of the cervix. *Gynescope,* 3:1.
———. (1975b). Origin of premalignant lesions of cervix uteri. In Taymor, M. L. and Green, T. H. (Eds.): *Progress in Gynecology.* New York, Grune, vol. 6, p. 517.
Coupez, F. (1970). La place de la colposcopie dans l'examen gynécologique actuel. *Rev Fr Gynecol,* 65:209.
Cramer, H. (1961). Kritisches zum Begriff der sogenannten atypischen Umwandlungszone. *Geburtshilfe Frauenheilkd,* 21:706.
Cramer, H. and Ohly, G. (1975). *Die Kolposkopie In Der Praxis.* Stuttgart, Thieme.
Crapanzano, J. T., Holmquist, N. D. and Mickal, A. (1966). Evaluation of superficial and intermediate cell dyskaryosis by colposcopy. *Am J Obstet Gynecol,* 94:405.
Creasman, W. T. and Rutledge, F. (1972). Carcinoma in situ of the cervix. An analysis of 861 patients. *Obstet Gynecol,* 39:373.
Creasman, W. T., Weed, J. G., Jr., Curry, S. L., Johnston, W. W., and Parker, R. T. (1973). Efficacy of cryosurgical treatment of severe intraepithelial neoplasia. *Obstet Gynecol* 41:501.
Crisp, W. E. (1972). Cryosurgical treatment of neoplasia of the uterine cervix. *Obstet Gynecol,* 39:495.
Crisp, W. E., Smith, M. S., Asadourian, L. A., and Warrenburg, C. B. (1970). Cryosurgical treatment of premalignant disease of the uterine cervix. *Am J Obstet Gynecol,* 107:737.
Crompton, A. C. (1976). The cervical epithelium during the menopause. In Jordan, J. A. and Singer, A. (Eds.): *The Cervix Uteri.* London, Saunders, p. 128.
Cunha, M. P. (1965). Colposcopic and colpocytologic study of 1350 patients clinically free of suspicion of malignant neoplasms. *An Brasil Ginecol,* 59:407.
Dabancens, A., Prado, R., Larraguibel, R., and Zanartu, J. (1974). Intraepithelial cervical neoplasia in women using intrauterine devices and long-acting injectable progestogens as contraceptives. *Am J Obstet Gynecol,* 119:1052.
Davidson, C. and Taylor, C. W. (1973). A study of patients previously treated for in situ carcinoma of the cervix. *J Obstet Gynaecol Br Commonw,* 80:654.
Davis, H. J. and Jones, H. W., Jr. (1969). Cervical cancer control with irrigation smears. *Obstet Gynecol Surv,* 24:927.
de Brux, J. A., and Dupre-Fremont, J. (1961). Interrelationship: Reserve cell hyperplasia, basal cell hyperplasia, dysplasia and cervical carcinoma. *Acta Cytol,* 5:265.
De Cenzo, J. A., Malo, T., and Cavanagh, D. (1971). Factors affecting cone-hysterectomy morbidity. *Am J Obstet Gynecol,* 110:380.

Decker, W. H. (1956). Minimal invasive carcinoma of the cervix with lymph node metastasis. *Am J Obstet Gynecol, 72*:1116.

Delgado, G. (1975). Diagnosis of cervical neoplasia by the nonspecialised colposcopist. *Gynecol Oncol, 3*:114.

Demin, U. N. (1968). Some aspects of carcinoma in situ of the uterine cervix. *Obstet Gynecol, 31*:288.

De Petrillo, A., Townsend, D. E., Morrow, C. P., Lickrish, G. M., DiSaia, P. J., and Roy, M. (1975). Colposcopic evaluation of the abnormal Papanicolaou test in pregnancy. *Am J Obstet Gynecol, 121*:441.

Devereux, W. P. and Edwards, C. L. (1967). Carcinoma in situ of the cervix. Applicability of diagnostic and treatment methods in 632 cases. *Am J Obstet Gynecol, 98*:497.

Dexeus, S. Jr., Casanelles, F., Carrera, J. M., y Font, V. (1968). La citologia y la colposcopia en el diagnóstico precoz del cancer uterino. *Acta Ginecol, 19*:881.

Dexeus, S., Jr., Fontane, F. J., and Carrera, J. M. (1964). Resultados obtenidos en neustras 500 primeras colposcopías. *Prog Obstet Ginecol, 7*:468.

Dilts, P. V., Elesh, R., and Greene, R. (1964). Re-evaluation of four quadrant punch biopsies of the cervix. *Am J Obstet Gynecol, 90*:961.

Dilworth, E. E. and Maxwell, G. E. (1962). Superficially invasive carcinoma and carcinoma in situ of the uterine cervix. *Am J Obstet Gynecol, 84*:83.

Di Paola, G. (1963). Investigations of the initial stages of cervical carcinoma. *Rev Colombia Obstet Ginecol, 14*:13.

Di Paola, G., Navratil, E., Blaikley, J. G., Way, S., Serebrov, A. I., Ulfelder, H., Hashimoto, K., Green, G. H., Magaro, N., Timonen, S., Louros, N. C., Brewer, J. I., and Chien-Tien Hsu. (1969). Which type of hysterectomy should be done in patients who have a proven diagnosis of carcinoma in situ of the cervix and who desire no more children? (Symposium). *Int J Gynecol Obstet, 7*:148.

DiSaia, P. J., Morrow, C. P., and Townsend, D. E. (1975). *Synopsis of Gynecologic Oncology.* New York, Wiley.

Dohnal, V. (1967). Schwangerschaft und Schleimhautveranderungen an der Cervix uteri. *Geburtshilfe Frauenheilkd, 27*:392.

Dolan, T. E., Boyce, J., Rosen, Y., and Lu, T. (1975). Cytology, colposcopy and directed biopsy: What are the limitations? *Gynecol Oncol, 3*:314.

Donohue, L. R. and Meriwether, W. (1972). Colposcopy as a diagnostic tool in the investigation of cervical neoplasia. *Am J Obstet Gynecol, 113*:107.

Fetherston, W. C. (1975). Squamous neoplasia of vagina related to DES syndrome. *Am J Obstet Gynecol, 122*:176.

Fegerl, H. E. (1964). Use of the colpophotogram. *Am J Obstet Gynecol, 89*:827.

Fegerl, H. E. and Ayre, J. E. (1970). Studies on cervical lesions in virgins: A combined cytological and colposcopic evaluation. *Cancer Cytol, 10*:39.

Feldman, M. J., Kent, D. R., Linzey, E. M., and Goldstein, A. I. (1976). The making of a colposcopist. A safe and sensible approach. *J Reprod Med, 16*:73.

Ferguson, J. H. (1967). Why some adolescents need cytologic screening. *Ann NY Acad Sci, 142*:654.

Ferguson, J. H. and Brown, G. C. (1960). Cervical conisation during pregnancy. *Surg Gynecol Obstet, 111*:603.

Feste, J. R., Kaufman, R. H., Skogland, H. L., and Topek, N. H. (1966). Management of abnormal cytology late in pregnancy. *Am J Obstet Gynecol, 95*:763.

Fidler, H. K. and Boyes, D. A. (1960). Occult invasive carcinoma of the cervix. *Cancer, 13*:764.

Fidler, H. K., Boyes, D. A., and Worth, A. J. (1968). Cervical cancer detection in British Columbia: A progress report. *J Obstet Gynaecol Br Commonw*, 75:392.
Fluhmann, C. F. (1959). The glandular structures of the cervix during pregnancy. *Am J Obstet Gynecol*, 78:990.
———. (1960). Carcinoma in situ and the transitional zone of the cervix uteri. *Obstet Gynecol*, 16:424.
———. (1961). *The Cervix Uteri and Its Diseases*. Philadelphia, Saunders.
———. (1963). Management of so-called erosions of the cervix uteri. *Clin Obstet Gynecol*, 6:344.
———. (1964a). The cervix uteri. In Gray, L. A. (Ed.): *Dysplasia, Carcinoma In Situ and Micro-invasive Carcinoma of the Cervix Uteri*. Springfield, Thomas, p. 6.
———. (1964b). Further observations on involvement of clefts and tunnels in carcinoma in situ of the cervix uteri. *Am J Obstet Gynecol*, 90:610.
Foote, F. W., Jr. and Stewart, F. W. (1948). The anatomical distribution of intraepithelial epidermoid carcinomas of the cervix. *Cancer*, 1:431.
Foraker, A. G. (1962). Histochemistry of the uterine cervix; Normal exocervical, metaplastic, dysplastic, intraepithelial and invasive squamous carcinomatous epithelium. *Ann NY Acad Sci*, 97:632.
Forsberg, J. G. (1965). An experimental approach to the problem of the derivation of the vaginal epithelium. *J Embryol Exp Morphol*, 14:213.
———. (1972). Estrogen, vaginal cancer and vaginal development. *Am J Obstet Gynecol*, 11:83.
———. (1976). Morphogenesis and differentiation of the cervicovaginal epithelium. In Jordan, J. A. and Singer, A. (Eds.): *The Cervix Uteri*. London, Saunders, p. 3.
Fox, C. H. (1968). Time necessary for conversion of normal to dysplastic cervical epithelium. *Obstet Gynecol*, 31:749.
Frick, H. C. II, Janovski, N. A., Gusberg, S. B., and Taylor, H. C., Jr. (1963). Early invasive cancer of the cervix. *Am J Obstet Gynecol*, 85:926.
Friedell, G. H. and Graham, J. B. (1959). Regional lymph node involvement in small carcinoma of the cervix. *Surg Gynecol Obstet*, 108:513.
Friedell, G. H., Hertig, A. T., and Younge, P. A. (1960). *Carcinoma In Situ of the Uterine Cervix*. Springfield, Thomas.
Frost, J. K. (1969). Diagnostic accuracy of "cervical smears." *Obstet Gynecol Surv*, 24:893.
Fujimori, H. and Noda, S. (1966). *Colpomicroscopy*. Osaka, Nagai.
Gall, S. A., Bourgeois, C. H., and Maguire, R. (1969). The morphologic effects of oral contraceptive agents on the cervix. *JAMA*, 207:2243.
Gallup, D. G. and Morley, G. W. (1975). Carcinoma in situ of the vagina. A study and review. *Obstet Gynecol*, 46:334.
Galvin, G. A., Jones, H. W., and TeLinde, R. W. (1955). The significance of basal cell hyperactivity in cervical biopsies. *Am J Obstet Gynecol*, 70:808.
Ganse, R. (1958). *Das normale und pathologische Gefass-Bild der Portio vaginalis uteri*. Berlin, Akad Verl.
———. (1963). *Einfuhrung in die Kolposkopie*. Jena, East Germany, Fischer.
———. (1966). *Initiation a la Colposcopie*. Paris, Librairie Maloine.
———. (1967). Veranderungen der atypischen Gefasse des Portiokarzinoms unter Telecobaltbestrahlung. *Geburtschilfe Frauenheilkd*, 27:476.
Ganse, R., Lang, W. R., Walz, W., and Zinser, H. K. (1961). Symposium on colposcopy of carcinoma in situ. Discussion: A. J. Bret, F. J. Coupez, C. I. do Amaral Ferreira,

H. Janisch, J. W. Jenny, A. Wacek, E. H. Kruger, and M. Marcov. *Acta Cytol,* 5: 401.
Garrett, W. J. (1964). Symptomless carcinoma of the cervix. *J Obstet Gynaecol Br Commonw,* 71:517.
Geelhoed, G. W., Henson, D. E., Taylor, P. T., and Ketcham, A. S. (1976). Carcinoma in situ of the vagina following treatment for carcinoma of the cervix: A distinctive clinical entity. *Am J Obstet Gynecol,* 124:510.
Gilotra, P. M., Lee, F. Y., Krupp, P. J., Batson, H. W., and Collins, J. H. (1976). Carcinoma in situ of the cervix uteri in pregnancy. *Surg Gynecol Obstet,* 142:396.
Glatthaar, E. (1955). Kolposkopie. *Seitz-Amreich: Biologie und Pathologie des Weibes.* Vienna, Urban, vol. 3.
Govan, A. D. T., Haines, R. M., Langley, F. A., Taylor, C. W., and Woodcock, A. S. (1969). The histology and cytology of changes in the epithelium of the cervix uteri. *J Clin Pathol,* 22:383.
Graham, J. B., Sotto, L. S., and Paloucek, F. P. (1962). *Carcinoma of the Cervix.* Philadelphia, Saunders.
Graham, R. M. (1972). *The Cytologic Diagnosis of Cancer.* Philadelphia, Saunders.
Gray, L. A. (Ed.). (1964a). *Dysplasia, Carcinoma In Situ and Micro-invasive Carcinoma of the Cervix Uteri.* Springfield, Thomas.
Gray, L. A. (1964b). Present knowledge of the preinvasive and very early invasive carcinomas of the cervix, the current approach to diagnosis and problems of the future. In Gray, L. A. (Ed.): *Dysplasia, Carcinoma In Situ and Micro-invasive Carcinoma of the Cervix Uteri.* Springfield, Thomas, p. 424.
———. (1969). The frequency of taking cervical smears. *Obstet Gynecol Surv,* 24:909.
Gray, L. A., Barnes, M. L. and Lee, J. J. (1960). Carcinoma in situ and dysplasia of the cervix. *Ann Surg,* 151:951.
Gray, L. A. and Christopherson, W. M. (1969). In situ and early invasive carcinoma of the vagina. *Obstet Gynecol,* 34:226.
Green, G. H. (1965). Cervical cytology and carcinoma in situ. *J Obstet Gynaecol Br Commonw,* 72:13.
———. (1966a). Pregnancy following cervical carcinoma in situ. A review of 60 cases. *J Obstet Gynaecol Br Commonw,* 73:897.
———. (1966b). The significance of cervical carcinoma in situ. *Am J Obstet Gynecol,* 94:1009.
———. (1970). Cervical carcinoma in situ. An atypical viewpoint. *Aust NZ J Obstet Gynaecol,* 10:41.
Green, G. H. and Donovan, J. W. (1970). The natural history of cervical carcinoma in situ *J Obstet Gynaecol Br Commonw,* 77:1.
Green, T. H., Jr. (1975). Surgical management of carcinoma of the cervix in pregnancy. In Taymor, M. L. and Green, T. H., Jr. (Eds.): *Progress in Gynecology.* New York, Grune, vol. 6, p. 607.
Griffiths, C. T., Austin, J. H., and Younge, P. A. (1964). Punch biopsy of the cervix. *Am J Obstet Gynecol,* 88:695.
Griffiths, C. T. and Younge, P. A. (1969). The clinical diagnosis of early cervical cancer. *Obstet Gynecol Surv,* 24:967.
Gronroos, M., Hautera, P., Jarvi, O., Kangas, S., and Rauramo, L. (1967). Cytology and colposcopy in mass screening for cervical cancer. *Acta Cytol,* 11:37.
Grunberger, V. (1963). Diagnosis and treatment of cancer in situ of the cervix uteri. *Acta Un Int Cancer,* 19:1419.

———. (1971). Prophylaxe des Collumcarcinoms durch Elektrokoagulation der Erythroplakie. *Minerva Ginecol, 23*:178.

Guhr, O. (1965). Kolposkopische, zytologische und histologische Portiobefunde bei ovulationshemmenden Medikamenten. *Arch Gynaekol, 202*:205.

Gunning, J. E. and Ostergard, D. R. (1976). Value of screening procedures for the detection of vaginal adenosis. *Obstet Gynecol, 47*:268.

Gusberg, S. B. (1969). Summary: Detection and diagnosis of early cervical neoplasia: Community methods. *Obstet Gynecol Surv, 24*:1041.

Gusberg, S. B. and Marshall, D. (1962). Intra-epithelial carcinoma of the cervix: A clinical reappraisal. *Obstet Gynecol, 19*:713.

Gusberg, S. B., Taylor, H. C., Jr., Reagan, J. W., and Ross, R. A. (1962). Symposium: Preinvasive lesions of the cervix. *Bull Sloane Hosp Wom, 8*:117.

Haam, E. von (1969). Summary: Concepts of genesis and development. *Obstet Gynecol Surv, 24*:879.

Haam, E. von and Old, J. W. (1964). Reserve cell hyperplasia, squamous metaplasia and epidermization. In Gray, L. A. (Ed.): *Dysplasia, Carcinoma In Situ and Microinvasive Carcinoma of the Cervix Uteri.* Springfield, Thomas, p. 41.

Hakama, M. and Rasanen, V. U. (1976). Effect of mass screening program in the risk of cervical cancer. *Am J Epidemiol, 103*:512.

Hall, J. E. and Walton, L. (1968). Dysplasia of the cervix: A prospective study of 206 cases. *Am J Obstet Gynecol, 100*:662.

Hamperl, H. and Kaufmann, C. (1959). The cervix uteri at different ages. *Obstet Gynecol, 14*:621.

Hamperl, H., Kaufmann, C., and Ober, K. G. (1954). Histologische Untersuchungen an der Cervix schwangerer Frauen. Die Erosion und das Carcinoma in situ. *Arch Gynaekol, 184*:181.

Hansen, L. H. and Collins, C. G. (1967). Multicentric squamous cell carcinoma of the lower female genital tract. Eleven cases with epidermoid carcinoma of both vulva and cervix. *Am J Obstet Gynecol, 98*:982.

Hansen, K. and Egholm, M. (1975). Diffuse vaginal adenosis. Three cases combined with imperforate hymen and haematocolpos. *Acta Obstet Gynecol Scand, 54*:287.

Hart, W. R., Townsend, D. E., Aldrich, J. O., Henderson, B. E., Roy, M. and Benton, B. (1976). Histopathologic spectrum of vaginal adenosis and related changes in stilbestrol-exposed females. *Cancer, 37*:763.

Hartmann, G. and Lau, H. (1973). Zur Diagnostik bei Vorstadien und Fruhformen des Zervixkarzinoms am kommunalen Klinikum. *Zentralbl Gynaekol, 95*:614.

Hartzell, J. M., Pratt, J. H., and Soule, E. H. (1963). In situ squamous cell carcinoma of the cervix with vaginal extension, recurrence and subsequent invasion: Report of a case. *Proc Mayo Clin, 28*:547.

Held, E., Schreiner, W., and Oehler, J. (1954). Bedeutung der Kolposkopie und Zytologie zur Erfassung des Genitalkarzinoms. *Schweiz Med Wochenschr, 84*:856.

Herbeck, G. (1976). Das Carcinoma in situ der Portio bei der Frau unter 30 Jahren. *Med Welt NF, 27*:1466.

Herbst, A. L., Cole, P., Colton, T., Robboy, S. J., and Scully, R. E. (1977). Age-incidence and risk of DES-related clear cell adenocarcinoma of the vagina and cervix. *Am J Obstet Gynecol,* in press.

Herbst, A. L., Kurman, R. J., and Scully, R. E. (1972). Vaginal and cervical abnormalities after exposure to stilbestrol in utero. *Obstet Gynecol, 40*:287.

Herbst, A. L., Kurman, R. J., Scully, R. E., and Poskanzer, D. C. (1972). Clear cell adenocarcinoma of the genital tract in young females. *N Eng J Med, 287*:1257.

Herbst, A. L., Poskanzer, D. C., Robboy, S. J., Friedlander, L., and Scully, R. E. (1975). Prenatal exposure to stilbestrol (A prospective comparison of exposed female offspring with unexposed controls). *N Eng J Med, 292*:334.

Herbst, A. L., Robboy, S. J., Macdonald, G. J., and Scully, R. E. (1974). The effects of local progesterone on stilbestrol-associated vaginal adenosis. *Am J Obstet Gynecol, 118*:607.

Herbst, A. L., Robboy, S. J., Scully, R. E., and Poskanzer, D. C. (1974). Clear cell adenocarcinoma of the vagina and cervix in girls: Analysis of 170 registry cases. *Am J Obstet Gynecol, 119*:713.

Herbst, A. L., Scully, R. E., and Robboy, S. J. (1975). Problems in the examination of the DES exposed female. *Obstet Gynecol, 46*:353.

Herbst, A. L., Scully, R. E., Robboy, S. J., Cole, P., and Welch, W. R. (1977). *Abnormal Development of the Human Genital Tract Following Exposure to Diethylstilbestrol*, in preparation.

Herbst, A. L., Scully, R. E., Robboy, S. J., Poskanzer, D. C., and Ulfelder, H. (1975). Stilbestrol-associated abnormalities of the genital tract in young women. In Taymor, M. L. and Green, T. H., Jr. (Eds.): *Progress in Gynecology*. New York, Grune, vol. 6, p. 647.

Herbst, A. L., Ulfelder, H., and Poskanzer, D. C. (1971). Adenocarcinoma of the vagina. Association of maternal stilbestrol therapy with tumour appearance in young women. *N Engl J Med, 284*:878.

Hilfrich, H. J. and Hofmann, P. (1973). Uber das Scheidenstumpfrezidiv des Carcinoma in situ der Zervix. *Geburtshilfe Frauenheilkd, 33*:212.

Hill, E. C. (1966). Preclinical cervical carcinoma, colposcopy and the "negative" smear. *Am J Obstet Gynecol, 95*:308.

Hillemans, H. G. (1964). *Enstehung und Wachstung des Zervix Karzinoms*. Basel, New York, S. Karger.

———. (1966). Kritische Bemerkungen zum Begriff der Dyskariose. *Gynaecologica, 161*: 224.

———. (1968). Biopsiemethoden und ihre selextive Anwendung in Diagnostik und Therapie des Zervixkarzinoms. *Geburtshilfe Frauenheilkd, 28*:1104.

———. (1969). *Das Cervixcarcinom aus "der Gynakologe."* Berlin, Springer-Verlag, vol. 1, p. 150.

Hillemanns, H. G., Sixtus-Klug, B., and Prestel, E. (1968). Cytoplasma-Kernrelationen den Malignitatsstufen des Cervix epithels, gemessen mit den Integrationsocular. I. *Arch Gynaekol, 206*:82.

Hinde, F. C. (1964). Cervical biopsy in pregnancy. *J Obstet Gynaecol Br Commonw, 71*:707.

Hinselmann, H. (1925). Verbesserung der Inspektionsmoglichkeit von Vulva, Vagina und Portio. *Munch Med Wochenschr, 77*:1733.

———. (1927). Zur Kenntnis der praekanzerosen Veranderungen der Portio. *Zentralbl Gynaekol, 51*:901.

———. (1955). *Colposcopy*. (With a section on colpophotography by A. Schmitt.) Girardet, Wuppertal-Elberfeld.

———. (1932). Beitrag zur Ordnung und Ableitung der Leukoplakien des weiblichen Geschlechstraktes. *Z Geburtshilfe Gynaekol, 101*:142.

———. (1933). *Einfuhrung in die Kolposkopie*. Hamburg, Hartung.

———. (1938). Die Essigsaureprobe, ein Bestandteil der erweiterton Kolposkopie. *Dtsch Med Wochenschr, 64*:40.

———. (1940a). Der Nachweis der aktiven Ausgestaltung der Gefasse beim jungen Portiokarzinom als neues differentialdiagnostiches Hilfsmittel. *Zentralbl Gynaekol*, 64:1810.

———. (1940b). Zur Theorie der kolposkopischen Fruhdiagnose und der Verhutung des Karzinoms am Muttermund. *Schweiz Med Wochenschr*, 70:320.

———. (1943). Vom werden des Kolposkopes bis zur Fluoreszenskolposkopie. *Schweiz Med Wochenschr*, 73:186.

———. (1952). Uber die Geschichte der Kolposkopie. *Z Aerztl Fortbild*, 23:702.

———. (1955). *Colposcopy*. (With a section on colpophotography by A. Schmitt.) Girardet, Wuppertal-Elberfeld.

Hohlbein, R. (1959). Ergebnisse von 127,000 kolposkopischen Untersuchungen. *Krebsforschung u. Krebsbekampfung*. Munich, Urban, vol. 3, p. 202.

Hollyock, V. E. and Chanen, W. (1972). The use of the colposcope in the selection of patients for cervical cone biopsy. *Am J Obstet Gynecol*, 114:185.

———. (1976). Electrocoagulation diathermy for the treatment of cervical dysplasia and carcinoma in situ. *Obstet Gynecol*, 47:196.

Holtorff, J. (1960). Kolposkopische Kriterien der atypischen Umwandlungszone. *Gerburtshilfe Frauenheilkd*, 20:931.

Hovadhanakul, P., Mehra, U., Terragano, A., Taylor, H. B., and Cavanagh, D. (1976). Comparison of colposcopy directed biopsies and cold knife conization in patients with abnormal cytology. *Sur Gynecol Obstet*, 142:333.

Huber, H. and Zechmann, W. (1974). Die zervikale Ektopie beim Kind und jungen Madchen. *Geburtshilfe Frauenheilkd*, 34:97.

Hummer, W. K., Mussey, E., Decker, D. G., and Dockerty, M. B. (1970). Carcinoma in situ of the vagina. *Am J Obstet Gynecol*, 108:1109.

International Federation of Gynecology and Obstetrics (1976). Kottmeier, H. L. (Ed.): *Annual Report on the Results of Treatment in Carcinoma of the Uterus, Vagina and Ovary*. Radiumhemmet, Stockholm, vol. 16.

Isaacs, J. H. and O'Connor, J. (1965). Recurrent carcinoma in situ of the cervix. *Obstet Gynecol*, 25:356.

Jakob, C. A., Benevenia, M., and Soler, M. (1965). Modifications of the uterine cervix in pregnant women and its colposcopic image. *An Brasil Ginecol*, 59:245.

Jakob, C. A. (1973). Geschichte der Kolposkopie in Argentinien. In Jakob, C. A. and Franco, M. (Eds.): *1 Weltkongress fur Kolposkopie und Zervixpathologie*. Sonderdrucksband. Rosario, Argentina, Molachino Establecimiento Gráfico.

Jeffcoate, T. N. (1966). Cervical cytology; Its value and limitations. *Br Med J*, 2:1091.

Jimerson, G. K. and Merrill, J. A. (1969). Multicentric squamous malignancy involving both cervix and vulva. *Cancer*, 26:639.

Johannisson, E., Kolstad, P., and Soderberg, G. (1966). Cytologic, vascular and histologic patterns of dysplasia, carcinoma in situ and early invasive carcinoma of the cervix. *Acta Radiol [Suppl. 258] (Stockh)*.

Johnson, L. D. (1969). The histopathological approach to early cervical neoplasia. *Obstet Gynecol Surv*, 24:735.

Johnson, L. D., Easterday, C. L., Gore, H., and Hertig, A. T. (1964). The histogenesis of carcinoma in situ of the uterine cervix: A preliminary report of the origin of carcinoma in situ in subcylindrical cell anaplasia. *Cancer*, 17:213.

Johnson, L. D., Hertig, A. T., Hinman, C. H., and Easterday, C. L. (1960). Preinvasive cervical lesions in obstetric patients. Method of diagnosis, course and clinical management. *Obstet Gynecol*, 16:133.

Johnson, L. D., Nickerson, R. J., Easterday, C. L., Stuart, R. S., and Hertig, A. T. (1968). Epidemiologic evidence for the spectrum of change from dysplasia through carcinoma in situ to invasive cancer. *Cancer, 22*:901.

Johnstone, N. R. (1974). Pregnancy following conservative management of dysplasia and carcinoma in situ of the uterine cervix. *Aust NZ J Obstet Gynaecol, 14*:9.

Jones, E. G., Schwinn, C. P., Bullock, W. K., Varga, A., Dunn, J. E., Freidman, H., Jr., and Weir, J. (1968). Cancer detection during pregnancy. *Am J Obstet Gynecol, 101*:298.

Jones, H. W., Jr. (1969). Summary: Detection and diagnosis of early cervical neoplasia: Laboratory techniques. *Obstet Gynecol Surv, 24*:993.

Jones, H. W., Jr., Davis, H. J., Frost, J. K., Park, I. J., Salimi, R., Tseng, P. Y., and Woodruff, J. D. (1968). The value of the assay of chromosomes in the diagnosis of cervical neoplasia. *Am J Obstet Gynecol, 102*:624.

Jones, H. W., Jr., Katayama, K. P., Stafl, A., and Davis, H. J. (1967). Chromosomes of cervical atypia, carcinoma in situ and epidermoid carcinoma of the cervix. *Obstet Gynecol, 30*:790.

Jordan, J. A. (1975). Vaginal and cervical neoplasia after exposure to stilboestrol in utero. *Br J Obstet Gynaecol, 82*:588.

———. (1976a). The diagnosis and management of premalignant conditions of the cervix. *Clin Obstet Gynecol, 3*:295.

———. (1976b). Scanning electronmicroscopy of cervical neoplasia. In Jordan, J. A. and Singer, A. (Eds.): *The Cervix Uteri.* London, Saunders, p. 372.

Jordan, J. A. and Singer, A. (1976a). *The Cervix.* London, Saunders.

———. (1976b). Effect of oral contraceptive steroids upon epithelium and mucus. In Jordan, J. A. and Singer, A. (Eds.): *The Cervix Uteri.* London, Saunders, p. 192.

Jordan, J. A. and Williams, A. E. (1971). Scanning electron microscopy in the study of cervical neoplasia. *J Obstet Gynaecol Br Commonw, 78*:940.

Jordan, M. J., Bader, G. M., and Day, E. (1964). Carcinoma in situ of the cervix and related lesions. An 11 year prospective study. *Am J Obstet Gynecol, 89*:160.

Josey, W. E., Nahmias, A. J., and Naib, Z. M. (1975). Relation of herpes simplex virus type 2 infection to cervical neoplasia. In Taymor, M. L. and Green, T. H., Jr. (Eds.): *Progress in Gynecology.* New York, Grune, vol. 6, p. 541.

Kaminetzky, H. A. and Swerdlow, M. D. (1965). Podophyllin and the mouse cervix: Assessment of carcinogenic potential. *Am J Obstet Gynecol, 93*:486.

Kanbour, A. I., Klionsky, B., and Murphy, A. I. (1974). Carcinoma of the vagina following cervical cancer. *Cancer, 34*:1838.

Kaplan, A. L. and Kaufman, R. H. (1967). Diagnosis and management of dysplasia and carcinoma in situ of the cervix in pregnancy. *Clin Obstet Gynecol, 10*:871.

Kaplan, I., Goldman, J., and Ger, R. (1973). The treatment of erosions of the uterine cervix by means of the CO_2 laser. *Obstet Gynecol, 41*:795.

Kaufman, R. H. (1967). Dysplasia and carcinoma in situ of the cervix. *Clin Obstet Gynecol, 10*:745.

———. (1967). Frozen section evaluation of the cervical conisation specimen. *Clin Obstet Gynecol, 10*:838.

Kaufman, R. H. and Conner, J. S. (1971). Cryosurgical treatment of cervical dysplasia. *Am J Obstet Gynecol, 109*:1167.

Kaufman, R. H., Gardner, H. L., Rawls, W. E., Dixon, R. E., and Young, R. L. (1973). Clinical features of herpes genitalis. *Cancer Res, 33*:1446.

Kaufman, R H., Janes, O. G., and Cox, H. A. (1965). Cervical conisation with frozen section diagnosis. *Am J Obstet Gynecol, 93*:71.

Kaufman, R. H., Johnson, W. A., Spjut, H. J., and Smith, A. A. (1967). A correlated cytohistopathologic approach to the rapid diagnosis of cervical atypias. *Acta Cytol*, 11:272.

Kaufman, R. H., Spjut, H. J., and Carrig, S. (1965). Cervico-vaginal cytology in the teenage patient. *Acta Cytol*, 9:314.

Kaufman, R. H., Strama, T., Norton, P. K., and Conner, J. J. (1973). Cryosurgical treatment of cervical intraepithelial neoplasia. *Obstet Gynecol*, 42:881.

Kaufmann, C. and Ober, K. G. (1959). The morphological changes of the cervix uteri with age and their significance in the early diagnosis of carcinoma. *Cancer of the Cervix, Diagnosis of Early Forms*. Ciba Foundation Study Group No. 3. London Churchill, p. 61.

Kaufmann, W. (1965). The use of colposcopy in a cancer screening program. *Acta Cytol*, 9:395.

Kay, S., Frable, W. J., and Hume, D. (1970). Cervical dysplasia and cancer developing in women on immunosuppression therapy for renal homotransplantation. *Cancer*, 26:1048.

Kehrer, B. and Kauser, G. A. (1968). Incidence and behaviour of cervical ectopia during treatment with ovulation inhibitors. *Gynaecologia (Basel)*, 165:209.

Kern, G. (1961). Colposcopic findings in carcinoma in situ. *Am J Obstet Gynecol*, 82:1409.

———. (1968). *Preinvasive Carcinoma of the Cervix*. Theory and Practice. R. M. Wynn, trans. Berlin, Springer-Verlag.

Kern, G. and Hofmann, W. D. (1972). Haufigkeit und Diagnostik des Kollumkarzinoms. *Med Klin*, 67:1197.

Kevorkian, A. Y. and Younge, P. A. (1963). Contemporary means of evaluation of the uterine cervix. *Clin Obstet Gynecol*, 6:334.

Kirkland, J. A. (1963). Atypical epithelial changes in the uterine cervix. *J Clin Pathol*, 16:150.

———. (1966a). Chromosomal and mitotic abnormalities in preinvasive carcinoma of the cervix. *Aust NZ J Obstet Gynaecol*, 6:35.

———. (1966b). The cytological and histological diagnosis of dysplasia, carcinoma in situ and early invasive carcinoma of the cervix. *Aust NZ J Obstet Gynaecol*, 6:15.

———. (1969). The study of chromosomes in cervical neoplasia. *Obstet Gynecol Surv*, 24:784.

Kirkland, J. A. and Stanley, M. A. (1970). Oral contraceptives and cervical neoplasia. *Cancer Cytol*, 10:9.

Kirkland, J. A., Stanley, M. A., and Cellier, K. M. (1967). Comparative study of histologic and chromosomal abnormalities in cervical neoplasia. *Cancer*, 20:1934.

Knapp, R. C. and Feldman, G. B. (1970). The problem of optimal management of cervical carcinoma in situ. *Clin Obstet Gynecol*, 13:889.

Kneale, B. (1966). Some pitfalls in the management of carcinoma in situ of the cervix. *Aust NZ J Obstet Gynaecol*, 6:57.

———. (1969). Surgical technique. Cone biopsy of the cervix. *Aust NZ J Obstet Gynaecol*, 9:93.

Koller, O. (1963). *The Vascular Patterns of the Uterine Cervix*. Oslo, Universitetsforlaget.

Koller, O. and Kolstad, P. (1963). A colpophotographic study of carcinoma in situ and of early invasive carcinoma of the cervix. *Acta Un Int Cancer*, 19:1390.

Kolstad, P. (1964). *Vascularisation, Oxygen Tension and Radiocurability in Cancer of the Cervix*. Oslo, Universitetsforlaget.

———. (1965). The development of the vascular bed in tumours as seen in squamous cell carcinoma of the cervix uteri. *Br J Radiol*, 38:216.

———. (1966). Carcinoma of the cervix. Stage O. Diagnosis and treatment. *Am J Obstet Gynecol*, 96:1098.

———. (1969). Carcinoma of the cervix. Stage 1A. Diagnosis and treatment. *Am J Obstet Gynecol*, 104:1015.

———. (1976). Colposcopic diagnosis of cervical neoplasia. In Jordan, J. A. and Singer, A. (Eds.): *The Cervix Uteri*. London, Saunders, p. 411.

Kolstad, P., Bergsjo, P., Koller, O., Pihl, A., and Sanner, T. (1967). Detection of preinvasive and early invasive cancer by 6-phosphogluconate dehydrogenase determination. *Am J Obstet Gynecol*, 98:804.

Kolstad, P. and Klem, V. (1976). Long-term follow-up of 1121 cases of carcinoma in situ. *Obstet Gynecol*, 48:125.

Kolstad, P. and Stafl, A. (1977). *Atlas of Colposcopy*, 2nd ed. Baltimore, Univ Park.

Korhanevick, E. V. and Ganina, K. P. (1967). Luminescent colpocervicoscopy in the diagnosis of cancer and precancerous changes of the uterine cervix. *Vopr Onkol*, 13:76.

Kos, J. (1960). Distribution of the vessels in the portio vaginalis cervix uteri under the normal non-diseased pavement epithelium. *Zentralbl Gynaekol*, 82:1849.

———. (1962). Demonstration of capillaries in excised tissue from the cervix uteri by histochemical methods. *Zentralbl Gynaekol*, 85:538.

Koss, L. G. (1964). Cytologic diagnosis of carcinoma of the uterine cervix. In Gray, L. A. (Ed.): *Dysplasia, Carcinoma In Situ and Micro-invasive Carcinoma of the Cervic Uteri*. Springfield, Thomas, p. 190.

———. (1968). *Diagnostic Cytology and Its Histopathologic Bases*, 2nd ed. Philadelphia, Lippincott.

———. (1969). Concepts of genesis and development of carcinoma of the cervix. *Obstet Gynecol Surv*, 24:850.

———. (1970). Significance of dysplasia. *Clin Obstet Gynecol*, 13:873.

Koss, L. G. and Melamed, M. R. (1970). Epithelial abnormalities on the ectocervix during pregnancy. *J Reprod Med*, 4:13.

Koss, L. G., Stewart, F. W., Foote, F. W., Jr., Jordan, M. J., Bader, G. M., and Day, E. (1963). Some histologic aspects of behaviour of in situ epidermoid carcinoma and related lesions of the uterine cervix. A long-term prospective study. *Cancer*, 16:1160.

Kottmeier, H. L. (1976) (Ed.). *Annual Report on the Results of Treatment in Carcinoma of the Uterus, Vagina and Ovary*. Stockholm, Radiumhemmet, vol. 16.

———. (1953). *Carcinoma of the Female Genitalia*. Baltimore, Williams & Wilkins.

———. (1959). Carcinoma of the cervix. A study of its initial stages. *Acta Obstet Gynecol Scand*, 38:522.

Kottmeier, H. L., Karlstedt, K., Santesson, L., and Moberger, C. (1959). Histopathological problems concerning the early diagnosis of carcinoma of the cervix. *Cancer of the Cervix. Diagnosis of Early Forms*. Ciba Foundation Study Group No. 3. London, Churchill, p. 20.

Kottmeier, H. L., Vasquez Ferro, E., Wacek, A., Jenny, J. W., and Wenner-Mangen, H. (1961). Schiller test in carcinoma in situ. (Symposium). *Acta Cytol*, 5:415.

Kramer, W. M. and Kay, S. (1967). "Anaplasia Clinic." Aid in the diagnosis and treatment of preinvasive cervical lesions. *Cancer*, 20:202.

Krantz, K. E. (1973). The anatomy of the human cervix, gross and microscopic. In

Blandau, R. I. and Moghissi, K. (Eds.): *The Biology of the Cervix*. Chicago, U of Chicago Pr, p. 57.

Krieger, J. S. (1964). Conservative treatment of carcinoma in situ of the uterine cervix. *Postgrad Med, 35:*124.

Krieger, J. S. and McCormack, L. J. (1958). The indications for conservative therapy for intra-epithelial carcinoma of the uterine cervix. *Am J Obstet Gynecol, 76:*312.

Krumholz, B. A. and Knapp, R. C. (1972). Colposcopic selection of biopsy sites. *Obstet Gynecol, 39:*22.

Krumholz, B. A. and Talebian, F. (1976). Colposcopy clinic: An evaluation of 500 new patients. *J Reprod Med, 16:*131.

Lane, V. (1960). The course of epithelialization of the cervix uteri after electrodiathermocoagulation and its significance for the prevention of carcinoma. Colpophotographic study. *Gynaecologia, 149:*89.

Lang, W. R. (1957a). Role of colposcopy in cervical atypism and cancer. *Proceedings of the Third National Cancer Conference*. Philadelphia, Lippincott.

———. (1957b). Benign cervical erosion in non-pregnant women of child-bearing age. Colposcopic study. *Am J Obstet Gynecol, 74:*993.

———. (1958). Colposcopy: Neglected method of cervical evaluation. *JAMA, 166:*893.

———. (1962). The cervical portio from menarche on: A colposcopic study. *Ann NY Acad Sci, 97:*653.

———. (1976). The respective roles of cytology and colposcopy in obstetric and gynecologic practice. *J Reprod Med, 16:*249.

Lang, W. R. and Rakoff, A. E. (1956). Colposcopy and cytology, comparative value in diagnosis of cervical atypism and malignancy. *Obstet Gynecol, 8:*312.

Langley, F. A. and Crompton, A. C. (1973). *Epithelial Abnormalities of the Cervix Uteri*. Recent Results in Cancer Research No. 40. Heidelberg, Springer.

Lanier, A. P., Noller, K. L., Decker, D. G., Elveback, L. R., and Kurland, L. T. (1973). Cancer and stilbestrol. A follow-up of 1719 persons exposed to estrogens in utero and born 1943-1954. *Mayo Clin Proc, 48:*793.

Lash, A. F. (1967). The therapy and follow-up of in situ and micro-invasive carcinoma of the cervix. *Int Surg, 47:*518.

Latour, J. P. (1961). Results in the management of preclinical carcinoma of the cervix. *Am J Obstet Gynecol, 81:*511.

Lee, R. A. and Symmonds, R. E. (1976). Recurrent carcinoma in situ of the vagina in patients previously treated for in situ carcinoma of the cervix. *Obstet Gynecol, 48:*61.

Leman, M. H., Benson, W. L., Kurman, R. J., and Park, R. C. (1976). Microinvasive carcinoma of the cervix. *Obstet Gynecol, 48:*571.

Lewis, G. C., Jr., Howson, J. Y., and Colwell, F. H. (1965). Cervical cancer detection. *Am J Obstet Gynecol, 91:*777.

Lewis, T. L. T. (1966). Management of carcinoma in situ of the cervix. *Proc R Soc Med, 59:*986.

Limburg, H. (1954). Erkennung und Behandlung des Oberflachenkarzinoms am Collum uteri an der Universitats-Frauenklinik, Hamburg in den Jahren 1936 bis 1953. *La Prophylaxie en Gynaecologie et Obstetrique*. Libraire de L'Universite, Georg. Geneve, p. 1175.

———. (1956). *Die Fruhdiagnose des Uteruskarzinoms, Histologie, Kolposkopie, Cytologie, Biochemische Methoden*, 3rd ed. Stuttgart, Thieme.

———. (1958). Comparison between cytology and colposcopy in the diagnosis of early cervical carcinoma. *Am J Obstet Gynecol,* 75:1298.
Limburg, H., Bret, A. J., Beritch, B., Cramer H., Kroemer, H., Lang, W. R., Mestwerdt, G., Navratil, E., Wespi, H. J., and Zinser, H. K. (1958). Symposium on comparison between cytology and colposcopy in the detection of early cancer. *Acta Un Int Cancer,* 14:321.
Linhartova, A. (1970). Congenital ectopy of the uterine cervix. *Int J Obstet Gynecol,* 8:653.
Loskant, G. and Heinen, G. (1968). Cytologic and colposcopic findings prior to or following administration of ovulation inhibitors. *Zentralbl Gynaekol,* 90:609.
Lundström, P. and Segerbrand, E. (1975). Therapeutische Resultate der kolposkopisch kontrollierten Entnahme von Kollumgewebe bei atypischem Zellabstrich der Frauen im alter bis zu 35 Jahren. *Zentralbl Gynakekol,* 97:449.
Lust, J. (1974). Die Aufgabe und Rolle der Kolposkopie und Zytologie in der onkologischen Organisation in Budapest. Vortrag auf der 2. Arbeitstagung der Arge. Cervix uteri. Wiesbaden (1974) referiert in *Geburtshilfe Frauenheilkd,* 34: 998.
McCann, S. W., Mickal, A., and Crapanzano, J. T. (1969). Sharp conisation of the cervix. Observations of 501 consecutive patients. *Obstet Gynecol,* 33:470.
McDonald, R. R. (1967). Cervical mucus: The picture so far. *Post Grad Med J Suppl,* 43:28.
McGarrity, K. A. (1966). A review of intra-epithelial carcinoma of the uterine cervix in New South Wales. *Aust NZ J Obstet Gynaecol,* 6:45.
Macgregor, J. E. (1967). Cervical carcinoma. The beginning of the end. *Lancet,* 2:1296.
McIndoe, W. A. (1968). Cytology or colposcopy. *Aust NZ J Obstet Gynaecol,* 8:117.
McIndoe, W. A. and Green, G. H. (1969). Vaginal carcinoma in situ following hysterectomy. *Acta Cytol,* 13:158.
Macivar, J. and Willcocks, J. (1968). The effect of diathermy conisation of the cervix on subsequent fertility, pregnancy and delivery. *J. Obstet Gynaecol Br Commonw,* 75:355.
McLaren, H. C. (1967). Conservative management of cervical pre-cancer. *J Obstet Gynaecol Br Commonw,* 74:487.
McLaren, H. C. (1969). Positive smear in pregnancy. *Br Med J,* 1:216.
———. (1976). The management of benign cervical abnormalities. In Jordan, J. A. and Singer, A. (Eds.): *The Cervix Uteri.* London, Saunders, p. 291.
McLaren, H. C., Jordan, J. A., Glover, M., and Attwood, M. E. (1974). Pregnancy after cone biopsy of the cervix. *J Obstet Gynaecol Br Commonw,* 81:383.
Madej, J. (1968). The vascular bed in squamous cell papilloma of the cervix and its significance for the colposcopical diagnosis of these lesions. *Gynaecologia (Basel),* 166:460.
Majewski, A. (1960). Die Noradrenalinprobe als neues Hilfsmittel der Kolposkopie. *Gerburtshilfe Frauenheilkd,* 20:983.
———. (1973). Die Bedeutung von Kolposkopie und Zytologie im Rahmen der Krebsvorsorgeuntersuchung der Frau. Rundtischgesprach. 1. Arbeitstagung der Arbeitsgemeinschaft. Cervix uteri, Wiesbaden. *GBK-Mitteilungsdienst,* 6:866.
Marcuse, P. M. (1971). Incipient micro-invasive carcinoma of the uterine cervix. *Obstet Gynecol,* 37:360.
Margulis, R. S., Ely, C. W., Jr., and Ladd, J. E. (1967). Diagnosis and management of Stage 1A (microinvasive) carcinoma of the cervix. *Obstet Gynecol,* 29:529.

Marlow, J. L. (1974). Colposcopic evaluation of stilbestrol exposed young women. *Med Ann DC, 43*:503.

Marsh, M. (1956). Original site of cervical carcinoma, topographical relationship of carcinoma of the cervix to the external os and to the squamocolumnar junction. *Obstet Gynecol, 7*:444.

Martin, C. E. (1966). *Marital and Coital Factors in Cervical Cancer.* Unpublished dissertation. Baltimore, The Johns Hopkins University.

Mattingly, R. F. and Stafl, A. (1976). Cancer risk in diethylstilbestrol exposed offspring. *Am J Obstet Gynecol, 126*:543.

Mayer, B., Nieminnen, U., and Timonen, S. (1969). Vergleichende Studie zwischen Kolposkopie, Zytologie und Histologie. *GBK-Mitteilungsdienst, 5*:475.

Meigs, J. V. (1964). The treatment of preclinical carcinoma or microcarcinoma or carcinoma with minimal invasion of the cervix. In Gray, L. A. (Ed.): *Dysplasia, Carcinoma In Situ and Micro-invasive Carcinoma of the Cervix Uteri.* Springfield, Thomas, p. 379.

Meisels, A. and Fortin, R. (1976). Condylomatous lesions of the cervix and vagina. I. Cytologic patterns. *Acta Cytol, 20*:505.

Melamed, M. R. and Kamentsky, L. A. (1969). An assessment of the potential role of automatic devices in cytology screening. *Obstet Gynecol Surv, 24*:914.

Melamed, M. R., Koss, L. G., Flehinger, B. J., Keslisky, R. P., and Dubrow, H. (1969). Prevalence rates of uterine cervical carcinoma in situ for women using the diaphragm or contraceptive oral steroids. *Br Med J, 3*:195.

Menken, F. (1955). *Photokolposkopie und Photodouglaskopie.* Girardet, Wuppertal-Elberfeld.

———. (1973). Moderne Aspekte de Kolposkopie. Vortrag auf der 1. Arbeitstagung der Arge. Cervix uteri, Wiesbaden, 1972. *GBK-Mitteilungsdienst, 6*:957.

Mestwerdt, G. (1970). Las displasias del cuello uterino. Limites entre la benignidad y la malignidad. *Rev Obstet Ginecol, 29*:331.

Mestwerdt, G. and Wespi, H. J. (1974). *Atlas der Kolposkopie,* 4th ed. Stuttgart, Fischer.

Mikolas, V., Stafl, A., and Linhartova, A. (1964). The terminal vascular network of cervix uteri in physiological conditions and in pre-cancer. *Acta Un Int Cancer, 20*: 729.

Mikuta, J. J., Enterline, H. T., and Braun, T. E., Jr. (1968). Carcinoma in situ of the cervix associated with pregnancy. A clinico-pathological review. *JAMA, 204*:763.

Moghissi, K. S. and Mack, H. C. (1968). Epidemiology of cervical cancer: Study of a prison population. *Am J Obstet Gynecol, 100*:607.

Moll, R. and Wagner-Kolb, D. (1973). Kolposkopische, zytologische und histologische Beziehungen. Vortrag auf der 1. Arbeitstagung der Arge. Cervix uteri, Wiesbaden, 1972. *GBK-Mitteilungsdienst, 6*:960.

Moore, J. G. (1952). Growth characteristics of normal and malignant cervical epithelium in tissue culture. *Am J Obstet Gynecol, 64*:13.

Moore, J. G., Morton, D. G., Applegate, J. W., and Hindle, W. (1961). Management of early carcinoma. *Am. J Obstet Gynecol, 81*:1175.

Moore, J. G., Wells, R. G., and Morton, D. G. (1966). Management of superficial cervical cancer in pregnancy. *Obstet Gynecol, 27*:307.

Murphy, J. F. (1976). The surface ultrastructure of exfoliated cervical cells. In Jordan, J. A. and Singer, A. (Eds.): *The Cervix Uteri.* London, Saunders, p. 376.

Murphy, J. F., Allen, J. M., Jordan, J. A., and Williams, A. E. (1975). Scanning electron microscopy of normal and abnormal exfoliated cervical squamous cells. *Br J Obstet Gynaecol, 82*:44.

Murphy, J. F., Jordan, J. A., and Williams, A. E. (1974). Correlation of scanning electron microscopy, colposcopy and histology in 50 patients presenting with abnormal cervical cytology. *J Obstet Gynaecol Br Commonw, 81*:236.

Mussey, E., Soule, E. H., and Welch, J. S. (1969). Microinvasive carcinoma of the cervix. *Am J Obstet Gynecol, 104*:738.

Muth, H. (1965). Die Bedeutung der Kolposkopie und Cytologie fur die Fruhdiagnostik des Kollum-Karzinoms. *Med Welt*, 2413.

Nagell, J. R. van, Parker, J. C., Jr., Hicks, L. P., Conrad, R., and England, G. (1976). Diagnostic and therapeutic efficacy of cervical conization. *Am J Obstet Gynecol, 124*:134.

Nagell, J. R. van, Roddick, J. W., Cooper, R. M., and Triplett, H. B. (1972). Vaginal hysterectomy following conization in the treatment of carcinoma in situ of the cervix. *Am J Obstet Gynecol, 113*:948.

Nahmias, A. J., Naib, Z. M., Josey, W. E., Franklin, E., and Jenkins, R. (1973). Association of genital herpes simplex infection and cervical anaplasia. A prospective study. *Cancer Res, 33*:1491.

Naib, Z. M., Nahmias, A. J., Josey, W. E., and Zaki, S. A. (1973). Relation of cytohistopathology of genital herpes virus infection to cervical anaplasia. *Cancer Res, 33*:1452.

Navratil, E. (1957). The value of simultaneous use of cytology and colposcopy in the diagnosis of early carcinoma of the cervix of the uterus. In Meigs, J. V. and Sturgis, S. H.: *Progress in Gynecology*. New York, Grune, vol. 3, p. 99.

———. (1964). Colposcopy. In Gray, L. A. (Ed.): *Dysplasia, Carcinoma In Situ and Micro-invasive Carcinoma of the Cervix Uteri*. Springfield, Thomas, p. 273.

———. (1965). Is there a place for the colposcope in an established cytologic screening program for uterine cancer? *Acta Cytol, 9*:391.

Navratil, E., Bajardi, F., and Burghardt, E. (1959). Weitere Ergebnisse der Krebsfahrtensuche an der Universitats-Frauenklinik. *Graz Wien Klin Wochenschr, 71*:781.

Navratil, E., Burghardt, E. and Bajardi, F. (1956). Ergebnisse der Erfassung praeklinischer Karzinome an der Universitats-Frauenklinik. *Graz Krebsarzt, 11*:193.

Navratil, E., Burghardt, E., Bajardi, F., and Nash, W. (1958). Simultaneous colposcopy and cytology used in screening for carcinoma of the cervix. *Am J Obstet Gynecol*, 75:1292.

Nebel, W., Shingleton, H. M., and Swanton, M. C. (1967). Cold knife conisation of the cervix uteri. *Surg Gynecol Obstet, 125*:780.

Nelson, J. H., Averette, H. E., and Richart, R. M. (1975). *Dysplasia and Early Cervical Cancer*. New York, Professional Education Publication, American Cancer Society.

Nelson, J. H. and Masterson, J. G. (1964). Confirmatory diagnostic procedures and definitive treatment following a positive cervical smear. *Ca J Clin, 14*:46.

Neumann, H. G., Seidenschnur, G., Buttner, H. H., and Bader, G. (1975). Organisation von Mass-Screening-Untersuchungen zur Erfassung der Vor–und Fruhstadien des Zervixkarzinoms. *Geburtshilfe Frauenheilkd, 85*:893.

Ng, A. B. P. and Reagan, J. W. (1969). Microinvasion of the uterine cervix. *Am J Clin Pathol, 52*:511.

Ng, A. B. P., Reagan, J. W., Nadji, M., and Greening, S. (1977). Natural history of vaginal adenosis in women exposed to diethylstilbestrol in utero. *J Reprod Med, 18*:1.

Niekerk, W. van (1972). Comparación de la citologia en la displasia en la carcinoma in situ y en la carcinoma infiltrante de cervix. In Jakob, C. A. and Franco, M. A. (Ed.): *Proceedings of the First World Congress in Colposcopy and Cervical Pathology.* Rosario, Argentina, Molachino, Establecimiento Gráfico, p. 161.

Noller, K. L., Decker, D. G., Lanier, A. P., and Kurland, L. T. (1972). Clear cell adenocarcinoma of the cervix after maternal treatment with synthetic estrogens. *Mayo Clin Proc, 47:*629.

Nunez-Montiel, J. T. (1966). Colposcopy as a method of exploring the endocervix. Technique and procedure. *Rev Obstet Ginecol Venezuela, 26:*431.

Nunez-Montiel, J. T., Rodriguez-Barboza, J., Molina, R. A., and Gamero, G. (1970). Colposcopic exploration of the endocervix. In Ariel, I. M. (Ed.): *Clinical Cancer.* New York, Grune.

Nyberg, R., Tornberg, G., and Westin, B. (1960). Colposcopy and Schiller's iodine test as an aid in the diagnosis of malignant and premalignant lesions of the squamous epithelium of the cervix uteri. *Acta Obstet Gynecol Scand, 39:*540.

Ober, K. G., Kaufmann, C., and Hamperl, H. (1961). Carcinoma in situ, beginnendes Karzinom und Klinischer Krebs der Cervix uteri. *Geburtshilfe Frauenheilkd, 21:*259.

Odeblad, E. (1976). The biophysical aspects of cervical mucus. In Jordan, J. A. and Singer, A. (Eds.): *The Cervix Uteri.* London, Saunders, p. 155.

Odell, L. D. (1976). The use of the colposcope in the detection and management of patients with early cervical neoplasia. *J Reprod Med, 16:*235.

Odell, L. D., Merrick, F. W., and Ortiz, R. (1968). A comparison between negative, slightly atypical and suspicious cervical smears and colposcopic observations. *Acta Cytol, 12:*305.

Odell, L. D., Rimkus, K., and Hagerty, C. (1971). Electrocautery for early cervical neoplasia. *J Reprod Med, 6:*143.

Odell, L. D. and Savage, E. W. (1974). Colposcopy. In Wynn, R. M. (Ed.): *Obstetrics and Gynecology Annual.* New York, Appleton.

Old, J. W., Wielenga, G., and Haam, E. Von (1963). Squamous carcinoma in situ of the uterine cervix. I. Classification and histogenesis. *Cancer, 18:*1598.

Olson, A. W. and Nichols, E. E. (1960). Colposcopic examination in a combined approach for early diagnosis and prevention of carcinoma of the cervix. *Obstet Gynecol, 15:*372.

―――. (1961). Leukoplakia of the cervix, the mosaic and papillary pattern. *Am J Obstet Gynecol, 82:*895.

Ortiz, R. and Newton, M. (1971). Colposcopy in the management of abnormal cervical smears in pregnancy. *Am J Obstet Gynecol, 109:*46.

Ortiz, R., Newton, M., and Langlois, P. L. (1969). Colposcopic biopsy in the diagnosis of carcinoma of the cervix. *Obstet Gynecol, 34:*303.

Ortiz, R., Newton, M., and Tsai, A. (1973). Electrocautery treatment of cervical intraepithelial neoplasia. *Obstet Gynecol, 41:*113.

Osborn, R. A. (1966). Early malignancies of the cervix: Their diagnosis and significance. *Aust NZJ Obstet Gynaecol, 6:*20.

Ostergard, D. and Gondos, B. (1973). Outpatient therapy of preinvasive cervical neoplasia. Selection of patients with the use of colposcopy. *Am J Obstet Gynecol, 115:*783.

Ostergard, D. R., Townsend, D. E., and Hirose, F. M. (1969). Comparison of electrocauterisation and cryosurgery for the treatment of benign disease of the uterine cervix. *Obstet Gynecol, 33:*58.

Palmer, R. (1961). Méthode d'examens des épitheliomas cervicaux sans signes fonctionels. Colposcopie et technique de prévèlement biopsique. *Rev Fr Gynecol,* 56: 745.

Papanicolaou, G. N. (1954). *Atlas of Exfoliative Cytology.* The Commonwealth Fund, Cambridge, Harvard U Pr, Suppl. 1, 1956; Suppl. 2, 1960.

Parker, R. T. (1969). The clinical problems of early cervical neoplasia. *Obstet Gynecol Surv,* 24:684.

Patten, S. F. (1969). *Diagnostic Cytology of the Uterine Cervix.* Monographs in Clinical Cytology No. 3. Basel, Karger.

Peckham, B. M. (1969). Summary: Laboratory methods of investigating early cervical neoplasia. *Obstet Gynecol Surv,* 24:837.

Perez, V. N., Weiner, E. A., and Tancer, M. L. (1976). Squamous cell carcinoma of the vagina associated with vaginal adenosis. *Obstet Gynecol,* 47:639.

Petersen, O. (1955). Precancerous changes of the cervical epithelium in relation to manifest cervical carcinoma. *Acta Radiol [Suppl. 127] (Stockh).*

———. (1956). Spontaneous course of cervical precancerous conditions. *Am J Obstet Gynecol,* 72:1063.

Pinkerton, J. H. M. (1963). Chronic inflammatory lesions of the cervix. *Clin Obstet Gynecol,* 6:365.

Pixley, E. C. (1967). Nature and fate of the cervical pseudo-erosion in the prepubertal female. A colposcopic and histological study. *Proceedings of the Fifth World Congress in Obstetrics and Gynaecology.* London, Butterworths, p. 855.

———. (1976a). Basic morphology of the prepubertal and youthful cervix. Topographic and histologic features. *J Reprod Med,* 16:221.

———. (1976b). Morphology of the fetal and prepubertal cervicovaginal epithelium. In Jordan, J. A. and Singer, A. (Eds.): *The Cervix Uteri.* London, Saunders, p. 75.

Plasse, G., Martin-Laval, J., and Dajoux, R. (1967). Colposcopy and colpophotography in gynaecologic practice. *Bull Fed Gynecol Obstet Fr,* 19:255.

Poulsen, H. E., Taylor, C. W., and Sobin, L. H. (1975). *Histological Typing of Female Genital Tumours.* Geneva, World Health Organization.

Probable or possible malignant cervical lesions—carcinoma in situ. (1961a). (Symposium). *Acta Cytol,* 5:331.

Probable or possible premalignant cervical lesions. II. Ectopy, ectropion and epidermisation. (1961b). (Symposium). *Acta Cytol,* 5:83.

Probable or possible premalignant cervical lesions. III. Leukoplakia. (1961c). (Symposium). *Acta Cytol,* 5:103.

Probable or possible premalignant cervical lesions. IV. Reserve cell hyperplasia, basal cell hyperplasia and dysplasia. (1961d). (Symposium). *Acta Cytol,* 5:133.

Przybora, L. A. and Plutowa, A. (1959). Histological topography of carcinoma in situ of the cervix uteri. *Cancer,* 12:263.

Purola, E. and Savia, E. (1977). Cytology of gynecologic condyloma acuminatum. *Acta Cytol,* 21:26.

Rawls, W. E., Laurel, D., Melnick, J. L., Glicksman, J. M., and Kaufman, R. H. (1968). A search for viruses in smegma, premalignant and early malignant cervical tissues. The isolation of herpes viruses with distinct antigenic properties. *Am J Epidemiol,* 87:647.

Reagan, J. W. (1964). Dysplasia of the uterine cervix. In Gray, L. A. (Ed.): *Dysplasia, Carcinoma In Situ and Micro-invasive Carcinoma of the Cervix Uteri.* Springfield, Thomas, p. 294.

———. (1977). Personal communication with the author.

Reagan, J. W., Bell, B. A., Newman, J. L., Scott, R. B., and Patten, S. F. (1961).

Dysplasia in uterine cervix during pregnancy: An analytic study of the cells. *Acta Cytol*, 5:17.

Reagan, J. W., Ng, A. B. P., and Wentz, B. (1969). Concepts of genesis and development in early cervical neoplasia. *Obstet Gynecol Surv*, 24:860.

Reagan, J. W., Siedemann, I. B., and Patten, S. F., Jr. (1962). Development stages of in situ carcinoma in uterine cervix: An analytical study of cells. *Acta Cytol*, 6:538.

Reagan, J. W. and Wentz, W. B. (1967). Genesis of carcinoma of the uterine cervix. *Clin Obstet Gynecol*, 10:883.

Reid, B. L. (1961-1962). The role of virus in the origin and progression of epithelial anomalies of the ectocervix. *Proceedings of the First International Congress in Exfoliative Cytology*. Vienna, Austria.

———. (1964a). Autoradiographic analysis of uptake of tritiated thymidine and S35 cystine by cultured human cervical explants undergoing metaplasia. *J Natl Cancer Inst*, 32:1059.

———. (1964b). The behaviour of human sperm toward cultured fragments of human cervix uteri. *Lancet*, 1:21.

———. (1965). Interaction between homologous sperm and somatic cells of the uterus and peritoneum in the mouse. *Exp Cell Res*, 40:679.

———. (1966). The fate of the nucleic acid of sperm phaged by regenerating cells. *Aust NZ J Obstet Gynaecol*, 6:30.

———. (1974). Integration of the living cell with its environment. Speculation of the function of the DNA content of surface mucoids. *Biosystems*, 5:207.

———. (1976). Current and future experimental approaches to aetiology. In Jordan, J. A. and Singer, A. (Eds.): *The Cervix Uteri*. London, Saunders, p. 442.

Reid, B. L. and Blackwell, P. M. (1967). Evidence for the possibility of nuclear uptake of polymerized deoxyribonucleic acid of sperm phagocytosed by macrophages. *Aust J Exp Biol Med Sci*, 45:323.

Reid, B. L. and Coppleson, M. (1964a). Autoradiographische untersuchungen an normalen und atypischem Plattenepithel der menschlichen Cervix und Vagina. *Arch Gynaekol*, 200:172.

———. (1964b). Physiological metaplasia on the human cervix uteri: A colposcopic and histological correlative study of the earliest stages. *Aust NZ J Obstet Gynaecol*, 4:49.

———. (1975). Recent researches on the origin of squamous carcinoma of the cervix uteri. *Mod Med Aust*, 18:11.

———. (1976). Natural history. Recent advances. In Jordan, J. A., and Singer, A. (Eds.): *The Cervix Uteri*. London, Saunders, p. 317.

———. (1978). The natural history of the origin of cervical cancer. In Macdonald, R. R. (Ed.): *Scientific Basis of Obstetrics and Gynaecology*. London, Churchill, 2nd ed.

Reid, B. L., Garrett, W. J., and Coppleson, M. (1963). Two types of squamous epithelium of the human ectocervix: A histological and colposcopic study. *Aust NZ J Obstet Gynaecol*, 3:1.

Reid, B. L., Singer, A., and Coppleson, M. (1967). The process of cervical regeneration after electrocauterization. Part 1. Histological and colposcopic study. Part 2. Histochemical, autoradiographic and pH study. *Aust NZ J Obstet Gynaecol*, 7:125.

Richart, R. M. (1964a). The correlation of Schiller positive areas on the exposed portion of the cervix with intraepithelial neoplasia. *Am J Obstet Gynecol*, 90:697.

———. (1964b). Evaluation of the true false negative rate in cytology. *Am J Obstet Gynecol*, 89:723.

———. (1965). Colpomicroscopic studies of the distribution of dysplasia and carcinoma in situ of the exposed portion of the human uterine cervix. *Cancer, 18*:950.

———. (1966). Influence of diagnostic and therapeutic procedures on the distribution of cervical intraepithelial neoplasia. *Cancer, 19*:1935.

———. (1967). Natural history of cervical intraepithelial neoplasia. *Clin Obstet Gynecol, 10*:748.

———. (1969). A theory of cervical carcinogenesis. *Obstet Gynec Surv, 24*:874.

Richart, R. M., Lerch, V., and Barron, B. A. (1966). Time lapse cinematographic observation of normal human cervical epithelium, dysplasia and carcinoma in situ. *J Natl Cancer Inst, 37*:317.

Richart, R. M. and Sciarra, J. J. (1968). Treatment of cervical dysplasia by outpatient electrocauterization. *Am J Obstet Gynecol, 101*:200.

Richart, R. M. and Wilbanks, G. D. (1966). The chromosomes of human intraepithelial neoplasia. *Cancer Res, 26*:60.

Rieper, J. P. (1941). Cancer incipiente de colo uterino descoberto pelo colposcopio. *An Brasil Ginecol, 11*:143.

———. (1969). Colposcopia um método indispensavel. *Ginecol Brasil, 1*:55.

———. (1972). Regeneración y carcinoma del cuello uterino. In Jakob, C. A. and Franco, M. A. (Eds.): *Proceedings of the First World Congress of Colposcopy and Cervical Pathology*. Rosario, Argentina, Molachino Establecimiento Gráfico, p. 87.

Ries, E. (1932). Erosion, leukoplakia and the colposcope in relation to carcinoma of the cervix. *Am J Obstet Gynecol, 23*:393.

Rocha, A. H. (1971). Die Differentialdiagnostik kolposkopischer Befunde mit der Albothylprobe. *Prophylaxe Zentralbl Soz*, Gesundheitsvors. Grenzgebiet, *103*:37.

Rocha, A. H., Meirelles Filho, R., and Pimenta Filho, R. (1965). Colposcopic status of the cervix uteri in pregnancy. *An Brasil Ginecol, 60*:1.

Roche, W. and Norris, H. J. (1975). Microinvasive carcinoma of the cervix. The significance of lymphatic invasion and confluent patterns of stromal growth. *Cancer, 36*:180.

Rogers, R. S. and Williams, J. H. (1967). The impact of the suspicious Papanicolaou smear on pregnancy—A study of nationwide attitudes and maternal and perinatal complications. *Am J Obstet Gynecol, 98*:488.

Roizman, B. and Frenkel, N. (1973). The transcription and state of herpes simplex virus DNA in productive infection and in human cervical cancer tissue. *Cancer Res, 33*:1402.

Rombout, R. P. (1966). Colposcopy for evaluation of cervical abnormalities. *Obstet Gynecol, 27*:404.

Rosenthal, A. H. and Hellman, L. M. (1967). Epithelial changes in fetal cervix including role of "reserve cell." *Am J Obstet Gynecol, 64*:260.

Rotkin, I. D. (1973). A comparison review of key epidemiological studies in cervical cancer related to current researches for transmissible agents. *Cancer Res, 33*:1353.

Rounds, D. E., Narayan, K. S., and Townsend, D. E. (1976). Prospects for a personal screening method for cervical carcinoma. *Gynecol Oncol, 4*:125.

Rubinstein, E. (1966). On the proliferation of the squamous epithelium on the portio vaginalis. A colposcopic, histologic and cytologic study. *Acta Obstet Gynecol Scand* [Suppl. 6].

Salgado, C. (1963). The teaching of colposcopy. *An Brasil Ginecol, 55*:149.

Salgado, C., Rieper, J. P., and Sanches, L. R. (1970). *Colposcopia*. Rio de Janeiro, Fename.

Salzer, R. B. (1959). Colposcopy. An aid in the detection of early cancer and precancerous conditions of the cervix. *Obstet Gynecol, 13*:451.

Sandberg, E. C. (1976). Benign cervical and vaginal changes associated with exposure to stilbestrol in utero. *Am J Obstet Gynecol, 125*:777.

Savage, E. W. (1972). Microinvasive carcinoma of the cervix. *Am J Obstet Gynecol, 113*:708.

———. (1975). Correlation of colposcopically directed biopsy and conization with histologic diagnosis of cervical lesions. *J Reprod Med, 15*:211.

Scheffey, L. C., Bolten, K. A., and Lang, W. R. (1955). Colposcopy. Aid in diagnosis of cervical cancer. *Obstet Gynecol, 5*:294.

Scheffey, L. C., Lang, W. R., and Tatarian, G. (1955). Experimental program with colposcopy. *Am J Obstet Gynecol, 70*:876.

Scheidt, Vom R. G. (1967). *A Course of Colposcopy*. Berlin, Leisegang.

Schiffer, M. A., Allen, A. C., Greene, H. J., and Mackles, A. (1968). Abnormal cytology of the cervix in pregnancy. *Am J Obstet Gynecol, 102*:597.

Schiffer, M. A., Greene, H. J., Pomerance, W., and Moltz, A. (1965). Cervical conisation for diagnosis and treatment of carcinoma in situ. *Am J Obstet Gynecol, 93*:889.

Schiffer, M. A., Mackles, A. M., and Greene, H. J. (1972). Carcinoma in situ of the vagina after hysterectomy. *Surg Gynecol Obstet, 134*:652.

Schmitt, A. (1957). The value of colposcopy in the diagnosis of cancer of the cervix. *Proceedings of the Third National Cancer Congress*. Philadelphia, Lippincott.

———. (1959). Colposcopy detection of atypical and cancerous lesions of the cervix. *Obstet Gynecol, 13*:665.

———. (1976). Practical application of colposcopy. *J Reprod Med, 16*:207.

Schonberg, L. A. (1975). A colposcopy referral service for family planning clinics. *Int J Gynaecol Obstet, 13*:174.

Schulman, H. and Cavanagh, D. (1961). Intraepithelial carcinoma of the cervix. The predictability of residual carcinoma in the uterus from microscopic study of the margins of the cone biopsy specimen. *Cancer, 14*:795.

Schulman, H. and Ferguson, J. H. (1962). Cone biopsy of the cervix. *J Obstet Gynaecol Br Commonw, 69*:474.

Scott, J. W. (1971). *Stereocolposcopic Atlas of the Uterine Cervix*. Florida, Zephyr.

———. (1972). Cytology, colposcopy, office biopsy and conization of the cervix; Their respective roles in practice to-day. *Obstet Gynecol Dig, 14*:18.

———. (1976). Colposcopy in private practice. *J Reprod Med, 16*:231.

Scott, J. W., Seckinger, D., and Puente-Duany, W. (1974). Colposcopic aspects of management of vaginal adenosis in DES children. *J Reprod Med, 12*:187.

Scott, J. W. and Vence, C. A. (1963). Colposcopy, cytology and biopsy in the office diagnosis of uterine malignancy. *Cancer Cytol, 5*:5.

Sedlis, A. (1975a). Cervical dysplasia. Diagnosis, prognosis, management. In Taymor, M. L. and Green, T. H., Jr. (Eds.): *Progress in Gynecology*. New York, Grune, vol. 6, p. 559.

———. (1975b). Cervical intraepithelial neoplasia; A continuing diagnostic and therapeutic challenge. *J Reprod Med, 14*:263.

Sedlis, A., Cohen, A., and Sall, S. (1970). The fate of cervical dysplasia. *Am J Obstet Gynecol, 107*:1065.

Seidl, S. (1973). Die diagnostische Konisation der Cervix uteri. *Gynaekol Rundsch, 13*:51.

———. (1974). Die suspekte Portio und das diagnostisch-therapeutische Vorgehen. Vortrag auf der 2. Arbeitstagung der Arge. Cervix uteri. 1974. Wiesbaden referiert in *Geburtshilfe Frauenheilkd, 34*:996.

Selim, M. A., So-Bosita, J. L., Blair, O. M., and Little, B. A. (1973). Cervical biopsy versus conisation. *Obstet Gynecol, 41*:177.

Seybolt, J. F. and Johnson, W. D. (1971). Cervical cytodiagnostic problems—A survey. *Am J Obstet Gynecol, 109*:1089.

Sherman, A. I., Goldrath, M., Berlin, A., Vakhariya, V., Banooni, F., Michaels, W., Goodman, P., and Brown, S. (1974). Cervical-vaginal adenosis after in utero exposure to synthetic estrogens. *Obstet Gynecol, 44*:531.

Shingleton, H. M. and Lawrence, W. D. (1976). Transmission electron microscopy of the physiological epithelium. In Jordan, J. A. and Singer, A. (Eds.): *The Cervix Uteri*. London, Saunders, p. 36.

Siegler, E. E. (1956). Microdiagnosis of carcinoma in situ of the uterine cervix. A comparative study of pathologists' diagnosis. *Cancer, 9*:463.

———. (1961). Histomorphology of carcinoma in situ. *Acta Cytol, 5*:275.

Silbar, E. L. and Woodruff, J. D. (1966). Evaluation of biopsy, cone and hysterectomy sequence in intraepithelial carcinoma of the cervix. *Obstet Gynecol, 27*:89.

Simcock, M. J. (1964). Papillomas of the uterine cervix. *Aust NZ J Obstet Gynaecol, 4*: 174.

Singer, A. (1967). Cervical regeneration. A histological and autoradiographic study. *J Coll Radiol Aust, 11*:46.

———. (1972). *The Effect of Physiological and Pathological Factors on the Cervix Uteri*. Unpublished dissertation. University of Sydney, Australia.

———. (1975a). The uterine cervix from adolescence to the menopause. *Br J Obstet Gynaecol, 82*:81.

———. (1975b). Cervical dysplasia in young women. *Proc R Soc Med, 68*:14.

———. (1976a). The cervical epithelium during puberty and adolescence. In Jordan, J. A. and Singer, A. (Eds.): *The Cervix Uteri*. London, Saunders, p. 87.

———. (1976b). The cervical epithelium during pregnancy and the puerperium. In Jordan, J. A. and Singer, A. (Eds.): *The Cervix Uteri*. London, Saunders, p. 105.

Singer, A. and Jordan, J. A. (1976). The anatomy of the cervix. In Jordan, J. A. and Singer, A. (Eds.): *The Cervix Uteri*. London, Saunders, p. 13.

Singer, A., Reid, B. L., and Coppleson, M. (1967). Process of cervical regeneration following electrodiathermy. *Proceedings of the Fifth World Congress in Obstetrics and Gynaecology*. London, Butterworths, p. 862.

———. (1968). The role of the peritoneal mononuclear cell in the regeneration of the uterine epithelium of the rat. *Aust NZ J Obstet Gynaecol, 8*:163.

———. (1976). A hypothesis: The role of a high-risk male in the etiology of cervical carcinoma. A correlation of epidemiology and molecular biology. *Am J Obstet Gynecol, 126*:111.

Singleton, W. P. and Rutledge, F. (1968). To cone or not to cone—The cervix. *Obstet Gynecol, 31*:430.

Skinner, G. R. B., Thouless, M. E., and Jordan, J. A. (1971). Antibodies to type 1 and type 2 herpes virus in women with abnormal cervical cytology. *J Obstet Gynaecol Br Commonw, 78*:1031.

Skipper, J. S. (1966). The conservative management of carcinoma in situ: Results 1963-4. *Aust NZ J Obstet Gynaecol, 6*:53.

Sonek, M., Bibbo, M. and Wied, G. L. (1976). Colposcopic findings in offspring of DES-treated mothers as related to onset of therapy. *J Reprod Med, 16*:65.

Sonek, M. and Newton, M. (1975). Colposcopy in the evaluation of patients with abnormal cytologic smears. In Taymor, M. L. and Green, T. H., Jr. (Eds.): *Progress in Gynecology*. New York, Grune, p. 217.

Song, J. (1964). *The Human Uterus, Morphogenesis and Embryological Basis for Cancer*. Springfield, Thomas.

Soost, H. and Jopp, H. (1968). Carcinoma in situ during pregnancy. *Acta Cytol, 10*:227.

Spjut, H. J. and Fechner, R. E. (1967). Cytologic diagnosis of cervical dysplasia and carcinoma in situ. *Clin Obstet Gynecol, 10*:785.

Spriggs, A. I. (1969). Oral contraceptives and carcinoma in situ. *Lancet, 1*:51.

———. (1974). Cytogenetics of cancer and precancerous states of the cervix uteri. In German, J. (Ed.): *Chromosomes and Cancer*. New York, Wiley, p. 423.

Spriggs, A. I., Bowey, E., and Cowdell, R. H. (1971). Chromosomes of precancerous lesions of the cervix uteri. *Cancer, 27*:1239.

Stafl, A. (1962). Use of the azocoupling method for identificiaton of alkaline phosphatase in study of the capillary network of the cervix uteri. *Cesk Morf, 10*:336.

———. (1971). Cryosurgery in the treatment of abnormal cervical lesions. An invitational symposium. *J Reprod Med, 7*:147.

———. (1976a). New nomenclature for colposcopy. Report of the Committee on Terminology. *Obstet Gynecol, 48*:124.

———. (1976b). Colposcopy. *Cancer [Suppl. 1], 38*:432.

Stafl, A., Friedrich, E. G., and Mattingly, R. F. (1973). Detection of cervical neoplasia. Reducing the risk of error. *Clin Obstet Gynecol, 16*:238.

Stafl, A., Dohnal, V., and Linhartova, A. (1963). On colposcopic, histological and vascular findings in the pathologically changed cervix. *Geburtshilfe Frauenheilkd, 23*:437.

Stafl, A. and Linhartova, A. (1967). Die Umwandlungzone und ihre Genese. *Arch Gynaekol, 204*:228.

Stafl, A., Linhartova, A. and Dohnal, V. (1963). The colposcopic picture of atypical epithelium and its pathogenesis. *Arch Gynaekol, 199*:223.

Stafl, A. and Mattingly, R. F. (1973). Colposcopic diagnosis of cervical neoplasia. *Obstet Gynecol, 41*:168.

———. (1974). Vaginal adenosis: A precancerous lesion? *Am J Obstet Gynecol, 120*:666.

———. (1975). Angiogenesis of cervical neoplasia. *Am J Obstet Gynecol, 121*:845.

———. (1976). Diethylstilboestrol and the cervicovaginal epithelium. In Jordan, J. A. and Singer, A. (Eds.): *The Cervix Uteri*. London, Saunders, p. 331.

Stafl, A., Mattingly, R. F., Foley, D. V., and Fetherston, W. C. (1974). Clinical diagnosis of vaginal adenosis. *Obstet Gynecol, 43*:118.

Stallworthy, J. (1962). Carcinoma of cervix. *Lancet, 2*:1165.

Stallworthy, J. and Bourne, G. L. (1966). Carcinoma of the cervix. *Recent Advances in Obstetrics and Gynaecology*. London, Churchill.

Stallworthy, J. and Wiernik, G. (1976). Management of cervical malignant disease—Combined radiotherapy and surgical techniques. In Jordan, J. A. and Singer, A. (Eds.): *The Cervix Uteri*. London, Saunders, p. 474.

Stanley, M. A. and Kirkland, J. A. (1975). Chromosome and histological patterns in preinvasive lesions of the cervix. *Acta Cytol, 19*:142.

Stening, M. (1964). The surgical treatment of carcinoma of the cervix. *J Coll Radiol, Aust, 8*:113.

Stern, E. (1969). Epidemiology of dysplasia. *Obstet Gynecol Surv, 24*:711.

Stern, E., Coffelt, C. F., Youkeles, L., and Forsythe, A. (1973). Steroid contraception and dysplasia of the cervix: An interim report. *J Reprod Med, 10*:177.

Stern, E. and Neely, P. M. (1963). Carcinoma and dysplasia of the cervix: A comparison of rates for new and returning populations. *Acta Cytol, 7*:357.

———. (1964). Dysplasia of the uterine cervix. Incidence of regression, recurrence and cancer. *Cancer, 17*:508.

Stoll, P. (1969). Möglichkeiten der früherkennung Bösartiger geschwulste in der Praxis (II). Gynäkologische Karzinome. *Z Allgemeinmed, 45*:1101.

———. (1974). Aufgaben der Krebsvorsorge-Untersuchungen bei der Frau. *Fortschr Med, 92*:353.

Talebian, F., Krumholz, B. A., Shayan, A., and Mann, L. I. (1976). Colposcopic evaluation of patients with abnormal cytologic smears during pregnancy. *Obstet Gynecol, 47*:693.

Thomison, J. B. and Tosh, R. H. (1962). Evaluation of punch biopsy in the diagnosis of carcinoma in situ of the cervix uteri. *Am J Obstet Gynecol, 84*:98.

Thompson, B. H., Woodruff, J. D., Davis, H. J., Julian, C. G., and Silva, F. G. (1972). Cytopathology, histopathology and colposcopy in the management of cervical neoplasia. *Am J Obstet Gynecol, 114*:329.

Thoms, G. and de Groot, R. J. (1969). The nuclear activity of lesions of the cervix. *Med J Aust, 13*:635.

Topek, N. A. (1967). Surgical treatment of carcinoma in situ of the cervix. *Clin Obstet Gynecol, 10*:853.

Torres, J. E. (1976). Colposcopy screening for cervical cancer in a family planning program. *J Reprod Med, 16*:246.

Torres, J. E., Holmquiat, N., and Pereira, C. (1964). Histological findings in the genital tract of female with class III smears. *Acta Cytol, 8*:284.

Tovell, H. M. (1976). Cone biopsy of the cervix. *Clin Obstet Gynecol, 19*:2.

Tovell, H. M., Banogan, P., and Nash, A. D. (1976). Cytology and colposcopy in the diagnosis and management of preclinical carcinoma of the cervix uteri: A learning experience. *Am J Obstet Gynecol, 124*:924.

Townsend, D. E. (1971). A cancer detection clinic in the United States. (Letter). *Med J Aust, 2*:113.

———. (1975). Cryosurgery in gynecology. In Taymor, M. L. and Green, T. H., Jr. (Eds.): *Progress in Gynecology.* New York, Grune, vol. 6, p. 583.

———. (1976). The management of cervical lesions by cryosurgery. In Jordan, J. A. and Singer, A. (Eds.): *The Cervix Uteri.* London, Saunders, p. 305.

Townsend, D. E. and Lickrish, G. (1971). Cryosurgery in the treatment of abnormal cervical lesions. An invitational symposium. *J Reprod Med, 7*:166.

Townsend, D. E. and Ostergard, D. R. (1971). Cryocauterization for preinvasive cervical neoplasia. *J Reprod Med, 6*:171.

Townsend, D. E., Ostergard, D. R., and Lickrish, G. M. (1971). Cryosurgery for benign disease of the uterine cervix. *J Obstet Gynaecol Br Commonw, 78*:667.

Townsend, D. E., Ostergard, D. R., Mishell, D. R., and Hirose, F. M. (1970). Abnormal Papanicolaou smears—Evaluation by colposcopy, biopsies and endocervical curettage. *Am J Obstet Gynecol, 108*:429.

Tredway, D. R., Townsend, D. E., Hovland, N. D., and Upton, R. T. (1972). Colposcopy and cryosurgery in cervical intraepithelial neoplasia. *Am J Obstet Gynecol, 114*:1020.

Trombetta, G. C. (1976). Colposcopic evaluation of cervical neoplasia in pregnancy. *J Reprod Med,* 16:243.

Tweeddale, D. N. (1970). Vascular involvement in microinvasive carcinoma of the cervix. *Obstet Gynecol News,* 5:7.

Tweeddale, D. N., Langenbach, S. R., Roddick, J. W., Jr., and Holt, M. L. (1969). The cytopathology of microinvasive squamous cancer of the cervix uteri. *Acta Cytol,* 13:447.

Ulfelder, H. (1973). Stilbestrol, adenosis and adenocarcinoma. *Am J Obstet Gynecol,* 117:794.

Ulfelder, H. (1976). The stilbestrol–adenosis–carcinoma syndrome. *Cancer [Suppl. 1],* 38:426.

Ullery, J. C., Boutselis, J., and Botschner, A. (1965). Microinvasive carcinoma of the cervix. *Obstet Gynecol,* 26:866.

Vacha, K., Rosol, M., and Kopecny, J. (1975). Prakanzerosen des Gebarmutterhalses bei jungen Frauen. *Zentralbl Gynaekol,* 97:525.

Vaillant, H. W., Cummins, G. T. M., and Richart, R. M. (1968). An island wide screening program for cervical neoplasia in Barbados. *Am J Obstet Gynecol,* 101: 943.

Wachtel, E. (1969). *Exfoliative Cytology in Gynaecological Practice.* London, Butterworths.

Wagner, D. and Fettig, O. (1961). Zytologische und histologische Untersuchungen zur atypischen Umwandlungszone. *Geburtshilfe Frauenheilkd,* 21:156.

Walz, W. (1958). Uber die Genese der sogenannten indirekten Metaplasie im Bereich des mullerschen gang Systems. *Z Geburtshilfe Gynaekol,* 151:1.

———. (1969). 16 Jahre klinische Erfahrungen in der Karzinom-Fruhdiagnose mittels der Kolposkopie, Zytologie und Kolpomikroskopie. *GBK-Mitteilungsdienst,* 5:544.

———. (1976). Colpomicroscopy in the diagnosis of cervical neoplasia in the cervix uteri. In Jordan, J. A. and Singer, A. (Eds.): *The Cervix Uteri.* London, Saunders, p. 422.

Way, S. (1963). *The Diagnosis of Early Carcinoma of the Cervix.* London, Churchill.

———. (1968). Management of cervical carcinoma in situ. *Lancet,* 2:637.

Way, S., Hennigan, M., and Wright, V. C. (1968). Some experiences with preinvasive and microinvasive carcinoma of the cervix. *J Obstet Gynaecol Br Commonw,* 75: 593.

Weese, W. H. (1976). A brief history of colposcopy. *J Reprod Med,* 16:209.

Wentz, W. B. and Reagan, J. W. (1970). Clinical significance of post irradiation dysplasia of the uterine cervix. *Am J Obstet Gynecol,* 106:812.

Wespi, H. J. (1949). *Early Carcinoma of the Uterine Cervix. Pathogenesis and Detection.* New York, Grune.

———. (1951). Kolpophotographie. *Arch Gynaekol,* 180:58.

———. (1970). Die Rolle der Kolposkopie bei der Diagnose und beim Ausschluss des Zervixkarzinoms. *Minerva Ginecol,* 22:1148.

———. (1973). Stereo-Kolpofotografie. Vortrag auf der 1. Arbeitstagung der Arge. Cervix uteri. 1972. Wiesbaden, *GBK-Mitteilungsdienst,* 6:950.

Wespi, H. J. and Lotmar, W. (1954). Fortschritte der Kolpophotographie und ihre Bedeutung. *Gynaecologia (Basel),* 137:300.

Wied, G. L. (1964a). Is there a place for the colposcope in an established cytologic screening program for uterine cancer? *Acta Cytol,* 8:321.

―――. (1964b). The meaning of Class III of the Papanicolaou classification of specimens from the female genital tract. *Acta Cytol, 8*:99.

Wied, G. L., Bartels, P. H., and Bahr, G. F. (1969). Laboratory organisation in the detection and diagnosis of early cervical neoplasia. *Obstet Gynecol Surv, 24*:935.

Wied, G. L., Legorreta, G., Mohr, D., and Rauzy, A. (1962). Cytology of invasive cervical carcinoma and carcinoma in situ. *Ann NY Acad Sci, 97*:759.

Wielenga, G., Old, J. W., and Haam, E. von (1965). Squamous carcinoma in situ of the uterine cervix II topography and clinical correlations. *Cancer, 18*:1612.

Wilbanks, G. D. (1973). A selective review of experimental studies in cervical carcinoma. *Cancer Res, 33*:1382.

―――. (1975). In vitro studies on human cervical epithelium, benign and neoplastic. *Am J Obstet Gynecol, 121*:771.

―――. (1976). In vivo and in vitro "markers" of human cervical intraepithelial neoplasia. *Cancer Res, 36*:2485.

Wilbanks, G. D. and Campbell, J. A. (1972). Effect of herpes virus hominis type 2 on human cervical epithelium; Scanning electron microscopic observations. *Am J Obstet Gynecol, 112*:924.

Wilbanks, G. D., Creasman, W. T., Kaufmann, L. A., and Parker, R. T. (1973). Treatment of cervical dysplasia with electrocautery and tetracycline suppositories. *Am J Obstet Gynecol, 117*:460.

Wilbanks, G. D. and Fink, C. G. (1976). Tissue and organ culture of cervical epithelium—Physiological and preinvasive. In Jordan, J. A. and Singer, A. (Eds.): *The Cervix Uteri*. London, Saunders, p. 429.

Wilbanks, G. D. and Richart, R. M. (1967). The puerperal cervix, injuries and healing. A colposcopic study. *Am J Obstet Gynecol, 97*:1105.

Wilds, P. L. (1962). Is colposcopy practical? *Obstet Gynecol, 20*:645.

Williams, A. E., Jordan, J. A., Allen, J. M., and Murphy, J. F. (1973). The surface ultrastructure of normal and metaplastic cervical epithelium and of carcinoma in situ. *Cancer Res, 33*:504.

Williams, T. J. and Turnbull, K. (1964). Carcinoma in situ and pregnancy. *Obstet Gynecol, 24*:857.

Woodruff, J. D. (1964). Eversion and eversive cervicitis. In Gray, L. A. (Ed.): *Dysplasia, Carcinoma In Situ and Micro-invasive Carcinoma of the Cervix Uteri*. Springfield, Thomas, p. 24.

Woodruff, J. D. (1965). Treatment of recurrent carcinoma in situ in the lower genital tract. *Clin Obstet Gynecol, 8*:757.

Worth, A. J., Boyes, D. A., and Fidler, H. K. (1967). The acceptance of the cervical cytology screening programme in the province of British Columbia. *J Obstet Gynaecol Br Commonw, 74*:479.

Worth, A. J. and Boyes, D. A. (1972). A case control study into the possible effects of birth control pills on preclinical carcinoma of the cervix. *J Obstet Gynaecol Br Commonw, 79*:673.

Wynder, E. L. (1969). Epidemiology of carcinoma in situ of the cervix. *Obstet Gynecol Surv, 24*:697.

Younge, P. A. (1957). The conservative treatment of carcinoma in situ of the cervix. *Proceedings of the Third National Cancer Conference*. Philadelphia, Lippincott, p. 682.

―――. (1962). Premalignant lesions of the cervix; Clinical management. *Clin Obstet Gynecol, 5*:1137.

———. (1964). Clinical findings in early lesions of the cervix. In Gray, L. A. (Ed.): *Dysplasia, Carcinoma In Situ and Micro-invasive Carcinoma of the Cervix Uteri.* Springfield, Thomas, p. 276.

———. (1965). The natural history of carcinoma in situ of the cervix uteri. *J Obstet Gynaecol Br Commonw,* 72:9.

Yule, R. (1964). Biopsy in the diagnosis of unsuspected carcinoma of the cervix. *Med J Aust,* 1:446.

Zilahi, Z., Nemes, J., and Bikkal, A. (1967). Follow-up study of cervical epithelial atypia of pregnancy. *Am J Obstet Gynecol,* 98:1154.

Youssef, A. F. (1957). Colposcopy. The results of its routine employment in 1000 gynaecological patients. *J Obstet Gynaecol Br Em,* 64:901.

Zinser, H. K. (1965). Colposcopy. *Acta Cytol,* 9:393.

Zinser, H. K. and Rosenbauer, K. A. (1960). Untersuchungen über die Angioarchitektonik der normalen und pathologisch en veranderten Cervix uteri. *Arch Gynaekol,* 194:73.

INDEX

A

Abnormal epithelium, 26, 385
Abnormal smear, *see* Cytology, exfoliative
Abnormal vessels, *see* Angioarchitecture
Abnormally differentiated epithelium, 385
Acetic acid solution in colposcopy, 44, 178, 179, 201, 203, 233, 262, 273, 277, 331, 334
Activated stromal cells, 81
Active and undifferentiated immature metaplasia, 25
Adenocarcinoma of cervix, 262, 414
Adenomatous hyperplasia, 25
Adenosis, *see* Vaginal adenosis
Adenosquamous carcinoma, 262
Adolescent nulliparous cervix, *see* Cervix of adolescent nullipara
Alkaline phosphatase studies, 123, 127, 141
Anaplasia, 25
Anatomical definitions, 16, 17
Angioarchitecture, 121, 123
    avascular areas, 236
    calibre of vessels, 121, 236, 242
        coarse, 141, 157, 236, 242, 261
        fine, 141, 236, 242, 261
        variations, 141, 157
    distorted by inclusion cysts, 133
    hyperaemia, 141, 278
    in atypical transformation zone
        atypical vessels, 44, 63, 78, 141, 142, 156, 157, 242, 261, 262, 277
        mosaic, 44, 78, 141, 226, 227, 242, 277, 313, 334, 357, 361, 366, 374
        punctation, 44, 78, 141, 226, 227, 236, 242, 277, 313, 334, 357, 361, 366, 374
        white epithelium, 44, 133, 141
    in colposcopically overt carcinoma, 142, 277
    in columnar epithelium, 127, 203
    in condyloma, 286
    in epithelia after cryosurgery and electrodiathermy, 180, 298, 361, 429
    in *neisseria gonorrhoeae* infection, 278
    in original squamous epithelium, 123, 194, 278
    in overt carcinoma, 262
    in papilloma, 286
    in *trichomonas vaginalis* infection, 278
    in typical transformation zone, 133, 210, 211
    in vaginocervicitis, 278
    intercapillary distance, 156, 236, 242, 261, 262, 334, 339
    modification of original vascular structures, 121
    pattern of vessels
        alterations with epithelial activity, 141
        irregular, 157, 242, 261
        linear, 298
        punctate, 141, 278
        regular, 236, 242, 261, 286
    prime morphological feature, 121, 194, 203, 211, 236, 277
    study
        alkaline phosphatase, 123, 127, 141
        colpophotographic, 123
        histological, 123
        special colpophotographic, 123
    subepithelial petechiae, 285
    types of vessels
        atypical, 44, 63, 78, 141, 142, 156, 157, 242, 261, 262, 277
        branching, 127, 133, 194, 210, 211, 357
        coiled, 141
        corkscrew, 242
        looped capillaries, 121, 123, 127, 141, 194, 236
        network capillaries, 121, 123, 194
        subepithelial, 121, 127, 133
        terminal capillaries, 211
        terminal circular, 211
Angiography, *see* Angioarchitecture
Arbor vitae, 203
Atrophic cervicitis, 45, 284, 285
    abnormal smear, 408
    oestrogen deficient vaginocervicitis, 284
    subepithelial petechiae, 285
    trauma of speculum, 285
Atypical colposcopic appearances of doubtful or physiological significance
    around gland openings in transformation zone, 361
    in adolescent cervix, 366

472   *Colposcopy*

in cervix following intrauterine exposure to synthetic oestrogens, 374
in oestrogen deficient post menopausal cervix, 361
in original transformation zone, 374
in regenerating epithelium after cryosurgery and electrodiathermy, 361
keratosis overlying original squamous epithelium, 361
persisting in physiological transformation zone, 361
transient during dynamic phases of metaplasia in adolescents and first pregnancy, 361
Atypical colposcopy, *see* Atypical transformation zone and Colposcopy
Atypical hyperplasia, 25
Atypical metaplasia, *see* Atypical transformation zone; Dysplasia; and Metaplasia
Atypical metaplastic epithelium, 25, 26, 44, 68, 74, 76, 80, 81, 92, 100, 101, 127, 209, *see also* Atypical transformation zone; Dysplasia; and Metaplasia
Atypical reserve cell hyperplasia, 25
Atypical transformation zone, 226-261
angioarchitecture, *see* Mosaic; Punctation
atypical vessels, 44, 78, 141, 156, 157, 242, 261
coarse dilated calibre, 236, 242, 261
coiled vessels, 141
corkscrew vessels, 242
fine calibre, 236, 242, 261
intercapillary relationships, 236, 242, 261
irregular pattern, 242, 261
looped capillaries, 236
regular pattern, 236, 242, 261
application of acetic acid solution, appearances after, 44, 233, 334
assessment of more serious lesions, 226, 397, 403
association with dysplasia, 76, 77, 226
with overt carcinoma, colposcopically suspect, 273
with preclinical carcinoma, 76, 77, 226
avascular areas, 236
colour, 233
colposcopic appearances, 226-261
atypical vessels, 44, 78, 141, 156, 157, 242, 261
combinations of mosaic and punctation, 242
keratosis, 142, 226, 233, 361, 374, 375
mosaic, 44, 141, 226, 227, 242, 313, 334, 357, 361, 366, 374
major grades, 141, 242, 277
minor grades, 141, 242
punctation, 141, 226, 227, 236, 242, 313, 334, 357, 361, 366, 374, 375
major grades, 141, 236, 242, 277
minor grades, 141, 236
white epithelium, 44, 133, 226, 227, 233, 236, 261, 313, 334, 357, 361, 366, 374
columnar epithelium, origin from, 227, 357, 375
combination with physiological appearances, 233
correlation with cytology, 396
correlation with histology, 157, 226, 357, 367, 396, 397, 408
cystic inclusions, 236
definition, 44
doubtful or physiological significance, 357, 361, 366, 367, 374
dynamic phases, 227
immature metaplastic epithelium, 227
early stages, 227
fragile epithelium, 286
grades, 121, 156, 157, 227, 242, 261, 391, 396, 397, 403, 408, 409, 412, 413, 416
correlation with histology, 79, 156, 157, 396, 397, 408
criteria for grading, 156, 157, 261
differences in prime morphological features, 121, 227, 242
discrepancy with histology, 157, 164, 226, 357, 367, 374, 385, *see also* Discrepancy between colposcopic and histological diagnosis
grade I, 156, 157, 261, 366, 391, 397, 403, 408, 409, 412
grade II, 156, 157, 261, 366, 391, 397, 403, 408, 409, 412
grade III, 156, 157, 261, 391, 397, 403, 408, 412, 416
guide to prognosis, 396, 397, 403
in management, 396, 397, 413, 416
in selection of cervical biopsy, 391
surface configuration, 156, 261
in DES exposed women, 334, 351, 374
in polyp, 298
in postmenopausal cervix, 114
diagnostic difficulty, 393
in pregnant cervix, 104, 361, 428
in prepubertal cervix, 100
in sexually active adolescent cervix, 101, 104, 366, 367, 374
in virgin cervix, 101, 366, 367

Index

intercapillary distance, 236, 242, 261
malignancy index of, 391
maturity, 92, 227
   arrest at intermediate stages, 92, 227, 334
opacity, 233
origin and development, 92, 227
   multifocal, 92
papillary elevations, 236, 261
physiological significance, 227, 357, 361, 366, 367, 374
precursors of cervical cancer, 76, 179, 226, 366, 374
prime morphological features, 227
selective biopsy of, 391, 397, 407, 408
site of dysplasia, 76, 226, 366, 367, 374
site of preclinical cancer, 76, 226
surface configuration, 236, 261
topography, 227
   new squamocolumnar junction, 233
   original squamocolumnar junction, limit of, 233
   outward extension, 233
   sharp delineation, 233
   vaginal site, 233, 330, 407, 426, 429
transient during dynamic phases of adolescence and first pregnancy, 361
true erosion, association with, 286
Atypical vessels, 44, 63, 78, 141, 142, 156, 157, 242, 261, 262, 277
Autoradiography, 6

B

Basal cell hyperplasia, 25, 385, see also Dysplasia
Basic colposcopic and histological correlations, see also Correlation between colposcopic and histological diagnosis
   atypical transformation zone, 133
   atypical vessels, 141
   colposcopically suspect overt carcinoma, 142
   columnar epithelium, 127
      angioarchitecture, 127
      colour, 127
      colposcopic counterparts, 127
      histology, 127
      surface configuration 127
   keratosis, 142
      histology, 142
   mosaic
      hyperaemia, 141
      vascular patterns, 141
   original squamous epithelium, 123
      colposcopic counterpart, 123
      histology, 123
      vascular patterns, 123
   punctation
      alkaline phosphatase studies, 141
      hyperaemia, 141
         marked degree, 141
         significance, 141
      vascular patterns, 141
   study
      alkaline phosphatase, 123
      colposcopy, 123
      histology, 123
      special colpophotography, 123
   typical transformation zone, 127
      angioarchitecture, 133
      colour, 127
      colposcopic counterparts, 81, 127, 133
      dynamic phases, 81, 209
      glandular structures, 133
      histology, 127
      mature phases, 127, 133, 209, 210
      vascular patterns, 133
   white epithelium, 133
      colour, 133
      keratin covering, 141
      surface changes, 133
      vascular patterns, 141
Behavioural aspects of metaplasia, see Metaplasia
   carcinogenesis, relation to, 79, 100, 116-119
   dynamic phase, 79-81, 88, 92, 101, 104
   initiation, see Dynamic phase
   maturation, 80, 88, 114
   natural history, 76, 79, 80, 88, 92
   sequential observation by colposcope, 79
Biopsy, cervical
   association with endocervical curettage, 397, 412-414
   association with fractional curettage, 409, 413, 414
   avoiding unnecessary biopsies, 391, 436
   colposcopically suspect overt carcinoma, 408, 416, 428
   cone
      as definitive treatment for CIN, 416, 424, 425, 426, 428
      avoidance of unnecessary, 413
      colposcopy in selection, 391, 407-413
      complications, 409, 412, 428
      in assessment of cervical canal, 413
      in pregnancy, 428
      indications, 408, 409

occasional use, 407
reduction in rate, 407
repeated abnormal smears, after, 414
residual lesions in cervix after, 418, 429
routine with positive and doubtful smears, 407
size, variation in, by use of colposcopy, 409
technique, 409
theoretical risks of lesser biopsies than, 407
correlation of colposcopy, expected histology and recommended biopsy, 408
in absence of colposcopy service, 407
in research, 436
in vaginal adenosis, 352, 432
punch, colposcopically directed, 407-409, 413
colposcopy appearances in selection of, 407
in pregnancy, 428
in vaginal lesions, 428
instruments, 186
use of Monsel's solution, 186, 413
rigid regimes, 407
Schiller's test, before, 180, 186, 407, 409
selection of sites by colposcopy, 407
size by colposcopy, 407
types by colposcopy, 407
selective, in atypical colposcopy, 391
wedge, 407, 408, 412

C

Capillaries, see Angioarchitecture
Carcinogenesis, 116-119
Carcinoma in situ of cervix
adenocarcinoma, 262, 414
adenosquamous, 262
association with dysplasia, 157, 233
biological significance, different, 164, 397, 403
colposcopic appearances, 133, 141, 157, 226, 233, 236, 242, see also Atypical transformation zone and Colposcopy, colposcopic grading; in assessment of
cone biopsy, see Diagnosis and Treatment
correlation between colposcopic findings and histology, 133, 156, 157, 226, 391, 392, 393, 397, 408
discrepancies, 157, 164, 226, 353, 385, 393, 397
cytology, see Cytology exfoliative
definition, 26
DES exposed women, in, 339, 340, 351, 352, 353
diagnosis
by biopsy, 391, 393, 396, 407, 408, 409, 413
by colposcopy, 133, 156, 157, 226, 391, 392, 393, 397, 408
by cytology, 390, 391, 396, 397
by unaided eye, 393
histology, 26
distinction from undifferentiated metaplastic epithelium, 26, 88, 133, 353
problems of, 88, 157, 164, 353, 357, 393, 397, 403
malignant potential, differences in, 397, 403
mass screening, detection by, 395
Papanicolaou smear, see Cytology, exfoliative
pathogenesis, scheme for, 79, 118
prognosis
prediction by colposcopy, 121, 164, 397, 403
prediction by histology, 164, 393, 396
residual "recurrent" lesions
after physical destruction, 418, 429, 432
in cervical canal after cone biopsy, 418, 429
in vaginal vault, 407, 426-429
significance of negative colposcopy, 393
topography, 68, 74, 393, 407
identity with physiological metaplasia and dysplasia, 74
treatment, see Carcinoma of cervix, preclinical
CO_2 laser, 418, 424
cone biopsy, see Biopsy, cone
definitive therapy, 416, 424-426, 428
follow up after, 418, 428, 429
indications, 408, 409
line of excision involved with CIN, 426
residual lesions following, 418, 429
conservative, 9, 417, 418
cryosurgery, 9, 409, 413, 418, 424, 426
electrocautery, 9, 418, 424, 426
electrodiathermy, 9, 409, 413, 418, 419, 426
hysterectomy, 9, 408, 409, 426, 429
in pregnancy, 428
local excision, see Conisation
recurrence
after cone biopsy, 418, 429
clinical invasive carcinoma after cone, 418
vaginal vault after hysterectomy, 407, 427-429

Index 475

vaginal cuff excision, 426
vaginal extension, 233, 407, 426-429
Carcinoma of cervix
 classification, FIGO, 27, 42, 43, WHO, 42
 epidemiology, 100
 etiology
  carcinogenesis, 116-119
  pathogenesis, scheme for, 79, 118
  youthful promiscuity, in, 100
 missed diagnosis by colposcopy, 10, 390
 natural history, 7, 118
 overt carcinoma, 27, 42, 43, 64, 92, see also Carcinoma in situ of cervix; Carcinoma; of cervix; preclinical; and Overt carcinoma
  adenocarcinoma, 262
  clear cell adenocarcinoma, 341, 343, 353
  colposcopy, 262-273
  distinction from colposcopically suspect overt carcinoma, 262
  in pregnancy, 428, 429
  squamous carcinoma, 262
  treatment, 10, 414, 415, 416
  verrucous carcinoma, 273
 stage 1A, see Carcinoma of cervix, preclinical invasive
 stage 1B, 42, 43, 415, 416
Carcinoma of cervix, preclinical
 atypical transformation zone, see Atypical transformation zone and Colposcopy
 classification
  complexity of, 27, 42, 43
  FIGO, 27, 42, 43
  WHO, 42
 colposcopic grading
  in forecasting histology, 156, 157, 391, 396, 397, 408
  in management, 396, 397, 413, 416
 colposcopic localisation of lesions, 403, 407
 colposcopically suspect overt carcinoma, 45, 142, 157, 262, 273-277, 397, 408, 409, 416, 428
 concepts, neither valid nor proven, 389
 conservative management, 9, 389
 correlation of histology with colposcopy, 133, 156, 157, 226, 391, 392, 393, 397, 408
 discrepancies, 157, 164, 226, 393, 397
 cytology, see Cytology, exfoliative
 cytology, and histopathology, combined use, subjectivity and fallibility of, 9
 definitions, 27, 42, 43
 diagnosis
  by biopsy, 391, 393, 396, 407, 408, 409, 413

  by colposcopy, 133, 156, 157, 226, 391, 392, 393, 397, 408
  by cytology, 64, 390, 391, 396, 397
  by unaided eye, 393
 histology, 27, 42, 43
 mass screening, detection by, 395
 origin in transformation zone, 76
 positive colposcopy with negative cytology, 390
 positive histology with negative colposcopy, 393
 predicament of histopathologist, 393
 prognosis, 121, 164, 393, 396, 397, 403
 relation to clinical cancer, 389
 rigid diagnostic and treatment schedules, 392
 significance of negative colposcopy, 393
 study of 321 patients, 392
 topography, 68, 74, 91, 393, 407
  identity with dysplasia and physiological metaplasia, 74
 treatment, see Carcinoma in situ, treatment; Carcinoma of cervix, preclinical invasive, treatment; and Treatment
  follow up after, 418, 426, 428, 429, 432
  in pregnancy, 428
  recurrence after treatment, 407, 418, 426-429, 432
  vaginal cuff excision, 426
Carcinoma of cervix, preclinical invasive
 classification, 27, 42, 43
 colposcopic findings, see Atypical transformation zone and Colposcopically suspect overt carcinoma
 colposcopically suspect overt carcinoma, 43, 45, 142, 157, 262, 273-277, 397, 408, 409, 416, 428
 curettage in diagnosis, 416
 definition, 27, 42, 43
 histopathology
  assessment of prognosis by, 397, 403, 415
  microinvasive carcinoma, 27, 43, 396, 415
  occult invasive carcinoma, 27, 43, 415
  parameters, 42, 43, 415
  problems, 27, 42, 43, 415
 in pregnancy, 428
 lymph node metastases, 415
 residual lesion, after conisation, 418
 treatment, see Carcinoma of cervix, preclinical
  aid of colposcopy, 409, 416, 428
  by less radical methods than for clinical cancer, 397, 409, 414-417

follow up, 429
in pregnancy, 428
radical, 397, 414, 416
recurrence after, 418, 429
results of, 414, 415
selection of treatment, based on histological report, 6, 415
Cervical canal
  evaluation
    colposcopy, 68, 74, 114, 180, 233, 393, 397
    cone biopsy, 397, 409, 414, 426
    endocervical curettage, 180, 397, 409, 412-414, 416
    endocervical speculum, 180, 412, 413, 426
    in presence of abnormal cytology, 412, 413
    speculum eversion, 17, 74, 179, 180, 403, 426
Cervical columnar epithelium, see Columnar epithelium
Cervical erosion, 15, 74, 194, 308, 434, 436
Cervical polyp, see Polyp
Cervical smear, see Cytology, exfoliative
Cervical ulcer, non-malignant, 288
  etiology, 288
  herpetic, 288
  syphilitic, 288
  traumatic, 288
  tuberculous, 288
Cervicitis, see Vaginocervicitis
  acute, 278, 397, 403
  atrophic, 45, 284, 285
  chronic, 15, 25, 26, 45, 194, 367, 434, 436
Cervix
  apparent and real views, 17, 74, 179, 180
  arbor vitae, 203
  atypical metaplastic epithelium, 25, 26, 74, 76, 80, 81, 88, 92, 114
  biopsy, see Biopsy
  carcinoma, see Carcinoma
  cervical intraepithelial neoplasia (CIN), 27, 286, 330, 340, 366, 432, see also Dysplasia and Carcinoma in situ
  chronic "cervicitis," 15, 25, 26, 45, 194, 434, 436
  "chronic inflammation," significance of, 26
  clefts, 25, 43, 88, 133, 156, 210, 236
  columnar epithelium, 25, 43, 127, 194, see also Columnar epithelium
  concepts
    false, 8
    present day, 7
    traditional, 7
  contraceptive pill, effects of, 116
  cysts, see Inclusion cysts
  diathermy coagulation and cryosurgery, colposcopic appearances after, 298
  dysplasia, see Dysplasia
  ectocervix, 16
  endocervical canal, 16, 17, 68, 74, 114, 179, 180, 233, 393, 397, 409, 412, 413, 414, 416
  endocervix, 16
  "erosion," 15, 74, 194, 308, 434
  erythroplakia, 15
  eversion
    apparent, 17, 74, 179, 180
    contraceptive pill, 116
    in pregnancy, 104
    real, 17, 180
  external os, 17, 100
  immature metaplastic epithelium, see Immature metaplastic epithelium
  inclusion cysts, 133, 156, 210, 211, 236
  infection, acute, 278, 397, 403
  "lacerations," 100
  metaplasia, see Metaplasia
  metaplastic epithelium, see Metaplasia
  nabothian follicles, 210, see also Inclusion cysts
  new squamocolumnar junction, 17, see also New squamocolumnar junction
  "normal," 74
  of adolescent nullipara, 100
    colposcopic and histological study, 100, 101
    columnar epithelium, 101
    immature metaplasia, 101, 334, 367
    in virgin, 101
    metaplasia, 101
      in sexually active adolescent, 101, 104, 366, 367, 374
    onset of sexual activity, 101
    topography, 101
    traditional virginal cervix, 101
  of foetus, 15, 92, 100
    colposcopic and histological study, 92, 374
    columnar epithelium, 92, 201, 378
    dynamic phase, 81, 378
    immature metaplasia, 101, 378, 385
    mature metaplasia, 378, 385
    original squamocolumnar junction, 100
    original squamous epithelium, 92
    original transformation zone, 100, 374, 378, 385
    physiological metaplasia, 100
    study, 92, 374

topographical variations, 92, 100
typical transformation zone, 92, 378
of postmenopause
  atypical metaplasia, 114
  colposcopic appearances, 114, 284, 285
  difficulty in examination of canal, 114
  ectocervical columnar epithelium, 114
  ectocervical metaplastic epithelium, 114
  effect of oestrogen, 114, 285
  eversion, 114
  immature forms of metaplasia, 92
  petechial haemorrhages, 114
  oestrogen deficient vaginocervicitis, 284, 285, 361
  reversion of transformation zone, 114, 393
  trauma of examination, 286
  true erosion, 286
  unsatisfactory colposcopic findings, 114, 393
  vaginocervicitis, 114
of pregnancy, see Pregnancy
  atypical metaplasia, 104
  dynamic phase, 80, 104, 361
  etiological importance, 104
  eversion, 104
  first pregnancy, 80
  physiological metaplasia, 104
  remodeling of, 104
  subsequent pregnancies, 80
  transient atypical colposcopic appearances, 361
of prepuberty
  atypical transformation zone, 100
  columnar epithelium, 100
  external os, 100
  "lacerations," 100
  metaplastic epithelium, 100, 378
  reversion after birth, 100
  typical transformation zone, 100
of reproductive years
  dynamic phase, 114
  maturity of metaplasia, 114
  permanency of metaplasia, 114
  study, 104
  "to" and "fro" movement, a false concept, 114
  transformation zone, mature, 114
of sexually active adolescent
  atypical transformation zone, 101, 366, 367, 374
  control group for DES exposed girls, 366
  dynamic phases, 101, 367
  histology, 104, 366, 367
  immature metaplastic epithelium, 104, 367
  mature metaplastic epithelium, 367
  original transformation zone, 367
  relationship to carcinoma, 374
  study, 100, 101, 366
  transient atypical colposcopic appearances, 361
  typical transformation zone, 101
of virgin
  atypical transformation zone, 101, 366, 367, 374
  columnar epithelium, 101
  control group for DES exposed girls, 366
  extent of metaplasia, 101
  immature metaplasia, 367
  mature metaplastic epithelium, 367
  study, 100, 101, 366
  traditional virgin cervix, 101
  typical transformation zone, 101, 367
original columnar epithelium, see Columnar epithelium
original squamocolumnar junction, 17, 25, see also Original squamocolumnar junction
original squamous epithelium, 25, 123, 193
physiological metaplastic epithelium, 25, 26, 76, 127, 133
precursors of cervical cancer, 74, 76, 179, 226, 366, 374
pseudoerosion, 15
squamo-squamous junction, 17, 308
topographical studies of epithelia, 68-74
undifferentiated metaplastic epithelium, 26, 81, 88, 227, 339
Chronic cervicitis, 15, 25, 26, 45, 367, 434, 436
Chronic endocervicitis, 25
"Chronic inflammation," significance of, 26
CIN—cervical intraepithelial neoplasia, 27, 286, 330, 340, 366, 432, see also Dysplasia and Carcinoma in situ
Classification stage 1 carcinoma of cervix, 27, 42, 43
Clear cell adenocarcinoma, 321, 330, 341
  age incidence, 343
  clinical appearance, 343
  colposcopy, 351
  cytology, 343
  DES, transplacental exposure, 341
  registry, 341
  risk of development, 339, 353
  site, 341
  treatment, 341, 343

Clinically overt carcinoma, *see* Overt carcinoma
"Colpitis," 45, *see also* Vaginocervicitis
Colpophotography, 189
Colposcopic and histological correlations, *see* Correlations between colposcopic and histological diagnosis; and Basic colposcopic and histological correlations
Colposcopic definitions, 43-63
Colposcopically suspect overt cancer, 43, 45, 142, 147, 153, 262, 273-277, 397, 408, 409, 416, 428, *see also* Overt carcinoma
Colposcopy
　acetic acid application, 44, 178, 179, 201, 203, 233, 262, 273, 277, 331, 334
　additional information available to gynaecologist, 9
　angioarchitecture, *see* Angioarchitecture
　appearances
　　atrophic cervicitis, 45, 284, 285
　　atypical, of doubtful or physiological significance, 357-385
　　atypical transformation zone, 44, 45, 133, 141, 142, 156, 226-261
　　atypical vessels, 44, 63, 78, 141, 142, 156, 157, 242, 261, 277
　　cervical polyp, 288, 298
　　colposcopically suspect overt carcinoma, 43, 45, 142, 157, 262, 273-277, 397, 408, 409, 416, 428
　　columnar epithelium, 127, 194-208, *see also* Columnar epithelium
　　combinations of mosaic and punctation, 242
　　condyloma, 286, 288
　　cryosurgery, after, 298, 361, 429
　　electrodiathermy coagulation, after, 298, 361, 429
　　inconspicuous iodine negative area, 45, 298
　　irradiation, after, 298
　　keratosis, 44, 142, 226, 233, 236, 313, 334, 361, 374, 375
　　mosaic, 44, 141, 226, 227, 242, 313, 334, 357, 361, 366, 374
　　oestrogen deficient cervicitis, 45, 284, 285
　　original epithelia, 193-208
　　original squamous epithelium, 123, 193, 194, *see also* Original squamous epithelium
　　original transformation zone, 44, 374, 378, 385
　　overt carcinoma, 262
　　papilloma, *see* Condyloma
　　punctation, 44, 141, 226, 227, 236, 242, 277, 313, 334, 357, 361, 366, 374
　　true erosion, 45, 285, 286
　　typical transformation zone, 127, 133, 209-225
　　　cystic inclusions, 133, 156, 210, 211
　　　early phases, 81, 88, 209
　　　gland openings (clefts), 133, 156, 210, 361
　　　mature phases, 127, 133, 142, 156, 209, 210, 211
　　　nabothian cysts, 210, *see also* Typical transformation zone
　　ulcer, non-malignant, 288
　　vagina, 180, 313, 331, 334, 339, 351, 374
　　vaginocervicitis, 278, 285, *see also* Vaginocervicitis
　　white epithelium, 44, 133, 141, 226, 227, 233, 236, 261, 313, 334, 357, 361, 366, 374
　atypical colposcopy, 393, *see also* Atypical transformation zone
　classification of atypical transformation zones
　　grading of quality, *see* Grading
　　recommended, 45, 63
　　traditional, 63
　colpophotography, 189
　complementary use with cytology, 390
　correlation with macroscopic findings, 393
　correlations with cytology, 390
　correlations with histology, 6, 7, 10, 43, 133, 156, 157, 226, 357, 367, 393, 396, 397, 408, 412, 413
　　absence of correlation, 157, 164, 226, 357, 367, 374, 385, 391, 393, 397
　　basic correlation, 123
　criticisms of, 8, 9
　definitions, 43-64
　disappointment with, 10
　false negative, 393
　　contact bleeding, 393
　　endocervical, 393
　　postmenopausal retraction and rigidity, 393
　field of neoplastic potential, 44, 76
　grading of quality of atypical transformation zones, *see* Atypical transformation zone and Grading
　history, *see* Preface
　identification of dysplasia, 403

in avoidance of unnecessary biopsies, 391, 436
in eradication of condylomata, 434
in evaluation of abnormal smear, 395-414
in evaluation of cervical canal, 9, 68, 179, 180, 413
in follow-up after treatment of preclinical carcinoma and CIN, 429
in guide to prognosis, 396, 397, 403
in identification and management of vaginal lesions, 426
in location of lesions, 403
   endocervical, 407, 409, 412, 413
   focal, 407, 408, 409, 412, 413
   no lesion seen, 407, 408, 409, 412
   vaginal, 307, 339, 340, 352, 353, 426-428
   vaginal extension, 407, 426, 429
in management of atypical transformation zones of doubtful significance, 432
in management of vaginal adenosis, 432
in mass screening for preclinical cancer, effectiveness, but impracticality, of, 390
in pregnancy, assessment of conditions, 428
in recognition of preclinical carcinoma, 390, 392
in research, 392, 436
in selection of women for vaginal cuff excision, 426
in selection of treatment for CIN, 6, 417
in selection of treatment for preclinical invasive carcinoma, 6, 414
in selection of type, size and site of cervical biopsy, 407, 408, 409, 412, 413
in understanding of cervical erosions, etc., 434
inconclusive findings, 397
indications for
   cancer detection clinic patients, 392
   follow-up after treatment, 429
   practical, 8, 390, 391
   routine screening, 8, 390, 391
   selective screening for research, 392
   students of colposcopy, 392
instruments, 167
malignancy index of atypias, 391
mismanagement frank cancer, 390
new, 5, 8
paramedical personnel, use of, 392
prime morphological features, *see* Prime morphological features
quality of atypical transformation zones, *see* Grading
recording of findings, 186, 187, 188, 189
satellite clinics, 392
study
   of adolescent cervix, 6, 72, 366
   of cervix of reproductive years, 104
   of dynamic phases of metaplasia, 80
   of foetal cervix, 6, 68
   of postmenopausal cervix, 6, 72
   of preclinical carcinoma, 392, 414
   of pregnant cervix, 6, 72, 80
   of prepubertal cervix, 6, 72
   of sexually active adolescent cervix, 6, 72, 366
   of 25,000 human cervices, 6
   of vaginal epithelia, 307
   of virgin cervix, 6, 72, 366
surface configuration, *see* Surface configuration
teaching of, 8, 10, 392
technique, 167-189
terminology
   new, 8
   recommended international, 45, 63
   traditional, 8
training, 10, 11, 392
unsatisfactory colposcopic findings, 63, 179, 397
uses of, *see* Uses of Colposcopy
Columnar epithelium, 194-208
   acetic acid solution, after application of, 201, 203
   angioarchitecture, 127, 203
      deep branching vessels, 127, 203
      large terminal vessels, 127, 203
      looped capillaries, 127, 203
      network capillaries, 127, 203
   arbor vitae, 203
   cranial zone, 203
   clefts (glands), 203
   clinical appearances and terms, 194
   colour, 127, 201
   colposcopic and histological correlation, 127, 142
   contact bleeding, 203
   contraceptive pill, effects of, 116
   cranial zone, 203
   cystic structures, 127, 133, 156, 210, 211, 236, 313
   definitions
      colposcopic, 43
      histological, 25
   ectopic, invalid term, 194
   embryologically determined extent, 201
   flat sheet, 203

histology, 25, 127
  in adolescent nulliparous cervix, 100
  in foetal cervix, 92, 201
  in postmenopausal cervix, 114
  in pregnancy, 104
  in prepubertal cervix, 100
  in virgin cervix, 101
  morphological zones, 203
  onset of metaplasia, 81
  origin, 201
  prime morphological features, 201
  reserve cells, 81
  surface configuration, 203
  topography
    asymmetrical arrangements, 201
    ectocervical site, 201
    "ectopic" columnar epithelium, invalid term, 194
    elliptic arrangement, 201
    endocervical, 201
    site of new squamocolumnar junction, 201
    site of original squamocolumnar junction, 201
    vaginal extension, 201
  variation in colposcopic features, 194
  villi, 25, 81, 127, 203
Condyloma
  abnormal smear, 408
  angioarchitecture, 286, 288
  coexistence with CIN, 286
  etiology, 286
  in transformation zone, 286, 288
  multiple, 288
  regularity of vessel spacing, 286
  resembling keratosis, 288
  resembling overt cancer, 286
  synonymous with papilloma, 45, 63, 286
  treatment, 434
Cone biopsy, see Biopsy, cone
Contraceptive pill, effects of, 116
Correlation between colposcopic and histological diagnosis, 6, 7, 10, 43, 156, 157, 226, 357, 367, 390, 391, 393, 396, 397, 408, 412, 413, see also Basic colposcopic and histological correlations; and Discrepancies between colposcopic and histological diagnosis
Criticisms of colposcopy, 8, 9
Cryosurgery, 9, 409, 413, 418, 424, 426, 428, 429, 432, 434, 436
Curettage in diagnosis, 397, 409, 412, 413, 414
Cystic cervicitis, 25

Cytochemistry, 6
Cytology, exfoliative, 8
  abnormal smear, 64, 395
    biopsy with, 407
    colposcopy as aid in selection of biopsy, 407
    colposcopy in avoidance of unnecessary biopsies, 391
    complementary use with colposcopy, 391, 392, 393
    correlation between colposcopy and histology in, 396, 397
  definition, 64
  in carcinoma in situ, 64, 390, 391, 396, 397
  in clear cell adenocarcinoma, 343
  in condyloma, 286
  in dysplastic epithelia, 64
  in vaginocervicitis, 64, 285
  management, 407
  repeated, with negative colposcopy, 409
  recognition of colposcopically suspect overt carcinoma with, 396
  with atypical colposcopy, 390
  doubtful smear, 64, 396
  fallibility, 9
  false negative, 9, 390, 396, 408
  false positive, 396, 397, 407, 409
  mass screening, use in, 64, 262, 395, 396
  negative smear, 64
  Papanicolaou classes I-V, 64, 396
  positive smear, 64
    after treatment CIN, 427
    prediction of carcinoma in situ, 64
    prediction of dysplasia, 64
    prediction of histology, 64, 396
    prediction of invasive carcinoma, 64
  prior to colposcopy, 176, 396
  repeat smears, 396
  subjectivity, 9
  suspicious smear, see Doubtful smear

D

Definitions, 15-65
  anatomical
    cervix, apparent view, 17
      real view, 17
    ectocervix, 16
    endocervical canal, 16
    endocervix, 16
    eversion, 17
      apparent, 17
      real, 17
    external os, 17

Index 481

new squamocolumnar junction, 17, 308
original squamocolumnar junction, 17, 308
original squamous epithelium, 25, 308
squamo-squamous junction, 17
vulvovaginal boundary, 308
clinical, 15
colposcopic
  atrophic cervicitis, 45
  atypical transformation zone, 44
  atypical vessels, 44
  cervical ulcer, non-malignant, 45
  colposcopically suspect overt carcinoma, 45
  columnar epithelium, 43
  condyloma, 45
  grading of atypical transformation zone, 44, 45
  ground structure, 63
  inconspicuous iodine-negative areas, 45
  keratosis, 44, 63
  leukoplakia, 63
  matrix areas, 63
  mosaic, 44
  oestrogen-deficient vaginocervicitis, 45
  original columnar epithelium, 43
  original squamous epithelium, 43
  original transformation zone, 44, 374
  papilloma, 45
  punctation, 44, 63
  true erosion, 45
  typical transformation zone, 44
    early phases, 44
  unsatisfactory colposcopic findings, 63
  vaginocervicitis, 45
  white epithelium, 44
cytological, exfoliative
  abnormal smear, 64
  doubtful smear, 64
  negative smear, 64
  Papanicolaou, classes I-V, 64
  positive smear, 64
histological
  abnormal epithelium, 26
  atypical metaplastic epithelium, 26
  carcinoma in situ, 26
  cervical columnar epithelium, 25
    clefts, 25
    "endocervical epithelium," 25
    glands, 25
    villi, 25
  cervical intraepithelial neoplasia (CIN), 27
  dysplasia, dysplastic epithelium, 26
  dysplasia major, 26
  dysplasia minor, 26
  endocervical epithelium, misleading term, 25
  immature metaplastic epithelium, 26
  metaplastic epithelium, 25
  microinvasive carcinoma, 27
  occult invasive carcinoma, 27
  original squamous epithelium, 25
  overt carcinoma, 27
  parakeratosis, 45
  physiological metaplastic epithelium, 25
  preclinical carcinoma, 27
  preclinical invasive carcinoma, 27
  stage O carcinoma, 26
  stage 1A carcinoma, 42, 415
  stage 1B carcinoma, 42
  undifferentiated metaplastic epithelium
DES, exposure in utero to, see Vaginal adenosis and Clear cell adenocarcinoma
Diagnosis
  biopsy, 391, 393, 396, 407, 408, 409, 413, see also Biopsy
  colposcopically directed punch biopsy, 186, 407, 408, 409, 413, 428
  colposcopy, 391, 393, 396, 407, 408, 409, 413, see also Colposcopy
  complementary use of cytology, colposcopy, 391, 392, 393
  cone biopsy, 407, 408, 409, 412, 413, 414
  cytology, see Cytology
  diagnostic curettage, 397, 409, 412, 413, 414
  during pregnancy, 428
  histopathology, see Histopathology
  miss frank cancer, 10
  problems of diagnosis, 26, 88, 133, 157, 164, 353, 357, 393, 397, 403
  punch biopsy, 407, see also Colposcopically directed punch biopsy
  rigid diagnostic regimes, 407
  Schiller's test, 407, 409, see also Schiller's test
  wedge biopsy, 407, 408, 412, see also Biopsy; Colposcopy; and Cytology
Discrepancy between colposcopic and histological diagnosis, 26, 88, 133, 157, 164, 226, 353, 357, 391, 393, 397, 403
Doubtful smear, 64, see also Cytology, exfoliative
Dynamic phases of metaplasia
  active phases, 79-88
  atypical, 92, 227
  colposcopic appearances, 81, 88, 209, 227

contraceptive pill, effect of, 116
further episodes, 80
histological appearances, 81, 88, 227
immature metaplastic epithelium, emergence of, 80, 81, 88, 334, 367
in adolescence, 81
in foetus, 81, 378
in pregnancy, 80, 81, 361
in reproductive years, 80, 114
in sexually active adolescents, 101, 367
methods of study, 80, 81, 100, 101, 366
neoplastic potential, acquirement of, 76
origin of cells, 81
physiological, 81, 88, 209
stages of early metaplasia (immature), 81, 88, 209, see also Metaplasia
Dysplasia, see also Carcinoma in situ; Cervical intraepithelial neoplasia (CIN); and Preclinical Carcinoma
"abnormal epithelium," 26, 385
abnormal smear, 396, 397
association with carcinoma in situ, 157, 233
atypical metaplasia, identity with, 26
atypical transformation zone, in, 76, 77, 226
biopsy, selection of, 397
cervical intraepithelial neoplasia (CIN), relationship to, 27
colposcopic appearances, see Atypical transformation zone
colposcopic-histological correlation, 157, 227
cytology, 64
definition, 26
difficulty in distinction from immature metaplastic epithelium, 88, 226, 385
dynamic phases of origin, 92
extension to vagina, 407
false negative colposcopy, 393
follow up, 429, 432
histopathology, 26
    as indicator of biological potential, 393
    subjectivity, 393
identification by colposcopy, 76, 77, 226
major, 26
management
    by cone biopsy, 424
    by hysterectomy, 426
    by physical destruction, 418
metaplasia, relationship to, 26, 68, 74
minor, 26
natural history, 79, 118
persistence, of, 92
prognosis
    based on colposcopy, 397, 403

selection of treatment, 417
topography
    cervical canal, 68, 74
    ectocervix, 74
    identity with carcinoma in situ, 26, 68, 74
    identity with physiological metaplasia, 26, 68, 74
    transformation zone development within, 76
    vaginal, 426
    vaginal vault, extension to, 426, 428

E

Ectopic columnar epithelium, see Columnar epithelium
Ectopy, 74
Electrocautery, 418, 424, 426
Electrodiathermy, 9, 409, 413, 418, 419, 426, 428, 429, 434, 436
Embryology of vagina, 307
Endocervical canal, see Cervical canal
Endocervical curettage, 180, 397, 409, 412, 413, 414, 416
Endocervical speculum, 180, 412, 413, 426
Endocervicitis, 25
Endometriosis of vagina, 323
Epidemiology of cervical carcinoma, 100
Epidermidalisation, 25
Epidermisation, 25
Epidermoid hyperplasia, 25
"Erosion," 15, 74, 194, 308, 434, 436
Erythroplakia, 15
Eversion
    apparent, 17, 74, 179, 180
    contraceptive pill, 116
    in pregnancy, 104
    real, 17, 180
Exfoliative cytology, see Cytology, exfoliative
External os, 17, 72, 100

F

Fallibility of histology, 9, 393, 415
False negative cervical smear, 9, 390, 396, 408
False negative colposcopy, 393
    contact bleeding, 393
    endocervical, 393
    postmenopausal retraction and rigidity, 393
False positive cervical smear, 396, 397, 407, 409
Field of neoplastic potential, 44
Foetal cervix, see Cervix of foetus
Follow up after treatment, 418, 426, 428, 429, 432

G

Glandular hyperplasia, 25
Grading of atypical transformation zone, 45, 121, 156, *see also* Atypical transformation zone
  correlation with expected histology and biopsy, 408
  correlation with histology, 79, 121, 156, 157, 396, 397, 408
  criteria for grading, 156
  differences in prime morphological features, 121, 227, 242
  discrepancy with histology, 157, 164, 366, *see also* Discrepancy between colposcopic and histological diagnosis
  grades
    Grade I, 156, 157, 261, 366, 391, 397, 403, 408, 409, 412
    Grade II, 156, 157, 261, 366, 391, 397, 403, 408, 409, 412
    Grade III, 156, 157, 261, 273, 391, 397, 403, 408, 412, 416
  in assessment of prognosis, 396, 397, 403
  in histological prediction, 121, 156, 391, 397
  in management, 396, 397, 413, 416
  in selection of cervical biopsy, 391
  major grades, 277
  subjectivity in, 156
  surface configuration, 156, 261

H

Herpes virus type 2 infection, 119, 288
Herpetic ulcer, 288
Histochemical studies, *see* Alkaline phosphatase studies
Histopathology
  abnormal epithelium, 26
  arrested immature metaplasia, 88, 92, 227, 309, 334, 339, 352, 353, 374
  assessment of prognosis by histomorphology, 164, 397, 403, 415
  atypical metaplastic epithelium, *see* Atypical metaplastic epithelium
  basal cell hyperplasia, 25, 385
  biological differences in histologically similar preclinical carcinoma, 158, 397
  carcinoma in situ, 26, 133, 392, 396
    distinction from other undifferentiated epithelia, 26, 88, 133, 353
    cervical intraepithelial neoplasia (CIN), 27, 286, 330, 340, 366, 432
    classifications of preclinical invasive carcinoma, 27, 42, 43
  clinical and histological subdivisions of Stage 1 cancer of the cervix, 27, 42, 43
  columnar epithelium, 25, 127, 142
  confused terminology, 17, 18, 26, 42, 415
  correlations with colposcopy, 6, 7, 10, 43, 133, 156, 157, 226, 357, 367, 391, 392, 393, 396, 397, 408, 412, 413, *see also* Correlation between colposcopic and histological diagnosis and Basic colposcopic and histological correlations
  deficiency in study, 120
  definitions, 17-27
  discrepancies with colposcopy, 157, 164, 226, 357, 367, 374, 385, 391, 393, 397
  dysplasia
    distinction from other undifferentiated epithelia, 26, 88, 133, 353
    dysplasia major, 26, 396
    dysplasia minor, 26, 396
  fallibility of, 9
  histologist as final arbiter, 120
  immature metaplastic epithelium, 26, 44, 76, 80, 81, 88, 101, 104, 142, 156, 180, 227, 334, 352, 353, 432
  information unavailable from, but available to colposcopy, 120
  keratosis, 142
  metaplastic epithelium, 25, 26, 44, 68, 74, 76, 79, 80, 81, 88, 92, 100, 101, 127, 133, 142, 156, 209
  microinvasive carcinoma, 27, 43, 396
  occult invasive carcinoma, 27, 43
  one step differences in diagnosis, 157
  original squamous epithelium, 25, 123, 142
  overt carcinoma, 27, 42, 43
  parakeratosis, 45
  physiological squamous metaplasia, 25, *see also* Metaplastic epithelium
  preclinical carcinoma, 27, 390
    correlation with colposcopy, 390, 392
  preclinical invasive carcinoma, 392
    complexity of terminology, 27, 42, 43, 415
    depth of penetration, 27, 42, 43, 415
    other parameters, 27, 42, 43, 415
  problems of, 26, 88, 157, 164, 353, 357, 393, 397, 403
  prognosis in assessment of, 164, 393, 396
  scheme for pathogenesis, 79, 118
  serial sectioning of cone biopsy, 407
  significance of negative colposcopy and positive histology in preclinical carcinoma, 393

simplified terminology, 25
stage 0, see Carcinoma in situ
stage 1A, see Preclinical invasive carcinoma
subjectivity of, 9, 27, 42, 43, 393, 415
typical transformation zone, 127, 142
undifferentiated metaplastic epithelium, see Immature metaplastic epithelium
vaginal adenosis, 313, 331, see also Vaginal adenosis
vaginal epithelia, 307, 308, 313
Hyperplasia
　atypical, 25
　atypical reserve cells, 25
　basal cell, 25
　glandular, 25
　intraglandular, 25
　prickle cell, 25
　prickle cell with dysplasia, 25
　pseudoepitheliomatous, 25
　reserve cell, 25
　subcylindrical cell, 25
Hysterectomy
　for in situ carcinoma, 9, 408, 409, 426, 429
　for preclinical invasive carcinoma, 409, 416, see also Treatment

I

Immature metaplasia, 26, 44, 76, 80, 88, 101, 104, 142, 156, 180, 227, 334, 339, 352, 353, 361, 367, 374
Inclusion cysts, 133, 156, 210, 211
Inconspicuous iodine non-staining area, 298
　definition, 45
　location, 298
　relation to original transformation zone, 45
　relation to parakeratosis, 298
Indications for colposcopy
　cancer detection clinic patients, 392
　follow up after treatment, 429
　practical, 8, 390, 391
　routine screening, 8, 390, 391
　selective screening for research, 392
　students of colposcopy, 392
Indirect metaplasia, 25
Inflammation, see Vaginocervicitis
Intercapillary distance, 156, 236, 242, 261, 262, 334, 339
Intraglandular hyperplasia, 25
Invasive cervical carcinoma, see Carcinoma of cervix and Carcinoma of cervix, preclinical invasive
Iodine, Lugol's see Schiller's test
Irradiation, 10, 416, 428
Irregular dysplasia, 25

J

Junction, see New squamocolumnar junction; Original squamocolumnar junction; and Squamo-squamous junction

K

Keratosis, 15, 44, 142, 226, 233, 236, 313, 334, 361, 374, 375
　condyloma, resembling, 236
　original transformation zone, 26, 378
　overlying original squamous epithelium, 236

L

"Laceration" of cervix, 100
Leukoplakia, see Keratosis and Atypical transformation zone
Location of lesions, see Topography
Lymph node metastases, in preclinical invasive carcinoma, 415

M

Malignancy index of colposcopic atypias, 391
　without grading, 391
　with grading, 391
Management, see Diagnosis and Treatment
Matrix areas, 63
Maturation of metaplastic epithelium, 25, 80, 81, 88, 92, 142, 227, 374, see also Metaplasia
Metaplasia, see also Atypical metaplasia; Atypical transformation zone; and Typical transformation zone
　atypical, 26, 92, see also Dysplasia and Carcinoma in situ
　atypical transformation zone, relation to, 76
　behavioural aspects
　　carcinogenesis, relation to, 76, 79, 116
　　dynamic phase, 80, 227
　　initiation, 80
　　maturation, 80
　　natural history, 76-119
　carcinogenesis, 116
　　initiation and promotion, 116, 118, 119
　　sperm DNA, 116, 117
　　sperm histones, 117
　　virus of herpes genitalis, 119
　colposcopic counterparts, see Typical and Atypical transformation zone
　contraceptive pill, effect of, 116
　dynamic phase
　　active phase, 79-88
　　atypical, 92, 227

Index

colposcopic appearances, 81, 88, 209, 227
contraceptive pill, effect of, 116
discrete patches, 209
fingerlike ridges, 209
further episodes, 80
histological appearances, 81, 88, 227
immature metaplastic epithelium
  emergence of, 80, 81, 88, 334, 367
in adolescence, 81
in foetus, 81, 378
in pregnancy, 80, 81, 361
in reproductive years, 80, 114
in sexually active adolescent, 101, 367
methods of study, 80, 81, 100, 101, 366
multifocal orgin, 88
neoplastic potential, acquirement of, 76, 79
origin of cells, 81
physiological, 81, 88, 209
stages of early metaplasia (immature) 81, 88, 209
early phases, 26, 81, 82
  colposcopic counterparts, 44, 88, 209, 227
histopathology, definitions
  atypical metaplastic epithelium, 26
  deficiencies in histological studies, 120
  immature metaplastic epithelium, 26, 80, 81
  mature metaplastic epithelium, 25, 127, 142
  physiological metaplastic epithelium, 25
  undifferentiated metaplastic epithelium, 81, 88 *see also* Dysplasia and Carcinoma in situ
immature metaplastic epithelium, 26, 80, 81, *see also* Immature metaplastic epithelium
in foetus
  colposcopic and histological study, 92, 374
  dynamic phase, 81, 378
  immature, 101, 378, 385
  mature, 92
  physiological, 100, 378, 385
in postmenopausal women
  atypical, 114
  ectocervical metaplastic epithelium, 114
  immature, 92
  reversion of transformation zone, 114, 393
in pregnancy
  atypical, 104
  dynamic phase, 80, 104, 361

eversion, 104
first pregnancy, 80, 81, 104
physiological, 104
subsequent pregnancies, 80, 104
in prepuberty
  atypical transformation, 100
  physiological, 100, 101
in reproductive years
  dynamic phase, 80, 114
  maturity, 80, 114
  permanency, 114
  static phase, 114
  study, 104
  "to" and "fro" movement, 114
in sexually active adolescent
  atypical transformation, 101, 366, 367, 374
  dynamic phase, 81, 101, 367
  immature, 104, 367
  mature, 367
  typical transformation, 101
in virgin
  atypical transformation, 101, 366, 367, 374
  extent, 101
  immature, 101, 367
  mature, 101, 367
  study, 100, 101, 366
  typical transformation, 101, 367
ingrowth or in situ development, 88, 209
interpreted as "cervicitis," 26
interpreted as "chronic inflammation," 26
maturation, 25, 80, 81, 88, 92, 142, 227, 374
multifocal origin, 92
permanency of, 114
physiological, 25, 26, 44, 68, 74, 76, 80, 81, 92, 100, 101, 127, 209, 321, 323, 331, 334, 374, 378, 385
origin from activated stromal cells, 81
origin from columnar reserve cells, 81
stages of early metaplasia
  colposcopic, 81, 88, 209, 227
  histological, 81, 88
stimulus to, acid pH, 88
"to" and "fro" movement, a false concept, 114
topography, 74, 76
  identity between physiological and atypical metaplasia, 74
  relation to new squamocolumnar junction, 76
  relation to original squamocolumnar junction, 76

relation to previous columnar epithelium, 194
relation to typical transformation zone, 25
vaginal site, 74
variations, 72, 74
transient atypical colposcopic appearances in first pregnancy and adolescence, 361
typical, *see also* Physiological
typical transformation zone, relation to, 76
vaginal, 321, 323
vaginal adenosis, 331, 334, 339, 352, 353, 374
Metaplastic epithelium, *see* Metaplasia
Microinvasive carcinoma
definition, 27, *see also* Carcinoma, invasive, preclinical
Mosaic, 44, 141, 226, 227, 242, 313, 334, 357, 361, 366, 374
major grades, 141, 242, 277
minor grades, 141, 242, *see also* Atypical transformation zone and Grading

N

Native columnar epithelium, *see* Columnar epithelium
Native squamous epithelium, *see* Original squamous epithelium
Natural history
of metaplasia, 76-118
of precursors of cervical cancer, 79, 118
Negative smear, *see* Cytology, exfoliative
Neisseria gonorrhoeae infection, 278, 397
New squamocolumnar junction, 17, 63, 74, 76, 179, 201, 210, 298, 308, 419

O

Occult invasive carcinoma, 27, 43, 415, *see also* Carcinoma, invasive, preclinical
Oestrogen deficient, vaginocervicitis, *see* Atrophic cervicitis
Original epithelia, *see also* Original squamous epithelium and Columnar epithelium
Original squamocolumnar junction, 17, 25, 26, 44, 72, 74, 76, 100, 127, 133, 179, 193, 201, 210, 233, 273, 298, 308, 313
Original squamous epithelium, 193, 194
angioarchitecture
deeper branching vessels, 194
looped capillaries, 127, 194
network capillaries, 127, 194
often obscure on colposcopy, 194
colour, 193
colposcopic and histological correlation, 142
colposcopy, 193, 194
definition, 25, 308
colposcopic, 43
histological, 25
histology, 25, 123
in foetal cervix, 92
in postmenopausal era, 114
in vagina, 308
keratosis, overlying, 236
not precursor of cancer, 193
origin, 193
prime morphological features, 193
surface configuration, 194
topography, 193
Original transformation zone, 45
colposcopic appearances, 378
definition, 44
development, 378
histological appearances, 45, 367, 378, 379
in cervix of DES exposed girl, 374
in cervix of sexually active adolescent, 104, 367
in cervix of virgin, 101
in cervix of foetus, 100
in vaginal transformation zone, 313
significance, 379
Overt carcinoma, *see also* Carcinoma of Cervix
clinically overt, 262-273
adenocarcinoma, 262
angioarchitecture, 262
association with Grade III atypical colposcopic transformation zone, 403
clear cell adenocarcinoma, 273
in pregnancy, 428
squamous, 262
surface configuration, 262
verrucous, 273
colposcopically suspect overt, 43, 45, 142, 157, 262, 273-277, 397, 408, 409, 416, 428
angioarchitecture, 142, 277
colour, 273
definition, 45
distinction from clinically overt, 273
in management of preclinical invasive carcinoma, 397, 416, 428
in pregnancy, 428
opacity, 273
surface configuration, 273, 277
topography, 273

Index

P

Papanicolaou smear, see Cytology, exfoliative
Papillary anaplasia, 25
Papilloma, see Condyloma
Parakeratosis, 45
Pathogenesis of carcinoma of cervix, scheme for, 79, 118
Physical destruction of CIN, 418-424
Physiological metaplasia, see Metaplasia and Typical transformation zone
Pill, contraceptive, effects of, 116
Polyp, cervical, 288
  adenomatous, 298
  atypical transformation zone, 298
  polypoidal, 298
  typical transformation zone, 298
Positive smear, see Cytology, exfoliative
Postmenopausal Cervix, see Cervix, of postmenopause
Precancerous metaplasia, 25
Preclinical cervical carcinoma, see Carcinoma of cervix, preclinical
Preclinical invasive carcinoma, see Carcinoma of cervix, preclinical invasive
Pregnancy
  assessment of abnormal smear, 428
  atypical metaplasia, 104
  biopsy in, 407, 428
  birth trauma, 104
  colposcopically suspect overt carcinoma, 428
  columnar epithelium, 203
  cone biopsy, 407, 429
  dynamic phase of metaplasia, 80, 361
  eversion, 104
  invasive carcinoma in, 428
  physiological metaplasia, 104
  remodeling of cervix, 104
  subsequent pregnancies, 104
  transient atypical colposcopic appearances, 361
Preinvasive carcinoma of cervix, see Carcinoma in situ of cervix
Prepubertal cervix, see Cervix of prepuberty
Prickle cell hyperplasia, 25
Prickle cell hyperplasia with dysplasia, 25
Prime morphological features
  angioarchitecture, 121, see also Angioarchitecture
  colour, 120
  grading, 121, see also Atypical transformation zone and Grading
  in atypical transformation zone, 227
  in colposcopically suspect overt carcinoma, 273
  in columnar epithelium, 201
  in original squamous epithelium, 193
  in typical transformation zone, 210
  information not available to histologist, but obvious to colposcopist, 120
  surface configuration, 120, 156
    embryonic variation, 121
    exophytia, 121
    microexophytic, 261
    neoplastic variation, 121
    "papillary," 261
    physiological variation, 121, 261, see also Surface configuration
  topography, 120, see also Topography
Prognosis, of cervical intraepithelial neoplasia, 121, 164, 393, 396, 397, 403
  of preclinical invasive carcinoma, 403, 415
Promiscuous adolescent cervix, see Cervix of sexually active adolescent
Pseudoepitheliomatous hyperplasia, 25
"Pseudoerosion," 25
Punch biopsy, see Biopsy
Punctation, 141, 226, 227, 236, 242, 313, 334, 357, 361, 366, 374, 375
  major grades, 141, 236, 242, 277
  minor grades, 141, 236, see also Atypical transformation zone and Grading

Q

Quality of atypical transformation zones, see Grading

R

Radium therapy, 416, 428
Recognition of preclinical carcinoma
  by colposcopy, 397, 403, 407
  relation to suspicious macroscopic features, 393
Recurrence after treatment, 407, 418, 426, 427, 428, 429, 432
Regenerating cervical epithelium following cryosurgery or electrodiathermy, 180, 298, 361, 429
Regular dysplasia, 25
Reproductive years, cervix of, see Cervix of reproductive years
Reserve cell anaplasia, 25
Reserve cell dysplasia, 25
Reserve cell hyperplasia, 25
Reserve cells, 81

Residual lesions
  after physical destruction, 418, 429, 432
  in cervical canal after cone biopsy, 418, 429
  vaginal vault, 407, 426, 427, 428, 429
Reversion of metaplastic squamous epithelium
  postmenopausal, 114, 393
  prepubertal, 100
  puerperium, 104

S

Saline technique, 178, 179, 334, see also Technique
Satellite colposcopy clinics, 392
Schiller's test, 45, 180, 186, 278, 298, 308, 313, 352, 378, 419
Special clinic for colposcopy, 392
Speculum, self-retaining, 176
  apparent and real view, 17, 179, 180
  cause of contact bleeding, 285
  cause of true erosion, 286
  effect on eversion, 179
  self-retaining, 176
Sperm DNA, 116, 117, 119
Sperm histones, 117
Squamocolumnar junction, see Original squamocolumnar junction and New squamocolumnar junction
Squamocolumnar prosoplasia, 25
Squamo-squamous junction, 17, 308
Squamous epithelium, metaplastic, see Metaplasia
Squamous epithelium, original, see Original squamous epithelium
Squamous metaplasia, see Metaplasia
Squamous prosoplasia, 25
Stage 1A Carcinoma of cervix, see Carcinoma of cervix, preclinical invasive
Stages of early metaplasia (stages 1, 2, 3), 81, 88, 209
Stromal cells
  activation of, 81
  as origin of metaplastic cells, 81
Subcylindrical cell hyperplasia, 25
Surface configuration, 120, 121, 127, 133, 142, 194, 203, 210, 236, 261, 262, 285, 286
Syphilitic ulcer, 288

T

Teaching of colposcopy, 8, 10, 392
Technique of colposcopy
  acetic acid application, 177, 178
    preference for, 178
  apparent and real views, 17, 179, 180
  biopsy instruments, 186
  biopsy technique, 186
  cervical smear, 176
  colpophotography, 179
    cinematography, 189
    still, 189
    television, 189
  colposcopes, various models, 167
  endocervical curettage, 180, 414
  endocervical speculum, 180
  examination of endocervix, 179, 180
  examination table, 176
  exposure of cervix, 176
  in operating theatre, 392
  in special clinic, 392
  instruments, 167
    focussing, 176
    green filters, 167, 334
    laser unit, 167
    magnification, 167
    photographic unit, 167
    stereoscopic viewing, 167
  iris hook, 186, 413
  Koller-Kolstad technique, 178
  Monsel's solution, 186, 413
  office requirements, 176
  position for examination, 176
  recording, 186
    forms, 187, 188
    photographic, 186, 189
  saline application, 178, 179
  Schiller's iodine solution, 180, 186, 278
  speculae, 176
  technique, 176
  tenaculum, 186
  unsatisfactory examination, 179
  vagina examination of, 180
Terminology (colposcopic)
  new, 8
  recommended international, 45, 63
  traditional, 8
Tissue culture, 6
Topography of cervical epithelia
  alteration after physical destruction, 298
  apparent and real views, 17, 74, 179, 180
  asymmetrical arrangement, 74
  atypical metaplasia, 74
  atypical transformation zone, 227, 228
  carcinoma in situ, see Intraepithelial neoplasia
  colposcopic inspection of cervical canal, see Cervical canal
  colposcopically suspect overt carcinoma, 273

colposcopy, misconceptions, 9, 403, 407
columnar epithelium, 201
discrete sites of metaplastic epithelium, 26
eversion by vaginal speculum, 17, 74, 179, 180
focal lesion, 407
haphazard arrangement, 74
identity of physiological metaplasia, dysplasia and carcinoma in situ, 68
in adolescent cervix, 100
in cervix of reproductive years, 104
in foetus, 92
in postmenopausal cervix, 114
in pregnant cervix, 104
in prepubertal cervix, 101
intraepithelial neoplasia
　ectocervical, 68
　endocervical, 68, 74
　vaginal, 74, 233, 307, 330, 339, 340, 352, 353, 426
in virgin cervix, 101
metaplastic epithelium, 74
methods of study (combined colpophotographic and histological), 68, 72
"normal cervix," 74
orientation of material, difficulties in, 68
original squamocolumnar junction, 76
　variations in level of
　　ectocervical, 74
　　endocervical, 72, 74
　　external os, 72
　　vaginal, 74
original squamous epithelium, 193
physiological metaplasia, 74
preclinical carcinoma
　ectocervical, 68
　endocervical, 68, 74
　vaginal, 74
precursors of cervical carcinoma, examined by colposcopy, 74
typical transformation zone, 201
transformation zone, 68, 74
vaginal site, 74, 233, 307, 330, 339, 340, 352, 353, 426
variations, 72
Topography of vaginal epithelia, 308
Transformation zone
　atypical, 76
　colposcopic features, see Colposcopy; Typical transformation zone; and Atypical transformation zone
　colposcopic-histological correlations, 127-157
　immature, 81, 88, 209, 227
　in nulliparous women, 81

natural history, 76-119
original, 374
pathological, 76
physiological, 76
relation to new squamocolumnar junction, 76
relation to original squamocolumnar junction, 76
relation to precursors of squamous cancer, 76
site of origin of preclinical squamous cancer, 76
site of origin of dysplasia, 76
topography, 76
typical, 76
vaginal, 313, see also Atypical transformation zone; Original transformation zone; and Typical transformation zone
Traumatic ulcer, of cervix, 286, 288
Treatment
　biopsy excision, 426
　carcinoma in situ, see Cervical intraepithelial neoplasia
　cervical intraepithelial neoplasia
　　cone biopsy, 416, 424, 425, 426, 428
　　conservative, 9, 417, 418
　　hysterectomy, 9, 408, 409, 426, 429
　　in pregnancy, 417
　　physical destruction, 418, 419, 424, 426, 429
　clear cell adenocarcinoma, 341, 343
　colposcopy
　　in eradication of condylomata, 434
　　in evaluation of abnormal smear, 395-414
　　in evaluation of cervical canal, 413
　　in identification and management of vaginal lesions, 426
　　in location of lesions, 403
　　in selection of biopsy, 407
　　in selection of treatment of preclinical invasive carcinoma, 414
　　in selection of treatment for CIN, 417
　　recognition of colposcopically suspect overt carcinoma in management, 397, 415, 428
　cone biopsy, see Biopsy, cone
　　definitive treatment for CIN, 416, 424, 425, 426, 428
　　line of excision involved, 426
　　residual carcinoma in cervix, following, 418, 429
　conservative approach, 69, 390, 396
　controversial, 389
　cryosurgery, 9, 409, 413, 418, 424, 426, 428, 429, 432, 434, 436

dysplasia, see Cervical intraepithelial neoplasia
electrocautery, 418, 424, 426
electrodiathermy, 9, 409, 413, 418, 419, 426, 428, 429, 434, 436
fluorourocil cream, 5FU, 428
follow-up, after treatment, 418, 426, 428, 429, 432
hysterectomy, 9
　conservative, 408, 409, 426, 429
　radical (Wertheim), 414, 416
　vaginal cuff excision, 426
inflexible regimes, 392
in pregnancy, 428
irradiation, 10, 416
laser, CO$_2$, 9, 409, 418, 424, 428, 434, 436
local excision, 428
overtreatment, 10, 415
preclinical, conservative management, 389
preclinical invasive carcinoma
　by less radical measures than for clinically overt carcinoma, 397, 409, 414, 416, 417
　in pregnancy, 428
　radical, 397, 414, 415, 416
　recognition of colposcopically suspect overt carcinoma, in management, 416, 428
　selection of treatment, based on histological report, 415
recurrence after treatment
　after cone biopsy, 418, 429
　after hysterectomy, 407, 427, 428, 429
　after physical destruction, 418, 429, 432
　lymph node metastases, 415, 416
results of treatment
　CIN by physical destruction, 418
　preclinical invasive carcinoma, 414, 415
　theoretically anticipated versus practical, 389
undertreatment, hazard of, 10
vaginal adenosis, 351
vaginal cuff extension, 426, 427
vaginal intraepithelial neoplasia, 428
vaginectomy, 428
Trichomonas vaginalis infection
　abnormal cytology, 408
　diagnostic problems, 278, see also Vaginocervicitis
True erosion, 285, 286
　biopsy, indication, 286
　definition, 45
　in postmenopausal woman, 286
　significance, 286
　traumatic, from speculum, 286

Tuberculous ulcer, 288
Typical metaplastic epithelium, see Metaplasia and Typical transformation zone
Typical transformation zone, 127, 133, 209-225
　angioarchitecture, 133, 210
　　branching vessels, 133, 210, 211
　　capillary network, 211
　　terminal circular vessels, 211
　　variable pattern, 133
　atypical appearances persisting in, 361
　benign significance, 76
　clefts, 133, 156, 210, 211
　colour, 210
　cystic structures, 127, 133, 156, 210, 211, 236, 313
　definitions, 25, 44
　　early, 44
　　mature, 44
　early stages, 81, 88, 209, see also Dynamic phases of metaplasia
　fully developed (healed) 210, 211
　fused villi, 209
　gland openings, 133, 156, 210, 211
　glandular structures, 127, 133, 156, 210, 211, 236, 313
　immature, 81, 88, 127, 133, 209
　in foetal cervix, 92, 378
　in prepubertal cervix, 100
　in sexually active adolescent cervix, 101
　in virgin cervix, 101, 367
　maturation, 209, 210, 227
　nabothian follicles, 210
　origin and development, 209, 227
　physiological metaplasia, relation to, 25, 76, 81, 82, 142, 209
　prime morphological features, 210
　stages I, II, III of early development, 81, 88, 209
　surface configuration, 210, 211
　topography, 210
　　new squamocolumnar junction, relation to, 210
　　original squamocolumnar junction, relation to, 210
　vaginal, 313
　variety of patterns, 210
　well-developed, 209

U

Ulcer, see Cervical ulcer, non-malignant
Ultrastructural studies, 6, 7
Undifferentiated metaplastic epithelium, 44, 81, 88, 92, 127, 227, see Immature metaplastic epithelium

Index

Undifferentiated regenerative epithelium, 25
Unruhig epithelium, 25
Unsatisfactory colposcopic findings, 63, 179, 397
Uses of colposcopy
  in avoidance of unnecessary biopsies, 391, 436
  in eradication of condylomata, 434
  in evaluation of abnormal smear, 395-414
  in evaluation of cervical canal, 9, 68, 179, 180, 413
  in follow-up after treatment of preclinical invasive carcinoma and CIN, 429
  in guide to prognosis, 396, 397, 403
  in identification and management of vaginal lesions, 426
  in locating lesions, 390, 403, 407, 408, 409, 412, 413, 426, 429
  in management of atypical transformation zones of doubtful significance, 432
  in management of vaginal adenosis, 432
  in pregnancy, assessment of abnormal smear, 428
  in recognition of preclinical carcinoma, 390, 392
  in research, 436
  in selection of patients for vaginal cuff excision, 426
  in selection of treatment for preclinical invasive carcinoma, 414
  in selection of treatment of Stage 0 and dysplasia (CIN), 417
  in selection of type, size and site of biopsy, 407, 408, 409, 412, 413
  in understanding of cervical erosion etc., 434

V

Vagina
  adenosis, 308, 321, 323, 331-340, 341, 344, 351, 352, 432, 434, see also Vaginal adenosis
  carcinoma in situ, 323, see also Intraepithelial neoplasia
  clear cell adenocarcinoma, 321, 330, 339, 341, 343, 351, 353
  clinical carcinoma, 321
  colposcopy
    atypical, 313, 321, 334, 351, 366, 374, 375
    atypical grading, 313
    examination, 180
    typical, 313
  columnar epithelium, 313, 321
    extension to vagina, 74, 201
  cysts, 323
  developmental disorders, 321
    atresia, 321
  dysplasia, 428, see also Intraepithelial neoplasia
  embryology, 307
  endometriosis, 323
  exposure to non-steroidal oestrogens (DES), 307, 321, 374
  glandular structures, 313, 323
  haematocolpos, 321
  histology, 313
  intraepithelial neoplasia, 307, 339, 340, 352, 353, 426-428
    extension from cervix to vagina, 74, 233, 330, 407, 426, 429
  junctions
    new squamocolumnar, 308
    original squamocolumnar, 74, 307, 308, 313, 321
    vulvovaginal, 308
  metaplasia, 321, 323
  multicentric carcinoma, 330
  neoplastic potential of vaginal epithelia, 323, 330
  original transformation zone, 313
  persistent or recurrent lesions, 330
  recurrent intraepithelial lesions after therapy, 407, 426, 427, 428, 429
  squamous carcinoma, 330
  study, 307
  teratogenic effects, 307
  transformation zone, 307, 313, 323
    atypical, 313, 321, 330
    original, 313
  treatment of intraepithelial neoplasia
    cryosurgery, 434
    electrodiathermy, 434
    5FU, 434
    laser, 434
    radium, 434
    vaginectomy, 434
Vaginal adenosis, see Vagina
  clear cell adenocarcinoma, relationship, 341
  cockscomb cervix, 344
  collar cervix, 344
  colposcopy
    atypical, 334, 351, 374
    columnar epithelium, 331, 334
    intercapillary distance, 334, 339
    saline technique and green filter, 334
    typical, 334
  colposcopic-histological-vascular correlation, 331, 332, 333
  contraception, 352

definition, 308, 331
development of metaplasia, 374
exposure to non-steroidal oestrogens (DES), 321, 334, 341
fertility, 341, 353
histology, 351
   arrested immature metaplasia, 334, 339, 352, 353, 374
   carcinoma in situ, 339, 340
   columnar epithelium, 331, 334
   immature metaplasia, 334, 352, 353, 374, 432
   intraepithelial neoplasia, 339, 340, 352, 353, 432
   metaplasia, 331, 334, 374
management, 340
   acidification, 352
   biopsy, 340, 432
   colposcopy, 352, 432, 434
   cryosurgery, 352, 434
   cytology, 352, 432
   electrodiathermy, 352, 434
   examination, 351, 352
   excision, 432
   follow-up, 340, 352
   iodine solution, 352
   laser, 352, 434
   progesterone, 352
natural history, 353
prognosis
   risk of clear cell adenocarcinoma, 339, 353
   risk of squamous carcinoma, 339, 340, 341, 353
vascular network, 331

Vaginal speculum, *see* Speculum, bivalve
Vaginal vault, residual lesions, 407, 426, 427, 428, 429
Vaginocervicitis, 278
   abnormal smear, 278, 408
   acute, 278, 393, 397, 403
   angioarchitecture, 278
   atrophic, *see* Atrophic cervicitis
   bacterial, 278
   candida albicans, 278
   "chronic cervicitis," 15, 25, 26, 45, 367, 434, 436
   definition, 45
   differential diagnosis from punctation, 278
   difficulty with colposcopic diagnosis, 284
   diffuse, 278, 284
   in false negative colposcopy, 393, 397
   localised, 278
   neisseria gonorrhoeae, 278, 397
   protozoal, 278
   Schiller's iodine in, 278
   trichomonas vaginalis, 278, 393, 397
   ulceration, 284
Vascular pattern, *see* Angioarchitecture
Villus of columnar epithelium, *see* Columnar epithelium
Virgin cervix, *see* Cervix of virgin
Vulvovaginal line, 308

W

Wedge biopsy, 407, 408, 412
Wertheim hysterectomy, 414, 416
White epithelium, 44, 133, 226, 227, 233, 236, 261, 313, 334, 357, 361, 366, 374, *see also* Atypical transformation zone